Handbook of DAIRY FOODS AND NUTRITION

Third Edition

Handbook of DAIRY FOODS AND NUTRITION

Third Edition

Gregory D. Miller
Judith K. Jarvis
Lois D. McBean

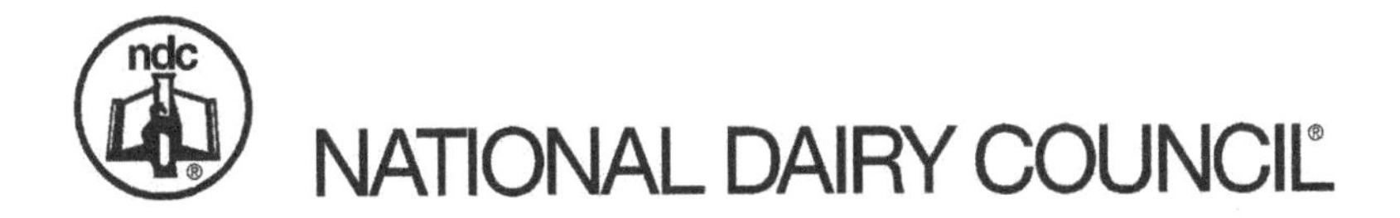

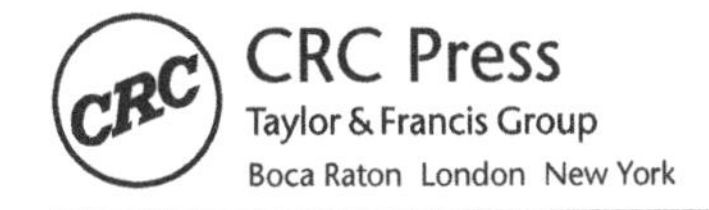

CRC Press is an imprint of the
Taylor & Francis Group, an informa business

CRC Press
Taylor & Francis Group
6000 Broken Sound Parkway NW, Suite 300
Boca Raton, FL 33487-2742

First issued in paperback 2019

ISBN-13: 978-0-8493-2828-2 (hbk)
ISBN-13: 978-0-367-38971-0 (pbk)

Library of Congress Cataloging-in-Publication Data

Miller, Gregory D.
Handbook of dairy foods and nutrition / National Dairy Council ; Gregory D. Miller, Judith K. Jarvis, Lois D. McBean. -- 3rd ed.
p. ; cm.
Includes bibliographical references and index.
ISBN-13: 978-0-8493-2828-2 (alk. paper)
ISBN-10: 0-8493-2828-4 (alk. paper)
1. Dairy products in human nutrition--Handbooks, manuals, etc. I. Jarvis, Judith K. II. McBean, Lois D. III. National Dairy Council. IV. Title.
[DNLM: 1. Dairy Products. 2. Nutrition. WB 428 M648h 2006]

QP144.M54M55 2006
613.2'6--dc22 2006021108

Visit the Taylor & Francis Web site at
http://www.taylorandfrancis.com

and the CRC Press Web site at
http://www.crcpress.com

Preface

America's dairy farmers participate in a national check-off program that provides financial support for promoting the consumption of dairy foods. A large portion of these funds is used to support nutrition research, communications, and education. Since 1915, the National Dairy Council has been committed to establishing programs and educational materials based on current scientific research.

This book is an update of the second edition of the *Handbook of Dairy Foods and Nutrition.* We have attempted to review the most current scientific information available on the role and value of dairy foods in a healthy diet. It is a part of our ongoing effort to provide state-of-the-art information on food and nutrition research to health professionals, educators, consumers, food processors, and other interested groups. We hope this new addition will continue to be a useful resource on the role of dairy foods in health and nutrition.

Acknowledgments

We would like to thank and acknowledge the many people who provided support in the development of this book. Special thanks are given to Agnieszka Kuzmicka in helping to prepare the manuscript and for obtaining permissions for reproduction of figures and tables; Fran Zimmerman for her assistance with copy editing; Lisa Spence for her assistance with technical information and review; and Lori Volp and Ann Horan for their help with literature searches.

Two experts reviewed each chapter. A list of the chapters and their reviewers is provided. We thank them for their helpful suggestions in the preparation of each chapter.

The Authors

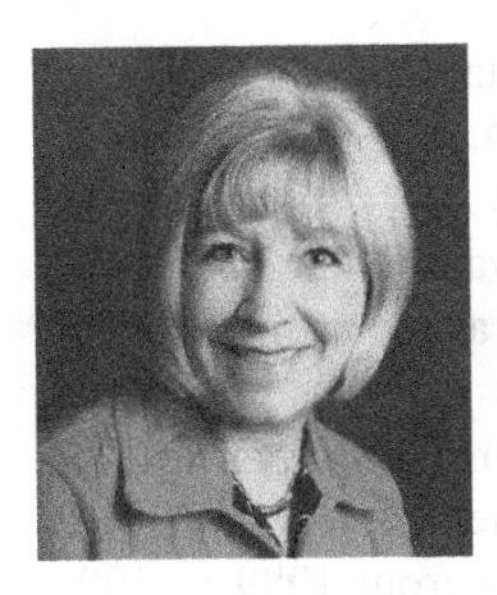

Judith K. Jarvis, M.S., R.D., is director of Nutrition and Scientific Affairs for the National Dairy Council (NDC), a division of Dairy Management, Inc. (DMI). She graduated in 1972 from the University of Illinois with a B.S. in communications. In 1989, she earned an M.S. degree from the University of Chicago in human nutrition and nutritional biology. She is a registered dietitian and an active member in the American Dietetic Association, the American College of Nutrition, and the Chicago Nutrition Association (CNA). She was president of CNA in 2000 and is currently serving as a board member. From 1995 to 1998, she served as the editor of the American College of Nutrition newsletter.

Jarvis is responsible for the management and implementation of communication and technical transfer activities, targeting core health professional groups for the National Dairy Council. Her activities include monitoring the nutrition and scientific literature and writing a research newsletter, summarizing dairy-relevant research for NDC staff, and managing NDC exhibits at health professional meetings. She leads the development of educational materials, including fact sheets, health professional presentations, book chapters, and Web site education as needed. She works closely with other groups at DMI to ensure that marketing and educational programs and materials are grounded in sound science and targeted and supported by the health professional community. Prior to joining the National Dairy Council, she worked as a clinical dietitian, providing nutritional care to cardiac and renal patients. Jarvis has authored several articles for scientific and nutrition journals and is a coauthor for all three editions of the *Handbook of Dairy Foods and Nutrition.*

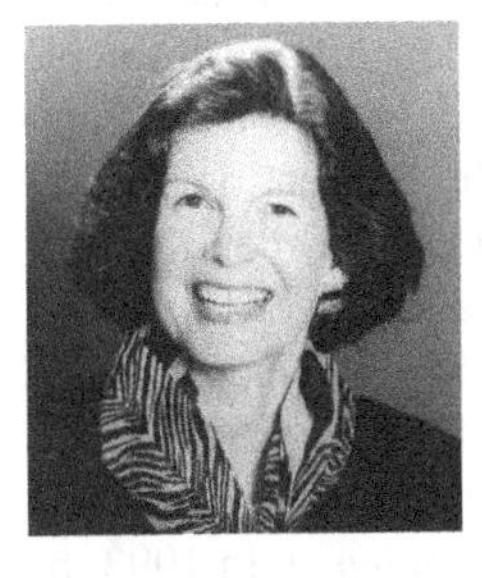

Lois D. McBean, M.S., R.D., is a nutrition consultant for the National Dairy Council. She is the author and editor of the NDC's *Dairy Council Digest*, a bimonthly review of nutrition research for health professionals and nutrition educators.

She has written extensively on many diet and health issues for the dairy and food industry. In addition to newsletters, she has authored numerous articles in peer-reviewed scientific journals, chapters in food and nutrition books, scientific backgrounders, fact sheets, educational materials (for example, the *Calcium Counseling Resource*), speeches, video conference scripts, and press releases. The *Dairy Council Digest*, the *Calcium Counseling Resource*, and several other materials can be obtained by visiting www.nationaldairycouncil.org. McBean also serves as a reviewer for government and health professional publications related to diet and nutrition. Prior to her career as a nutrition writer, editor, and consultant, she was a research nutritionist for the federal government in Washington, D.C., where she was involved in research studies, establishing zinc as an essential nutrient. She also worked at NDC where she participated in the nutrition research program.

McBean received a B.A. from the University of Toronto, Toronto, Ontario, Canada, and she earned an M.S. degree in nutrition from Cornell University, Ithaca, New York. She is a registered dietitian and an active member of the American Dietetic Association, the American Society for Nutrition, Inc., and the Institute of Food Technology. She is a recipient of several APEX (Awards for Publication Excellence) (*Dairy Council Digest*) and received honorable mention for the 1999 Huddleson Award for the article, "Allaying Fears and Fallacies about Lactose Intolerance," published in the *Journal of the American Dietetic Association.* She is a coauthor for all three editions of the *Handbook of Dairy Foods and Nutrition.*

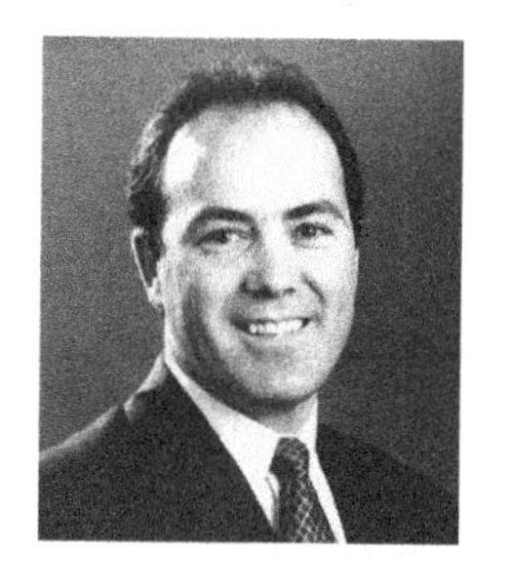

Gregory D. Miller, Ph.D., MACN, is the executive vice president for innovation for the National Dairy Council and is an adjunct associate professor in the Department of Food Science and Nutrition at the University of Illinois.

Dr. Miller graduated in 1978 from Michigan State University with a B.S. degree in nutrition, and in 1982, he earned an M.S. degree in nutrition (toxicology) from The Pennsylvania State University. In 1986, he received a Ph.D. in nutrition (toxicology) from The Pennsylvania State University.

Dr. Miller served as an undergraduate research assistant in nutrition–toxicology at Michigan State University in 1978 and was a graduate research assistant at the Center for Air Environment Studies and Nutrition Department of The Pennsylvania State University from 1979 to 1986. He was a research scientist for Kraft, Inc., Glenview, Illinois, from 1986 to 1989, and was a senior research scientist from 1989 to 1992. He was vice president of nutrition research for the National Dairy Council from 1992 to 2001. From 2001 to 2004, he was senior vice president for Nutrition and Scientific Affairs. In 2004, he became senior vice president for nutrition and product innovation, and he was promoted in 2005 to executive vice president for Science & Innovation.

Dr. Miller was a scientific advisory panel member for the Office of Technology Assessment for the development of several reports to the U.S. Congress on issues in the treatment and prevention of osteoporosis. He has chaired or cochaired more than 35 workshops and symposia for national organizations including the American College of Nutrition, the American Society for Nutritional Sciences, and the International Life Sciences Institute.

He is a member of the Editorial Board for the *Journal of the American College of Nutrition*, the *Journal of Nutritional Biochemistry*, *Current Nutrition & Food Science*, and *Mature Medicine Canada*. He has served as a symposium editor for the *Journal of Nutrition*, *American Journal of Clinical Nutrition*, and the *Journal of the American College of Nutrition*. He is an editorial advisor for *Dairy Foods* magazine. He has served as a member of the Board of Directors as secretary/treasurer, vice president, president-elect, and president for the American College of Nutrition. He was president of the International Dairy Federation's Commission on Science, Nutrition and Education. He is a past member of the Program Coordination Committee for the International Dairy Federation and the Board of the U.S. National Committee of the International Dairy Federation. Dr. Miller served as president of The Pennsylvania State University Nutrition and Dietetics Alumni Society. He is a member of the Board of Directors for the International Society of Nutrigenetics/Nutrigenomics.

Among other awards, he has received the 1989 Kraft Basic Science Award and was listed in the 1992 *American Men and Women of Science*, and the 1992 *Who's Who in Science*. In 1993, he was elected as a Fellow of the American College of Nutrition, and in 2003, he was awarded a Master of the College. He was selected as an Outstanding Alumni by the College of Human Ecology at Michigan State University in 1996, and received the College of Health and Human Development Alumni Recognition Award in 1996 from The Pennsylvania State University. In 2000, he was recognized as an Outstanding Alumni by the Department of Food Science and Human Nutrition of Michigan State University. He was also named one of the dairy industries "Movers & Shakers" of 2000 by *Dairy Foods* magazine. In 2002, he was named an Alumni Fellow by The Pennsylvania State University, the highest award given by the alumni society. The Pennsylvania State University Nutrition and Dietetics Alumni Society named him an Outstanding Alumni in 2006.

He has presented more than 100 invited lectures at national and international meetings and has published more than 130 research papers, reviews, articles, and abstracts. He has coedited three books on diet, nutrition, and toxicology, and he has contributed chapters to nine books. He is coauthor of all three editions of the *Handbook of Dairy Foods and Nutrition*.

He has appeared on the *NBC Today Show*, CNBC, CNN, and *CBS Evening News* as well as other national and local television programs. He has also appeared on National Public Radio, WABC-NY, and other radio programs. He has been quoted in the *New York Times*, *USA Today*, the *Chicago Tribune*, the *Los Angeles Times*, *Financial Times* (London), *Redbook*, and other publications.

List of Reviewers

Dominick P. DePaola, D.D.S., Ph.D.
Forsyth Dental Center
Boston, Massachusetts

William H. Bowen, B.D.S., Ph.D.
University of Rochester
Rochester, New York

David A. McCarron, M.D.
Academic Network
Portland, Oregon

Marlene Most, Ph.D., R.D., LDN, FADA
Pennington Biomedical Research Center
Baton Rouge, Louisiana

Peter R. Holt, M.D.
St. Luke's and Roosevelt Hospital
New York, New York

David M. Klurfeld, Ph.D.
U.S. Department of Agriculture
Beltsville, Maryland

Ronald M. Krauss, M.D.
University of California, Berkeley
Oakland, California

David Kritchevsky, Ph.D.
The Wistar Institute
Philadelphia, Pennsylvania

Manfred Kroger, Ph.D.
The Pennsylvania State University
University Park, Pennsylvania

Louise A. Berner, Ph.D.
California Polytech State University
San Luis Obispo, California

Robert P. Heaney, M.D.
Creighton University
Omaha, Nebraska

Connie M. Weaver, Ph.D.
Purdue University
West Lafayette, Indiana

Michael B. Zemel, Ph.D.
University of Tennessee
Knoxville, Tennessee

Marta D. Van Loan, Ph.D., FACSM
University of California, Davis
Davis, California

Table of Contents

Chapter 7

Chapter 8

Chapter 9

1 The Importance of Milk and Milk Products in the Diet

1.1 INTRODUCTION

Milk and other dairy foods were recognized as important foods as early as 4000BC, evidenced by rock drawings from the Sahara depicting dairying. Remains of cheese have been found in Egyptian tombs dating back to 2300BC [1]. About 3000 years ago, milk and its products were familiar enough to be used as metaphors or analogues. An example is reference to the Biblical Promised Land as a land "flowing with milk and honey." During the Middle Ages, dairy products were important foods throughout Europe, although preferences for specific dairy foods varied geographically. In Greece and Rome, cheese, but not fresh milk or butter, was popular. In contrast, fresh milk and butter, but not cheese, were popular in northern Europe and Asia. Writings by Marco Polo, who traveled to China between 1271 and 1295, describe the drying of milk and drinking of a fermented milk (probably koumiss) by nomadic tribes. From the Middle Ages through the eighteenth century, changes in the handling of milk came slowly, and milking, churning, and cheese-making were largely done by hand [1].

In North America, milk and milk products were introduced with the arrival of the Europeans. In the early 1600s, the first dairy herd was established in the United States. With the Industrial Revolution, which brought railroads, steam engines, and refrigeration, fresh milk became available to a large population. Milking machines and automatic churns to make butter from cream appeared in the 1830s, followed by specialized cheese factories in the 1850s. As a result of continued advances and improvements in the dairy industry over the years, a wide variety of types of milk and other dairy products is available today [2].

This chapter presents an overview of specific nutrients — such as energy, protein, carbohydrate, fat, vitamins, and minerals — in milk and dairy foods, their nutritional contribution to Western diets, and dietary recommendations to include milk and milk products in the diet. Protecting the quality of milk and other dairy foods, trends in dairy food consumption, and the wide variety of dairy foods available, including flavored milk, cheeses, cultured and culture-containing dairy foods, and whey products are also discussed. For additional information on this subject, readers are referred to several publications [2–9].

1.2 NUTRIENT COMPONENTS OF MILK AND MILK PRODUCTS

Although fluid whole cow's milk is a liquid food (87% water), it contains an average of 13% total solids and 9% solids-not-fat, an amount comparable to the solids content of many other foods (Figure 1.1) [10]. More than 100 different components have been identified in cow's milk. Important nutritional contributions of milk and milk products are calcium, vitamin D (if fortified), protein, potassium, vitamin A, vitamin B_{12}, riboflavin, niacin (or niacin equivalents), and phosphorus [2,11,12]. As a result of new technologies in genetics, molecular biology, and analytical chemistry,

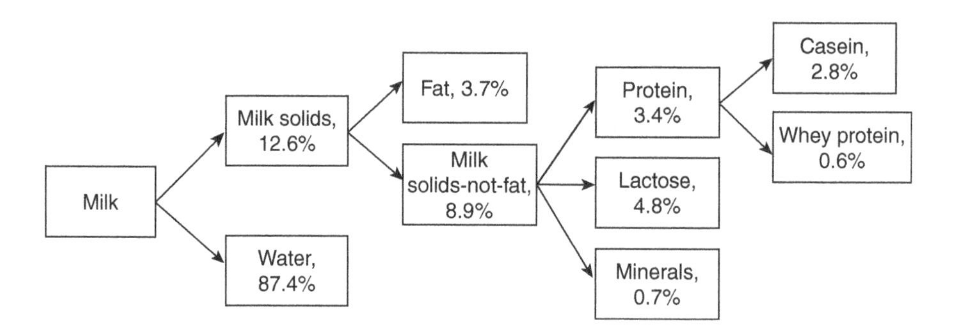

FIGURE 1.1 Major constituents of milk. (From Chandan, R., *Dairy-Based Ingredients*, Eagan Press, St. Paul, MN, 1997.)

a number of milk constituents with physiological benefits beyond milk's traditional package of nutrients are being recognized [13].

1.2.1 Energy

The energy (calorie) content of milk and other dairy foods varies widely and depends mostly on the fat content of the milk, but also on the addition of nonfat milk solids, sweeteners, and other energy-yielding components [12]. For example, whole milk (3.25% milk fat) provides about 150 kcal per cup; reduced-fat (2%) milk provides 120 kcal per cup; low-fat (1%) milk provides 100 kcal per cup; and nonfat (skim) milk provides 80 kcal per cup [12]. As mentioned above, milk is considered to be a food of high nutrient density, providing a high concentration of nutrients in relation to its energy content. There is no scientific evidence that the intake of specific foods such as dairy foods contributes to obesity. On the contrary, emerging science indicates a beneficial role for calcium-rich dairy foods in weight management when consumed as part of an energy-reduced diet (see Chapter 7). The 2005 *Dietary Guidelines for Americans* [14] states that "adults and children should not avoid milk and milk products because of concerns that these foods lead to weight gain." Weight loss is achieved by reducing total caloric intake and/or increasing physical activity. For individuals concerned about reducing their body weight, there is a wide variety of dairy products of different energy content available [12].

1.2.2 Protein

Cow's milk is recognized as an excellent source of high-quality protein [15–17]. In 2000, milk and other dairy foods (excluding butter) contributed 19% of the protein available in the nation's food supply [18]. Cow's milk contains about 3.5% protein by weight, which accounts for about 38% of the total solids-not-fat content of milk, and contributes about 21% of the energy of whole milk [3,9]. As shown in Table 1.1, cow's milk protein is a heterogeneous mixture of proteins [3]. Milk also contains small amounts of various enzymes and traces of nonprotein nitrogenous materials [3]. Of the total protein in cow's milk, about 80% is casein and 20% is whey protein [3]. Casein, the dominant protein in cow's milk, can be fractionated electrophoretically into four major components: alpha-, beta-, gamma-, and kappa-casein. Casein is generally defined as the protein precipitated at pH 4.6, a property used in the manufacturing of cheese. Whey protein, which is more heterogeneous than casein, consists predominantly of beta-lactoglobulin and alpha-lactalbumin. Alpha-lactalbumin has a high content of the amino acid tryptophan, a precursor of niacin. Because of milk's tryptophan content, this food is an excellent source of niacin equivalents. One niacin equivalent is defined as 1 mg of niacin or 60 mg of tryptophan. Other whey proteins present in smaller amounts are serum albumin, immunoglobulins (e.g., IgA, IgG, IgM), protease peptones,

TABLE 1.1
Protein Fractions Isolated from Cow's Milk

Protein and Protein Fraction	Concentration in Milk g/L
Total protein	36
Casein	29.5
α_{s1}-Casein	11.9
α_{s2}-Casein	3.1
β-Casein	9.8
κ-Casein	3.5
γ-Casein	1.2
Whey proteins	6.3
β-Lactoglobulin	3.2
α-Lactalbumin serum	1.2
Serum Albumin	0.4
Immunoglobulins	0.8
Proteose-Peptones	1.0

Source: From Jensen, R. G. Ed., *Handbook of Milk Composition*, Academic Press, New York, p. 465, 1995.

lactoferrin, and transferrin. Each of these proteins has unique characteristics and biological functions [19]. Whey protein concentrates and isolates are used as ingredients in a number of formulated food products [20].

Nutritionally, cow's milk protein is considered to be high-quality or a "complete protein," because it contains, in varying amounts, all nine of the essential amino acids that human bodies cannot synthesize, and in proportions resembling amino acid requirements [5,12,15,17]. Table 1.2 lists the amino-acid distribution in milk and selected cheeses as compared to the Recommended Dietary Allowance (RDA) for essential amino acids. Because of its high quality, cow's milk protein is used as a standard reference protein to evaluate the nutritive value of food proteins [15]. The quality of a protein is determined by any one of the several parameters indicated in Table 1.3.

Individual milk proteins have been shown to exhibit a wide range of beneficial functions [21–23]. A symposium on the emerging role of dairy proteins and bioactive peptides in nutrition and health addressed the benefits of bovine milk-derived peptides and amino acids in glycemic control and weight management, food intake regulation, muscle metabolism, hypertension, and reduction of dental caries [23]. Dairy foods are rich in the branched-chain amino acid leucine, which has been demonstrated to stimulate recovery of muscle protein synthesis during food restriction (dieting) or after endurance exercise and to modulate the use of glucose by exercising muscles, which is important in endurance exercise [24]. Milk proteins, such as casein and whey protein, are a rich source of peptides that inhibit the vasoconstrictor angiotensin-I-converting enzyme and significantly lower systolic and diastolic blood pressure [21,25]. Other dairy proteins, such as caseinphosphopeptides and glycomacropeptides, as well as lactoferrin, help to reduce the risk of dental caries [26]. Both whey and casein proteins, such as alpha-lactalbumin, cholecystokinin, casomorphin, caseinomacropeptide, and leucine, may help contribute to satiety and regulate food intake [27]. However, further study is needed to clarify the role of dairy proteins in satiety or energy metabolism [28].

Evidence from *in vitro* and experimental animal studies indicates that milk proteins may protect against cancer [29–31]. McIntosh et al. [29] demonstrated that dairy protein-based diets reduced the development of cancer in Sprague Dawley male rats that received a chemical carcinogen. As reviewed by Parodi [31], whey proteins in particular appear to be anticarcinogenic.

TABLE 1.2
Amino Acid Distribution in Milk and Selected Cheeses

Amino Acids	RDA for Adults[a] g/day	2% Reduced Fat Fluid Milk g/1 cup (8oz. 244 g)	Pasteurized Process American Cheese g/oz (28 g)	Cheddar Cheese g/oz (28 g)	Swiss Cheese g/oz (28 g)	Cottage Cheese g/oz (113 g) (2% Milk Fat)
Essential (Indispensable)						
Histidine	0.98	0.230	0.256	0.248	0.302	0.516
Isolecine	1.3	0.517	0.290	0.438	0.436	0.913
Leucine	2.9	0.835	0.555	0.676	0.839	0.597
Lysine	2.7	0.676	0.623	0.587	0.733	1.255
Methionine[b]	1.3	0.213	0.162	0.185	0.222	0.467
Phenylalanine[c]	2.3	0.412	0.319	0.372	0.471	0.837
Threonine	1.4	0.385	0.204	0.251	0.294	0.688
Tryptophan	0.35	0.120	0.092	0.091	0.114	0.173
Valine	1.68	0.571	0.376	0.471	0.606	0.962
Nonessential (Dispensable)						
Alanine		0.294	0.157	0.199	0.259	0.806
Arginine		0.309	0.263	0.267	0.263	0.709
Aspartic acid		0.647	0.386	0.454	0.445	1.051
Cystine		0.078	0.040	0.035	0.082	0.144
Glutamic acid		1.786	1.303	1.727	1.617	3.363
Glycine		0.181	0.103	0.122	0.144	0.338
Proline		0.826	0.639	0.796	1.046	1.799
Serine		0.463	0.303	0.413	0.465	0.871
Tyrosine		0.412	0.344	0.341	0.480	0.827

[a] Values calculated for 70 kg adult male.
[b] Value for total S-containing amino acids (methionine + cystine).
[c] Value for total aromatic amino acids (phenylalanine + tyrosine).

Source: From Institute of Medicine, Dietary Reference Intakes for Energy, Carbohydrate, Fiber, Fat, Fatty Acids, Cholesterol, Protein, and Amino Acids, 2002 and USDA National Database for Standard Reference, Release 17.

Whey proteins are rich in substrates (e.g., the sulfur amino acids cysteine and methionine) for the synthesis of glutathione, which has been demonstrated to prevent cancer under experimental conditions. The ability of casein- and whey-derived peptides to enhance immunity in *in vitro* and laboratory animal studies may also explain the anticancer activity of bovine milk proteins [19–21,32]. Alternatively, the presence of high-affinity binding proteins in the whey protein fraction may bind potential cocarcinogens, rendering them unavailable. In the 1990s, researchers hypothesized that the A1 form of beta-casein, the second-most abundant protein in cow's milk, is a risk factor for type-1 diabetes, coronary heart disease (CHD), and possibly schizophrenia and autism, whereas A2 beta-casein does not have these adverse effects. However, a recent critical review of the A1/A2 hypothesis by Professor Truswell at the University of Sydney in Australia led to the conclusion that "there is no convincing or even probable evidence that the A1 B-casein of cow milk has any adverse effect in humans" [33]. This review is independent of a separate, unpublished review conducted by the New Zealand food standard and food safety authorities that concluded in 2003 that "no relationship has been established between A1 or A2 milk and

TABLE 1.3
Average Measures of Protein Quality for Milk and Milk Proteins

	BV[a]	PD	NP-U	PER	PDCAAS
Milk	91	95	86.45	3.1	1.21
Casein	77	100	76	2.9	1.23
Whey protein	104	100	92	3.6	1.15
Biological value (BV)	Proportion of absorbed protein that is retained in the body for maintenance and/or growth				
Protein digestibility (PD)	= Proportion of food protein absorbed				
Net protein utilization (NPU)	= Proportion of protein intake that is retained (calculated as BV x PD)				
Protein efficiency ratio (PER)	= Gain in body weight divided by weight of protein consumed				
Protein digestibility corrected amino acid score (PDCAAS)	= The amino acid score multiplied by a digestibility factor				

[a] The BV of egg protein is defined as 100.
Source: Adapted from *Nutritional Quality of Proteins,* European Dairy Association, 1997. With permission.

diabetes, CHD, or other diseases" [33]. A limited number of infants and young children exhibit allergic responses to cow's milk protein, primarily beta-lactoglobulin, casein, alpha-lactalbumin, and bovine serum albumin [34,35]. The prevalence of cow's milk protein allergy or sensitivity (i.e., an abnormal immunological response to one or more of cow's milk proteins) is often overestimated, particularly by parents, and estimates vary widely [35–37]. When strict diagnostic tests are used to diagnose the condition, the prevalence in infants is estimated to be 2.2% to 2.8% [38]. The incidence is somewhat higher in infants who are fed cow's milk very early in life (i.e., before 3 to 4 months of age) or have a family history of allergies. In the majority of cases, this condition is temporary, and 80% to 90% of children outgrow their sensitivity to cow's milk or develop tolerance by 3 to 5 years of age [34,35,38]. Crittenden and Bennett [35] report that the prevalence of cow's milk allergy in adults is 0.1% to 0.5%, compared to 2% to 6% in infants. Although some researchers have suggested that milk proteins, particularly bovine serum albumin (BSA), trigger an autoimmune response that destroys pancreas beta cells in genetically susceptible children, causing type-I or insulin-dependent diabetes (IDDM) [39–41], scientific evidence to date fails to support a causal association between cow's milk proteins and IDDM [42–51]. When the feeding practices of more than 250 children with IDDM were compared to those of nondiabetic children, no association was found between early introduction of cow's milk during infancy and IDDM [44]. In another investigation involving 253 children (aged 9 months to 7 years) from 171 families of persons with IDDM, researchers found that children who developed B-cell autoimmunity (BCA), an early predictor of IDDM, were no more likely to have been exposed to cow's milk protein than children without BCA [45]. Blood levels of antibodies to BSA do not predict diabetes, according to several researchers [42,46]. Evidence to date does not support a recommendation to avoid cow's milk during childhood or change current feeding guidelines to reduce the risk of type-1 diabetes [50,51]. A review of research related to infant feeding practices and type-1 diabetes concludes that "there is no causal relationship between early exposure to cow's milk and the development of autoimmune diabetes mellitus in children" [50].

There is no scientific evidence that intake of dairy foods causes type-2 diabetes, which is characterized by a decrease in insulin secretion. On the contrary, dietary patterns characterized by high dairy-food intake may lower the risk of this disease [52,53]. When the relationship between dairy food intake and the incidence of type-2 diabetes was examined in 41,254 men over a 12-year period, intake of dairy foods, especially low-fat dairy foods, was associated with a lower risk of type-2 diabetes [53].

1.2.3 Carbohydrate

Lactose, the principal carbohydrate in milk, is synthesized in the mammary gland. Lactose accounts for approximately 54% of the total solids-not-fat content of milk and contributes about 30% of the energy (calories) of whole milk. Cow's milk contains about 4.8% lactose (12 to 12.5 g lactose/cup) compared with 7% (15 to 18 g lactose/cup) in human milk [54,55]. Refer to Table 8.6 in Chapter 8, Lactose Content of Dairy Products.

In infants, some lactose enters the distal bowel (colon), where it promotes the growth of certain beneficial lactic-acid-producing bacteria that may help combat gastrointestinal disturbances resulting from undesirable putrefactive bacteria [38]. In addition, lactose favors the intestinal absorption of calcium and perhaps phosphorus in infants [56]. However, there is no scientific evidence that lactose improves calcium absorption in adults [57].

Minor quantities of glucose, galactose, and oligosaccharides are also present in milk. Glucose and galactose are the products of lactose hydrolysis by the enzyme lactase [3]. Researchers speculate that galactose may have a unique role in the rapidly developing infant brain [3]. Some individuals have difficulty digesting lactose because of reduced lactase levels, a condition called *lactase nonpersistence*. However, research findings indicate that most persons with lactase nonpersistence are able to consume the amount of lactose in up to 2 cups of milk a day if taken with meals, one at breakfast and the other at dinner (see Chapter 8) [58,59]. Other dairy foods, such as aged cheeses and yogurts with live active cultures, are also well-tolerated [58,59]. In cheese-making, lactose is converted to lactic acid by select microorganisms. A number of low-lactose and lactose-reduced milks and milk products are available. Commercial lactase hydrolyzes lactose in milk when added prior to processing. Lactose-reduced milk contains about 70% less lactose than regular milk. Lactose-free milk has about 99.9% of its lactose hydrolyzed. Another alternative is lactase enzyme tablets that individuals can consume with lactose-containing foods to improve the digestion of lactose [60]. The National Medical Association [61] recommends that African Americans, many of whom are lactase maldigesters, consume 3 to 4 servings per day of low-fat milk, cheese, or yogurt to improve their health. The 2005 *Dietary Guidelines for Americans* [14] states "If a person wants to consider milk alternatives because of lactose intolerance, the most reliable and easiest ways to derive the health benefits associated with milk and milk product consumption is to choose alternatives within the milk food group, such as yogurt or lactose-free milk, or to consume the enzyme lactase prior to the consumption of milk products."

1.2.4 Fat

Milk fat contributes unique characteristics to the appearance, texture, flavor, and satiability of dairy foods, and is a source of energy, essential fatty acids, fat-soluble vitamins, and several other potential health-promoting components [62,63].

Milk fat, the most complex of dietary fats, exists in microscopic globules in an oil-in-water emulsion in milk. Milk's lipids are mainly triglycerides (triacylglycerols) or esters of fatty acids with glycerol (97% to 98% of total lipid), with phospholipids, cholesterol and cholesterol esters, diacylglycerols, monoacylglycerols, and free fatty acids, along with varying amounts of the fat-soluble vitamins A, D, E, and K making up the remaining 2% to 3% [63]. The fat contributes about 49% of the energy of whole milk, 35% of the energy of 2% reduced-fat milk, and 21% of the energy in 1% low-fat milk [12]. More than 400 different fatty acids and fatty-acid derivatives have been identified in milk fat, ranging from butyric acid — with four carbon atoms — to fatty acids with 26 carbon atoms [3,62,64]. Milk fat is unique among animal fats, because it contains a relatively high proportion of short-chain and medium-chain saturated fatty acids (i.e., those with 4 to 12 carbons in length). The composition of milk fat varies somewhat according to the breed of the cow, stage of lactation, season, geographical location, and feed composition [63,64]. In whole milk (3.25% fat), approximately 57% of the fat is saturated fatty acids, 25% is monounsaturated fatty acids, and 6% is polyunsaturated fatty acids [12]. The saturated fatty acids present in the largest amount in milk fat are palmitic, stearic, and myristic acids. Although saturated fatty acids generally contribute to an increase in blood cholesterol levels, individual saturated fatty acids differ in their blood cholesterol-raising effects (see Chapter 2). Long-chain saturated fatty acids, such as lauric, myristic, and palmitic acids, raise blood total and low-density lipoprotein (LDL, or "bad" cholesterol) levels, whereas stearic acid and short-chain saturated fatty acids such as butyric, caproic, caprylic, and capric acids have either a neutral effect or may lower blood cholesterol levels [65,66]. Oleic acid is the main monounsaturated fatty acid in milk fat [3]. Polyunsaturated fatty acids, such as arachidonic acid, are present in trace amounts. Arachidonic acid is required, but can be made from its precursor, linoleic acid, an essential fatty acid. Linoleic and linolenic acids are not synthesized in the human body or are synthesized at such a slow rate that they must be supplied by the diet. The essential polyunsaturated fatty acid linoleic acid is present in milk fat in a form that favors conversion to arachidonic acid. Omega-3-linolenic acid and its products, eicosapentaenoic acid (EPA) and docosahexaenoic acid (DHA), are also present in small but significant amounts.

Trans fatty acids are naturally present in very small amounts in milk and dairy foods as a result of biohydrogenation in ruminants [12]. In most cases, the amount of *trans* fatty acids in a serving of dairy foods is less than the U.S. Food and Drug Administration's (FDA) labeling threshold of 0.5 g per serving [67,68]. Cow's milk contains an estimated 0.22 g *trans* fatty acids per serving, whereas traditional stick margarine contains ten times this amount [67]. The main source of *trans* fatty acids in the U.S. diet is partially-hydrogenated vegetable oils used in crackers and other baked goods, margarines, and fried snack foods [69]. Although intake of *trans* fatty acids from industrial sources is associated with increased risk of atherosclerosis, there is no scientific evidence that *trans* fatty acids in dairy foods are harmful to health [70]. On the contrary, the predominant *trans* fatty acid in milk fat, *trans*−11-18:1 (vaccenic acid), is converted to conjugated linoleic acid (CLA), specifically *cis*-9, *trans*-11 CLA (rumenic acid) [63,70]. As discussed below, several potential health benefits of CLA have been identified [63,70]. See Chapter 2 for information on the effect of individual fatty acids in milk fat on risk of coronary heart disease. Current dietary recommendations advise moderation in total fat intake (20% to 35% of calories), less than 10% of calories from saturated fatty acids, and intake of *trans* fatty acids as low as possible. When selecting milk or milk products, low-fat or fat-free choices are recommended [14,17,66].

Cholesterol is a normal constituent in milk, although milk contains relatively little cholesterol (less than 0.5% of milk fat) [12]. Because cholesterol occurs in the fat-globule membrane, its concentration in dairy foods is related to the fat content. A one-cup serving (8 fluid ounces) of whole (3.25% fat), 2%, 1%, and nonfat (skim) milk contains 24 mg, 20 mg, 12 mg, and 5 mg cholesterol, respectively [12]. Cholesterol in the body is the precursor of many important substances, such as adrenocortical hormones, vitamin D, bile salts, and sex hormones. Milk and other dairy foods contributed about 16% of the cholesterol available in the food supply in 2000 [18]. This share of cholesterol from dairy foods has remained about the same since the early 1900s, although the contribution of individual dairy foods to the availability of cholesterol has varied over the years. Today, more low-fat milks, yogurts, and cheeses contribute to the availability of cholesterol than earlier in the century, whereas less cholesterol now comes from whole milk and cream than in the past. Not only do dairy foods make a relatively small contribution to total cholesterol intake, but dietary cholesterol, regardless of source, has a modest effect on blood cholesterol levels. Moreover, individuals vary widely in their blood cholesterol response to dietary cholesterol (see Chapter 2).

Emerging scientific findings indicate that milk fat contains several components, such as CLA, sphingomyelin, and butyric acid, that may potentially protect against major chronic diseases (see Chapter 4 on Dairy Foods and Cancer and Chapter 2 on Dairy Foods and Cardiovascular Health) [63,71]. Milk fat is the richest natural dietary source of CLA, containing 2.4 to 28.1 mg CLA per g of milk fat [71,72]. The CLA content of most dairy products ranges from 2.5 to 9.1 mg/g of milk fat. In cheeses, the CLA content is reported to range from 3.6 to 8 mg/g fat; in fluid milks, from 3.3 to 6.4 mg/g fat; and in butter, from 5.5 to 6.5 mg/g fat. Moreover, 90% of the CLA in dairy foods is in the *cis*-9, *trans*-11-18:2 isomeric form (called *rumenic acid*), which is believed to be the biologically-active CLA isomer [63,71]. The CLA content of dairy foods is influenced primarily by the CLA content of the starting raw milk and the final fat content. In addition, the protein content, type of fermentation bacteria, and processing procedures (such as agitation) may make a small contribution to differences in the CLA content among and within dairy foods [73]. Pasteurization increases the CLA content of dairy foods and differences in protein content, and the type of fermentation bacteria used in some dairy foods influences their CLA content [72].

Numerous health benefits have been attributed to CLA [63,70,74–80]. Findings from experimental animal, cell culture, and limited human studies demonstrate that CLA may help reduce the risk of several types of cancer (e.g., colorectal, breast, lung, prostate, ovarian) (see Chapter 4 on Dairy Foods and Cancer), heart disease (see Chapter 2 on Dairy Foods and Cardiovascular Disease), and diabetes, enhance bone formation and immune function.

Sphingomyelin, the most common sphingolipid, makes up about one-third of total milk phospholipids, although it can vary according to season and a cow's stage of lactation [63,80]. Sphingomyelin is present in cow's milk at a concentration of 0.1 mg/mL or about 0.2% to 1.0% of the total lipids of milk, or one-fourth to one-third of total milk phospholipids. Because sphingolipids are found mainly in the milk fat globule membrane, low-fat and nonfat, as well as traditional, dairy products are good sources of sphingolipids [80]. *In vitro* and experimental animal studies indicate that dietary sphingolipids may have a protective role in some cancers and possibly cardiovascular disease [63,81]. Schmelz and coworkers [82] found that intake of dairy sphingomyelin reduced the proliferation of colonic cells and the appearance of aberrant crypt foci in mice treated with a chemical carcinogen. Milk sphingomyelin has been shown to inhibit the absorption of cholesterol, fat, and other lipids in laboratory rats [83]. A unique feature of milk fat is the presence of butyric acid, which is found at a level of more than 3% of the major fatty acids in milk fat. No other common food contains this four-carbon short-chain fatty acid. Most butyric acid in the human body is derived from the fermentation of fiber in the digestive tract. Findings from cell culture and experimental animal studies indicate that butyric acid may protect against some cancers [63,80,84,85]. In a variety of cancer cell lines (colon, leukemia, prostate, breast), butyric acid inhibits the proliferation and induces differentiation and programmed cell death (apoptosis). At the molecular level, butyric acid is associated with down-regulation or inactivation of the expression of cancer genes [80,84]. Butyric acid may also inhibit tumor invasiveness and metastasis [80,84].

The question of whether or not milk fat favorably influences satiety is currently being entertained. Numerous studies under varying conditions have examined whether specific macronutrients — such as fat, carbohydrate, and protein — improve satiety or a feeling of fullness following intake. Compared to low-fat meals, a high-fat meal empties more slowly from the stomach and decreases intestinal mobility, which delays the onset of hunger and contributes to a postmeal feeling of satiety [63]. Little is known about the effect of specific fatty acids or different sources of fats, such as milk fat, on satiety. Research is needed to determine the satiety value of milk fat and certain fatty acids in milk fat. If milk fat, as compared to other sources of fat, is demonstrated to have a unique effect on satiety, this finding could support recommendations to include milk fat in the diet to help control hunger and food intake. A preliminary study involving healthy adults found that dairy fat affected satiety differently than nondairy fat [86]. Compared to nondairy fat, a meal consumed with dairy fat resulted in higher initial blood glucose levels and lower blood glucose levels 4 to 6 hours following the meal. The researchers acknowledge that the link between blood glucose and satiety is complex and recommend that additional research be conducted to determine the potential of dairy fat to influence satiety [86]. In a study of healthy young men in France, a pasta lunch containing butter delayed the desire for the next meal by approximately 30 minutes, compared with the same meal containing a low-energy butter substitute despite no change in energy intake [87].

Milk fat may have a beneficial effect on bone health, according to experimental animal studies [88,89]. In a study in young chicks, intake of different dietary fats influenced changes in prostaglandin E2 (PGE2), which is associated with bone resorption and other bone growth factors [89]. Saturated fat (butter or butterfat) lowered bone levels of the essential unsaturated fatty acid, arachidonic acid, which is a precursor of PGE2, raised insulin-like growth factor (IGF-1), which is associated with bone growth, moderated PGE2 production, and increased bone formation rate [89]. Additionally, in chicks fed saturated fat (butter), the higher bone formation rate was accompanied by an increase in blood levels of hexosamines, a component of bone matrix protein, reflective of increased bone turnover [89]. The chicks fed the saturated-fat diet (butter) also maintained the highest blood levels of vitamin E. In a previous investigation, high blood levels of vitamin E were associated with increased bone formation rate [90]. A saturated-fat diet increases the saturated/polyunsaturated fat ratio in bone and may spare vitamin E to enhance the formation of bone. These findings indicate that saturated fat (butter) may optimize bone formation by its effects on bone growth factors.

The potential to modify milk fat to provide a specific nutritional or health advantage has been investigated [91]. Manipulating the fatty acid content of milk fat by altering the feed of cows has been demonstrated to have a favorable effect on blood lipid levels in humans [92,93]. By modifying the diet of dairy cows, researchers produced a milk fat with a reduced concentration of saturated fatty acids and an increased content of unsaturated fatty acids [93]. Compared to regular milk fat, intake of this fat-modified milk had positive effects on blood lipids (i.e., LDL/high-density lipoprotein [HDL] ratio and Lp(a) concentrations) in humans [93]. The monounsaturated fat content of milk can be increased by increasing the monounsaturated content of cows' feed [94]. According to a study involving 30 adults with type-IIa hyperlipidemia, intake of butter and cheese that contained a higher content of monounsaturated fat content increased blood levels of HDL cholesterol, the "good" cholesterol [95]. The monounsaturated fat-rich dairy foods were produced by feeding cows full-fat soybeans. The cholesterol-raising properties of milk fat can be reduced by removing cholesterol, fractionating milk fat, or altering the fatty acid profile of milk fat by changing cows' feed. Manipulating the diets of dairy cows can also increase the content of beneficial dietary fatty acids (CLA, vaccenic acid, omega-3 fatty acids) in milk [96].

1.2.5 Vitamins

Almost all of the vitamins known to be essential to humans have been detected at some level in milk. Vitamins A, D, E, and K are associated with the fat component of milk. Vitamin A plays important roles in vision, gene expression, cellular differentiation, embryonic development, growth, reproduction, and immunocompetence [97]. Both vitamin A and its precursors, called *carotenoids* — principally beta-carotene — are present in variable amounts in milk fat [3]. The carotenoids are the yellow pigments in milk fat responsible for the color of butter and, along with the green riboflavin vitamin, for milk's characteristic creamy color. About 11% to 50% of total vitamin A activity in milk is derived from carotenoids, the specific proportion depending on the breed and feed of the cow and season of year, among other factors [7]. Milk and milk products are an important dietary source of vitamin A, providing about 22.1% of this vitamin in the U.S. food supply (Table 1.4) [18]. Whole cow's milk (3.25% fat) provides about 249 International Unit (IU) (68 retinol activity equivalents [RAE]) of vitamin A per 8-ounce serving [12]. Three cups of whole milk, therefore, provide 23% and 29% of the RDA for vitamin A for adult males and females, respectively [12,97]. Not only is cow's milk a good source of vitamin A, but β-lactoglobulin, the

TABLE 1.4
Nutrient Contribution of Dairy Foods, Excluding Butter, to the U.S. per Capita Food Supply, 2000

Nutrient	%
Energy	9.1
Protein	19.4
Fat	11.8
Carbohydrate	4.5
Minerals	
Calcium	72.2
Phosphorus	32.7
Zinc	16.8
Magnesium	15.8
Iron	1.9
Vitamins	
Riboflavin	26.3
Vitamin A	22.1
Vitamin B_{12}	20.3
Vitamin B_6	8.7
Thiamin	4.7
Folate	2.6
Ascorbic Acid	2.5
Vitamin E	2.4
Niacin	1.2
Electrolytes	
Sodium	32.6
Potassium	18.1

Source: From Gerrior, S., Bente, L., and Hiza, H., Nutrient Content of the U.S. Food Supply, 1909 to 2000, Home Economics Research Report No. 56, U.S. Department of Agriculture, Center for Nutrition Policy and Promotion, Washington, D.C., 2004.

major protein component of bovine milk whey, may enhance vitamin A absorption [98]. Because vitamin A and carotene exist in the fat portion of milk, lower-fat and fat-free (nonfat or skim) milks contain little of this vitamin. Consequently, fluid lower-fat and fat-free (nonfat or skim) milks must be fortified with chemically-derived vitamin A (retinyl palmitate) to a level found in whole milk or 300 IU (6% Daily Value [DV]) per 8-fluid-ounce serving. However, dairy processors are encouraged to continue to fortify low-fat milks to the current level of 500 IU of vitamin A per cup (10% DV), or 2000 IU per quart [99]. If vitamin A is added to whole milk or other milks for which it is not required, the label must state this fact [100].

Vitamin D, a fat-soluble vitamin that enhances the intestinal absorption of calcium and phosphorus, is essential for the maintenance of a healthy skeleton throughout life [101]. A deficiency of this vitamin results in inadequate mineralization of bone and leads to the development of rickets in children and osteomalacia in adults [101]. In addition, vitamin D deficiency leads to secondary hyperparathyroidism, which enhances mobilization of calcium from the skeleton, resulting in osteoporosis [101]. Vitamin D is present in low concentrations in unfortified milk (47 to 105 IU vitamin D per L) [3,7]. However, although optional, nearly all fluid milk marketed in the United States — irrespective of its fat content — is fortified with vitamin D to obtain the standardized amount of 400 IU (10 μg/quart) [99,101,102]. One cup (8 ounces) of vitamin

D-fortified milk provides 25% of the AI [101] for this vitamin for adults aged 51–70 years. When a food is fortified with vitamin D, vitamin D must be listed on the nutrition label [99]. Fortification of fluid milk with vitamin D is supported by health professional organizations [103,104]. Although vitamin D fortification of milk is considered to be an important public health measure and has been largely responsible for the virtual elimination of rickets (a disease characterized by soft and deformed bones) in the United States [105,106], this disease has recently made an unexpected comeback among young children [103,107]. Further, subclinical vitamin D deficiency has been identified in otherwise relatively healthy children, adolescents, and adults [108,109]. Experts attribute the recent increase in rickets in children and subclinical vitamin D deficiency in adolescents and adults in part to low intake of vitamin D-fortified milk [109]. Data from national surveys reveal that intake of vitamin D from food sources and supplements falls short of recommended intake levels and dairy products are the primary source of vitamin D [11,110,111]. Consuming a sufficient intake of vitamin D-fortified milk and milk products is especially important for individuals at risk of vitamin D deficiency, such as those who have limited exposure to sunlight (e.g., housebound older adults) and people with darker skin [14,101]. To help ensure that milk contains the amount of vitamin D specified on the label, milk is monitored primarily by state governments in cooperation with the federal FDA [112]. The FDA recommends that the vitamin D content of milk be measured by a certified laboratory and determined to be acceptable by this regulatory agency [112]. According to good manufacturing practices (GMP), the acceptable range allowed for vitamin D fortification of milk is not less than 100% and not more than 150% of label claims (i.e., 400 to 600 IU vitamin D) [112]. Milk remains an important and carefully monitored source of vitamin D in the diets of all who consume this food. In addition to vitamin D-fortified milk, vitamin D-fortified process cheese may be another option to improve vitamin D status [113]. Johnson et al. [113] found that vitamin D in fortified process cheese is bioavailable and that older adults absorb vitamin D from this dairy food just as efficiently as do younger adults. Dairy food manufacturers are now adding vitamin D to some cheeses and yogurt. Check the nutrition facts panel on the label to see if the product has added vitamin D.

Vitamin E (mainly tocopherol) is an antioxidant, protecting cell membranes and lipoproteins from oxidative damage by free radicals [7,114]. This vitamin also helps to maintain cell membrane integrity and stimulate the immune response [7,114]. Some studies also support a protective role for vitamin E in cardiovascular disease and possibly some cancers [114]. Although widely available in the US food supply, vitamin E is present in low concentrations in milk (0.06 mg alpha-tocopherol equivalents/100 g or 0.150 mg alpha-tocopherol equivalents per 1 cup) [12]. The RDA for vitamin E is 15 mg alpha-tocopherol for males and females 14 years of age and older [114]. Vitamin K, which is necessary for blood clotting, is found in low concentrations in milk (0.2 μg/100 g) [12,97]. This vitamin may have a protective role in bone health [97].

In addition to the essential fat-soluble vitamins, milk and other dairy foods also contain all of the water-soluble vitamins in varying amounts required by humans. Significant amounts of thiamin (vitamin B_1), which acts as a coenzyme for many reactions in carbohydrate metabolism, are found in milk (0.04 mg/100 g or 0.11 mg/cup). Three 8-ounce glasses of milk provide about 29% and 27% of the thiamin recommended for adult males and females, respectively [12,115]. Milk is also an excellent source of riboflavin, or vitamin B_2. This vitamin functions as a precursor for certain essential coenzymes important in the oxidation of glucose, fatty acids, amino acids, and purines [115]. The average riboflavin content of fluid whole milk is about 0.18 mg/100 g. Three 8-ounce glasses of milk would supply 122 and 100%, respectively, of the 1.1 and 1.3 mg/day of riboflavin recommended for adult females and males aged 19 years and older, respectively [12,115]. Niacin (nicotinic acid and nicotinamide) functions as part of a coenzyme in fat synthesis, tissue respiration, and utilization of carbohydrate [115]. This vitamin promotes healthy skin, nerves, and digestive tract, as well as aiding in digestion and fostering a normal appetite. The average content of niacin in milk is 0.107 mg/100 g. The presence of the amino acid tryptophan in milk protein can be used by the body for the synthesis of niacin. A dietary intake of 60 mg tryptophan is considered to be equivalent to 1 mg of niacin in the body [3]. The niacin equivalents in three 8-ounce glasses of milk, therefore, equal 9.93 (0.783 mg preformed niacin plus 9.15 mg from tryptophan). This provides 71% and 62%, respectively, of the 14 mg and 16 mg of niacin per day recommended for adult females and males, respectively [12,115].

Milk is a good source of pantothenic acid, a component of the coenzyme A involved in fatty acid metabolism [115]. The average amount of pantothenic acid in milk is 0.36 mg/100 g [12]. Three glasses of milk provide 53% of the 5 mg of pantothenic acid per day recommended for adults [115]. Vitamin B_6 (pyridoxine, pyridoxal, pyridoxamine) functions as a coenzyme for more than 100 enzymes involved in protein metabolism [115]. On the average, about 0.04 mg of vitamin B_6 are found in 100 g of milk. Three glasses of milk provide about 23% and 18%, respectively, of the 1.3 mg and 1.7 mg of vitamin B_6 per day recommended for adults [115].

Folate (folic acid) is a growth factor and functions as a coenzyme in the transfer of one-carbon units in the de novo synthesis of nucleotides necessary for DNA synthesis [115]. Cow's milk contains a high-affinity folate binding protein (FBP), a minor whey protein that promotes retention and increases the bioavailability of folate by slowing the rate of absorption [116]. The ability of cow's milk to enhance the bioavailability of folate contained in other foods was demonstrated in a study of 31 young women who were fed low-folate diets with or without cow's milk for 8 weeks [117]. Adequate folate nutrition is especially important for women of childbearing age to reduce the risk of neural tube defects in infants. The average level of folate in milk is 5 μg/100 g [12]. Three glasses of milk would supply 9% of the 400 μg folate/day recommended for nonpregnant, nonlactating adults [115].Vitamin B_{12} is necessary for growth, maintenance of nerve tissues, and normal blood formation [115]. Milk provides 0.44 μg vitamin B_{12}/100 g [12]. Three glasses of milk would furnish all of the 2.4 μg vitamin B_{12} recommended for most adults [12,115]. Ascorbic acid (vitamin C), which forms cementing substances such as collagen in the body, is important in wound healing and increasing resistance to infections [114]. This vitamin also enhances the absorption of nonheme iron and may protect against some cancers and cardiovascular disease [114]. Milk contains an insignificant amount of vitamin C [12].

1.2.6 Minerals

Milk and other dairy foods are important sources of major minerals, particularly calcium, phosphorus, magnesium, potassium, and trace elements such as zinc [12]. The mineral content of cow's milk is influenced by several factors, including the stage of lactation, environmental influences, and genetics. For this reason, there may be wide variation in the content of specific minerals in milk.

Milk (whole, low-fat, fat-free, flavored) and other dairy products (yogurt, cheese) are an excellent source of readily bioavailable calcium, providing approximately 300 mg per serving [12]. About 99% of the body's calcium is found in bone and teeth, with the remaining one percent in body fluids, nerves, heart, and muscle [101]. Throughout life, calcium is continually being removed from bones and replaced with more calcium. Consequently, the need for an adequate supply of dietary calcium is important throughout life, not only during the years of skeletal development. In addition to calcium's beneficial role in bone health, this mineral fulfills several other important physiological functions in human metabolism, as evidenced by its role in blood coagulation, myocardial function, muscle contractility, and integrity of intracellular cement substances and various membranes [101].

Unfortunately, calcium is one nutrient for which dietary intake is likely to be below recommended levels [118]. Prolonged calcium deficiency is one of several factors contributing to osteoporosis, a disease characterized by low bone mass and increased risk of fractures (see Chapter 5 on Dairy Foods and Bone Health). An adequate intake of calcium helps to protect against hypertension (see Chapter 3 on Dairy Foods and Hypertension) and some cancers (see Chapter 4 on Dairy Foods and Cancer), and may have a beneficial role in weight management (see Chapter 7 on Dairy Foods and Weight Management).

Calcium in milk may also reduce the risk of kidney stones [119–123]. In a four-year prospective study involving 45,000 male health professionals with no history of kidney stones, those who consumed a calcium-rich diet (1326 mg calcium) experienced a 44% lower risk of symptomatic kidney stones than men who consumed 516 mg calcium/day [119]. Calcium-rich foods, such as nonfat and low-fat milk, cottage cheese, and ricotta cheese, had the strongest association with decreased risk of kidney stones, whereas calcium supplements (above 500 mg a day) offered no protective effect [119]. Similar findings have been found in women [120,122,123]. In a prospective study of 90,000 women aged 34 to 59 years who were followed for 12 years, those who consumed more than 1119 mg calcium/day from foods such as dairy foods were 35% less likely to develop stones than those who consumed 430 mg calcium a day or less. In contrast to food sources of calcium, calcium supplements increased the risk of kidney stones [120]. More recently, another prospective study of more than 96,000 women aged 27 to 44 years who were followed for 8 years found that those who consumed the highest intake of calcium (greater than 1129 mg/day) were 27% less likely to develop kidney stones than women consuming the lowest calcium intakes (less than 626 mg/day) [123]. Dietary calcium, but not calcium supplements, was associated with reduced risk of developing kidney stones [123]. The researchers stated that, although calcium from all food sources can be singled out as protective, "dairy products may be a source of some other, as yet, unidentified, protective factor" [123].

Researchers speculate that a diet high in calcium may reduce the risk of kidney stones by decreasing the intestinal absorption and excretion of oxalate, a substance found in many plants, including spinach. An investigation involving 21 adults with a history of calcium oxalate kidney stones and normal urine calcium levels found that substituting 1.5 cups of fat-free milk for apple juice increased urine calcium levels and decreased urine oxalate levels by an average of 18% [121]. The researchers recommend that milk be consumed simultaneously with oxalate-containing foods to bind the oxalate in the diet and reduce the risk of calcium oxalate kidney stones. Based on an analysis of the data, researchers estimated that if high-risk individuals increased their dairy food intake to 3 to 4 servings per day, kidney stones would be reduced by 25% from year 1 through year 5, resulting in estimated health care cost savings of $2.5 billion over 5 years [124].

An analysis of government consumption data (Continuing Survey of Food Intakes by Individuals, 1994 to 1996, 1998 and the National Health and Nutrition Examination Survey (NHANES), 1999 to 2000) led researchers to conclude that: "Taken together, these data indicate that recommending 3 to 4 servings from the milk group for all individuals greater than 9 years of age is reasonable, practical, and necessary in order to ensure adequate intakes of calcium" [125]. The results indicated that at least 2 servings of dairy per day are necessary to meet the calcium needs of children ages 2 to 8 years [125]. These recommendations are consistent with those recently issued by the 2005 *Dietary Guidelines for Americans* [14], *MyPyramid* [126], and *MyPyramid for Kids* [127]. The absorption of calcium is facilitated by vitamin D [101]. For this reason, vitamin D-fortified milk is an important source of dietary calcium.

Milk is also an important source of phosphorus, providing 222 mg per 8-ounce serving [12]. This essential mineral plays a central role in metabolism and is a component of lipids, proteins, and carbohydrates [101]. Current dietary recommendations for phosphorus are not tied to calcium [101]. Instead, phosphorus recommendations are based on the amount of dietary phosphorus to maintain serum inorganic phosphate levels consistent with cellular and bone formation needs [101]. Three cups of milk will supply about 95% of the 700 mg phosphorus recommended per day for adults 19 years and older and 53% of the 1250 mg phosphorus per day recommended for 9- to 18-year-olds [12,101].

Magnesium, a required cofactor for over 300 enzyme systems in the body, is related to calcium and phosphorus in function. This mineral activates many of the body's enzymes, participates in the synthesis of protein from amino acids, and plays a role in the metabolism of carbohydrate and fat

[101]. Because magnesium is widely distributed in foods, particularly those of vegetable origin, a deficiency of this nutrient is rare. The Institute of Medicine recommends 420 mg and 320 mg magnesium per day for adult males and females 31 years and older, respectively [101]. Milk contains about 10 mg magnesium per 100 g [12]. Three 8-ounce glasses of milk will, therefore, provide 17% of the magnesium recommended for adult males and 22% for adult females [12,101].

Potassium contributes to the transmission of nerve impulses and helps to control skeletal muscle contraction. Accumulating scientific evidence supports a beneficial role for potassium in blood pressure control or prevention of hypertension (see Chapter 3 on Dairy Foods and Hypertension). Milk contains about 150 mg potassium per 100 g [12]. Three 8-ounce glasses of milk provide about 55% of the 4700 mg potassium per day recommended for persons aged 14 years and over [12,128]. Milk is ranked as the top food source of potassium among U.S. adults, according to the U.S. Department of Agriculture (USDA) national food intake surveys [14,129]. To help meet potassium recommendations, the Dietary Guidelines Advisory Committee increased the amount of milk and milk products recommended for all age groups 9 years of age and older to 3 cups or equivalent [130]. The 2005 *Dietary Guidelines for Americans* encourages a diet adequate in potassium-rich foods, such as fruits, vegetables, and dairy products [14].

Milk and other dairy foods contain many trace elements or nutrients needed by the body at levels of only a few milligrams per day. Of the more than 100 known trace elements, dietary recommendations have been established for relatively few trace elements (e.g., those considered to be of nutritional importance, such as iron, zinc, selenium, iodine, fluoride, boron, chromium, copper, manganese, molybdenum, nickel, and vanadium) [97,101,114]. Trace elements in cow's milk are highly variable and depend on the stage of lactation, season, milk yield, amount of the trace element in each cow's diet, postpasteurization handling of milk, storage conditions, and accuracy of analysis.

Iron is found in low concentrations in milk, providing 0.03 mg per 100 g [12]. Increasing the iron intake of cows does not increase milk's iron content. In addition to its low iron content, the bioavailability of iron from cow's milk is low. To reduce the risk of iron deficiency anemia, cow's milk is not recommended for infants during the first year of life [38,131]. However, when cow's milk is fed as recommended (i.e., after 12 months of age), there is little risk of iron deficiency anemia.

Zinc is a constituent of nearly 100 enzymes involved in most major metabolic pathways, such as the synthesis of ribonucleic acid, deoxyribonucleic acid, and protein [3,97]. This trace element is essential for growth and development, wound healing, immunity, and other physiological processes [97]. Zinc is also a regulator of gene expression and helps maintain the integrity of cell membranes [97]. Dairy foods such as milk, cheese, and yogurt are good sources of zinc [12]. Milk contains about 0.40 mg zinc per 100 g. The level of zinc in milk is mostly related to milk's protein content. Because only about 1% to 3% of zinc in cow's milk is in the lipid fraction, the zinc concentration of low-fat and fat-free milk is virtually identical to that of whole milk. Three servings of milk provide about 27% and 37% of the zinc RDA [12,97] for adults (i.e., 11 mg per day for males, 8 mg per day for females). Milk and milk products provide 16.5% of the zinc available in the nation's food supply [18].

Selenium functions largely through an association with proteins or selenoproteins [114]. For example, selenium is an integral component of the selenoprotein glutathione peroxidase which helps to protect cell components from oxidative damage [114]. The selenium content of cow's milk varies widely depending on the selenium intake of the cow [3]. Most of the selenium is found in the skim or serum portion of milk, with only 2% to 10% in the fat fraction [3]. The selenium content of whole cow's milk is 3.7 μg per 100 g [12]. Three 8-ounce servings of whole milk provide about half (49%) of the 55 μg selenium per day recommended for adults [12,114].

Iodine, which occurs naturally in milk, is an essential component of the thyroid hormones thyroxine and triiodothyronine, which regulate growth and metabolism [97]. The iodine content of cow's milk varies widely, depending on the geographical area and iodine intake of the cow. Low concentrations of iodine are used as a sanitizer in the dairy industry on equipment and to sanitize cows' udders prior to the milking process [3]. The iodine products used by the dairy industry are formulated with ingredients that have been approved by the FDA as safe to use. All other sanitizers and their specific uses are also approved by the FDA [112]. To avoid residues of these unpleasant-tasting substances, the dairy industry makes special efforts to educate dairy farmers about the proper use of iodine as a sanitizer at the farm and in the dairy processing plant. The tolerable upper intake level for iodine for adults is 1100 μg/day, which is almost 10 times the recommended intake of 150 μg iodine/day for adults [97]. In general, iodine deficiency is a more likely occurrence than iodine excess. A deficiency of iodine can cause enlargement of the thyroid gland (goiter) [97].

1.3 NUTRIENT CONTRIBUTION OF MILK AND MILK PRODUCTS

1.3.1 Nutrient Contribution to the Food Supply

Since 1909, the U.S. government has reported the amounts of nutrients per capita per day in food available for consumption [18]. Milk and other dairy products make a significant contribution to the nation's supply of nutrients (Table 1.4) [18]. As estimated for 2000, dairy foods (excluding butter) contributed only 9% of the total calories available in the nation's food supply. Yet, these foods provided 72% of the calcium, 26% of the riboflavin, 33% of the phosphorus, 19% of the protein, 16% of the magnesium, 20% of the vitamin B_{12}, 22% of the vitamin A, 9% of the vitamin B_6, and 5% of the thiamin, in addition to appreciable amounts of vitamin D and niacin equivalents available in the U.S. food supply [18].

Milk and other dairy foods are naturally nutrient-dense foods, supplying a high concentration of many nutrients in relation to their energy (caloric) value. Considering the obesity epidemic in the United States and shortcomings in dietary intakes of nutrients such as calcium, recent attention has focused on the importance of consuming naturally nutrient-rich foods [132]. A key recommendation in the 2005 *Dietary Guidelines for Americans* [14] is to "consume a variety of nutrient-dense foods and beverages within and among the basic food groups."

1.3.2 Dairy Food Intake Improves Nutrient Intake

Milk and other dairy foods are the major contributors of dietary calcium intake [11,18,129,133]. An investigation of calcium intakes of over 18,000 people aged 2 years and older in the USDA's 1994 to 1996, 1998 Continuing Survey of Food Intakes by Individuals (CSFII) found that milk, cheese, and yogurt alone and in mixed foods (e.g., macaroni and cheese, pizza) contributed 63% of dietary calcium intake [133]. Without consuming dairy foods, it is difficult to meet recommended intakes of calcium and vitamin D [134–139]. According to the U.S. Department of Health and Human Services' (DHHS) *Healthy People 2010* [137], "with current food selection practices, use of dairy foods may constitute the difference between getting enough calcium in one's diet or not."

An investigation of approximately 800 high school students revealed that 79% of the students' calcium intake came from milk and other dairy foods [140]. In another study involving adolescents, calcium intake was positively associated with milk intake [141]. Milk intake was shown to be a primary determinant of calcium intake for white, Hispanic, and Asian adolescents aged 10 to 18 years [142]. Similarly, adult women who met their calcium recommendations consumed significantly more servings of milk and milk products than women whose diets did not meet their calcium needs [143].

Consuming milk and milk products improves the overall nutritional quality of the diet [11,129,138,144–156]. Studies in children and adolescents demonstrate that consumption of dairy products increases calcium intake and improves the overall nutritional quality of the diet [144,147,149,151–153]. When school-aged children included milk as part of their noon meal, intake of calcium, as well as vitamin A, vitamin E, and zinc, increased [144]. Researchers have found that intake of flavored milk positively affects calcium intake and overall diet quality [152,153].

Studies of children's beverage choices suggest that milk intake is a marker for a better-quality diet. When beverage choices of over 4000 children aged 2 to 17 years were examined, milk consumption was shown to be positively associated with the likelihood of achieving recommended intakes of vitamin A, folate, vitamin B_{12}, calcium, and magnesium [156]. In another study using data from USDA's 1994-96 CSFII to assess trends in beverage choices and the impact on nutrient intakes in over 700 young females aged 12 to 19 years, milk drinkers had a more nutritious diet than non-milk drinkers [151]. The girls who did not drink milk had inadequate intakes of vitamin A, calcium, phosphorus, folate, and magnesium [151]. Studies in adults also support dairy foods' favorable impact on nutrient intakes [129,143,145,146,148,150,154,155]. When the contribution of specific foods to nutrient intake was examined among more than 10,000 U.S. adults, milk and cheese were ranked among the top sources of several nutrients, such as calcium, riboflavin, phosphorus, potassium, zinc, magnesium, and protein [129]. When the nutritional impact of dairy product consumption was examined in 1266 young adults participating in the Bogalusa Heart Study between 1995 and 1996, researchers found that the greater number of dairy servings consumed, the higher the intakes of calcium, magnesium, potassium, zinc, sodium, folate, thiamin, riboflavin, and vitamins B_6, B_{12}, A, D, and E [150]. In an investigation in Oregon, adults who included more dairy foods in their diets for at least 12 weeks increased their intake of calcium as well as other nutrients such as magnesium, riboflavin, potassium, phosphorus, and vitamin D [146]. A longitudinal study in postmenopausal women in Australia found that women who increased their calcium intake by 1000 mg/day by consuming fat-free milk powder also increased their intake of other essential nutrients, such as protein, potassium, phosphorus, magnesium, riboflavin, thiamin, and zinc [148]. In contrast, the women who took calcium supplements (calcium lactate gluconate) increased only their intake of calcium and sodium [148]. A randomized open trial in the United States found that increasing milk intake improved the overall nutritional quality of older adults' diets [155]. In this investigation of adults who typically consumed a low intake of dairy foods (1.5 servings/day or less), those who increased their fluid milk intake by three 8-ounce servings/day for 12 weeks significantly increased their intake of calcium, as well as other nutrients, such as protein, vitamins A, D, and B_{12}, riboflavin, phosphorus, magnesium, zinc, and potassium [155]. Increasing milk intake reduced the prevalence of dietary shortcomings for several nutrients. Another investigation found that yogurt intake contributed to improving the nutritional quality of adults' diets [154]. The 2005 *Dietary Guidelines for Americans* [14] recognizes that consuming milk products is associated with overall diet quality and adequacy of intake of many nutrients, including calcium, potassium, magnesium, zinc, iron, riboflavin, vitamin A, folate, and vitamin D. A study that used data from USDA's CSFII 1994 to 1996, 1998 to quantify the impact of dairy foods on nutrient intakes found that total dairy and milk intakes were associated with statistically-significant and often large increases in the intake of essential nutrients, includingcalcium, magnesium, potassium, zinc, iron, vitamin A, riboflavin, and folate [11]. Not only was intake of total dairy food and milk associated with higher micronutrient intakes, but there was also no adverse effect on fat or dietary cholesterol intake [11]. Findings from other studies demonstrate that consumption of dairy foods improves the nutritional quality of the diet without significantly increasing total calorie or fat intake, body weight, or percent body fat [146–149,151,153,155]. In fact, emerging science indicates that consuming calcium-rich dairy foods as part of a reduced-calorie diet can have a beneficial effect on body weight (see Chapter 6).

1.4 RECOMMENDATIONS TO INCLUDE MILK AND MILK PRODUCTS IN THE DIET

1.4.1 Dietary Recommendations

Official recommendations, including the USDA *MyPyramid* [126], *MyPyramid for Kids* [127], and the DHHS and USDA's 2005 *Dietary Guidelines for Americans* [14], recognize milk and other milk products as one of the major food groups. USDA's *MyPyramid*, like the 2005 *Dietary Guidelines for Americans*, recommends daily consumption of 3 cups of fat-free or low-fat milk or an equivalent amount of yogurt or cheese for Americans 9 years of age and older [14,126]. This recommendation is consistent with other recent reports issued by health professional organizations. The National Medical Association, the nation's oldest and largest organization representing African-American physicians, recommends that the American public in general and African Americans in particular consume 3 to 4 servings of low-fat milk, cheese, or yogurt a day to help reduce the risk of nutrient-related chronic diseases and improve health [61]. The 2004 U.S. Surgeon General's report on *Bone Health and Osteoporosis* recommends 3 daily servings of low-fat milk to help build better bodies and strong bones [157].

To help meet daily calcium needs, Health Canada [158], the American Academy of Pediatrics [159,160], and the American Heart Association [161] recommend up to 4 servings of dairy a day. The American Academy of Pediatrics, in its report on optimizing bone health and calcium intakes of infants, children, and adolescents, recommends 3 servings of milk or equivalent (i.e., flavored milk, cheese, or yogurt) each day for children 4 to 8 years of age and 4 servings of milk or equivalent for adolescents [160]. Using data from the 1994 to 1996, 1998 CSFII and from 1999 to 2000 NHANES, researchers determined that 3 to 4 servings of dairy foods a day was the optimal level to ensure an adequate intake of calcium by Americans [125]. Specifically, 2 servings of dairy/day are needed for children 2 to 8 years, 4 servings of dairy/day for children 9 to 18 years, and 3 servings/day for adults 19 years of age and over to meet calcium recommendations [125]. Foods naturally rich in calcium, such as dairy products, are the preferred source of calcium [14,134–138,158,160,162,163]. According to a renowned medical expert, "While it is possible to arrange an adequate diet using available Western foods, it is usually difficult to do so without including dairy products. Few individuals succeed, and, in general, a diet low in dairy foods means a diet that is poor in several respects beyond insufficiency of calcium. Additionally, a high dairy food intake is described as cost-efficient as well as cost-effective" [136].

1.4.2 Intake of Milk and Milk Products throughout Life

Intake of cow's milk and milk products contributes to health throughout life (see Chapter 9). According to the American Academy of Pediatrics [38], the nutritional adequacy of diets for children should be achieved by consuming a wide variety of foods, and children should be provided with sufficient energy to support their growth and development and to reach or maintain desirable body weight. Dairy foods are nutrient-dense foods providing abundant amounts of protein, vitamins, and minerals necessary for growth and development. Studies indicate that intake of calcium-rich foods, such as milk and other dairy foods, during childhood and adolescence is an important determinant of peak bone mass and future risk of osteoporosis (see Chapter 5 on Dairy Foods and Bone Health). Unfortunately, many children are not consuming recommended servings of dairy foods. Boys aged 6 to 11 years consume 2.2 servings of dairy/day and girls in the same age range consume only 1.9 servings of dairy/day [164]. During adulthood, intake of dairy foods provides essential nutrients needed for body maintenance and protection against major chronic diseases. For example, milk and other dairy foods are an important source of calcium, which helps to reduce the risk of osteoporosis (see Chapter 5), hypertension (see Chapter 3), and some cancers (see Chapter 4), as well as playing a beneficial role in weight management (see Chapter 7). For older adults in particular, milk and other dairy foods furnish a generous supply of nutrients in relation to calories. Adults, similar to children, are not consuming recommended servings of dairy foods [164]. A survey conducted by the USDA found that males and females aged 20 and over are consuming an average of only 1.8 and 1.4 servings of dairy/day, respectively, compared to the recommended 3 servings of dairy/day [14,164]. According to a recent analysis of the medical literature, McCarron and Heaney [124] concluded that there is adequate scientific evidence that if American adults increased their dairy food intake to 3 to 4 servings/day, the incidence of obesity, hypertension, stroke, coronary artery disease, type 2 diabetes, osteoporosis, kidney stones, and colorectal cancer would be substantially reduced. The accompanying reductions in health care costs were conservatively estimated to be $26 billion in the first year and more than $200 billion in 5 years [124]. In addition to reducing the risk of disease, dairy food consumption has been linked to increased longevity [165]. A study of Japanese centenarians found that survival was higher among those who preferred dairy products (i.e., milk, yogurt) than among those who had a preference for other dietary patterns (i.e., of vegetables, or beverages, or cereals) [165].

1.4.3 Government Feeding Programs/Child Nutrition Programs

Milk and other dairy foods are an important component of the meals and snacks offered in the federal government's child nutrition programs [2]. In 2003, an estimated 5400 million half-pints of fluid milk were served in child nutrition programs in schools: 4000 million half-pints in the National School Lunch Program (NSLP), 1216 million half-pints in the School Breakfast Program (SBP), and 108 million half-pints in the School Milk Program (SMP) (Table 1.5) [2]. In addition to milk, other dairy foods such as cheese and yogurt are consumed as part of the child nutrition programs. Yogurt may be used to meet all or part of the meat/meat alternate requirements for breakfasts and lunches served under any of the child nutrition programs [166]. Four ounces of yogurt equal one ounce of the meat/meat alternate requirement [166]. In the metric system, as used in Canada and Europe as well as elsewhere, 3 ounces is about 100 grams. Nationally representative evaluations of USDA's NSLP and SBP indicate that participation in these programs significantly increases children's intake of a range of nutrients, especially those such as calcium, phosphorus, riboflavin, and protein found in milk and other dairy products [167–171]. Much of the beneficial effect of consuming NSLP and SBP meals is attributed to the increased intake of milk and milk products [144,172]. According to a USDA analysis, NSLP participants consumed four times more milk at lunch than nonparticipants (0.8 servings vs. 0.2 servings) and larger amounts of cheese than nonparticipants [171]. Total dairy consumption at school lunch was greater for participants

TABLE 1.5
Milk Consumed through Federal School Programs: 1990 to 2003

	School Lunch Program (Half-Pints)	School Breakfast Program (Half-Pints)	Special Milk Program (Half-Pints)	Total Half-Pints Served	Total Gallons	% of U.S. Fluid Milk Sales
1990	3407.7	594.3	181.2	4183.2	261.5	4.1
1991	3443.3	648.6	177.0	4268.8	266.8	4.1
1992	3486.6	716.2	174.4	4377.2	273.6	4.3
1993	3517.0	775.8	167.3	4460.2	278.8	4.3
1994	3571.5	841.3	158.8	4571.7	285.7	4.5
1995	3615.4	906.3	151.4	4673.1	292.1	4.5
1996	3666.2	945.6	144.3	4756.1	297.3	4.5
1997	3747.7	1000.6	140.6	4888.9	305.6	4.6
1998	3761.2	1025.6	133.6	4920.4	307.5	4.8
1999	3836.2	1064.8	126.9	5027.9	314.2	4.9
2000	3888.8	1094.9	120.1	5103.8	319.0	5.0
2001	3896.9	1121.0	116.3	5134.2	320.9	5.0
2002[a]	4009.3	1180.0	112.9	5302.2	331.4	5.2
2003	4048.8	1216.2	107.8	5372.8	335.8	5.3

[a] Revised.

Source: USDA, National Agricultural Statistics Service; Food and Nutrition Service.

(1.1 servings) than for nonparticipants (0.4 servings). The higher consumption of dairy foods by NSLP participants resulted in higher intakes of several nutrients, including calcium, vitamin D, vitamin A, and magnesium, among others [171,173]. The significant differences in dairy product consumption and calcium intake based on participation in the NSLP were similar to differences found over a 24-hour period [171]. An examination of the nutrient contributions of five meal components of school lunches revealed that milk contributed the most calcium and protein per 100 calories and per penny, making milk a nutrient-dense and cost-effective component of school lunches [172]. Johnson et al. [144] found that children who drank milk instead of other beverages (e.g., soft drinks, juice, tea, fruit drinks) at lunch consumed more calcium (for that meal as well as the whole day), vitamin A, and zinc. Likewise, studies have shown that children who participate in the SBP have higher intakes of milk and several nutrients (e.g., calcium, phosphorus, magnesium, protein, thiamin, and riboflavin) at breakfast and over a 24-hour period than nonparticipants who have breakfast at home or who skip the meal [171,173]. Children who participated in both the NSLP and SBP consumed more dairy products (2.2 servings vs. 0.9 servings), more calcium, and fewer soda and fruit drinks than nonparticipants for these meals combined and over 24 hour [171,173]. In an effort to increase milk consumption in child nutrition programs, National Dairy Council and the American School Food Service Association (now called the School Nutrition Association) sponsored a School Milk Pilot Test (SMPT) [174]. This test was designed to learn how a combination of upgrades in milk packaging (e.g., kid-appealing plastic resealable containers in various sizes), flavor variety (e.g., a minimum of three flavors offered: white, chocolate, and a third flavor, usually strawberry), refrigeration (i.e., served cold), and merchandising locations (e.g., offered in three locations: lunch line, à la carte, and vending machines) impact students' selection and consumption of milk and their participation in the NSLP [174]. The test involved more than 100,000 students enrolled in 146 elementary and secondary schools (47 control, 99 test) from 18 school districts in different parts of the United States. Findings from this SMPT indicate that the combination of milk enhancements increases students' selection and consumption of milk and their participation in the NSLP [174]. If this combination of milk enhancements were adopted by schools nationally, the nutritional intake of millions of children could be significantly improved [175]. As a result of a new USDA regulation, schools have increased flexibility in their milk offerings [176]. This regulation removes the previous requirement that schools must offer the same milk types that were consumed in the previous school year. This change increases schools' options regarding the type of milk to serve, including flavored and unflavored milk, lactose-reduced milk, and milks at different fat levels [176]. Also, a provision gives schools the authority to offer milk at anytime and anywhere on school premises or at school events [176]. Dairy foods, such as milk and cheese, are also an important component of other government feeding programs such as the Women, Infants, and Children (WIC) program [177]. This program provides specified amounts of milk (flavored or unflavored whole, 2% reduced fat, low-fat, or fat-free milk, or fluid buttermilk, as well as reduced-lactose milk), cheese, and other foods to eligible low-income, nutritionally-at-risk pregnant, breast-feeding, and nonbreast-feeding postpartum women, and infants and children up to 5 years of age [177,178]. WIC regulations do not allow the substitution of yogurt or soy- or rice-based beverages for milk in the WIC food package. Only cheese is an approved substitute for milk. However, proposed changes to the WIC food package include offering only milk that contains no more than 2% fat for women and children over 2 years, allowing tofu and soy beverages as alternatives to milk for women, and permitting yogurt as a substitute for some of the milk for both women and children [179]. However, soy foods are not appropriate substitutes for dairy foods. Because soy beverages do not have the nutritional profile of milk, soy beverage processors must add nutrients such as calcium to the native soy beverage to compensate for inherent nutrient deficiencies [180]. Calcium-fortified soy beverages do not have a standard of identity, which allows variability in their nutrient content. Additionally, studies show that calcium-fortified soy beverages can contain poorly bioavailable calcium [180,181].

1.5 PROTECTING THE QUALITY OF MILK AND OTHER DAIRY FOODS

Throughout the years, dairy farmers and processors have worked closely with the Food and Drug Administration and state regulatory officials to establish safety regulations and practices including the Pasteurized Milk Ordinance [112] and the Hazard Analysis and Critical Control Point system (HACCP) [182]. As a result, American milk and dairy products are among the safest and most highly-regulated foods in the world.

1.5.1 Who Is Responsible for the Quality of Milk?

Quality relates to the chemical, microbiological, physical, organoleptic, and safety properties of milk. Rigid sanitary conditions are employed to assure this food's quality or result in milk with a low bacterial count, good flavor and appearance, satisfactory keeping quality, high nutritive value, and freedom from disease-producing microorganisms and foreign constituents. Cow's milk is among the most perishable of all foods because of its excellent nutritive composition and fluid form. As it comes from the cow, milk provides a good medium for the growth of bacteria. Unless milk is constantly protected against contamination and adverse environmental conditions, it may also develop flavor changes. Milk is relied upon as an important source of many nutrients. For this reason, maximum retention of these nutrients must be assured at every stage of production, processing (e.g., pasteurization), and distribution of milk and milk products.

Protecting the quality of milk is everyone's responsibility — public health officials, the dairy and dairy-related industries, and consumers. Progress in dairy technology and public health over the years has resulted in milk that can be depended upon as a safe, nutritious, pleasing food, even though it may be produced hundreds or thousands of miles away from the point of consumption. Vigilance is continuously exercised in maintaining this quality as new challenges arise in the environment. Numerous controls and treatments are in place to ensure the quality of milk.

1.5.2 Pasteurized Milk Ordinance

The Pasteurized Milk Ordinance (PMO) [112] continues to be one of the most effective instruments for protecting the quality of the American milk supply. It is a set of requirements for milk product hauling, pasteurization, product safety, equipment sanitation, and labeling established by the U.S. Public Health Service (USPHS)-FDA for voluntary adoption by states and other jurisdictions. Recognized by state and local milk regulatory agencies and the dairy industry, the PMO describes the steps necessary to protect the milk supply and the reasons for the procedures [112]. Although the PMO is a recommended standard for sanitary Grade-A milk, legal responsibility for the provision of milk quality is exercised mostly by state and local governments whose requirements are, in some instances, even more stringent than the PMO guidelines. Since the first guidelines were established in 1924, the PMO has been revised periodically along with technological advances in processes and equipment, as based on new research. Milk is routinely sampled and tested by state regulatory authorities, according to procedures outlined in the PMO. The HACCP system is a structured and scientific process used throughout the food industry to help ensure food safety [182]. Processing plants follow critical steps throughout the manufacturing process and establish schemes to monitor and minimize any risks. HACCP plans are reviewed, approved, and enforced by food safety agencies.

1.5.3 Unintentional Microconstituents

The dairy industry has stringent regulations and programs in place from the farm to the marketplace to ensure the public of safe and wholesome products. However, almost every food, including milk and dairy products, may contain trace residues of contaminants, either naturally or from external sources. While it is impossible to completely eliminate these residues, risk of adverse health effects is minimal as a result of a strong regulatory system [9].

Milk from cows given an antibiotic, primarily penicillin or tetracycline, to treat temporary bacterial infections such as mastitis, is withheld from the market until the milk is demonstrated to be free of the antibiotic or the level of the antibiotic is below an established safe level [3,9,112]. There is little concern regarding antibiotic residues in food, particularly because the public is protected from these residues as a result of regulatory actions. Every tank load of milk entering dairy processing plants is strictly tested for animal drug residues to ensure that this requirement is observed [112,183]. The U.S. dairy industry conducts more than 3.5 million tests each year to ensure that antibiotics are kept out of the milk supply [183]. In 2003, less than one-tenth of one percent (0.067%) of loads tested positive for animal drug residues, including antibiotics [183]. The milk in any tanker that tests positive is disposed of immediately, never reaching the public.

Pesticide residues in most U.S. foods pose minimal, if any, health risk because of federal regulations which limit human exposure to these contaminants [9]. All pesticides sold in the United States must be approved for safety by the U.S. Environmental Protection Agency (EPA) before they can be used. Tolerance or action levels for allowable pesticide residues in foods such as milk have been established by regulatory agencies [9]. The FDA, under its pesticide monitoring program and "Total Diet Study," collects and samples food nationwide for pesticide and other chemical contaminants [184]. This surveillance has demonstrated that pesticide contamination of foods in the United States is extremely low [184]. In 2002, 96% of domestic samples of milk/dairy products/eggs analyzed had no pesticide residues detected, and none contained residues in amounts over tolerance levels [184].

The dairy industry extensively tests any new procedures and technologies before widespread adoption to assure that they are safe for both cows and milk consumers. An example of such a technology is a milk production-enhancing hormone, bovine somatotropin (bST), which was approved by FDA in 1993 for commercial use in the United States [185]. This hormone, when added to the already-existing bST in the cow, increases milk output by up to 20% and thus improves a dairy farm's milk production efficiency. Before its approval, bST and milk produced from bST-treated cows underwent extensive testing for its safety by the FDA, the National Institutes of Health (NIH), and numerous independent groups. Based on the scientific findings, regulatory agencies worldwide have independently concluded that milk produced by bST-treated cows is safe for human consumption and indistinguishable from milk produced by untreated cows. There are several reasons why bST, which is naturally present in trace amounts in cow's milk, does not have any physiological effect on humans consuming the milk. bST is species-specific (of use in bovines only), which means that it is biologically inactive in humans. In addition, pasteurization destroys 90% of bST in milk. The remaining trace amounts of bST in milk are broken down into inactive fragments (i.e., constituent amino acids by enzymes in the human gastrointestinal tract, similar to any other protein) [186,187]. Because there are no differences in milk from bST-treated cows and milk from cows not treated with this hormone, the FDA has established that dairy products from cows treated with bST do not need to be labeled.

1.5.4 Milk Treatments

Most market milk in the United States is homogenized, although this is an optional process. Homogenization results in milk or milk products in which the fat globules are reduced in size to such an extent that no visible cream separation occurs in the milk. This process basically results in milk of uniform composition or consistency and palatability without removing or adding any constituents. Homogenization increases the whiteness of milk, because the greater number of fat globules scatters light more effectively. Homogenized milk is less susceptible to oxidized flavor, and the softer curd formed by it when entering the stomach aids digestion [3,9,10].

Pasteurization is required by law for all fluid milk and milk products moved in interstate commerce for retail sale. Even under the best sanitary dairy practices, disease-producing organisms may enter raw milk accidentally from environmental and human sources. However, as a result of pasteurization and other safeguards, illness related to milk intake has decreased dramatically during the past six decades [112]. Today, milk and fluid milk products are associated with less than 1% of all disease outbreaks due to infected food and contaminated water compared to 25% in 1938 [112]. The PMO outlines procedures for the proper pasteurization of milk and milk products. Basically, pasteurization is the heating of raw milk to 63°C (145°F) for at least 30 minutes or 72°C (161°F) for 15 seconds, followed by rapid cooling to 4°C (40°F). Pasteurization destroys pathogenic bacteria, yeasts, molds, and almost all other nonpathogenic bacteria. It also inactivates most enzymes that might cause spoilage through the development of off-flavors. Pasteurization makes milk bacteriologically safe and increases its shelf life to 10 to 14 days without significantly changing its nutritive value [3].

Some milk and milk products undergo ultrapasteurization (UP). This process involves thermal heating of milk and cream to at least 138°C (280°F) for at least 2 seconds [188]. Because of less stringent packaging, UP products must be refrigerated. The shelf life of milk is extended 60 to 90 days. The levels of most nutrients in milk are not significantly affected by UP processing and storage. With appropriate controls on the quality of milk, as well as on the processing and packaging, UP milk tastes very much like conventionally pasteurized milk. Ultrahigh temperature (UHT) pasteurization typically involved heating milk or cream to 138°C to 150°C (280°F to 302° F) for 1 or 2 seconds [188]. The milk is then packaged in sterile, hermetically-sealed (airtight) containers and can be stored without refrigeration for up to 90 days. After opening, the product must be refrigerated.

1.5.5 Storage and Handling

Proper handling of dairy products and open dating are designed to assure consumers of dairy products with a good shelf life, or the length of time after processing that the product will retain its quality. Open dating on milk and milk product containers indicates when the product should be withdrawn from retail sale. It is used by the dairy industry to reflect the age of individual packages, not the shelf life of products. Generally, depending upon storage conditions and care in the home, a product will remain fresh and usable for a few days beyond this "pull date" or "sell-by date." Regulation of open dating varies among states and other municipalities [9].

To preserve the quality of milk and dairy products, consumers are advised to:

- Use proper containers to protect milk from exposure to sunlight, bright daylight, and strongfluorescent light to prevent the development of off-flavor and a reduction in riboflavin, vitamin A, and vitamin B_6 content.
- Store milk at refrigerated temperatures (7°C) or below as soon as possible after purchase.
- Keep milk containers closed to prevent absorption of other food flavors in the refrigerator. An absorbed flavor may alter the taste, but the milk is still safe.
- Use milk in the order purchased.
- Serve milk cold.
- Return milk containers to the refrigerator immediately to prevent bacterial growth. Never return unused milk to the original container.
- Keep canned milk in a cool, dry place. Once opened, it should be transferred to a clean, opaque container and refrigerated.
- Store dry milk in a cool, dry place and reseal the container after opening. Humidity causes dry milk to lump and may also cause flavor and color changes. Once reconstituted, dry milk should be treated like any other fluid milk (i.e., covered and stored in the refrigerator).
- Serve UHT milk and other dairy products cold and store in the refrigerator after opening.

Freezing may be used to preserve some dairy foods. However, for milk and other fluid dairy products, freezing is not recommended. While freezing has little impact on the nutritional value of milk, it does decrease milk's quality somewhat in that the delicate texture is affected. This also holds true for many other dairy products. The dairy industry is aggressively investigating new technologies, for example, the use of carbon dioxide gas or bacteriocins (organic compounds such as lactate and acetate that inhibit the growth of spoilage microorganisms) produced by lactic acid bacteria to extend the shelf life of dairy foods [189]. For example, carbon dioxide gas is used in more than 15 commercial cottage cheese operations nationwide and one particular bacteriocin, nisin, has been approved by FDA for use in pasteurized cheese and processed cheese spreads to control the growth of pathogenic microorganisms [189].

1.6 KINDS OF MILK AND MILK PRODUCTS

1.6.1 Consumption Trends

Between 1960 and 2003, total milk production in the United States increased 47,000 million pounds (i.e., from 123,000 to 170,000 million pounds) [2]. Nearly 70% of the milk produced in 2003 was used to make either cheese (37.9%) or fluid milk, cream, and related products (32.3%) (Figure 1.2) [2]. Per capita consumption of total dairy products was 594 pounds in 2003, an increase of 55 pounds from 1975, but down 7 pounds from 1987 [190]. In recent decades, the consumption pattern of individual milk and milk products has changed dramatically [190–193]. Noteworthy trends include more use of low-fat milk, fluid cream products, yogurt, and cheese, and less use of whole milk [192]. Consumption of low-fat milk has increased, while that of whole milk has declined (Figure 1.3) [193]. By 2001, Americans were consuming less than 8 gallons per person of whole milk, compared to nearly 41 gallons in 1945 and 25 gallons in 1970. In contrast, per capita consumption of total lower-fat milks was 15 gallons in 2001, up from 4 gallons in 1945 and 6 gallons in 1970 [193]. The decline in the per capita consumption of total milk is attributed in part to competition from other beverages, especially carbonated soft drinks, as well as fruit juices, fruit drinks, bottled water, and flavored teas. In 1945, Americans drank at least four times more milk than carbonated soft drinks [191]. In contrast, in 1998, they consumed 2⅓ times more soft drinks than milk. Yen and Lin [194], in an analysis of USDA food consumption survey data, found that, on average, for each 1-ounce reduction in milk consumption, a child consumes 4.2 ounces of soft drinks, resulting in a net gain of 31 calories and a decline in calcium of 34 mg. Although Americans are switching to lower-fat milks, they are consuming more fluid cream products and cheese [18,190,193]. The per capita consumption of fluid cream products increased from 5.0 pounds per capita in 1975 to 10 pounds per capita in 2000 [18]. In 2001, Americans consumed 30 pounds of cheese per person, eight times more than they did in 1909 and more than twice as much as they did in 1975 (Figure 1.4) [194]. The growth in cheese consumption is attributed in large part to the demand for time-saving convenience foods (e.g., demand for cheese needed in pizza-making and prepared foods), the increase in ethnic diversity, and the greater variety of cheeses available [18,193]. An estimated 300 different varieties of cheese are available in the United States marketplace [2]. In addition to cheese, the demand for yogurt has increased, from 0.8 pounds per capita in 1970 to 5 pounds per capita in 2000 [18].

1.6.2 Wide Range of Milk and Milk Products

An ever-increasing variety of milk and other dairy products is available to meet the taste, nutrition, health, and convenience demands of consumers [2]. For example, dairy products of varied fat content, of low- or reduced-lactose content, fortified with nutrients such as vitamins A, D, and calcium, and processed to improve keeping quality (e.g., ultrapasteurized) are available. These products include milks (unflavored, flavored, evaporated, condensed, sweetened condensed, dry, nonfat dry), cultured or culture-containing dairy foods (yogurt, kefir, acidophilus milk, cultured buttermilk, sour cream), creams (heavy, light, whipping, half-and-half), butter, ice cream, and

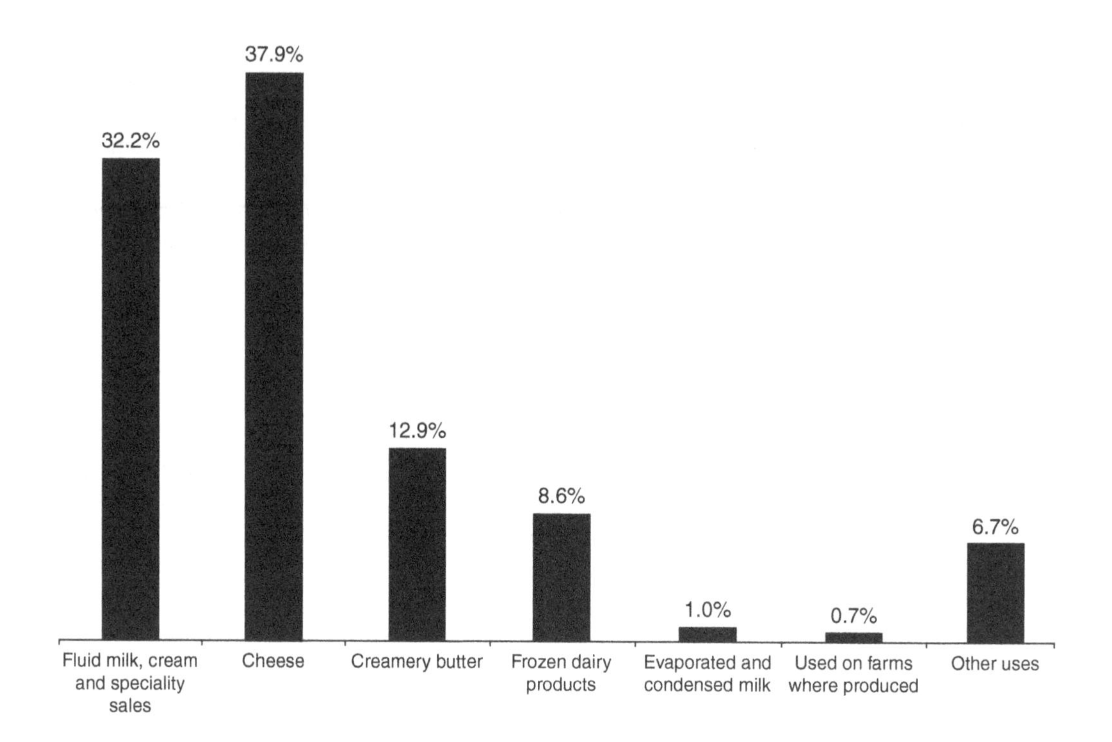

FIGURE 1.2 2003 U.S. milk supply utilization by product. (From International Dairy Foods Association, *Dairy Facts 2004 Edition*, Washington, D.C., 2004.)

cheeses, among other products. For a description of some of these dairy products, refer to Table 1.6 and other publications [2,102]. As a result of comprehensive food labeling regulations, consumers can readily choose foods such as dairy foods that meet their specific needs [100]. All dairy products are required to carry a food label headed by the title "Nutrition Facts" which lists mandatory and optional dietary components per serving in a specified order (Figure 1.5). This label is required to include information on total calories and calories from fat and on amounts of total fat, saturated fat, cholesterol, sodium, total carbohydrate, dietary fiber, sugars, protein, vitamin A, vitamin C, calcium, and iron, in this order [100]. Other dietary components that may be listed voluntarily include: calories from saturated fat, amounts of polyunsaturated and monounsaturated fat,

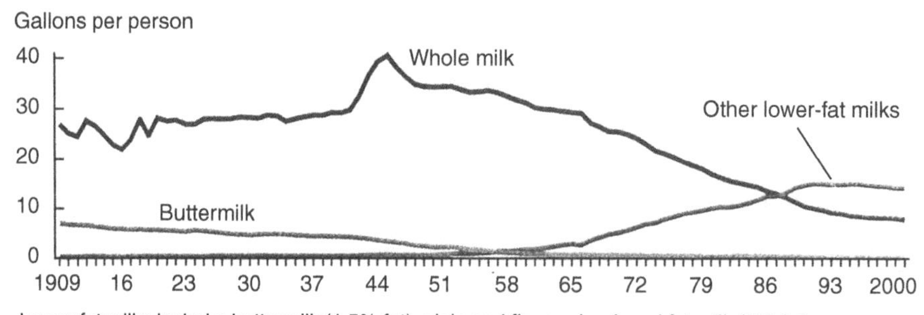

FIGURE 1.3 Milk consumption 1909 to 2000. (From Putnam, J. and Allshouse, J., Trends in U.S. per capita consumption of dairy products, 1909 to 2001, *Amber Waves*, 1, 12, 2003.)

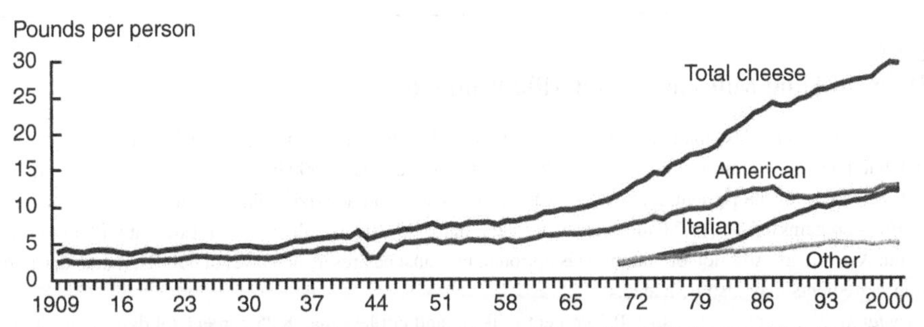

Amercian cheese includes Cheddar, Colby, Washed or Stirred Curd, Monterey, and Jack; Italian cheese includes Mozzarella, Ricotta, Provolone, Romano, Parmesan, and other Italian cheeses. Other natural cheese includes Swiss (including imports of Gruyere and Emmenthaler), Brick, Cream, Neufchatel, Blue, Gorgonzola, Edam, Gouda, and all others.

FIGURE 1.4 Cheese consumption 1909 to 2000. (From Putnam, J. and Allshouse J., Trends in U.S. per capita consumption of dairy products, 1909 to 2001, *Amber Waves*, 1, 12, 2003.)

potassium, soluble and insoluble fiber, sugar alcohol, other carbohydrate, and other essential vitamins and minerals. If a claim is made about any of these components, or if a dairy food is fortified or enriched with any of them, listing of the optional component becomes mandatory. The quantitative amount per serving (e.g., grams, milligrams) of total fat, saturated fat, *trans* fat, cholesterol, sodium, total carbohydrate, dietary fibers, sugars, and protein is listed on the label. The amount of each of the above, as well as of vitamins and minerals (e.g., vitamins A and C, calcium, iron), also is presented as a percentage of the Daily Value (% Daily Value). Some labels list the Daily Values for a daily diet of 2000 and 2500 calories. Daily Values can help consumers

Nutrition Facts

Serving size 1 cup (236ml)
Servings per container 1

Amount per serving	
Calories 120	Calories from Fat 45
	% Daily value*
Total Fat 5g	8%
Saturated Fat 3g	15%
Trans Fat 0g	
Cholesterol 20mg	7%
Sodium 20mg	5%
Total Carbohydrate 11g	4%
Dietary Fiber 0g	0%
Sugars 11g	
Protein 9g	17%

Vitamin A 10% • Vitamin C 4%
Calcium 30% • Iron 0% • Vitamin D 25%

*Percent Daily Values are based on a 2,000 calorie diet. Your daily values may be higher or lower depending on your calorie needs.

FIGURE 1.5 Nutrition Facts label for 2% reduced-fat milk. (Adapted from How to Understand and Use the Nutrition Facts Label, http://www.cfsan.fda.gov/~dms/foodlab.html.)

TABLE 1.6
Definitions of Fluid Milks and Fluid Milk Products

Whole Milk — contains not less than 3.25 percent milk fat and 8.25 percent solids-not-fat. Addition of vitamins A and D is optional, but if added, vitamin A must be present at a level of not less than 2000 International Units (IU) per quart; vitamin D is optional, but must be present at a level of 400 IU, if added. Characterizing flavor ingredients may also be added.

Low-fat Milk — contains 0.5,1.5, or 2.0 milk fat and not less than 8.25 percent solids-not-fat. Low-fat milk must contain 2000 IU vitamin A per quart. Addition of vitamin D is optional, but must be present at a level of 400 IU, if added. Characterizing flavoring ingredients may also be added.

Skim or Nonfat Milk — contains less than 0.5 percent milk fat and not less than 8.25 percent solids-not-fat. Skim or nonfat milk must contain 2000 IU of vitamin A per quart. Addition of vitamin D is optional, but must be present at a level of 400 IU, if added. Characterizing flavoring ingredients may be added.

Cultured Milks — are produced by culturing any of the milks listed above with appropriate characterizing bacteria. The addition of certain characterizing ingredients and lactic-acid producing bacteria may permit, for example, the product to be labeled "cultured buttermilk," "cultured low-fat buttermilk," or "cultured skim milk (nonfat) buttermilk" depending upon the level of milk fat in the finished product.

Half-and-Half — consists of a mixture of milk and cream containing not less than 10.5 percent milk fat, but less than 18 percent milk fat.

Light Cream — contains not less than 18 percent milk fat, but less than 30 percent. Light cream may also be called "coffee cream" or "table cream."

Light Whipping Cream — contains not less than 30 percent milk fat, but less than 36 percent milk fat. Light whipping cream may also be called "whipping cream."

Heavy Cream — contains not less than 36 percent milk fat. Heavy cream may also be called "heavy whipping cream."

Sour Cream — is the product resulting from the addition of lactic acid-producing bacteria to pasteurized cream containing not less than 18 percent milk fat. Sour cream may also be called "cultured sour cream."

Sour Half-and-Half — is the product resulting from the addition of lactic acid-producing bacteria to half-and-half. Sour half-and-half contains not less than 18 percent milk fat. The product may or may not contain lactic acid-producing bacteria.

Dry Curd Cottage Cheese — is a soft, unripened cheese made from skim milk and/or reconstituted nonfat dry milk. The cheese curd is formed by the addition of either lactic acid-producing bacteria or acidifiers. The latter process is called direct acidification. Rennet and/or other suitable enzymes may be used to assist cured formation. Dry curd cottage cheese contains less than 0.5 percent milk fat and not more than 80 percent moisture. The product may also be called "cottage cheese dry curd."

Cottage Cheese — is the product resulting from the addition of a creaming mixture (dressing) to dry curd cottage cheese. Cottage cheese contains not less than 4 percent milk fat and not more than 80 percent moisture.

Low-fat Cottage Cheese — is the product resulting from the addition of a creaming mixture (dressing) to dry curd cottage cheese. Low-fat cottage cheese contains either 0.5,1.0 or 2 percent milk fat and not more than 82.5 percent moisture.

Yogurt — is the product resulting from the culturing of a mixture of milk and cream products with the lactic acid-producing bacteria, *Lactobacillus bulgaricus* and *Streptococcus thermophilus*. Sweeteners, flavorings and other ingredients may also be added. Yogurt contains not less than 3.25 percent milk fat and 8.25 percent solids-not-fat.

Low-fat Yogurt — is similar in composition to yogurt except that it contains either 0.5,1,1.5 or 2 percent milk fat.

Nonfat Yogurt — is similar in composition to yogurt and low-fat yogurt except that it contains less than 0.5 percent milk fat.

Source: From International Dairy Foods Association, *Dairy Facts 2004 Edition*, Washington, D.C., 2004 and U.S. Department of Health and Human Services, Food and Drug Administration, Code of Federal Regulations, Title 21, Part 131, Milk and Cream, Washington, D.C., 2004.

determine how a food fits into an overall diet. These labeling regulations also provide consistent serving sizes and standard definitions for descriptive terms on food labels. Serving sizes, given in both household and metric measures (e.g., 1 cup [240 mL] for milk; 225 g [1 cup] yogurt), replace those previously set by manufacturers.

Uniform definitions for descriptive terms such as "free," "low," "high," "good source," "reduced," "less," "light," "more," and "% fat-free" are now provided (Table 1.7). For example,

TABLE 1.7
Nutrient Content Descriptions for Dairy Products in the United States

1	Free (without, no, zero)	Based on Value of Nutrient per Reference Amount and per Labeled Serving Size
	Fat-free	Less than 0.5 g fat
	Calorie-free	Less than 5 calories
	Sodium-free	Less than 5 mg sodium
	Cholesterol-free	Less than 2 g saturated fat and 2 mg cholesterol.
2	Low (little, few, low source)	3 g or less of fat per serving
	Low-fat	1 g or less of saturated fat per serving
	Low saturated fat	40 calories or less per serving
	Low calorie	Less than 140 mg per serving
	Low sodium	Less than 140 mg per serving
	Low cholesterol	Less than 20 mg cholesterol and no more than 2 g saturated fat per serving
3	High	Food contains 20% or more of RDI of a nutrient per serving
4	Good source	Food contains 10 to 14% of RDI of a nutrient per serving
5	Reduced	Food contains 25% less of a nutrient or calories per serving than reference product. For cholesterol an additional requirement is maximum 2 g saturated fat per serving. The term reduced is used for nutritionally altered foods.
6	Less (fewer)	Food contains a minimum of 25% less of a nutrient or calories per serving. Additional requirement for cholesterol is maximum of 2 g saturated fat per serving. Food need not be nutritionally altered.
7	Light (lite)	If less than 50% of calories are from fat, calories should be reduced by 1/3 or fat content should be reduced by 50%. If 50% or more of calories come from fat, reduction must be 50% of fat. May also denote physical and organoleptic attributes, e.g., color.
8	More	Food, not necessarily nutritionally altered, contains at least 10% more of RDI of a nutrient.
9	Percent fat-free	Food must be low-fat or fat-free. If a food contains 2 g fat per 50 g, it may be called 96% fat free.

Source: From Kosikowski, F.V. and Mistry, V.V., *Cheese and Fermented Milk Foods*, p. 558, 1997. With permission.

"free" is defined as <5 calories; or <5 mg sodium; or <2 mg cholesterol; or <0.5 g saturated fat; or <2 mg cholesterol; or <0.5 g sugar [100]. The terms "light" and "reduced" (calorie, fat) are always used with a comparison to the reference food. The term "healthy" can be used on the label if the food is low in fat and saturated fat, has limited amounts of cholesterol and sodium, and contains at least 10% of the Daily Value for one or more of vitamins A or C, or iron, calcium, protein, or fiber [195,196]. Some dairy foods may also carry a health claim [196]. The FDA defines a health claim as any statement that characterizes the relationship of a substance in food or dietary supplement to a disease or health-related condition [196]. For example, some dairy foods may carry a food label with a health claim related to calcium and osteoporosis such as, "Regular exercise and a healthy diet with enough calcium helps teen and young adult white and Asian women maintain good bone health and may reduce their high risk of osteoporosis later in life" [100,196]. To carry a health claim, a food must contain no more than 20% of the Daily Value of fat (13 g), saturated fat (4 g), cholesterol (60 mg), and sodium (480 mg). For a calcium-osteoporosis claim, a food must also provide at least 20% of the reference daily intake of 1000 mg calcium (i.e., 200 mg calcium per serving). Also, for foods that might be fortified with large amounts of calcium, FDA requires a disclaimer indicating that a calcium intake of about 2000 mg per day is unlikely to provide any additional benefit [100]. Fat free (skim, nonfat), low-fat (1%), and reduced-fat (2%) milk and milk products (e.g., low-fat/fat-free yogurt) qualify for the calcium-osteoporosis health claim. Another example of a health claim is one for potassium, "diets containing foods that are good sources of potassium and low in sodium may reduce the risk of high blood pressure and stroke" [196,197]. A food making this claim must contain at least 350 mg of potassium per serving, have no more than 140 mg of sodium per serving, and be low in fat [197]. Nonfat milk qualifies to make this claim [197]. Other potential health claims for dairy products are shown in Table 1.8 [197].

Some dairy foods may carry a "structure/function" claim [196]. Structure/function claims describe the role of a nutrient that maintains the "structure" or "function" of the human body, but does not affect a disease state [196]. These claims do not require FDA approval. A food manufacturer is responsible for ensuring that structure/function claims be truthful and not misleading. Examples of structure/function claims on dairy products include "3-A-Day of Dairy for Stronger Bones" and "3-A-Day of Dairy Increases Weight Loss When Part of a Reduced-Calorie Diet" [196]. A number of traditional foods, including whole milk, sour cream, cottage cheese, and yogurt, have a standard of identity (i.e., the ingredients are fixed by law). Beginning January 1, 1998, the standards of identity for 12 lower-fat dairy products, including low-fat milk, skim (nonfat) milk, low-fat cottage cheese, sweetened condensed skimmed milk, sour half-and-half, evaporated skimmed milk, low-fat dry milk, and the lower-fat versions of all cultured dairy products, with the exception of yogurt, were eliminated [198]. These foods are subject to the requirements of FDA's "general standard," which permits foods to be named by use of a defined nutrient content claim (e.g., reduced fat or low-fat) and a standardized term (e.g., "milk" or "cottage cheese"). This change was made to help consumers better understand the fat content of milk and other dairy foods and to make the low- and reduced-fat terminology consistent from one food category to the next. Under these rules, skim milk may be called fat-free or nonfat milk; 1% low-fat milk may be labeled "low-fat" or "light;" and 2% low-fat milk is called 2% reduced-fat milk. Labeling for whole milk (often referred to as vitamin D or homogenized milk) is unchanged (Table 1.9) [198].

1.6.3 Flavored Milk

Although a variety of flavored milks (e.g., chocolate, vanilla, banana, orange, strawberry) are available locally and nationally, chocolate milk is by far the most popular flavored milk [2]. Chocolate milk is milk to which chocolate or cocoa and sweetener has been added. Similar to unflavored milks, chocolate milk has an excellent nutritional profile, providing significant amounts of high-quality protein, calcium, riboflavin, magnesium, phosphorus, niacin equivalents, vitamin B_{12}, vitamin A, and (when added) vitamin D, as well as several other essential nutrients [12]. Chocolate milk is a rich source of calcium. Each 8-ounce serving of chocolate milk provides 35% of the 800 mg recommended for this nutrient for children 4 through 8, 23% of the 1300 mg recommended for those 9 through 18 years, and 30% of the 1000 mg recommended for adults 19 through 50 [12,101]. The nutrient content of chocolate milk — whole, 1% low-fat, 2% reduced-fat,

TABLE 1.8
Potential Helath Claims for Dairy Products[a]

Health Claim[b]	Reduced Fat Milk (2% Milk Fat)	Low-Fat Milk (1% Milk Fat)	Fat-Free Milk (Skim)	Yogurt Plain (Low-Fat)	Yogurt Plain (Fat-Free)	Cottage Cheese (Fat-Free)	Cottage Cheese (1% Milk Fat)	Cottage Cheese (2% Milk Fat)
Calcium and osteoporosis *"Regular exercise and a healthy diet with enough calcium help teens and young adult white and Asian women maintain good bone health and may reduce their high risk of osteoporosis later in life."*	Yes	Yes	Yes	Yes	Yes	No	No	No
Sodium and hypertension *"Diets low in sodium may reduce the risk of high blood pressure, a disease associated with. many factors."* *OR* *"Development of hypertension or high blood pressure depends on many factors. [This product] can be a part of a low sodium, low salt diet that might reduce the risk of hypertension or high blood pressure."*	Yes	Yes	Yes	No	No	No	No	No
Dietary fat and cancer *"Development of cancer depends on many factors. A diet low in total fat may reduce the risk of some cancers."*	No	Yes	Yes	Yes	Yes	Yes	Yes	No
Dietary saturated fat and cholesterol and risk of coronary heart disease *"Willie many factors affect heart disease, diets low in saturated fat and cholesterol may reduce the risk of this disease."*	No	No	Yes	No	Yes	Yes	No	No

(continued)

TABLE 1.8 ***(Continued)***

Health Claim[b]	Reduced Fat Milk (2% Milk Fat)	Low-Fat Milk (1% Milk Fat)	Fat-Free Milk (Skim)	Yogurt Plain (Low-Fat)	Yogurt Plain (Fat-Free)	Cottage Cheese (Fat-Free)	Cottage Cheese (1% Milk Fat)	Cottage Cheese (2% Milk Fat)
Potassium and the risk of high blood pressure and stroke *"Diets containing foods that are a good source of potassium and that are low in sodium may reduce the risk of high blood pressure and stroke."*	No	No	Yes	No	No	No	No	No

[a] Claims based on values taken from the U.S. Department of Agriculture, Agricultural Research Service. 2005. USDA National Nutrient Database for Standard Reference, Release 18. Nutrient Data Laboratory Home Page: http://www.nal.usda.gov/fnic/foodcomp. Individual products may vary based on independent lab analysis. This list is for illustration purposes only. Consult the Code of Federal Regulations for specific nutrition labeling requirements for making health claims.

[b] Whole milk, whole milk yogurts and whole milk cottage cheese do not qualify for health claims as they exceed the levels of the disqualifying nutrients specified by the claim and, hence, are not included (see subsequent pages for disqualifying nutrient levels for specific health claims).

TABLE 1.9
Fluid Milk Products

	(One Serving is 1 Cup or 8 Fluid Ounces)			
Name	**Calories**	**Fat (g)**	**Sat. Fat (g)**	**Calcium (mg)**
Fat free milk or skim or nonfat milk	83	0	0	306
1%[a] Lowfat milk, or light milk	102	2.5	1.5	290
2%[a] Reduced-fat milk	122	5	3	285
Whole milk	146	8	5	276

[a] The milk fat percentages on labels are optional.

Source: USDA National Nutrient Database for Standard Release 18 (2005). http://www.ars.usda.gov/ba/bhnrc.ndl

and fat-free (skim or nonfat) — is similar to that of the corresponding unflavored milk. The main exceptions are the higher contents of carbohydrate and calories in chocolate milk, due to the addition of sucrose and other nutritive sweeteners [12]. In general, chocolate-flavored milks have about 60 calories more than their unflavored counterpart. An 8-ounce serving of chocolate low-fat (1%) milk contains 158 calories, 2% reduced-fat chocolate milk contains 179 calories, and chocolate whole milk contains 208 calories [12].

Chocolate milk is a highly nutritious, well-liked beverage. An investigation of how children view milk served at school found that milk flavor strongly influences milk-drinking behavior and that the majority of children prefer chocolate milk [199]. A study of nearly 4000 school-aged children and adolescents found that those who drank flavored milk, such as chocolate milk, consumed more total milk and fewer soft drinks and fruit drinks than children who did not drink flavored milk [153]. In addition, flavored milk consumers had higher calcium intakes, but not a higher percent of energy from total fat and added sugars intake than nonconsumers of flavored milk [153]. A retrospective analysis of diets of more than 3000 children ages 6 to 17 years found a positive effect on children's overall diets when they chose flavored milks and yogurts instead of sodas and sweetened drinks [152]. The American Academy of Pediatrics has published a policy statement recommending that pediatricians work to eliminate sweetened drinks in schools and encourage alternatives such as low-fat white or flavored milk [200]. In its report on optimizing bone health and calcium intakes of infants, children, and adolescents, the American Academy of Pediatrics recommends flavored milk containing reduced fat or no fat and modest amounts of added sweeteners as an option to help meet calcium needs [160]. For the first time, schools are encouraged to offer flavored milk, as a result of the Child Nutrition and WIC Reauthorization Act signed into law (P.L. 108 to 265) on June 30, 2004 and effective July 2005 [176].

There is no scientific evidence that chocolate milk, because of its increased sugar content, contributes to dental caries (see Chapter 7 on Dairy Foods and Oral Health). In fact, chocolate milk may contribute less to dental caries than other foods with similar sugar content. Because it is a liquid, chocolate milk is cleared from the mouth relatively quickly and therefore may be less cariogenic than many other foods, such as raisins or candies, that adhere to tooth surfaces. Moreover, several components in chocolate milk, such as cocoa, milk fat, calcium, and phosphorus, have been suggested to protect against dental caries. The American Academy of Pediatric Dentistry states that "chocolate milk is OK for children's teeth" [201]. A briefing paper concludes that the cariogenicity of flavored milk is "negligible to low" [202]. Likewise, there is no scientific evidence that sugar — per se or in foods such as chocolate milk — contributes to obesity or behavioral and learning disorders [203,204]. Chocolate milk contains a small amount (0.5 to 0.6%)

of oxalic acid, a compound occurring naturally in cocoa beans and other plants. Although oxalic acid can combine with calcium to form an insoluble salt, there is no scientific evidence that oxalic acid in chocolate milk impairs calcium absorption [205]. The absorption of calcium from chocolate milk has been found to be similar to that of unflavored milk and other calcium-containing foods [205].

A single-blind, randomized study of nine male endurance-trained cyclists found that those who drank chocolate milk after an intense bout of exercise were able to work out longer and with more power during a second workout compared to the cyclists who drank a carbohydrate beverage [206]. The researchers concluded that chocolate milk, with is high carbohydrate and protein content, may be an effective alternative to commercial sports drinks in helping athletes recover from strenuous, energy-depleting exercise [206].

1.6.4 Cheese

According to an ancient legend, cheese was discovered several thousand years ago by an Arabian merchant who placed milk in a pouch made from a sheep's stomach as he set out for a day's journey across the desert [2]. The rennet in the lining of the pouch, combined with the heat of the sun, caused the milk to separate into the curd of cheese and thin liquid now called whey. The art of cheese-making is thought to have come to Europe from Asian travelers. During the Middle Ages, cheese-making flourished in countries such as Italy and France. In 1620, when the Pilgrims made their voyage to America, cheese was included in the *Mayflower*'s supplies. In North America, cheese-making remained a local farm industry until 1851, when the first cheese (Cheddar) factory opened in New York State. Shortly thereafter, in 1868, a Limburger cheese factory was opened in Wisconsin [2]. Since these early years, the cheese industry has grown phenomenally, both in total production and in the varieties of cheese products offered to consumers.Total natural cheese production in the United States grew from 418 million pounds in 1920, to 2200 million pounds in 1970, to more than 6000 million in the early 1990s, to more than 8600 million pounds in 2003 [2]. Similarly, the production of processed cheese has increased over the years, to nearly 2,500 million pounds in 2003 [2]. Per-capita consumption of natural cheese also has risen, specifically to 30.6 pounds in 2003, a 17% increase over the last 10 years (Figure 1.6). American varieties, which include Cheddar, Colby, and Monterey Jack, account for the largest percent, closely followed by

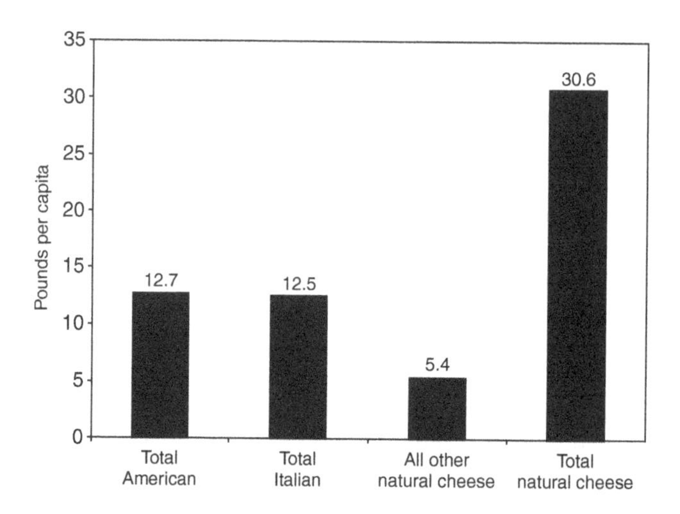

FIGURE 1.6 U.S. natural cheese per capita consumption, 2003. (From International Dairy Foods Association, *Dairy Facts 2004 Edition*, Washington, D.C., 2004.)

Italian varieties (e.g., Mozzarella, Ricotta, etc.). This increase in cheese consumption may be explained by cheese's pleasing taste, excellent nutritional value, versatility, economy, and — more recently — the introduction of innovative new products, a wider availability of specialty cheeses, more-convenient packaging, and new ideas on how to use the product.

Cheese is a concentrated dairy product made by draining off the whey after coagulation of casein, the major milk protein [4,9,10,12]. Casein is coagulated by acid produced by select microorganisms and/or coagulating enzymes, resulting in curd formation. Milk may also be acidified by adding food-grade acidulants in the manufacture of certain varieties of cheese, such as cottage cheese. In fresh, unripened cheese (e.g., creamed cottage cheese, cream cheese), the curd, separated from the whey, can be used immediately, whereas in matured or ripened cheeses (e.g., Cheddar, Swiss), the curd is treated further by the action of beneficial select strains of bacteria, mold, yeasts, or combinations of any of these ripening agents, to produce a cheese of a specific flavor, texture, and appearance [4]. Natural cheese is produced directly from milk. Pasteurized blended cheese, processed cheese, cheese foods, cheese spreads, and cold-pack cheeses are made by blending one or more different kinds of natural cheese with suitable emulsifying agents into a homogeneous mass. These cheeses are processed to produce uniform, safe, longer-keeping products.

Most cheeses produced in the United States have a standard of identity [102]. These federal standards define cheeses by specifying the ingredients used, the composition (maximum moisture content and minimum percentage of fat in the cheese solids or in the total mass of cheese), the requirements regarding pasteurization of the milk or an alternate minimum ripening period, production procedures, and any special requirements unique to a variety or class of cheese. However, manufacturers may list nutrient content claims on the labels of standardized foods (e.g., reduced-fat cheese) if certain conditions are met [100]. The nutrient content claim (e.g., reduced fat) must meet FDA's definition, which — in the case of reduced fat — is at least 25% less fat than in the standard product. Additionally, the modified food cannot be nutritionally inferior to the traditional standardized food, and the new food must have performance characteristics similar to those of the standardized food. If not, the label must state the difference in performance. A modified food that uses a standardized term (e.g., Swiss cheese), but does not comply with the standard of identity, must be labeled either as an "imitation" if it is nutritionally inferior (e.g., imitation Swiss cheese), or as a "substitute," "alternative," or other appropriate term (e.g., Swiss cheese alternative) if it is not nutritionally inferior. The majority of imitation cheeses are imitation or alternate process cheeses. The dairy industry administers a program for identifying real dairy foods. The REAL Seal on a carton or package identifies cheese, milk, and other qualified dairy foods made from U.S.- produced milk that meets federal and state standards [4]. This seal assures consumers that the food is not an imitation or substitute.

More than one-third of all the milk produced in the United States each year is used to make cheese (Figure 1.2) [2]. About 10 pounds (5 quarts) of milk are required to make one pound of Cheddar cheese and nine pounds of whey. During the typical cheese — making process, there is a significant partitioning of milk's nutrients with separation of the curds from the whey and changes in milk's nutrients during ripening of the cheese. The water-insoluble components of milk (casein, fat) remain primarily in the curd, whereas most of the water-soluble constituents (carbohydrates, salts, proteins smaller than casein) are in the whey. The amount of various nutrients retained in the curd and whey largely depends on the type of cheese manufactured, the milk (whole, low-fat, reduced fat, nonfat), and manner of coagulation. During ripening, microorganisms and enzymes which transform the fresh curd into a cheese of specific flavor, texture, and appearance can also alter the nutrient content of the product. Cheese makes an appreciable contribution to the amount of nutrients available in the U.S. food supply (Table 1.10). In 2000, cheese contributed 8.5% of the protein, 25.5% of the calcium, and 4.5% of the riboflavin available [18]. In addition, cheese supplies many other nutrients in significant amounts. The protein of cheese is largely casein, with small amounts of alpha-lactalbumin and beta-lactoglobulin. Together, these proteins in the curd amount to about four-fifths of the protein of the original milk. One-fifth of milk's protein,

TABLE 1.10
Percent Total Nutrients Contributed by Cheese to the U.S. per Capita Food Supply, 2000

	Total Cheese (%)
Food energy	3.3
Protein	8.5
Fat	5.7
Carbohydrate	0.2
Minerals	
Calcium	25.5
Phosphorus	10.6
Zinc	7.1
Magnesium	2.5
Potassium	1.0
Iron	0.9
Vitamins	
Vitamin A activity	6.9
Riboflavin	4.5
Vitamin B_{12}	4.4
Vitamin B_6	1.2
Vitamin E	0.9
Folate	0.6
Thiamin	0.3
Niacin	0.1
Ascorbic acid	0.0

Source: From Gerrior, S., Bente, L., and Hiza, H., *Nutrient Content of the U.S. Food Supply, 1909–2000*, Home Economic Research Report No. 56, U.S. Department of Agriculture, Center for Nutrition Policy and Promotion, Washington, D.C., 2004.

mostly the soluble albumins and globulins, remains in the whey. The method of coagulation of milk, as well as the degree of ripening (i.e., enzyme-coagulated or acid-coagulated), influence the protein content of cheese. In hard ripened cheeses, such as Cheddar and Swiss, relatively little hydrolysis of protein occurs, whereas in soft ripened cheeses, such as Camembert, protein is broken down to water-soluble compounds, including peptides, amino acids, and ammonia. Cheese protein is classified as a high-quality protein because of its unique amino acid composition. Cheese contains all of the amino acids commonly found in food protein, and in significant amounts. The relative surplus of one of the dietary essential amino acids, lysine, in cheese protein (as in the proteins of milk) makes cheese, as well as milk, valuable in supplementing vegetable proteins, especially those of grain products, which are low in lysine.

The carbohydrate content, namely lactose, in ripened cheese is not nutritionally significant. Lactose is largely removed with the whey during cheese-making [4,9]. The presence of small amounts (about 2%) of lactose in cheese depends on the quantity of entrapped whey in the curd. During ripening, this lactose is generally transformed to lactic acid and other products by the bacteria, molds, yeasts, and enzymes that produce the characteristic flavor of specific cheeses. After 21 to 28 days of ripening, generally no lactose remains [4]. The legal addition of optional ingredients, such as fat-free milk and cheese whey, during the manufacture of process cheese products may increase the carbohydrate content of these products. Because most varieties of cheese contain an insignificant amount of lactose, this food is well-tolerated by consumers who are lactase nonpersistent (see Chapter 8 on Dairy Foods and Lactose Intolerance).

The milk fat content of cheese is partly responsible for this food's satiety value, flavor, and texture. During curing or ripening, milk fat in cheese undergoes a certain amount of hydrolysis, which results in the release of volatile fatty acids (e.g., butyric, caproic, and caprylic acids and higher-carbon-chain fatty acids), which, in turn, contribute to the flavor of cheese. Cheeses vary widely in milk fat content, from almost 0% in plain cottage cheese dry curd (made with nonfat milk) to at least 33% in cream cheese made from whole cow's milk and cream. A higher-fat cheese, such as cream cheese, is always enriched with cream and, therefore, contains a greater proportion of fat than protein. Cheeses such as Cheddar, Swiss, and Gouda generally have about the same amount of fat and protein. A reduced-fat cheese has a higher protein-to-fat ratio. When fat is reduced, the taste and texture of cheese may be negatively altered. Numerous reduced-fat cheeses have been introduced, and much progress has been made to overcome some of these drawbacks [4].

As mentioned above, the minimum milk fat (and maximum moisture) content of most cheeses is governed by federal and state regulations. Generally, natural cheeses such as Cheddar, Swiss, and Roquefort contain about 8 to 9 g of fat per ounce. Processed cheeses have a fat content closely related to the cheese or mixtures of cheeses from which they are made. Generally, these processed cheeses contain about 7 to 9 g of fat per ounce. Cheese foods and spreads have 6 to 7 g of fat per ounce. Numerous processed cheeses with reduced or less fat or labeled light or "lite" are available on the market [4]. In addition, a fat-free product called nonfat pasteurized process cheese product is available. Nutrient content descriptors are defined by law. The Nutrition Facts label on the cheese product indicates its fat and calorie content (Figure 1.7).

Although fat in cheese is similar to that of milk fat, the composition of fatty acids in cheese differs from the original milk fat because of the ripening action which cheese undergoes. However, the fatty acid patterns for specific cheeses are not appreciably different from one another. A variety of cheeses, including Cheddar, are good sources of the anticancer agent CLA (see Chapter 4 on Dairy Foods and Cancer). CLA has been demonstrated to protect against both cancer and coronary heart disease in laboratory animals. In humans, intake of 112 g (or 4 ounces) of Cheddar cheese increased blood levels of CLA by 19% to 27%, according to a study of nine healthy men [207]. The cholesterol content of cheese varies with the fat content. Full-fat cheeses, such as Cheddar cheese and cream cheese, contain approximately 30 mg cholesterol per ounce. A one-third-fat-reduced Cheddar cheese has approximately 21 mg of cholesterol per serving, and fat-free cheeses contain about 5 mg of cholesterol per serving [4]. The vitamin content of cheese depends on the vitamins in the milk used, the manufacturing of the cheese, the cultures or microorganisms employed, and the conditions and length of the curing period. Wide variations in the vitamin content occur among individual samples of the same variety of cheese, as well as among different varieties. As most of the fat in milk is retained in the curd, cheese contains the fat-soluble vitamins of the milk used. Cheese such as Cheddar, which is made with whole milk, is a good source of vitamin A activity (265 RAE or 1002 IU per 100 g), whereas low-fat Cheddar cheese contains a relatively smaller amount of this vitamin (60 RAE or 207 IU per 100 g) [12]. Water-soluble vitamins such as thiamin, riboflavin, niacin, vitamin B_6, pantothenic acid, biotin, and folate remain largely in the whey. The more whey retained in the cheese, the greater the content of these vitamins in the cheese. Generally, any cheese variety high in one B vitamin is high in most of the other B vitamins. In surface-ripened cheeses, such as Brie and Camembert, and mold-ripened cheese varieties, such as blue cheese and Gorgonzola, a higher concentration of B-complex vitamins may occur on the outer layers of the cheese.

Cheese is a good source of minerals (Table 1.10) [12]. However, similar to vitamins, the mineral content of cheese varies both within and among varieties. In 2000, cheeses contributed about 25.5% of the calcium available in the food supply [18]. The calcium content of cheese is largely influenced by the acidity at coagulation and by extent of expulsion of the whey from the curd. In ripened whole-milk cheeses made with a coagulating enzyme (e.g., Cheddar cheese), the

Nutrition Facts

Serving size 1 ounce 28g (28g)

Amount per serving

Calories 80	Calories from Fat 47
	% Daily value*
Total Fat 5g	8%
Saturated Fat 3g	16%
Trans Fat	
Cholesterol 16mg	5%
Sodium 205mg	9%
Total Carbohydrate 1g	0%
Dietary Fiber 0g	0%
Sugars 0g	
Protein 8g	

Vitamin A	4%	• Vitamin C	0%
Calcium	26%	• Iron	0%

*Percent daily values are based on a 2,000 calorie diet. Your daily values may be higher or lower depending on your calorie needs.

	Calories	2,000	2,500
Total Fat	Less than	65g	80g
Sat Fat	Less than	20g	25g
Cholesterol	Less than	300mg	300mg
Sodium	Less than	2,400mg	2,400mg
Total carbohydrate		300g	375g
Fiber		25g	30g

Calories per gram:
Fat 9 • Carbohydrate 4 • Protein 4

Nutritiondata.com

FIGURE 1.7 Sample label for Cheddar cheese. (From Nutritional Data and Images Courtesy of www.NutritionData.com.)

calcium and phosphorus of milk remain in the curd for the most part. In contrast, cheese coagulated by lactic acid alone (e.g., cottage or cream cheese) contains less calcium and phosphorus, because the calcium salts are removed from the casein as casein is precipitated [4]. Cheddar cheese contains 721 mg calcium per 100 g, whereas dry-curd cottage cheese contains 36 mg calcium per 100 g [12]. The calcium content of cottage cheese may be increased by adding calcium-containing creaming mixtures. Generally, cheeses that are high in calcium contain other minerals, such as magnesium, in appreciable amounts. Cheese contributes small, but variable, amounts of specific trace elements, such as zinc, to the diet.

The sodium content of cheese is variable because of the addition of sodium chloride (salt) as an optional ingredient during manufacturing. On average, one ounce of natural Cheddar cheese contributes only 7.6% of the daily sodium intake limit of 2300 mg/day and a similar amount of natural Swiss cheese contributes about 2% [128]. Although Americans are advised to decrease their intake of sodium to reduce their risk of hypertension, only some individuals are salt-sensitive (see Chapter 3 on Dairy Foods and Hypertension). Other factors, such as excess body weight and reduced physical activity, may play a more important role in the development of high blood pressure. However, for salt-sensitive individuals, sodium-free (5 mg or less per serving), low-sodium (140 mg or less per serving), very-low-sodium (35 mg or less), reduced-sodium (at least 25% less sodium), and light (reduced in sodium by 50% or more) cheeses are available.

Cheese is an important source of essential nutrients throughout life. Research indicates that certain cheeses may protect against dental caries (see Chapter 6 on Dairy Foods and Oral Health). Studies in experimental animals and in humans demonstrate that intake of natural and processed cheeses reduce the risk of tooth decay. Components in cheese, such as calcium and possibly phosphorus, may inhibit demineralization and favor remineralization of teeth. As mentioned above, because of its low lactose content, cheese is an important source of many nutrients found in milk, particularly calcium, for individuals with lactase nonpersistance.

1.6.5 Cultured and Culture-Containing Dairy Foods

Cultured (fermented) dairy foods are milk products that result from the fermentation of milk or its products by starter cultures (selected specific microorganisms) that produce lactic acid under controlled conditions [4]. In culture-containing dairy products, concentrated cultures of bacteria — such as *Lactobacillus acidophilus* or bifidobacteria — are added to pasteurized and other types of heat-treated milk with no subsequent incubation or fermentation. There is a variety of cultured dairy foods differing in flavor and consistency, such as acidophilus milk, Bulgarian buttermilk, cultured buttermilk, cultured or sour cream, kefir, and yogurt [4]. All of these fermented milk products are characterized by the presence of lactic acid. Yogurt is made from milk fermented by a mixed culture of *Lactobacillus bulgaricus* and *Streptococcus thermophilus*. This dairy product may be plain, sweetened, flavored, or even frozen. Culturing or fermenting dairy foods is a method of preserving these foods as well as improving taste, digestibility, and increasing the variety of dairy foods available. In recent decades, the production and availability of cultured and culture-containing dairy foods have increased dramatically, in part because of their healthy image, trendy flavors, milder cultures, and convenience (availability in cups, drinkable forms, tubes) [208]. Per-capita sales of yogurt increased 10.7% between 2002 and 2003 [2]. Cultured and culture-containing dairy foods are important sources of many of milk's nutrients, including protein, calcium, phosphorus, magnesium, riboflavin, vitamin B_{12}, and niacin equivalents [4,12]. In general, the nutrient content of cultured and culture-containing foods is similar to that of the milk from which these products are made. However, factors such as the type and strain of bacteria, milk (whole, low-fat, nonfat) used, fermentation conditions, storage, and other treatments, such as the addition of milk solids-not-fat, sweeteners, and fruits (in yogurts, for example), can influence the nutrient composition of cultured and culture-containing dairy foods [4]. Some lactic acid-producing bacteria require vitamins for growth, whereas others synthesize some vitamins. The mineral content of milk is unchanged by fermentation. The fermentation of milk results in partial breakdown and better absorption of milk's protein, carbohydrate (lactose), and fat [209]. These changes are thought to result in a food of improved digestibility. Similar to their noncultured counterparts, cultured dairy foods of varied fat and energy contents are available. For example, in the United States, three categories of yogurt exist: yogurt ($>$3.25% fat, $>$8.25% milk solids-not-fat), low-fat yogurt ($>$0.5 to $<$2.0% fat, $>$8.25% milk solids-not-fat), and nonfat yogurt ($<$0.5% fat, $>$8.25% milk solids-not-fat) [102].

Since the early 1900s, when Elie Metchnikoff associated the consumption of large quantities of Bulgarian fermented milk with a long life in his book *The Prolongation of Life*, numerous health benefits have been attributed to cultured dairy foods [4]. These include improved lactose utilization, control of intestinal infections, reduced blood cholesterol levels, and anticarcinogenic activity. In recent years, probiotic or health-promoting bacteria have been added to an array of dairy foods. Probiotics are defined as "live microorganisms administered in adequate amounts that confer a health effect on the host" [210]. Dairy foods containing probiotics are a major and growing segment of the world's market for functional foods (i.e., foods fortified with ingredients capable of producing health benefits) [211,212]. As discussed below, some promising health benefits are attributed to specific strains of probiotics consumed at adequate levels. For more information about probiotics, readers are referred to reviews [210,213–217], proceedings of symposia [218–220], and books [212,221] on this subject. In addition, the Web site http:/www.usprobiotics.org provides up-to-date information on probiotics and dairy foods in the United States Intake of yogurt and some probiotics is beneficial for individuals with lactase nonpersistance (see Chapter 8 on Lactose Intolerance). This beneficial effect is explained by the lower lactose content of cultured dairy foods such as yogurt compared to milk, and the ability of starter cultures used in the manufacture of yogurt with live active cultures to produce the enzyme lactase, which hydrolyzes lactose [209,222]. Yogurt and probiotics may also improve tolerance to lactose by their positive effects on intestinal functions and colonic microflora or by reducing individuals' sensitivity to symptoms [222]. Although yogurt with live active cultures is particularly advantageous for lactose-intolerant individuals, unfermented or sweet acidophilus milk (pasteurized milk with *Lactobacillus acidophilus* added but not incubated), cultured buttermilk (pasteurized nonfat or low-fat milk cultured with *Streptococcus lactis* culture), and yogurt without live active cultures are tolerated about the same as milk. Yogurts with live active cultures can be identified by the National Yogurt Association's "Live & Active Cultures" seal [209]. Only yogurt products meeting specific requirements (i.e., at least 108 million organisms per gram at the time of manufacture) may carry this seal.

An extensive body of research supports a beneficial role for probiotics and fermented dairy foods such as yogurt in the prevention and treatment of a variety of diarrheal illnesses, such as acute diarrhea caused by rotavirus infections, antibiotic-associated diarrhea, and travelers' diarrhea [209,217,223]. According to a meta-analysis of randomized controlled studies, therapy using lactobacilli offers a safe and effective means to treat acute infectious diarrheal diseases in children [224]. Two meta-analyses of placebo-controlled clinical trials support a strong benefit of probiotics in reducing the risk of antibiotic-associated diarrhea [225,226]. Probiotics may help prevent or treat infections such as postoperative infections, respiratory infections, and the growth of *Helicobacter pylori*, a bacterial pathogen responsible for type B gastritis, peptic ulcers, and perhaps stomach cancer [216,227,228]. A 7-month, randomized, double-blind placebo-controlled study of more than 570 healthy children aged 1 to 6 years in day-care centers found that intake of a probiotic milk containing *L. rhamnosus* GG reduced the number and severity of respiratory infections and the need for antibiotics [227]. Some evidence, primarily from *in vitro* and experimental animal studies, indicates that culture-containing dairy foods, such as yogurt and specific probiotic cultures, may reduce the risk of some cancers, such as those of the colon and breast [209,214,217]; see Chapter 4 on Dairy Foods and Cancer). Although some epidemiological studies in humans link intake of yogurt or other fermented milk products to decreased cancer risk, a recent review of the evidence led researchers to conclude that the protective role of milks fermented with probiotic cultures in colon cancer risk reduction in humans is promising, but as yet inconclusive [229]. Findings from experimental animal and mostly short-term human studies indicate that yogurt and probiotics, such as lactobacilli and bifidobacteria, stimulate certain cellular and antibody functions of the immune system, which may in turn increase resistance to immune-related diseases (e.g., infections, gastrointestinal disorders, cancer, allergies) [209,214,217,230]. In older adults, especially those with poorly-functioning immune systems, consumption of milk supplemented with a relatively-low dose of the probiotic *B. lactis* HN019 enhanced some aspects of cellular immunity, including total, helper, and activated T-cells, leukocyte phagocytosis, and tumor-killing cells [230]. The addition of *L. casei* to a repletion diet improved resistance to pneumococcal respiratory infection in malnourished mice [231].Because probiotics can influence the intestinal flora, they may have beneficial effects for patients with inflammatory bowel disease, which includes ulcerative colitis, Crohn's disease, and pouchitis [209,213–215,232]. Probiotics may also reduce symptoms of irritable bowel syndrome [217]; help prevent allergic reactions in individuals at high risk of allergies such as food allergies [233]; reduce the risk of heart disease by their beneficial effects on blood lipid levels and blood pressure [217,234]; help prevent and treat urinary tract infections, bacterial vaginosis, and yeast vaginosis in women [215,235]; alleviate kidney stones [215]; and protect against dental caries [215]. Although potential health benefits of cultured dairy foods and probiotics have been identified, many of these benefits must be confirmed by well-controlled human studies [209,210,214,217]. As a result of increased understanding of probiotics' mechanisms and functions and new gene technologies that can lead to the development of probiotic strains with specific characteristics, an increasing number of dairy foods with probiotic bacteria can be expected [210,212]. Probiotic bacteria have long been associated with dairy foods, and these foods are considered a desirable natural vehicle to deliver probiotic bacteria. Consuming probiotics with dairy foods buffers stomach acid and increases the likelihood that the bacteria will survive into the intestine [212]. Dairy products containing probiotics also provide a number of essential nutrients, including calcium and protein, as well as components such as bioactive peptides, sphingolipids, and CLA. Researchers are investigating the possibility of syngergistic effects between components in dairy foods and probiotic cultures and whether components in milk can trigger beneficial genes in probiotic cultures.

1.6.6 Whey Products

Whey is the portion of milk remaining after casein and fat are formed into cheese curd, usually by acid, heat, or rennet [4,10]. Once regarded mainly as an animal feed product, today the uses of whey and whey products for human consumption have greatly expanded as a result of the recognition of whey's excellent nutritional and functional properties [20,236,237]. As used for human food, whey is concentrated by evaporation to condensed products or maximally concentrated by drying into powder. All whey for human use must be pasteurized. The food industry uses whey and its products in baked goods, beverages, flavorings (sauces, salad dressings), canned goods (fruits and vegetables), cheese products (dips, spreads, process cheese, confections), dry mixes, frozen foods, jams and jellies, fat substitutes, and meat, pasta, and milk products [20]. Whey and modified whey products are an acceptable substitute for nonfat dry milk (NFDM) in some foods and may partially replace NFDM in frozen desserts. Whey cheese, such as traditional Italian Ricotta cheese, is made by concentrating whey and coagulating the whey protein with heat and acid, with or without the addition of milk and milk fat.

Whey is recognized for its high nutritional quality. This coproduct of the cheese industry contains protein, lactose, minerals (e.g., calcium, phosphorus, magnesium, zinc), vitamins, and traces of milk fat [12,20]. There are two basic types of whey: sweet whey and acid whey [12]. Sweet whey (pH greater than or equal to 5.6) is mainly obtained from milk used in the manufacture of natural enzyme-produced cheeses, such as Cheddar, Mozzarella, and Swiss cheese. Acid whey (pH less than or equal to 5.1) is mainly obtained from nonfat milk used in the manufacture of cottage, ricotta, or similar cheeses. An average composition of sweet and acid dry wheys is provided in Table 1.11 [12]. Wide ranges in the nutrient content of these wheys are recognized because of diverse manufacturing processes presently used for the cheese from which sweet and acid whey products are obtained.

Fresh-pasteurized liquid whey is rarely used as such for foods or feeds because of high transporting costs and susceptibility to deterioration during storage. Consequently, whey is processed to provide a wide range of products, including condensed whey, dry whey, and modified whey products, each with unique functional characteristics (e.g., whipping/foaming, emulsification, high solubility, gelation, viscosity). These whey products contain a high concentration of whey solids that are easily transported, have enhanced storage stability, blend well with other foods, and are economical sources of milk solids [4].

Condensed whey is the liquid food obtained by removing some of the moisture from whey. The whey may be condensed about tenfold, but all constituents other than moisture remain in the same relative proportions as in the original whey. Condensed whey may be directly added to processed cheese foods. Sweet condensed whey is used in candy formulas. Acid whey has a more limited use for humans. Dry whey, the most suitable form for use in foods or feeds, is the food obtained by removing about 95% of the moisture from whey but which contains all other constituents in the

TABLE 1.11
Average Composition of Sweet and Acid Dry Wheys[a]

Constituent	Sweet	Acid
Protein, Nx6.38 (%)	12.9	11.7
Fat (%)	1.1	0.5
Lactose (%)	74.5	73.4
Total ash (%)	8.3	10.8
Vitamins[b]		
Vitamin A (IU)	30	59
Vitamin C (mg)	1.5	0.9
Vitamin E (mg)	0.03	0.00
Thiamin (B1) (mg)	0.5	0.62
Riboflavin (B2) (mg)	2.2	2.06
Pyridoxine (B6) (mg)	0.6	0.62
Vitamin B12 (meg)	2.4	2.5
Pantothenic Acid (mg)	5.6	5.6
Niacin (mg)	1.3	1.2
Folate (meg)	12.0	0.33
Minerals		
Calcium (mg)	796	2050
Phosphorus (mg)	932	1349
Sodium (mg	1079	968
Potassium (mg)	2080	2289
Magnesium (mg)	176	199
Zinc (mg)	1.97	6.3
Iron (mg)	0.9	1.2
Copper (mg)	0.07	0.05
Selenium (meg)	27.2	27.3

[a] Values per 100 g dry whey.

Source: From USDA Nutrient Database for Standard Reference, Release 17, 2004 (www.nal.usda.gov.fnic/foodcomp).

same relative proportions as in whey. This form of whey can be stored almost indefinitely under reasonable conditions without harm to its physical or nutritional properties.Modified whey products may be obtained by various processes and procedures, such as ultrafiltration and reverse osmosis. Examples of modified whey products include partially-delactosed whey, demineralized and partially-demineralized whey, whey protein concentrate, and whey protein isolates [10,20]. Partially-delactosed whey contains no more than 60% lactose on a solids basis. Lactose (62% to 75% of dry whey) is removed by crystallization for use in many products, such as a carrier or extender in pharmaceuticals. Partially-demineralized whey contains a maximum of 7% mineral matter on a solids basis, and demineralized whey contains a maximum of 1½% on a solids basis. The minerals in whey (7% to 10% total in dry whey) are removed because they may contribute to an off-taste. Whey protein concentrate contains a minimum of 25% protein on a solids basis and little, if any, lactose or fat. Whey protein concentrates may be added to coffee whiteners, soups, and infant formula because of their emulsification properties; to desserts and whipped toppings because of their ability to form and stabilize foams; to meats and baked goods for texture and structure because of their gelling properties; and to low-fat cheeses because of their ability to soften cheese texture [4,20]. Whey-protein edible coatings may be used to extend the shelf life of oxygen-sensitive foods such as nuts or fresh fruits and vegetables. Whey protein isolate, which is less common than whey protein concentrate, contains at least 90% protein on a dry weight basis and little, if any, lactose or fat. In addition, whey protein isolates can be heated with acid or treated with proteolytic enzymes to form hydrolyzed whey proteins. As a result of new technologies, a variety of biologically-active amino acids, peptides, and fractions can be isolated from whey protein [236]. Emerging research indicates that whey-derived bioactive components, particularly whey proteins, have antimicrobial and antiviral properties; enhance immune defense; possess antioxidative activity; may help protect against cancer and cardiovascular disease; and enhance the performance of physically active individuals, among other benefits [20,236,237]. The majority of studies examining potential health benefits of whey/whey components are tissue culture and experimental animal studies, with limited human trials.

Whey proteins have proportionately more sulfur-containing amino acids (cysteine, methionine) than casein, which is almost devoid of sulfur amino acids. The amino acid cysteine is important for the biosynthesis of glutathione, a tripeptide with antioxidant, anticarcinogen, and immune stimulatory properties [236,237]. Whey proteins are also a good source of branched-chain amino acids, isoleucine, leucine, and valine [236]. Branched-chain amino acids are unique because they help minimize muscle wasting under conditions of increased protein breakdown, which makes whey particularly beneficial for athletes. Whey protein consists of several different proteins, including beta-lactoglobulin, alpha-lactalbumin, immunoglobulins, bovine serum albumin, lactoferrin, and lactoperoxidase, as well as glycomacropeptide (a casein-derived protein released into whey during cheese manufacturing), each of which has specific biological activities [20,236]. Several whey proteins may protect against toxins, bacteria, and viruses [20,236–239]. For example, lactoferrin has been shown to inhibit the growth of some harmful food-borne pathogens, such as *E. coli* and *Listeria monocytogenes*, and has significant antiviral activity against human immunodeficiency virus (HIV) [238,239]. Lactoferrin is most effective during the early stage of HIV infection [239]. In suckling mice, intake of a whey protein concentrate product reduced symptoms (i.e., diarrhea) associated with rotavirus infection [240].A number of whey proteins modulates immune activity [237]. Lactoferrin can stimulate the growth of various cells of the immune defense system, including lymphocytes, macrophages, monocytes, humoral immune response, and antibody response [31,236,237,241]. A study in mice found that whey protein concentrate enhanced humoral immune responses to a variety of antigens, such as influenza and poliomyelitis vaccines [241]. Increasing evidence from cellular and animal models indicates that whey, whey protein (e.g., lactoferrin, lactoperoxidase, alpha-lactalbumin, bovine serum albumin) and peptides, as well as other whey components, may protect against some cancers (e.g., intestinal, mammary, colon) [236,237,242,243]. Researchers in Australia reported decreased levels of aberrant crypt foci, precancer markers, in the proximal colon of rats fed whey protein concentrate and treated with a chemical carcinogen [243]. In addition to whey protein, other components, such as sphingomyelin and CLA, in whey lipids and the calcium content of whey may contribute to whey's cancer protective property (see Chapter 4 on Dairy Foods and Cancer) [63,77]. In addition to whey's potential anticancer properties, whey contains bioactive components that may help protect against cardiovascular disease. For example, whey-derived peptides may protect against hypertension, inhibit platelet aggregation, and reduce blood cholesterol or have a favorable effect on blood lipid levels [25,244,245]. Whey and whey components offer several benefits for individuals with physically active lifestyles, according to a review by Ha and Zemel [246]. Whey proteins are easily-digested high-quality proteins with a relatively high proportion of branched-chain amino acids such as leucine [20,236,246]. These amino acids provide an energy source during endurance exercise, allowing athletes to train more extensively for longer periods of time. The abundance of leucine in whey plays a role in the synthesis of muscle protein [247]. Additionally, whey proteins are rich in the amino acids arginine and lysine, which may increase the release of growth hormone, a stimulator of muscle growth. In addition, bioactive compounds isolated from whey protein (e.g., lactoferrin and lactoferricin) may improve immune function and gastrointestinal health, as well as reduce excess free radical production in athletes when intensive training compromises these systems [246]. Because of their favorable effect on body composition, whey protein may be important for individuals trying to maintain or lose weight [247,248]. Whey proteins may also increase satiety [249–251]. Accumulating evidence indicates that other whey components, particularly calcium, may have a beneficial role in weight management (see Chapter 7 on Dairy Foods and Weight Management).Additional potential health benefits of whey and whey components include their effect on bones and cognitive performance and alertness. Findings that some whey proteins (lactoferrin, for example) may increase bone-forming cells and inhibit cells responsible for bone resorption suggest that whey may have a potential therapeutic use in the treatment of osteoporosis [252,253]. Alpha-lactalbumin, a whey protein in cow's milk with a high content of tryptophan (a precursor of serotonin), has been shown to improve cognitive performance (i.e., memory) in stress-vulnerable individuals [254] and, when consumed in the evening, improves alertness and attention the next morning in subjects with mild sleep complaints [255]. Increasing knowledge of the potential health benefits of whey and whey components offers to expand their use in a variety of functional foods designed to meet the health concerns of specific population groups.

1.7 SUMMARY

The nutritional and health benefits of milk and other dairy foods are well-documented, and sound scientific evidence supports their importance in the diet. In fact, these foods have a long history of contributing to health and well-being. Today, milk and other dairy foods are recognized as nutrient-dense foods. Although they contribute only 9% of the total calories (energy) available in the U.S. food supply, these foods provide 72% of the calcium, 26% of the riboflavin, 32% of the phosphorus, 19% of the protein, 15% of the magnesium, 20% of the vitamin B_{12}, 23% of the vitamin A, 9% of the vitamin B_6, and 4.6% of the thiamin, in addition to appreciable amounts of vitamin D and niacin equivalents [18]. Dairy foods contribute to nutrient intake and health from childhood through older adult years. Unfortunately, many people fail to consume recommended servings of these foods, thereby making it difficult for them to meet nutrient recommendations [174]. Consuming milk and other dairy foods improves the overall nutritional quality of the diet without necessarily increasing total energy or fat intake, body weight, or percent body fat [146–149,151,153,155].

With respect to specific nutrients, cow's milk is an excellent source of high-quality protein which contains, in varying amounts, all of the essential amino acids required for humans [15]. Because of its content of the amino acid tryptophan, milk is an excellent source of niacin equivalents. Experimental studies indicate that cow's milk protein may help to increase bone strength, enhance immune function, reduce blood pressure and risk of some cancers, and protect against dental caries. The prevalence of cow's milk protein allergy or sensitivity is generally overestimated and, if present in high-risk children, is usually outgrown by three years of age [34,35,38]. Scientific findings fail to confirm the suggestion that cow's milk protein contributes to the development of type I (insulin-dependent) diabetes in genetically susceptible children [42–51,256]. Although the primary carbohydrate in cow's milk is lactose, its amount varies widely among different dairy foods. As discussed in Chapter 8, those who are lactase-nonpersistent can comfortably consume the amount of lactose in up to 2 cups of milk per day when taken with meals. Fat in milk contributes to the appearance, texture, and flavor of dairy foods. Milk fat is also a source of energy, essential fatty acids (linoleic and linolenic), fat-soluble vitamins (A, D, E, and K), and several health-promoting components such as CLA, sphingomyelin, and butyric acid [63,80]. For example, emerging scientific findings reveal that CLA may protect against certain cancers and cardiovascular disease, enhance immune function, and reduce body fatness/increase lean body tissue [63,74–80]. Milk and other dairy foods are an important source of many vitamins and minerals [11,129]. Vitamin A in whole milk, and added to fluid lower-fat and fat-free milks, plays a key role in vision, cellular differentiation, and immunity. Nearly all fluid milks in the

United States are fortified with vitamin D. Vitamin D enhances the intestinal absorption of calcium and phosphorus and is essential for the maintenance of a healthy skeleton. In addition to these fat-soluble vitamins, milk and other dairy foods contribute appreciable amounts of water-soluble vitamins, such as riboflavin, vitamin B_{12}, and vitamin B_6. Milk and milk products provide almost three-quarters of the calcium available in the nation's food supply [18]. A sufficient intake of calcium helps to reduce the risk of osteoporosis (see Chapter 5), hypertension (see Chapter 3), some cancers (see Chapter 4), and some types of kidney stones, and may have a beneficial role in weight management (see Chapter 7). The high nutritional value of milk, as well as its overall quality, is ensured by rigid sanitary conditions employed from farm to marketplace. Protecting the quality of milk is everyone's responsibility, from government health officials to the dairy industry to consumers. The Pasteurized Milk Ordinance [112] is an example of an effective instrument for protecting the quality of the nation's milk. To improve milk's quality, most milk is homogenized and pasteurized. Homogenization results in milk of uniform consistency, which is less susceptible to off-flavors. Pasteurization is required by law for all fluid milk and milk products moved in interstate commerce for retail sale. As a result of pasteurization, milk and milk products are now associated with less than 1% of all disease outbreaks due to infected food and contaminated water, compared to 25% in 1938 [112].

Today, consumers have a wide variety of dairy foods to choose from to meet their taste, nutrition, health, and convenience needs. Dairy foods of varied fat content, of low or reduced lactose content, fortified with nutrients such as vitamin A, vitamin D, and calcium, and processed to improve the keeping quality are readily available. These foods include milks (unflavored, flavored, evaporated, condensed, sweetened condensed, dry, nonfat dry), cultured and culture-containing dairy foods (yogurts, acidophilus milk, cultured buttermilk, sour cream), creams, butter, ice cream, and cheeses [12,102]. Over the years, consumption of individual milks and milk products has changed dramatically. Noteworthy trends include more use of reduced-fat milks, yogurt, creams, and cheese, and less use of whole milk [193]. As a result of comprehensive food labeling regulations, consumers can readily choose dairy foods that meet their specific needs by referring to the Nutrition Facts label on product packages [100]. To help consumers better understand the fat content of milk and other dairy foods, standards of identity for 12 lower fat dairy foods have been removed and new labels introduced. For example, skim (nonfat) milk is now labeled fat-free as well as nonfat and skim [99].

The nutritional and health benefits of specific dairy foods, such as flavored milk, cheese, cultured and culture-containing dairy products, and whey products have been reviewed. Intake of chocolate milk, a highly nutritious, well-liked beverage, has been demonstrated to improve children's overall nutrient intake [152,153]. Cheese is a concentrated source of many of milk's nutrients [4,12]. Because of their insignificant amount of lactose, most cheeses are well-tolerated by individuals with lactase nonpersistence (see Chapter 8). Cheeses are also a good source of CLA, and several varieties of cheese may protect against dental caries (see Chapter 7). Not only are cultured (fermented) and culture-containing dairy foods such as yogurt an excellent source of many of milk's nutrients, but they may offer health benefits including improved lactose digestion, control of intestinal infections, reduced blood cholesterol levels, and anticancer activity [209,210,217]. These beneficial effects depend on the type and strain of bacteria, fermentation condition, type of milk, and other factors. Similar to cultured dairy foods, whey, a coproduct of the cheese industry, is being recognized for its excellent nutritional and functional properties [20,236,237]. Clearly, consumers today are presented with an abundant array of safe, nutritious dairy foods tailored to meet their specific health and other needs.

The 2005 *Dietary Guidelines for Americans* [14] and *MyPyramid* [126] acknowledge the important role of dairy foods in the diet and recommend that Americans 9 years of age and older consume 3 cups per day of fat-free or low-fat milk or equivalent milk products (cheese, yogurt, etc.) as part of a healthful diet. This recommendation is consistent with other reports, such as those issued by the National Medical Association [61], the Surgeon General's report on

Bone Health and Osteoporosis [157], and the American Academy of Pediatrics [160]. An analysis of government food and nutrient consumption data determined that 3 to 4 servings of dairy foods a day for all individuals 9 years of age and older is the optimal amount to ensure adequate calcium intake [125]. If American adults increased their intake of dairy foods to 3 to 4 servings per day, researchers conservatively estimated that health care cost savings associated with several common medical conditions (obesity, hypertension, type 2 diabetes, osteoporosis, kidney stones, certain outcomes of pregnancy, and some cancers) would be approximately $26 billion in the first year, with 5-year cumulative savings in excess of $200 billion [124]. Dairy foods are an affordable, convenient, and great-tasting way to enhance the nutritional quality of a diet.

REFERENCES

1. McGee, H., *On Food and Cooking: The Science and Lore of the Kitchen*, Macmillan, New York, 1984.
2. International Dairy Foods Association, *Dairy Facts 2004 Edition*, International Dairy Foods Association, Washington, D.C., September 2, 2004..
3. Jensen, R. G., Ed., *Handbook of Milk Composition*, Academic Press, New York, 1995.
4. Kosikowski, F. V. and Mistry, V. V., *Cheese and Fermented Milk Foods, Vol. 1. Origins and Principles,* Vol. 11, *Procedures and Analysis*, 3rd ed., F.V. Kosikowski and Associates, Brooktondale, NY, 1997.
5. Fox, P. F., Ed., *Advanced Dairy Chemistry,* Vol. 1, *Proteins*, Chapman & Hall, New York, 1992.
6. Fox, P. F., Ed., *Advanced Dairy Chemistry,* Vol. 2, *Lipids,* 2nd ed., Chapman & Hall, New York, 1995.
7. Fox, P. F., Ed., *Advanced Dairy Chemistry,* Vol. 3, *Lactose, Water, Salts, and Vitamins,* 2nd ed., Chapman & Hall, New York, 1997.
8. CAST (Council for Agricultural Science and Technology), *Contribution of Animal Products to Healthful Diets.* Task Force Report No. 131, Council for Agricultural Science and Technology, Ames, IA, October 1997.
9. National Dairy Council, *Newer Knowledge of Dairy Foods*, National Dairy Council, Rosemont, IL, 2000, http://www.nationaldairycouncil.org (Nutrition and Product Information/Dairy Products/Supportive Science).
10. Chandan, R., *Dairy-Based Ingredients*, Eagan Press, St. Paul, MN, 1997.
11. Weinberg, L. G., Berner, L. A., and Groves, J. E., Nutrient contributions of dairy foods in the United States, Continuing Survey of Food Intakes by Individuals, 1994–1996, 1998, *J. Am. Diet. Assoc.*, 104, 895, 2004.
12. U.S. Department of Agriculture, Agricultural Research Service, USDA Nutrient Database for Standard Reference, Release 18, Nutrient Data Laboratory Home Page, http://www.ars.usda.gov/ba/bhnrc/ndl.
13. German, J. B., Dillard, C. J., and Ward, R. E., Bioactive components in milk, *Curr. Opin. Clin. Metab. Care*, 5, 653, 2002.
14. U.S. Department of Health and Human Services and U.S. Department of Agriculture. *Dietary Guidelines for Americans, 2005*, 6th ed., U.S. Government Printing Office, Washington, D.C., January 2005, http://www.healthierus.gov/dietaryguidelines.
15. European Dairy Association, *Nutritional Quality of Proteins*, European Dairy Association, Brussels, Belgium, 1997.
16. International Dairy Federation, *Milk Protein Definition & Standardization*, International Dairy Federation, Brussels, Belgium, 1994.
17. Institute of Medicine of the National Academies, *Dietary Reference Intakes for Energy, Carbohydrate, Fiber, Fat, Fatty Acids, Cholesterol, Protein, and Amino Acids*, The National Academies Press, Washington, D.C., 2002.
18. Gerrior, S., Bente, L., and Hiza, H., *Nutrient Content of the U.S. Food Supply, 1909–2000 Home Economics Research Report No. 56*, U.S. Department of Agriculture, Center for Nutrition Policy and Promotion, 2004.
19. Pihlanto, A. and Korhonen, H., Bioactive peptides and proteins, *Adv. Food Nutr. Res.*, 47, 175, 2003.

20. U.S. Dairy Export Council, *Reference Manual for U.S. Whey and Lactose Products*, June 2004, http:/ www.usdec.org/publications/PubDetail.cfm?itemNumber = 587.
21. Shah, N. P., Effects of milk-derived bioactives: an overview, *Br. J. Nutr.*, 84 (suppl.), 3s, 2000.
22. Wolfe, R. R. and Miller, S. L., Protein metabolism in response to ingestion pattern and composition of proteins, *J. Nutr.*, 132, 3207s, 2002.
23. Huth, P. J., Layman, D. K., and Brown, P. H., The emerging role of dairy proteins and bioactive peptides in nutrition and health, *J. Nutr.*, 134 (suppl. 4), 961s, 2004.
24. Layman, D. K. and Baum, J. I., Dietary protein impact on glycemic control during weight loss, *J. Nutr.*, 134 (suppl. 4), 968s, 2004.
25. FitzGerald, R. J., Murray, B. A., and Walsh, D. J., Hypotensive peptides from milk proteins, *J. Nutr.*, 134 (suppl. 4), 980s, 2004.
26. Aimutis, W. R., Bioactive properties of milk proteins with particular focus on anticariogenesis, *J. Nutr.*, 134 (suppl. 4), 989s, 2004.
27. Anderson, G. H. and Moore, S. E., Dietary proteins in the regulation of food intake and body weight in humans, *J. Nutr.*, 134 (suppl. 4), 974s, 2004.
28. Noakes, M., Bowen, J., and Clifton, P., Dairy foods or fractions for appetite and weight control, *Aust. J. Dairy Technol.*, 60, 152, 2005.
29. McIntosh, G. H. et al., Dairy proteins protect against dimethylhydrazine-induced intestinal cancers in rats, *J. Nutr.*, 125, 809, 1995.
30. MacDonald, R. S., Thornton, W. H. Jr., and Marshall, R. T., A cell culture model to identify biologically active peptides generated by bacterial hydrolysis of casein, *J. Dairy Sci.*, 77, 1167, 1994.
31. Parodi, P. W., A role for milk proteins in cancer prevention, *Aust. J. Dairy Technol.*, 53, 37, 1998.
32. Gill, H. S. et al., Immunoregulatory peptides in bovine milk, *Br. J. Nutr.*, 84 (suppl. 1), 111s, 2000.
33. Truswell, A. S., The A2 milk case: a critical review, *Eur. J. Clin. Nutr.*, 59, 623, 2005.
34. Bock, S. A., Prospective appraisal of complaints of adverse reactions to foods in children during the first 3 years of life, *Pediatrics*, 79, 683, 1987.
35. Crittenden, R. G. and Bennett, L. E., Cow's milk allergy: a complex disorder, *J. Am. Coll. Nutr.*, 24, 582s, 2005.
36. Eggesbo, M. et al., The prevalence of CMA/CMPI in young children: the validity of parentally perceived reactions in a population-based study, *Allergy*, 56, 393, 2001.
37. Host, A., Frequency of cow's milk allergy in childhood, *Ann. Allergy Asthma Immunol.*, 89 (6) (suppl. 1), 33, 2002.
38. Kleinman, R. E., Ed., *Pediatric Nutrition Handbook,* 5th ed., American Academy of Pediatrics, Elk Grove Village, IL, 2004.
39. Karjalainen, J. et al., A bovine albumin peptide as a possible trigger of insulin-dependent diabetes mellitus, *N. Engl. J. Med.*, 327, 302, 1992.
40. Ahmed, T. et al., Circulating antibodies to common food antigens in Japanese children with IDDM, *Diabetes Care*, 20 (1), 74, 1997.
41. Cavallo, M. G. et al., Cell-mediated immune response to B casein in recent-onset insulin-dependent diabetes: implications for disease pathogenesis, *Lancet*, 348, 926, 1996.
42. Atkinson, M. A. and Ellis, T. M., Infant diets and insulin-dependent diabetes: evaluating the "cows' milk hypothesis" and a role for anti-bovine serum albumin immunity, *J. Am. Coll. Nutr.*, 16, 334, 1997.
43. Paxson, J. A., Weber, J. G., and Kulczycki, A. Jr., Cow's milk-free diet does not prevent diabetes in NOD mice, *J. Am. Diabetes Assoc.*, 46 (11), 1711, 1997.
44. Bodington, M. J., McNally, P. G., and Burden, A. C., Cow's milk and Type I childhood diabetes: no increase in risk, *Diabetic Med.*, 11, 663, 1994.
45. Norris, J. M. et al., Lack of association between early exposure to cow's milk protein and B-cell immunity: Diabetes Autoimmunity Study in the Young (DAISY), *JAMA*, 276, 609, 1996.
46. Fuchtenbusch, M. et al., Antibodies to bovine serum albumin (BSA) in type 1 diabetes and other autoimmune disorders, *Exp. Clin. Endocrinol. Diabetes*, 105, 86, 1997.
47. Schatz, D. A. and Maclaren, N. K., Cow's milk and insulin-dependent diabetes mellitus. Innocent until proven guilty, *JAMA*, 276, 647, 1996.
48. Scott, F. W., AAP recommendations on cow milk, soy, and early infant feeding, *Pediatrics*, 95, 515, 1995.

49. Ellis, T. M. and Atkinson, M. A., Early infant diets and insulin-dependent diabetes, *Lancet*, 347, 1464, 1996.
50. Berdanier, C. D., Diabetes mellitus: is there a connection with infant-feeding practices? *Nutr. Today*, 36, 241, 2001.
51. Schrezenmeir, J. and Jagla, A., Milk and diabetes, *J. Am. Coll. Nutr.*, 19 (suppl.), 176s, 2000.
52. Pereira, M. A. et al., Dairy consumption, obesity, and the insulin resistance syndrome in young adults, The CARDIA study, *JAMA*, 287, 2081, 2002.
53. Choi, H. K. et al., Dairy consumption and risk of Type 2 diabetes mellitus in men, *Arch. Intern. Med.*, 165, 997, 2005.
54. Filer, L. J. and Reynolds, W. A., Lessons in comparative physiology: lactose intolerance, *Nutr. Today*, 32, 79, 1997.
55. Suarez, F. L. and Savaiano, D. A., Diet, genetics, and lactose intolerance, *Food Technol.*, 51, 74, 1997.
56. Ziegler, E. E. and Fomon, S. J., Lactose enhances mineral absorption in infancy, *J. Pediatr. Gastroenterol. Nutr.*, 2, 288, 1983.
57. Nickel, K. P. et al., Calcium bioavailability from bovine milk and dairy products in premenopausal women using intrinisic and extrinsic labeling techniques, *J. Nutr.*, 126, 1406, 1996.
58. McBean, L. D. and Miller, G. D., Allaying fears and fallacies about lactose intolerance, *J. Am. Diet. Assoc.*, 98, 671, 1998.
59. Jarvis, J. K. and Miller, G. D., Overcoming the barrier of lactose intolerance to reduce health disparities, *J. Natl. Med. Assoc.*, 94, 55, 2002.
60. Dobler, M. L., *Lactose Intolerance Nutrition Guide*, American Dietetic Association, Chicago, IL, 2003.
61. Wooten, W. J. and Price, W. P. Consensus Report of the National Medical Association, The role of dairy and dairy nutrients in the diet of African Americans, *J. Natl Med. Assoc.*, 96 (suppl.), 1s, 2004.
62. German, J. B. and Dillard, C. J., Fractionated milk fat: composition, structure, and functional properties, *Food Technol.*, 52, 33, 1998.
63. Parodi, P. W., Milk fat in human nutrition, *Aust. J. Dairy Technol.*, 59, 3, 2004.
64. Jensen, R. G. and Lammi-Keefe, C. J., Current status of research on the composition of bovine and human milk lipids, in *Lipids in Infant Nutrition*, Huang, Y. S. and Sinclair, A. J., Eds., AOCS Press, Champaign, IL, pp. 168–191, 1998.
65. Katan, M. B., Zock, P. L., and Mensink, R. P., Dietary oils, serum lipoproteins, and coronary heart disease, *Am. J. Clin. Nutr.*, 61 (suppl.), 1368s, 1995.
66. Krauss, R. M. et al., AHA dietary guidelines. Revision 2000: a statement for healthcare professionals from the Nutrition Committee of the American Heart Association, *Circulation*, 102, 2284, 2000.
67. Institute of Medicine, Food and Drug Administration, Letter Report on Dietary Reference Intakes for *Trans* Fatty Acids. Drawn from the Report on Dietary Reference Intakes for Energy, Carbohydrate, Fiber, Fat, Fatty Acids, Cholesterol, Protein, and Amino Acids. Report of the Panel on Macronutrients, Subcommittees on Upper Reference Levels of Nutrients and on Interpretation and Uses of Dietary Reference Intakes, and the Standing Committee on the Scientific Evaluation of Dietary Reference Intakes, July 2002.
68. Food and Drug Administration, Department of Health and Human Services, Food labeling; *trans* fatty acids in nutrition labeling; consumer research to consider nutrient content and health claims and possible footnote or disclosure statements; final rule and proposed rule, *Fed. Regist.* 68 (No. 133), July 11, 41434, 2003.
69. Hunter, J. E., Dietary levels of *trans*-fatty acids: basis for health concerns and industry efforts to limit use, *Nutr. Res.*, 25, 499, 2005.
70. Lock, A. L., Parodi, P. W., and Bauman, D. E., The biology of *trans* fatty acids: implications for human health and the dairy industry, *Aust. J. Dairy Technol.*, 60, 134, 2005.
71. Chin, S. F. et al., Dietary sources of conjugated dienoic isomers of linoleic acid, a newly recognized class of anticarcinogens, *J. Food Comp. Anal.*, 5, 185, 1992.
72. Lin, H. et al., Survey of the conjugated linoleic acid contents of dairy products, *J. Dairy Sci.*, 78, 2358, 1995.
73. Shantha, N. C. et al., Conjugated linoleic acid concentrations in dairy products as affected by processing and storage, *J. Food Sci.*, 60 (4), 695–720, 1995.

74. Yurawecz, M. P. et al., Eds., *Advances in Conjugated Linoleic Acid Research*, Vol. 1, AOCS Press, Champaign, IL, 1999.
75. Sebedio, J.-L., Christie, W. W., and Adlof, R., Eds., *Advances in Conjugated Linoleic Acid Research*, Vol. 2, AOCS Press, Champaign, IL, 2003.
76. Belury, M. A., Dietary conjugated linoleic acid in health: physiological effects and mechanisms of action, *Annu. Rev. Nutr.*, 22, 505, 2002.
77. Parodi, P. W., Anti-cancer agents in milk fat, *Aust. J. Dairy Technol.*, 58, 114, 2003.
78. Angel, A., The role of conjugated linoleic acid in human health, *Am. J. Clin. Nutr.*, 79, 1131, 2004.
79. Rainer, L. and Heiss, C. J., Conjugated linoleic acid: health implications and effects on body composition, *J. Am. Diet. Assoc.*, 104, 963, 2004.
80. Parodi, P. W., Cows' milk fat components as potential anticarcinogenic agents, *J. Nutr.*, 127, 1055, 1997.
81. Merrill, A. H. Jr. et al., Importance of sphingolipids and inhibitors of sphingolipid metabolism as components of animal diets, *J. Nutr.*, 127, 830s, 1997.
82. Schmelz, E. M. et al., Colonic cell proliferation and aberrant crypt foci formation are inhibited by dairy glycosphingolipids in 1,2-dimethylhydrazine-treated CF1 mice, *J. Nutr.*, 130, 522, 2000.
83. Noh, S. K. and Koo, S. I., Milk sphingomyelin is more effective than egg sphingomyelin in inhibiting intestinal absorption of cholesterol and fat in rats, *J. Nutr.*, 134, 2611, 2004.
84. Smith, J. G. and German, J. B., Molecular and genetic effects of dietary derived butyric acid, *Food Technol.*, 49, 87, 1995.
85. Aukema, H. M. et al., Butyrate alters activity of specific CAMP-receptor proteins in a transgenic mouse colonic cell line, *J. Nutr.*, 127, 18, 1997.
86. Burton-Freeman, B., Davis, P. A., and Schneeman, B. O., Dairy products as dietary fat sources: effects on postprandial glucose and insulin, *FASEB J.*, Feb. 28, 1997, A372 (Abstr. 2157).
87. Himaya, A. et al., Satiety power of dietary fat: a new appraisal, *Am. J. Clin. Nutr.*, 65, 1410, 1997.
88. Seifert, M. F. and Watkins, B. A., Role of dietary lipid and antioxidants in bone metabolism, *Nutr. Res.*, 17 (7), 1209, 1997.
89. Watkins, B. A. et al., Dietary lipids modulate bone prostaglandin E2 production, insulin-like growth factor-1 concentration and formation rate in chicks, *J. Nutr.*, 127, 1084, 1997.
90. Xu, H., Watkins, B. A., and Seifert, M. F., Vitamin E stimulates trabecular bone formation and alters epiphyseal cartilage morphometry, *Calcif. Tissue Int.*, 57, 293, 1995.
91. Kaylegian, K. E., Functional characteristics and nontraditional applications of milk lipid components in food and nonfood systems, *J. Dairy Sci.*, 78, 2524, 1995.
92. Noakes, M., Nestel, P. J., and Clifton, P. M., Modifying the fatty acid profile of dairy products through feedlot technology lowers plasma cholesterol of humans consuming the products, *Am. J. Clin. Nutr.*, 63, 42, 1996.
93. Seidel, C., Deufel, T., and Jahreis, G., Effects of fat-modified dairy products on blood lipids in humans in comparison with other fats, *Ann. Nutr. Metab.*, 49, 42, 2005.
94. Lin, M.-P. et al., Modification of fatty acids in milk by feeding calcium-protected high oleic sunflower oil, *J. Food Sci.*, 61 (1), 24, 1996.
95. O'Callaghan, D. et al., Are butter and cheese rich in monounsaturates beneficial in hyperlipidaemic patients?, *J. Cardiovasc. Risk*, 3, 441, 1996.
96. Allred, S. L. et al., Milk and cheese from cows fed calcium salts of palm and fish oil alone or in combination with soybean products, *J. Dairy Sci.*, 89, 234, 2006.
97. Institute of Medicine, *Dietary Reference Intakes for Vitamin A, Vitamin K, Arsenic, Boron, Chromium, Copper, Iodine, Iron, Manganese, Molybdenum, Nickel, Silicon, Vanadium, and Zinc*, National Academy Press, Washington, D.C., 2001.
98. Said, H. M., Ong, D. E., and Shingleton, J. L., Intestinal uptake of retinol: enhancement by bovine milk B-lactoglobulin, *Am. J. Clin. Nutr.*, 49, 690, 1989.
99. Food and Drug Administration, U.S. Department of Health and Human Services, Low-fat and skim milk products, low-fat and nonfat yogurt products, low-fat cottage cheese: revocation of standards of identity; food labeling; nutrient content claims for fat, fatty acids, and cholesterol content of food, *Fed. Regist.*, 61 (225), 58991 (November 20), 1996.

100. Food and Drug Administration, U.S. Department of Health and Human Services, Food labeling; general provisions; nutrition labeling; label format; nutrient content claims; health claims; ingredient labeling; state and local requirements; and exemptions; final rules, 21 CFR Parts 101&102, *Fed. Regist.* 58, 2065 (January 6), 1993.
101. Institute of Medicine, *Dietary Reference Intakes for Calcium, Phosphorus, Magnesium, Vitamin D, and Fluoride*, National Academy Press, Washington, D.C., 1997.
102. U.S. Department of Health and Human Services, Food and Drug Administration, *Code of Federal Regulations, Title 21, Part 131, Subpart B, Milk and Cream, Part 133, Subpart B, Cheeses and Related Cheese Products,* U.S. Government Printing Office, Washington, D.C., April 2004.
103. Gartner, L. M. and Greer, F. R., and the Section of Breastfeeding and Committee on Nutrition, American Academy of Pediatrics Prevention of rickets and vitamin D deficiency: new guidelines for vitamin D intake, *Pediatrics*, 111, 908, 2003.
104. American Medical Association, The nutritive quality of processed foods: general policies for nutrient additives, *Nutr. Rev.*, 40, 93, 1982.
105. American Medical Association, Council on Foods and Nutrition, importance of vitamin D milk, *JAMA*, 159, 1018, 1955.
106. Anderson, J. J. B. and Toverud, S. U., Diet and vitamin D: a review with an emphasis on human function, *J. Nutr. Biochem.*, 5, 58, 1994.
107. Weisberg, P. et al., Nutritional rickets among children in the United States: review of cases reported between 1986 and 2003, *Am. J. Clin. Nutr.*, 80 (suppl.), 1697s, 2004.
108. Gordon, C. M. et al., Prevalence of vitamin D deficiency among healthy adolescents, *Arch. Pediatr. Adolesc. Med.*, 158, 531, 2004.
109. Raiten, D. J. and Picciano, M. F., Vitamin D and health in the 21st century: bone and beyond, executive summary, *Am. J. Clin. Nutr.*, 80 (suppl.), 1673s, 2004.
110. Moore, C. et al., Vitamin D intake in the United States, *J. Am. Diet. Assoc.*, 104, 980, 2004.
111. Moore, C. E., Murphy, M. M., and Holick, M. F., Vitamin D intakes by children and adults in the United States differ among ethnic groups, *J. Nutr.*, 135, 2478, 2005.
112. U.S. Department of Health and Human Services, Public Health Service, Food and Drug Administration, *Grade "A" Pasteurized Milk Ordinance, 2003 Revision*, PHS/FDA Pub. No. 229, USDHHS, PHS, FDA, Washington, D.C., 2005, http://www.cfsan.fda.gov/~ear/pmo03toc.html.
113. Johnson, J. L. et al., Bioavailability of vitamin D from fortified process cheese and effects on vitamin D status in the elderly, *J. Dairy Sci.*, 88, 2295, 2005.
114. Institute of Medicine, *Dietary Reference Intakes for Vitamin C, Vitamin E, Selenium, and Carotenoids*, National Academy Press, Washington, D.C., 2000.
115. Institute of Medicine, *Dietary Reference Intakes for Thiamin, Riboflavin, Niacin, Vitamin B_6, Folate, Vitamin B_{12}, Pantothenic Acid, Biotin, and Choline*, National Academy Press, Washington, D.C., 1998.
116. Parodi, P. W., Cows' milk folate binding protein: its role in folate nutrition, *Aust. J. Dairy Technol.*, 52, 109, 1997.
117. Picciano, M. F. et al., Effect of cow milk on food folate bioavailability in young women, *Am. J. Clin. Nutr.*, 80, 1565, 2004.
118. Moshfegh, A., Goldman, J., and Cleveland, L., What We Eat in America, NHANES 2001–2002: Usual Nutrient Intakes from Food Compared to Dietary Reference Intakes, U.S. Department of Agriculture, Agricultural Research Service, 2005, http://www.ars.usda.gov/foodsurvey.
119. Curhan, G. C. et al., A prospective study of dietary calcium and other nutrients and the risk of symptomatic kidney stones, *N. Engl. J. Med.*, 328, 833, 1993.
120. Curhan, G. C. et al., Comparison of dietary calcium with supplemental calcium and other nutrients as factors affecting the risk for kidney stones in women, *Ann. Intern. Med.*, 126, 497, 1997.
121. Massey, L. K. and Kynast-Gales, S. A., Substituting milk for apple juice does not increase kidney stone risk in most normocalciuric adults who form calcium oxalate stones, *J. Am. Diet. Assoc.*, 98, 303, 1998.
122. Curhan, G. C. et al., Beverage use and risk for kidney stones in women, *Ann. Intern. Med.*, 128, 534, 1998.
123. Curhan, G. C. et al., Dietary factors and risk of incident kidney stones in younger women. Nurses' Health Study II, *Arch. Intern. Med.*, 164, 885, 2004.

124. McCarron, D. A. and Heaney, R. P., Estimated health care savings associated with adequate dairy food intake, *Am. J. Hypertens.*, 17, 88, 2004.
125. Fulgoni, V. L. III et al., Determination of the optimal number of dairy servings to ensure a low prevalence of inadequate calcium intake in Americans, *J. Am. Coll. Nutr.*, 23, 651, 2004.
126. U.S. Department of Agriculture, *MyPyramid. Steps to a Healthier You*, U.S. Department of Agriculture, Washington, D.C., 2005, www.mypyramid.gov.
127. U.S. Department of Agriculture, *MyPyramid for Kids*, www.mypyramid.gov.kids/index.html.
128. Institute of Medicine of the National Academies, *Dietary Reference Intakes for Water, Potassium, Sodium, Chloride, and Sulfate*, The National Academies Press, Washington, D.C., 2004.
129. Cotton, P. A. et al., Dietary sources of nutrients among U.S. adults, 1994 to 1996, *J. Am. Diet. Assoc.*, 104, 921, 2004.
130. 2005 Dietary Guidelines Advisory Committee, *Report of the Dietary Guidelines Advisory Committee on the Dietary Guidelines for Americans, 2005*, August 2004, www.health.gov/dietaryguidelines/dga2005/report.
131. American Academy of Pediatrics, Committee on Nutrition, The use of whole cow's milk in infancy, *Pediatrics*, 89, 1105, 1992.
132. Zelman, K. and Kennedy, E., Naturally nutrient rich...putting more power on Americans' plates, *Nutr. Today*, 40, 60, 2005.
133. Cook, A. J. and Friday, J. E., Food mixture or ingredient sources for dietary calcium: shifts in food group contributions using four grouping protocols, *J. Am. Diet. Assoc.*, 103, 1513, 2003.
134. National Institutes of Health, *Optimal Calcium Intake*, NIH Consensus Statement 12, 4, NIH, Bethesda, MD, 1994.
135. American Medical Association, Council on Scientific Affairs, intake of dietary calcium to reduce the incidence of osteoporosis, *Arch. Fam. Med.*, 6, 495, 1997.
136. Heaney, R. P., Calcium, dairy products, and osteoporosis, *J. Am. Coll. Nutr.*, 19 (suppl.), 83s, 2000.
137. U.S. Department of Health and Human Services, *Healthy People 2010* (Conference Edition, in Two Volumes), Washington, D.C., January 2000, www.health.gov/healthypeople.
138. Miller, G. D., Jarvis, J. K., and McBean, L. D., The importance of meeting calcium needs with foods, *J. Am. Coll. Nutr.*, 20 (suppl.), 168s, 2001.
139. Fleming, K. H. and Heimbach, J. T., Consumption of calcium in the U.S.: food sources and intake levels, *J. Nutr.*, 124 (suppl.), 1426s, 1994.
140. Barr, S. I., Associations of social and demographic variables with calcium intakes of high school students, *J. Am. Diet. Assoc.*, 94, 260, 1994.
141. Albertson, A. M., Tobelmann, R. C., and Marquart, L., Estimated dietary calcium intake and food sources for adolescent females: 1980–1992, *J. Adol. Health*, 20, 20, 1997.
142. Novotny, R. et al., Calcium intake of Asian, Hispanic and white youth, *J. Am. Coll. Nutr.*, 22, 64, 2003.
143. Guthrie, J. E., Dietary patterns and personal characteristics of women consuming recommended amounts of calcium, *Family Econ. Nutr. Rev.*, 9, 33, 1996.
144. Johnson, R. K., Panely, C., and Wang, M. Q., The association between noon beverage consumption and the diet quality of school-age children, *J. Child. Nutr. Management*, 22, 95, 1998.
145. Barger-Lux, M. J. et al., Nutritional correlates of low calcium intake, *Clin. Appl. Nutr.*, 2 (4), 39, 1992.
146. Karanja, N. et al., Impact of increasing calcium in the diet on nutrient consumption, plasma lipids, and lipoproteins in humans, *Am. J. Clin. Nutr.*, 59, 900, 1994.
147. Chan, G. M., Hoffman, K., and McMurray, M., Effects of dairy products on bone and body composition in pubertal girls, *J. Pediatr.*, 126, 551, 1995.
148. Devine, A., Prince, R. L., and Bell, R., Nutritional effect of calcium supplementation by skim milk powder or calcium tablets on total nutrient intake in postmenopausal women, *Am. J. Clin. Nutr.*, 64, 731, 1996.
149. Cadogan, J. et al., Milk intake and bone mineral acquisition in adolescent girls: randomized, controlled intervention trial, *Br. Med. J.*, 315, 1255, 1997.
150. Rajeshwari, R. et al., The nutritional impact of dairy product consumption on dietary intake of young adults (1995–1996): The Bogalusa Heart Study, *J. Am. Diet. Assoc.*, 105, 1391, 2005.

151. Bowman, S. A., Beverage choices of young females: changes and impact on nutrient intakes, *J. Am. Diet. Assoc.*, 102, 1234, 2002.
152. Frary, C. D., Johnson, R. K., and Wang, M. Q., Children and adolescents' choices of foods and beverages high in added sugars are associated with intakes of key nutrients and food groups, *J. Adol. Health*, 34, 56, 2004.
153. Johnson, R. K., Frary, C., and Wang, M. Q., The nutritional consequences of flavored milk consumption by school-aged children and adolescents in the United States, *J. Am. Diet. Assoc.*, 102, 853, 2002.
154. Heaney, R. P., Rafferty, K., and Dowell, M. S., Effect of yogurt on a urinary marker of bone resorption in postmenopausal women, *J. Am. Diet. Assoc.*, 102, 1672, 2002.
155. Barr, S. I. et al., Effects of increased consumption of fluid milk on energy and nutrient intake, body weight, cardiovascular risk factors in healthy older adults, *J. Am. Diet. Assoc.*, 100, 810, 2000.
156. Ballew, C., Kuester, S., and Gillespie, C., Beverage choices affect adequacy of children's nutrient intakes, *Arch. Pediatr. Adolesc. Med.*, 154, 1148, 2000.
157. U.S. Department of Health and Human Services, *Bone Health and Osteoporosis: A Report of the U.S. Surgeon General,* U.S. Department of Health and Human Services, Office of the Surgeon General, Rockville, MD, 2004, www.surgeongeneral.gov/library.
158. Health Canada, *Using the Food Guide*, www.hc-sc.gc.ca/hpfb-dgpsa/onppbppn/using_food_-guide_e.html.
159. American Academy of Pediatrics, *Calcium and You: Facts for Teens, Brochure*, 2001.
160. Greer, F. R. and Krebs, N. F., Optand the Committee on Nutrition, American Academy of Pediatrics Optimizing bone health and calcium intakes of infants, children, and adolescents, *Pediatrics*, 117, 578, 2006.
161. American Heart Association, *Eating Plan: Milk Products*, www.americanheart.org/presenter.jhtml?identifier = 1080.
162. NIH Consensus Development Program, Consensus Statements, *Osteoporosis Prevention, Diagnosis, and Therapy*, Vol. 17, No. 1, March 27–29, 2000, http://consensus.nih.gov.
163. North American Menopause Society, The role of calcium in peri- and postmenopausal women: consensus opinion of the North American Menopause Society, *Menopause*, 8, 84, 2001.
164. Cook, A. J. and Friday, J. E., Pyramid Servings Intakes in the United States 1999–2002, 1 Day, Agricultural Research Service, Community Nutrition Research Group, CNRG Table Set 3.0, 2004, www.ba.ars.usda.gov/cnrg.
165. Shimizu, K. et al., Dietary patterns and further survival in Japanese centenarians, *J. Nutr. Sci. Vitaminol.*, 49, 133, 2003.
166. U.S. Department of Agriculture, Food and Consumer Service, National School Lunch Program, School Breakfast Program, Summer Food Service Program for Children, and Child and Adult Care Food Program, Meat Alternates Used in the Child Nutrition Programs, final rule, *Fed. Regist.*, 62 (44), 10187, 1997.
167. Devaney, B., Gordon, A. R., and Burghardt, J. A., Dietary intakes of students, *Am. J. Clin. Nutr.*, 61 (suppl.), 205, 1995.
168. Fox, M. K., Hamilton, W., and Lin, B.-H., *Effects of Food Assistance and Nutrition Programs on Nutrition and Health,* Vol. 4, *Executive Summary of the Literature Review*. Food Assistance and Nutrition Research Report No. 19-4, USDA, Economic Research Service, Washington, D.C., November 2004.
169. U.S. Department of Agriculture, *School Nutrition Dietary Assessment Study II*, January 2001, www.fns.usda.gov/oane.
170. Bhattacharya, J., Currie, J., and Haider, S. J., *Evaluating the Impact of School Nutrition Programs, Final Report*, July 2004, www.ers.usda.gov/publications/efan04008.
171. Gleason, P. and Suitor, C., *Children's Diets in the Mid-1990s: Dietary Intake and its Relationship with School Meal Participation*, Nutrition Assistance Programs Report Series, Report No. CN-01-CD1, January 2001, www.fns.usda.gov/oane.
172. Shanklin, C. W. and Wie, S., Nutrient contribution per 100 kcal and per penny for the 5 meal components in school lunch: entrée, milk, vegetable/fruit, bread/grain, and miscellaneous, *J. Am. Diet. Assoc.*, 101, 1358, 2001.

173. Nicklas, T. A., Calcium intake trends and health consequences from childhood through adulthood, *J. Am. Coll. Nutr.*, 22, 340, 2003.
174. National Dairy Council, *New Look of School Milk Fact Sheet*, www.nationaldairycouncil.org (Nutrition & Product Information/Child Nutrition).
175. Promar International, *School Milk Pilot Test: Estimating the Effects of National Implementation*, A Report prepared for National Dairy Council and the American School Food Service Association, November 22, 2002, www.nationaldairycouncil.org (Nutrition & Product Information/Child Nutrition).
176. Child Nutrition and WIC Reauthorization Act of 2004 (P.L. 108–265, signed June 30, 2004), Sec. 102.
177. U.S. Department of Agriculture, Food and Nutrition Service, Child Nutrition Home Page, www.fns.usda.gov/cnd.
178. WIC Food Package, www.fns.usda.gov/wic/benefitsandservices/foodpkg.htm.
179. Committee to Review the WIC Food Packages, *WIC Food Packages: Time for a Change*, The National Academies Press, Washington, D.C., 2005, www.nap.edu/catalog/11280.html.
180. Heaney, R. P. et al., Bioavailability of the calcium in fortified soy imitation milk, with some observations on method, *Am. J. Clin. Nutr.*, 71, 1166, 2000.
181. Heaney, R. P. et al., Not all calcium-fortified beverages are equal, *Nutr. Today*, 40, 39, 2005.
182. U.S. Food and Drug Administration, Center for Food Safety and Applied Nutrition, *Dairy Grade A Voluntary HACCP*, www.cfsan.fda.gov/~comm/haccpdai.html.
183. U.S. Food and Drug Administration, Center for Food Safety and Applied Nutrition, *National Milk Drug Residue Data Base Fiscal Year 2003*, Annual Report, February 2004, www.cfsan.fda.gov/~ear/milkrp03.html.
184. Food and Drug Administration, FDA Pesticide Program Residue Monitoring, 1993–2002, Food and Drug Administration, Center for Food Safety and Applied Nutrition, Washington, D.C., March 2004, www.cfsan.fda.gov.
185. Ropp, K. L., New animal drug increases milk production, *FDA Consumer*, 28 (4), 24, 1994.
186. Juskevich, J. C. and Guyer, C. G., Bovine growth hormone: human food safety evaluation, *Science*, 249, 875, 1990.
187. Technology Assessment Panel, NIH Technology Assessment Conference statement on bovine somatotropin, *JAMA*, 265, 1423, 1991.
188. U.S. Food and Drug Administration, Food Safety A to Z Reference Guide, List of Terms: P, www.cfsan.fda.gov/~dms/a22-p.html.
189. Dairy Management Inc., Extending shelf life in dairy foods, in *Innovations in Dairy*, April 1998.
190. U.S. Department of Agriculture, Dairy: data tables, www.ers.usda.gov/briefing/dairy/data.htm.
191. Putnam, J., Major trends in U.S. food supply, 1909–1999, *Food Rev.*, 23, 8, 2000.
192. Putnam, J., Allshouse, J., and Kantor, L. S., U.S. per capita food supply trends: more calories, refined carbohydrates, and fats, *Food Rev.*, 25 (3), 2, 2002.
193. Putnam, J. and Allshouse, J., Trends in U.S. per capita consumption of dairy products, 1909 to 2001, *Amber Waves*, 1 (3), 12, 2003.
194. Yen, S. T. and Lin, B.-H., Beverage consumption among U.S. children and adolescents: full-information and quasi maximum likelihood estimation of a censored system, *Eur. Rev. Agric. Econ.*, 29, 85, 2002.
195. Food and Drug Administration, Food labeling: nutrient content claims, definition of terms, healthy, final rule, *Fed. Regist.*, 59, 24232, 1994, (May 10).
196. National Dairy Council, *Quick Reference Guide for Nutrition Claims on Dairy Products*, Dairy Management Inc., Rosemont, IL, 2005.
197. US Food and Drug Administration, Center for Food Safety and Applied Nutrition, Health Claim Notification for Potassium Containing Foods, October 31, 2000, http://vm.cfsan.fda.gov/~dms/hclm-k.html.
198. Food and Drug Administration, Low-fat and skim milk products, low-fat and nonfat yogurt products, low-fat cottage cheese: revocation of standards of identity; food labeling, nutrient content claims for fat, fatty acids, and cholesterol content of food, final rule, *Fed. Regist.*, 61, 58991, 198. (November 20), 1996.

199. Conners, P., Bednar, C., and Klammer, S., Cafeteria factors that influence milk-drinking behaviors of elementary school children: grounded theory approach, *J. Nutr. Educ.*, 33, 31, 2001.
200. American Academy of Pediatrics, Policy statement: soft drinks in schools, *Pediatrics*, 113, 152, 2004.
201. The American Academy of Pediatric Dentistry, Diet and Dental Health, American Academy of Pediatric Fast Facts, 2002–2003.
202. Levine, R. S., Milk, flavored milk and caries, *Br. Dent. J.*, 191, 20, 2001.
203. The American Dietetic Association, Position of The American Dietetic Association on use of nutritive and nonnutritive sweeteners, *J. Am. Diet. Assoc.*, 104, 255, 2004.
204. White, J. W. and Wolraich, M., Effect of sugar on behavior and mental performance, *Am. J. Clin. Nutr.*, 62 (suppl.), 242, 1995.
205. Recker, R. R. et al., Calcium absorbability from milk products, an imitation milk, and calcium carbonate, *Am. J. Clin. Nutr.*, 47 (1), 93, 1988.
206. Karp, J. R. et al., Chocolate milk as a post-exercise recovery aid, *Int. J. Sports Nutr. Exerc. Metab.*, 16, 78, 2006.
207. Huang, Y.-C., Luedecke, L. O., and Shultz, T. D., Effect of Cheddar cheese consumption on plasma conjugated linoleic acid concentrations in men, *Nutr. Res.*, 14 (3), 373, 1994.
208. Berry, D., Cultured dairy foods. A world of opportunity, *Dairy Foods*, 105, 28, 2004.
209. Adolfsson, O., Meydani, S. N., and Russell, R. M., Yogurt and gut function, *Am. J. Clin. Nutr.*, 80, 245, 2004.
210. Sanders, M. E., Probiotics: considerations for human health, *Nutr. Rev.*, 61, 91, 2003.
211. American Dietetic Association, Position of the American Dietetic Association: functional foods, *J. Am. Diet. Assoc.*, 104, 814, 2004.
212. Mattila-Sandholm, T. and Saarela, M., Eds., *Functional Dairy Products*, CRC Press, Boca Raton, FL, 2003.
213. Kopp-Hoolihan, L., Prophylactic and therapeutic uses of probiotics: a review, *J. Am. Diet. Assoc.*, 101, 229, 2001.
214. Goossens, D. et al., Probiotics in gastroenterology: indications and future perspectives, *Scand. J. Gastroenterol.*, 38 (suppl. 239), 15, 2003.
215. Reid, G. et al., New scientific paradigms for probiotics and prebiotics, *J. Clin. Gastroenterol.*, 37, 105, 2003.
216. Broussard, E. K. and Surawicz, C. M., Probiotics and prebiotics in clinical practice, *Nutr. Clin. Care*, 7, 104, 2004.
217. Brown, A. C. and Valiere, A., Probiotics and medical nutrition therapy, *Nutr. Clin. Care*, 7, 56, 2004.
218. DiRienzo, D. B., Symposium: probiotic bacteria: implications for human health, *J. Nutr.*, 130, 382s, 2000.
219. Schrezenmeir, J., de Vrese, M., and Heller, K., Probiotics and prebiotics, *Am. J. Clin. Nutr.*, 73 (suppl. 2), 361, 2001.
220. Walker, W. A., Probiotics in health and disease, *Am. J. Clin. Nutr.*, 73 (suppl.), 1118s, 2001.
221. Tannock, G. W., Ed., *Probiotics. A Critical Review*, Horizon Press, Norfolk, England, 1999.
222. DeVrese, M. et al., Probiotics — compensation for lactase insufficiency, *Am. J. Clin. Nutr.*, 73 (suppl.), 421s, 2001.
223. Heyman, M., Effect of lactic acid bacteria on diarrheal diseases, *J. Am. Coll. Nutr.*, 19 (suppl.), 137s, 2000.
224. Van Niel, C. W. et al., *Lactobacillus* therapy for acute infectious diarrhea in children: a meta-analysis, *Pediatrics*, 109, 678, 2002.
225. D'Souza, A. L. et al., Probiotics in prevention of antibiotic associated diarrhea: meta-analysis, *Br. Med. J.*, 324, 1, 2002.
226. Cremonini, F. et al., Meta-analysis: the effect of probiotic administration on antibiotic-associated diarrhea, *Aliment. Pharmacol. Ther.*, 16, 1461, 2002.
227. Hatakka, K. et al., Effect of long term consumption of probiotic milk on infections in children attending day care centres; double blind, randomized trial, *Br. Med. J.*, 322, 1327, 2001.
228. Wang, K.-Y. et al., Effects of ingesting Lactobacillus- and Bifidobacterium-containing yogurt in subjects with colonized *Helicobacter pylori*, *Am. J. Clin. Nutr.*, 80, 737, 2004.
229. Saikali, J. et al., Fermented milks, probiotic cultures, and colon cancer, *Nutr. Cancer*, 49, 14, 2004.

230. Gill, H. S. et al., Enhancement of immunity in the elderly by dietary supplementation with probiotic *Bifidobacterium lactis* HN019, *Am. J. Clin. Nutr.*, 74, 833, 2001.
231. Villena, J. et al., *Lactobacillus casei* improves resistance to pneumococcal respiratory infection in malnourished mice, *J. Nutr.*, 135, 1462, 2005.
232. Ishikawa, H. et al., Randomized controlled trial of the effect of Bifidobacteria-fermented milk on ulcerative colitis, *J. Am. Coll. Nutr.*, 22, 56, 2003.
233. Kalliomaki, M. et al., Probiotics in primary prevention of atopic disease: a randomized placebo-controlled trial, *Lancet*, 357, 1076, 2001.
234. Pereira, D. I. and Gibson, G. R., Effects of consumption of probiotics and prebiotics on serum lipid levels in humans, *Crit. Rev. Biochem. Mol. Biol.*, 37, 259, 2002.
235. Kontiokari, T. et al., Dietary factors protecting women from urinary tract infection, *Am. J. Clin. Nutr.*, 77, 600, 2003.
236. Walzem, R. L., Dillard, C. J., and German, J. B., Whey components: millennia of evolution create functionalities for mammalian nutrition: what we know and what we may be overlooking, *Crit. Rev. Food Sci. Nutr.*, 42, 353, 2002.
237. Harper, W. J., *Biological Properties of Whey Components, A Review, Update 2004*, prepared for and published by: The American Dairy Products Institute, Elmhurst, IL, 2004.
238. Floris, R. et al., Antibacterial and antiviral effects of milk proteins and derivatives thereof, *Curr. Pharmaceut. Design*, 9, 1257, 2003.
239. Berkhout, B. et al., The antiviral activity of the milk protein lactoferrin against the human immunodeficiency virus type 1, *Biometals*, 17, 291, 2004.
240. Wolber, F. M. et al., Supplemental dietary whey protein concentrate reduces rotavirus-induced disease symptoms in suckling mice, *J. Nutr.*, 135, 1470, 2005.
241. Low, P. P. et al., Effect of dietary whey protein concentrate on primary and secondary antibody responses in immunized BALB/C mice, *Immunopharmacology*, 3, 393, 2003.
242. Gill, H. S. and Cross, M. L., Anticancer properties of bovine milk, *Br. J. Nutr.*, 84 (suppl. 1), 161s, 2000.
243. Belobrajdic, D. P., McIntosh, G. H., and Owens, J. A., Whey proteins protect more than red meat against azoxymethane induced ACF in Wistar rats, *Cancer Lett.*, 198, 43, 2003.
244. Rutherfurd, K. J. and Gill, H. S., Peptides affecting coagulation, *Br. J. Nutr.*, 84 (suppl. 1), 99s, 2000.
245. Kawase, M. et al., Effect of administration of fermented milk containing whey protein concentrate to rats and healthy men on serum lipids and blood pressure, *J. Dairy Sci.*, 83, 255, 2000.
246. Ha, E. and Zemel, M. B., Functional properties of whey, whey components, and essential amino acids: mechanisms underlying health benefits for active people (review), *J. Nutr. Biochem.*, 14 (suppl.), 251, 2003.
247. Layman, D., The role of leucine in weight loss diets and glucose homeostasis, *J. Nutr.*, 133 (suppl.), 261s, 2003.
248. Zemel, M. B., The role of dairy foods in weight management, *J. Am. Coll. Nutr.*, 24, 537s, 2005.
249. Anderson, G. H. et al., Protein source, quantity, and time of consumption determine the effect of proteins on short-term food intake in young men, *J. Nutr.*, 134, 3011, 2004.
250. Belobrajdic, D. P., McIntosh, G. H., and Owens, J. A., A high-whey-protein diet reduces body weight gain and alters insulin sensitivity relative to red meat in Wistar rats, *J. Nutr.*, 134, 1454, 2004.
251. Hall, W. L. et al., Casein and whey exert different effects on plasma amino acid profiles, gastrointestinal hormone secretion and appetite, *Br. J. Nutr.*, 89, 239, 2003.
252. Toba, Y. et al., Milk basic protein promotes bone formation and suppresses bone resorption in healthy adult men, *Biosci. Biotechnol. Biochem.*, 65, 1353, 2001.
253. Cornish, J. et al., Lactoferrin is a potent regulator of bone cell activity and increases bone formation in vivo, *Endocrinology*, 145, 4366, 2004.
254. Markus, C. R., Olivier, B., and deHaan, E. H. F., Whey protein rich in alpha-lactalbumin increases the ratio of plasma tryptophan to the sum of the other large neutral amino acids and improves cognitive performance in stress vulnerable subjects, *Am. J. Clin. Nutr.*, 75, 1051, 2002.
255. Markus, C. R. et al., Evening intake of α-lactalbumin increases plasma tryptophan availability and improves morning alertness and brain measures of attention, *Am. J. Clin. Nutr.*, 81, 1026, 2005.
256. Goldberg, J. P., Folta, S. C., and Must, A., Milk: can a "good" food be so bad? *Pediatrics*, 110, 826, 2002.

2 Dairy Foods and Cardiovascular Health

2.1 INTRODUCTION

Coronary heart disease (CHD), the most common and serious form of cardiovascular disease, is the leading cause of death in developed industrialized countries. Despite the dramatic decline in age-adjusted CHD mortality in the United States since the 1950s, CHD still accounts for more deaths than any other disease or groups of diseases [1,2]. In 2003, 13.2 million people in the United States. had CHD, and more than 653,000 people died from this disease (i.e., 1 out of every 5 deaths in the United States) [2]. The estimated direct and indirect cost of CHD in 2006 is $142.5 billion [2]. Considering the high incidence of CHD mortality and morbidity, as well as its economic toll, prevention or early management of risk factors for CHD is a major public health goal for both developed and developing countries [3–6].

Many risk factors, both genetic and environmental, contribute to the development of CHD [1,2,5]. Major modifiable risk factors for CHD include cigarette smoking, high blood pressure, and elevated blood cholesterol levels, particularly high low-density lipoprotein (LDL) cholesterol [4,5]. Other risk factors for CHD include diabetes mellitus, physical inactivity, low blood levels of high-density lipoprotein (HDL) cholesterol, elevated blood triglyceride levels, and overweight/obesity [2,4,5]. Some persons have a constellation of risk factors, known as metabolic syndrome, that increases the risk of cardiovascular disease (4). Metabolic syndrome is identified by the presence of three or more of the following: abdominal obesity, elevated triglyceride levels, low HDL cholesterol levels, elevated blood pressure, and high fasting glucose levels [4,5,7]. To reduce the risk of heart disease, the National Cholesterol Education Program (NCEP) Adult Treatment Panel III focuses on LDL cholesterol as the primary target and metabolic syndrome as a secondary target [4]. Psychosocial factors, lipoprotein (a), homocysteine, oxidative stress, and prothrombotic and proinflammatory factors may also influence CHD risk [4,5]. Advancing age (45 years and older for men; 55 years and older for women), race (e.g., African American), and a family history of premature CHD are risk factors which cannot be modified [1,5].

The multifactorial nature of CHD is recognized by numerous federal government agencies, health professional organizations, and health experts [1–6,8–14]. However, a high blood total cholesterol level — particularly LDL cholesterol — is regarded as one of the major modifiable risk factors. The NCEP's Adult Treatment Panel III [4] classifies desirable total blood cholesterol levels as levels below 200 mg/dl, borderline-high as values between 200 and 239 mg/dl, and high as total cholesterol levels 240 mg/dl and above. Optimal levels of LDL cholesterol are <100 mg/dl; desirable levels of HDL cholesterol are 60 mg/dl or higher; and optimal levels of triglycerides are less than 150 mg/dl (Table 2.1) [4].

The positive association between elevated blood cholesterol and CHD risk is supported by extensive epidemiological, laboratory, and clinical findings [4,5,11]. Blood lipid-protein agglomerates, collectively called lipoproteins, are associated with CHD risk [7,9,11]. The four classes of lipoproteins, based on density as well as lipid and apolipoprotein (apo) composition, include

TABLE 2.1
NCEP Classification of Blood Lipid Levels

Blood Lipid Ranges (mg per deciliter)	
Total Cholesterol	
<200	Desirable
200 to 239	Borderline high
⩾240	High
LDL Cholesterol	
<100	Optimal
100 to 129	Near or above optimal
130 to 159	Borderline high
160 to 189	High
⩾190	Very high
HDL Cholesterol	
<40	Undesirable
⩾60	Desirable
Triglycerides	
<150	Normal
150 to 199	Borderline high
200 to 499	High
⩾500	Very high

Source: Adapted from NCEP/Adult Treatment Panel III Report, *JAMA*, 285, 2486, 2001.

chylomicrons, very-low density lipoproteins (VLDL), LDL, and HDL. In addition, there are various subclasses of lipoproteins, such as intermediate-density lipoproteins (IDL), small dense LDL (LDL subclass pattern B), and HDL2 and HDL3.

An elevated level of blood LDL cholesterol, the major cholesterol-carrying lipoprotein, is associated with increased risk of CHD [5]. In contrast, a low level of HDL cholesterol constitutes a CHD risk factor. Lipoprotein subclasses are also predictive of CHD [15]. High blood concentrations of small, dense LDL and lipoprotein (a) are associated with increased risk of CHD [16]. In addition, small HDL particles and large, VLDL particles may play a role in the development of CHD [15]. Routine lipid testing may, therefore, fail to accurately predict CHD risk. Elevated blood triglyceride level is an independent risk factor for CHD [4]. Factors that contribute to higher-than-normal triglyceride levels include obesity and overweight, physical inactivity, cigarette smoking, high carbohydrate diets (>60% of energy intake), some diseases, certain drugs, and genetic disorders [4].

Numerous studies indicate that lowering total and LDL cholesterol levels can reduce the risk of CHD [5,11,16]. Evidence indicates a role for both diet and genetics in influencing blood cholesterol and lipoprotein levels [4,5,8,10,16–20]. Of all the dietary factors studied, fat intake has received the most attention. Extensive research has established that different types and amounts of dietary fats influence blood cholesterol levels. High intakes of total and saturated fat, and, to a lesser extent, cholesterol, can increase blood total and LDL cholesterol levels [4,5,8,11,21–23]. However, whether everyone can benefit from reduced intake of total and saturated fat is questioned by some [19,24–27]. As discussed below, dietary fat intake also affects HDL cholesterol and LDL and HDL subclasses with varying atherogenic potential. The effects of decreasing total and saturated fat on these markers of CHD risk, as well as the differential effects of dietary fat/saturated fat in subgroups of the population and in individuals with a specific genetic make-up, justify some caution in the widespread application of low-fat/low-saturated fat diets to reduce the risk of CHD.

There is increasing support for tailoring dietary fat/saturated fat recommendations to individuals to reduce CHD risk [5,19,20,28].

Some public health recommendations for U.S. adults advise a reduction in total fat intake to 30% or less of calories to reduce the incidence of CHD. The NCEP's Step 1 diet for the general healthy population recommends restriction of total fat to 30% or less of calories [4]. Likewise, the American Heart Association (AHA) advises a reduction in fat intake to 30% or less of total calories [5]. However, it has been recognized that very-low-fat diets (<20% of calories) may lead to nutrient shortcomings and potentially be harmful to cardiovascular health (e.g., by decreasing HDL cholesterol and increasing blood triglyceride levels) [5,13,29]. More-recent dietary fat recommendations, such as those issued by the Institute of Medicine (IOM) [11] and the federal government's 2005 *Dietary Guidelines for Americans* [13] advise a range of total fat intake of 20% to 35% of calories for all Americans age 18 years and over. Total fat intake can comprise up to 35% of calories, while saturated fat intake should be less than 10% of calories, and intake of *trans* fatty acids as low as possible [11,13].

Dietary recommendations consistently advise healthy American adults to reduce their saturated fat intake to 10% or less of calories [4,5,11,13]. For adults with elevated LDL cholesterol levels or with cardiovascular disease, a lower intake of saturated fat (for example, <7% of calories) is recommended. The IOM's report [11] recommends that intake of saturated fat be as low as possible while consuming a nutritionally-adequate diet. However, the lower safe level of saturated fat or specific saturated fats remains to be established [24]. Population-based guidelines also recommend that healthy Americans 2 years of age and older consume a diet containing 300 mg or less of cholesterol a day [5,13]. Lower intakes of cholesterol (<200 mg/day) are recommended as part of a therapeutic diet for adults with elevated LDL blood cholesterol [4].

To help ensure that children readily meet their nutrient needs for growth and development, flexible guidelines are recommended [5,13,14,30,31]. The American Academy of Pediatrics (AAP) [30] advises that between the ages of 2 and 5 years, children should gradually adopt a diet that meets 30% of calories from fat. The AAP does not recommend diets containing less than 30% of calories from fat for children, because of the difficulty in meeting sufficient calories and other nutrients for optimal growth and development [30]. A Working Group convened by Health Canada and the Canadian Paediatric Society recommends a gradual decrease in fat intake from the high-fat diet of infancy to a diet that provides no more than 30% of energy from fat by the time linear growth (i.e., adolescence) is reached [31]. The 2005 *Dietary Guidelines for Americans* [13] recommends a total fat intake between 30% and 35% of calories for children aged 2 to 3 years and a fat intake of 25% to 35% of calories for children and adolescents aged 4 to 18 years. Similar recommendations for total fat intake for children are recommended by the AHA and endorsed by the AAPs [14].

With respect to intake of total fat, saturated fat, and cholesterol, data from the Third National Health and Nutrition Examination Survey (NHANES III) and from NHANES 1999 to 2000 indicate that for all ages of the U.S. population, 32.7% of calories came from total fat and 11.2% from saturated fat [32]. For adults age 20 to 74, age-adjusted mean dietary cholesterol intake was 341 mg for men and 242 mg for women (above the recommended level of 300 mg per day for adult males and below it for adult females) [32]. As reported by the IOM [11], data from the Continuing Survey of Food Intakes by Individuals (CSFII) 1994 to 1996, 1998 indicates that approximately 25% of children and adults have total fat intakes greater than 35% of calories. To help Americans meet dietary fat recommendations, the Department of Health and Human Services, Food and Drug Administration [33] has authorized the use of health claims relating to an association between dietary lipids, specifically fat and cholesterol, and CHD on the labels of certain foods. Such foods may bear the following health claim, "While many factors affect heart disease, diets low in saturated fat and cholesterol may reduce the risk of this disease" [33].

To meet current dietary guidelines for fat and cholesterol, increased consumption of foods low in these nutrients is advised. With respect to dairy products, lower-fat dairy foods are generally recommended [4,5,13,14]. While the fat, saturated fat, and cholesterol content of many dairy foods [34] might be expected to increase blood cholesterol levels, there is no direct evidence that consumption of whole-fat dairy foods in moderation within the context of a total diet increases the risk of CHD [35]. In fact, several components in milk (e.g., calcium, bioactive peptides, conjugated linoleic acid) may have effects that could help reduce the risk of CHD [35–37].

2.2 CONTRIBUTION OF MILK AND MILK PRODUCTS TO FAT, SATURATED FAT, AND CHOLESTEROL INTAKE

According to the most recent U.S. Department of Agriculture (USDA) food disappearance data, in 2000, dairy foods, excluding butter, contributed 12% of total dietary fat, 23% of saturated fat, and 16% of the cholesterol available in the U.S. food supply (Figure 2.1 through Figure 2.3) [38]. To put this data into perspective, the contribution of dairy foods to total fat availability is far less than that provided by fats and oils (56%) or meat, poultry, and fish (23%) (Figure 2.1 through Figure 2.3) [38]. Similarly, meat, poultry and fish contribute more to the saturated fat and cholesterol available in the U.S. food supply than do dairy foods (Figure 2.2 and Figure 2.3) [38]. Butter contributed an estimated 3% of total fat, 5% of saturated fat, and 3% of the cholesterol available in the food supply in 2000 [38]. In terms of actual intake, data from nearly 18,000 respondents in the 1994 to 1996, 1998 CSFII indicate that dairy foods/ingredients contributed an average of 19% of total fat, 32% of saturated fat, and 22% of cholesterol consumed [39].

2.3 DAIRY NUTRIENTS, DAIRY FOODS, AND CORONARY HEART DISEASE

2.3.1 SINGLE NUTRIENTS

Nutrients in dairy foods, particularly dietary fatty acids, total fat and cholesterol, and (to a lesser extent) protein and calcium, have been examined for their roles in influencing blood lipid and lipoprotein levels and CHD risk.

2.3.1.1 Dietary Fatty Acids

The quality (type) and quantity (amount) of dietary fatty acids affect blood total and lipoprotein cholesterol levels and CHD risk [5,8,9,11,16–18]. The quality or type of dietary fat has a greater

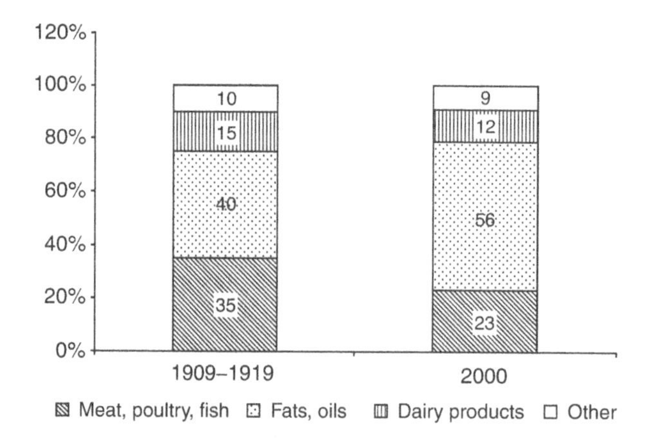

FIGURE 2.1 Sources of fat in the United State food supply. (Adapted from Gerrior, S., Bente, L., and Hiza, H., *Nutrient Content of the U.S. Food Supply, 1909–2000*, Home Economics Research Report No. 56, U.S. Department of Agriculture, Center for Nutrition Policy and Promotion, 2004.)

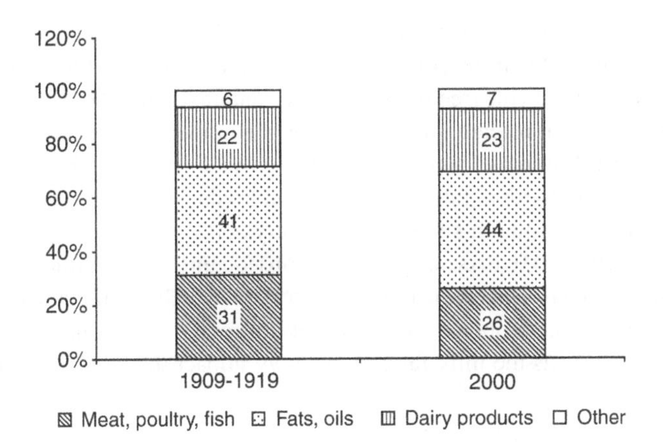

FIGURE 2.2 Sources of saturated fatty acids (SFA) in the U.S. food supply. (Adapted from Gerrior, S., Bente, L., and Hiza, H., *Nutrient Content of the U.S. Food Supply, 1909–2000*, Home Economics Research Report No. 56, U.S. Department of Agriculture, Center for Nutrition Policy and Promotion, 2004.)

influence on CHD risk than the quantity or amount of fat consumed [11,40]. Both the degree of unsaturation and the chain length of a specific type of fatty acid influence blood total cholesterol and specific lipoprotein fractions. Fatty acids also may be classified as saturated fatty acids (SFA) (no double bonds), monounsaturated fatty acids (MUFA) (one double bond), or polyunsaturated fatty acids (PUFA) (2 or more double bonds). Polyunsaturated fatty acids are further subdivided according to the position of the first double bond as omega-6 PUFAs or omega-3 PUFAs [5,8,9,11]. When classified by length, fatty acids are short-chain (<6 carbon atoms), medium-chain (6 to 12 carbon atoms), or long-chain (12 or more carbon atoms).

In whole milk (3.25% fat), approximately 57% of the fat is SFAs, 25% is MUFAs, and 6% is PUFAs [34]. With respect to chain length, short- and medium-chain SFAs generally constitute about 20% of the weight of total SFAs, whereas long-chain SFAs make up approximately 80% of the total weight of SFAs [34]. *Trans* fatty acids are found in very small amounts in milk and dairy foods [34]. In most cases, the amount of *trans* fatty acids in a serving of dairy foods is less than the labeling threshold of 0.5 g per serving set by the U.S. Food and Drug Administration (FDA) [41].

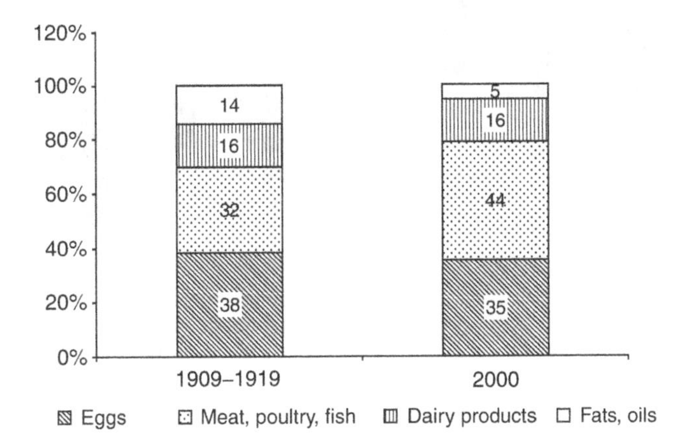

FIGURE 2.3 Sources of cholesterol in the U.S. food supply. (Adapted from Gerrior, S., Bente, L., and Hiza, H., *Nutrient Content of the U.S. Food Supply, 1909–2000*, Home Economics Research Report No. 56, U.S. Department of Agriculture, Center for Nutrition Policy and Promotion, 2004.)

With respect to cholesterol, one 8-ounce serving of whole (3.25% fat) milk contains 24 mg cholesterol, whereas 2% reduced-fat milk contains 20 mg cholesterol, 1% reduced-fat milk contains 12 mg cholesterol, and nonfat (fat-free or skim) milk contains 5 mg cholesterol [34].

A considerable amount of research has focused on the influence of specific fatty acids on blood lipid levels [9,11,16,40]. Findings from this research provide information regarding the direction and differential effects of individual fatty acids on blood lipids. However, it is important to appreciate that dietary studies examining a single class of fatty acids often use liquid formula diets with high levels of either SFAs, MUFAs, or PUFAs. Consequently, it is difficult to extrapolate the findings from these studies to the typical American diet, which contains a mixture of different types of fat in more moderate amounts from a variety of foods. Additionally, the unique physical forms of fats in foods, such as the milk fat globule, may impact the effects of fats on blood lipids.

2.3.1.1.1 Saturated Fatty Acids

Saturated fatty acids (SFA) intake is one of the strongest predictors of blood total, LDL, and HDL cholesterol levels [4,5,8,9,17,18,37,40]. Mathematical equations developed for groups predict that a 1% decrease in SFAs as energy will lower blood LDL cholesterol by 1% to 2% [4,16]. These prediction equations assume constant levels of protein and carbohydrate intakes, and may not be valid if protein or carbohydrate levels are changed (20). In addition to this, individuals vary in their blood lipid response to changes in saturated fat intake [20,24,37]. Individuals with elevated LDL cholesterol levels are reported to be more responsive to dietary SFAs than expected, and overweight or obese individuals are reported to be less responsive [42,43]. Additionally, it has long been known that not all SFAs have the same effect on blood cholesterol levels (Figure 2.4) [5,9,11,21,22,40,44]. Specifically, palmitic (C16:0), myristic (C14:0), and lauric (C12:0) acids raise blood total and LDL

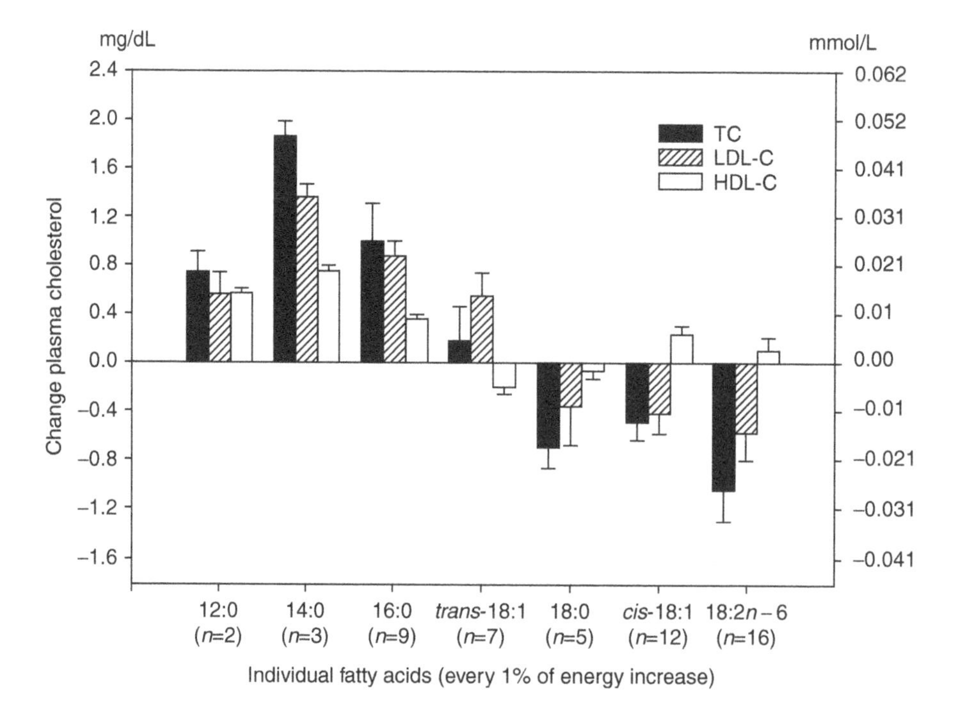

FIGURE 2.4 Effects of lauric (12:0), myristic (14:0), palmitic (16:0), elaidic (*trans*-18:1), stearic (18:0), oleic (*cis*-18:1), and linoleic (18:2*n*−6) acids compared with 18:1, TC, plasma total cholesterol. (From Kris-Etherton, P. M. and Yu, S., *Am. J. Clin. Nutr.*, 65 (suppl.), 1628s, 1997. With permission.)

cholesterol levels, whereas stearic (C18:0) and medium-chain SFAs have little or no effect on blood total and LDL cholesterol levels [37,44–46]. Individual SFAs also differ in their effects on HDL cholesterol levels [44,47]. A study in young men found that HDL cholesterol levels were higher after intake of myristic acid than stearic acid [47]. According to a meta-analysis of 35 studies, stearic acid has no effect on HDL cholesterol, whereas other long-chain SFAs, such as lauric acid, increase HDL cholesterol levels [44].

Although palmitic acid is the major SFA in the diet, findings regarding its hypercholesterolemic effect relative to lauric acid are inconsistent [9,45,46,48]. Palmitic acid has been shown to be hypercholesterolemic compared with lauric, stearic, and oleic fatty acids [9]. Well-controlled studies indicate that myristic acid is the most hypercholesterolemic SFA [9,35], although further studies are necessary to substantiate this conclusion. Given the relatively-low intake of myristic acid, especially in comparison with palmitic acid, in the American diet, its potential contribution to high blood cholesterol is considered to be small [8].

Stearic acid, compared with other long-chain SFAs such as palmitic, myristic, and lauric acids, lowers blood total and LDL cholesterol levels when substituted for these SFAs [9,16,35,44,45,49,50]. In a strictly-controlled metabolic study in Denmark involving healthy young men, a diet high in stearic acid (15% of total energy intake) favorably affected blood lipids compared with a diet high in palmitic acid or myristic and lauric acids (Figure 2.5) [45]. A meta-analysis of 35 studies indicates that, when substituted for carbohydrate, stearic acid has a minimal effect on LDL cholesterol and no effect on HDL cholesterol [44].

Short- and medium-chain SFAs are absorbed directly from the intestine into the portal circulation and are not transported through the bloodstream to the liver by chylomicrons; consequently, these SFAs would be expected to have different effects on blood lipids than long-chain fatty acids [8]. Despite limited data, the effects of medium-chain fatty acids on blood lipids are considered to be minimal [8,9].

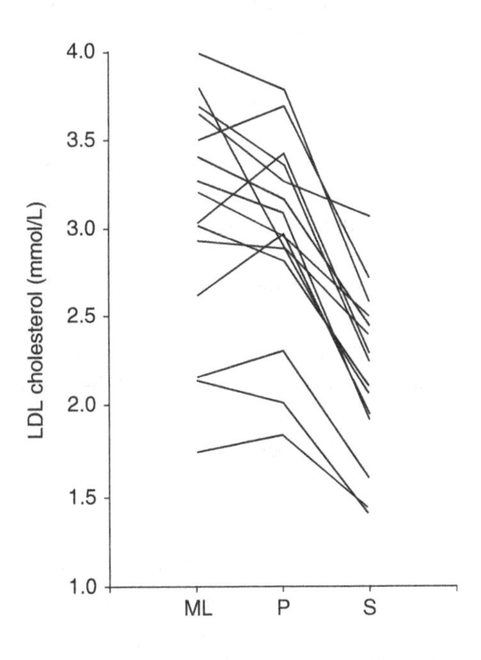

FIGURE 2.5 Plasma concentrations of low-density lipoprotein (LDL) cholesterol in 15 subjects during three diets. ML is a diet high in myristic and lauric acids, P is a diet high in palmitic acid, and S is a diet high in stearic acid. Each point represents the mean of three determinations at the end of the 3-week diet intervention. To convert values for LDL cholesterol to milligrams per deciliter, multiply by 88.54. (From Tholstrup, T. et al., *Am. J. Clin. Nutr.*, 59, 371, 1994. With permission.)

2.3.1.1.2 Monounsaturated Fatty Acids

Monounsaturated fatty acids (MUFAs), particularly oleic acid (C18:1), are found in fats of both plant (olive oil) and animal (25% to 30% of the fatty acids in milk fat) origin. Olive oil, rapeseed oil (canola oil), vegetable shortening, and beef fat are the major sources of MUFAs in the diet [16].

Monounsaturated fatty acids (i.e., *cis*-MUFAs) appear to have a neutral effect on blood cholesterol levels or to be mildly hypocholesterolemic [9,16,18,22,23]. As reviewed by Kris-Etherton and Yu [9], oleic acid reduces total and LDL cholesterol levels when substituted for lauric, myristic, or palmitic SFAs. A meta-analysis of metabolic feeding studies indicates that isocaloric replacement of carbohydrate with MUFAs slightly increases HDL cholesterol levels [18]. Although a high-MUFA/low-SFA diet has been shown to result in a more favorable metabolic profile with respect to total cholesterol, HDL cholesterol, and triglyceride concentrations than a conventional diet or a low-fat/high-carbohydrate diet, some evidence indicates that a high intake of MUFAs may increase the risk of CHD [51]. Atherosclerosis has been shown to be greater in monkeys fed a diet rich in MUFAs than in those fed a diet rich in PUFAs, even though blood LDL and HDL cholesterol levels were similar [52,53]. In addition, some evidence in humans demonstrates that a single high-fat meal rich in MUFAs (or SFAs) adversely affects endothelial function, which may be an early event in the atherogenic process [54].

2.3.1.1.3 Polyunsaturated Fatty Acids

There are two major classes of polyunsaturated fatty acids (PUFAs): *n*-3 fatty acids, found in fish oils and as minor constituents of some vegetable oils; and *n*-6 fatty acids — including the essential fatty acid linoleic acid — found in vegetable oils such as corn, cottonseed, and soybean oils [5,11,16]. A number of studies indicate that substitution of *n*-6 PUFAs for SFAs in the diet lowers blood total and LDL cholesterol levels [9,11,17,18,21]. In a review of the effects of individual fatty acids on plasma lipids in humans, Kris-Etherton and Yu [9] concluded that of all the fatty acids, PUFAs have the most potent hypo-cholesterolemic effect. Every 1% increase in PUFAs is predicted to lower total blood cholesterol levels by 0.9 mg/dl and LDL cholesterol levels by 0.5 mg/dl [17]. However, diets very high in linoleic acid reduce HDL as well as LDL cholesterol levels.

The American diet contains 5% to 8% of energy as PUFAs, an intake below the upper level of 10% of total energy recommended by the federal government and other health professional organizations [11]. No data is available regarding the long-term effects of diets high in PUFAs (i.e., $>10\%$) [11].

Evidence indicates that consumption of omega-3 fatty acids (i.e., eicosapentaenoic acid and docosahexaenoic acid) reduces the risk of mortality from cardiovascular disease by decreasing arrhythmia, lowering blood triglyceride levels, and reducing blood-clotting tendency [5]. Because of the beneficial effects of omega-3 fatty acids on risk of heart disease, and because fish — especially fatty fish such as salmon — is the major food source of omega-3 fatty acids, the AHA [5,14] recommends 2 servings of fish per week.

2.3.1.1.4 Trans Fatty Acids

The majority (80% to 90%) of dietary *trans* fatty acids in the U.S. diet originates from partially-hydrogenated vegetable oils used in cooking and preparation of processed foods [41,55,56]. In contrast to these "man-made" *trans* fatty acids, a small percentage of *trans* fatty acids occurs naturally in dairy and meat products as a result of biohydrogenation of pasture and feed linoleic and linolenic acids by rumen microorganisms in animals [35]. Cow's milk contains an estimated 0.22 g *trans* fatty acids per serving, whereas traditional stick margarine contains ten times this amount [41]. It is important to recognize that structural differences between man-made and naturally-occurring *trans* fatty acids can result in different biological and health outcomes [55].

Most of the available data examining *trans* fatty acids and CHD relates to *trans* fatty acids from partially-hydrogenated vegetable oils [37,55]. In contrast, the predominant *trans* fatty acid in milk fat, *trans* 11-18:1 (vaccenic acid), is converted to conjugated linoleic acid (CLA), specifically *cis*-9, *trans*-11 (rumenic acid), which may have several potential health benefits [35,55].

In the United States about 2% to 3% of total calories comes from *trans* fatty acids [5,56]. The average *trans* fat intake from animal sources is approximately 0.5% of energy. Based on findings that dietary intake of *trans* fat at sufficiently-high levels increases LDL cholesterol levels similarly to those achieved with SFAs, and — unlike SFAs — reduces HDL cholesterol, as well as increases other cardiovascular disease risk factors (i.e., serum Lp (a) and triglycerides), dietary recommendations encourage all population groups to keep *trans* fatty acid consumption as low as possible (~1% of energy intake or less) [5,11,13,55].

To help people reduce their intake of *trans* fatty acids, the FDA issued a final regulation, effective January 1, 2006, requiring food manufacturers to list the amount of *trans* fatty acids on the Nutrition Facts Panel of most food products and some dietary supplements [57]. Under the regulation, manufacturers are allowed to label certain foods as "*trans* fat-free" (i.e., less than 0.5 g per serving). Because milk and most dairy products, including full-fat dairy products, contain very low levels of naturally-occurring *trans* fats, they will fall below this threshold of 0.5 g per serving, and thus will have zero grams listed on the nutrition label. Exceptions include some super-premium ice creams with various mix-ins and possibly some butter products. It is important to note that *trans* fatty acid information on food labels in the United States does not distinguish between the different types of *trans* fatty acids. In some countries, ruminant-derived food products are exempt from *trans* fatty acid labeling, in recognition that *trans* fatty acids from ruminants do not have an adverse effect on heart disease risk as do industrially-produced *trans* fatty acids [55].

There is no scientific evidence that *trans* fatty acids in dairy foods are harmful to health. Not only are *trans* fatty acids present in very low amounts in dairy foods, but the major *trans* fatty acids in dairy foods (i.e., vaccenic and rumenic acids) are not the same as those used in most studies (e.g., elaidic acid) [35,55]. For example, data from the Nurses' Health Study reveals that *trans* fatty acids derived from vegetable fat increase the risk of CHD, whereas risk of CHD decreases with increasing intake of *trans* fatty acids from animal sources [58]. Pietinen et al. [59] also found that intake of *trans* fatty acids from vegetable sources, but not animal sources, was associated with increased risk of CHD in a cohort of Finnish men.

2.3.1.1.5 Conjugated Linoleic Acid and Sphingolipids

Other fatty acids present in dairy foods, such as CLA and sphingolipids, may have effects that protect against CHD. Conjugated linoleic acid, a mixture of positional and geometric isomers of linoleic acid, is present in foods from ruminant animals and especially rich in milk products. Although most CLA-related research thus far has focused on a potential anticarcinogenic effect of this substance (see Chapter 4 on Dairy Foods and Cancer), studies, primarily in experimental animals, indicate that CLA may also reduce the risk of CHD [35,60–68].

When rabbits received 0.5 g CLA per day in food, marked reductions were observed in plasma total and LDL cholesterol, the LDL/HDL cholesterol ratio, and triglyceride levels [60]. In addition, lower degrees of atherosclerosis were detected in the aortas of CLA-fed rabbits. An investigation by Nicolosi et al. [61] supports the above observations. In this study, hamsters were equally divided into five groups: a control group, which received no CLA, and either low (0.06% of energy), medium (0.11% of energy), or high (1.1% of energy) CLA or 1.1% of energy as linoleic acid for 11 weeks [61]. Compared to the control animals, the CLA-fed animals exhibited lower levels of plasma total cholesterol, non-HDL cholesterol (combined very low and LDL), and triglycerides. An antioxidant effect of CLA was suggested by determination of plasma tocopherol/total cholesterol ratios. In addition, measurement of the aortic fatty streak areas revealed less early atherosclerosis in the CLA-fed hamsters [61]. The findings led the researchers to conclude that CLA has the ability to reduce atherosclerosis risk factors and fatty streak formation [61]. When researchers examined the effect of a diet containing butter enriched with vaccenic and rumenic acids on blood lipids in cholesterol-fed hamsters, they found significantly lower blood total and LDL cholesterol levels in the animals fed the enriched butter diet than in those fed the control diet (20% standard butter diet) [68].

Other studies have shown that feeding a mixture of CLA isomers or individual isomers (i.e., *cis*-9, *trans* 11 and *trans* 10, *cis* 12) reduces the severity of cholesterol-induced atherosclerotic lesions in rabbits [65,66]. When individual CLA isomers and a mixture of these isomers were fed as part of a semipurified diet containing 0.2% cholesterol to rabbits with pre-established atheromatous lesions, atherogenesis was reduced by 50% [66]. When fed as part of a cholesterol-free diet to rabbits with established atherosclerosis, these individual CLA isomers and the CLA mix reduced lesions by 26%. The individual isomers had effects on atherosclerosis similar to those observed with the CLA mix. In ApoE knockout mice with pre-established atherosclerosis, a dietary supplement of *cis*-9, *trans*-11 CLA (the predominant CLA isomer in milk fat) not only reduced further development of atherosclerotic lesions, but also induced regression of aortic lesions [67]. Using this same mouse model, researchers found that different forms of CLA have unique effects on HDL cholesterol particles [69]. Specifically, *trans*-10, *cis*-12 CLA modified HDL to form more atherosclerosis-promoting apoA-II particles and other changes compatible with the metabolic syndrome, whereas *cis*-9, *trans*-11 CLA did not promote this effect [69].

In humans, intake of dairy products naturally enriched in *cis*-9, *trans*-11 CLA in amounts similar to habitual intakes of these foods (milk, cheese, butter) has been shown to increase *cis*-9, *trans*-11 CLA content of plasma and cellular lipids [70]. When the effects of CLA isomers were investigated in healthy normolipidemic males, the *cis*-9, *trans*-11 isomer modestly improved blood lipid profiles, whereas the *trans*-10, *cis*-12 isomer had a relatively detrimental effect [71]. Although it has yet to be clearly established whether CLA has a major effect on blood lipid levels in humans [72,73], several mechanisms by which CLA could reduce atherosclerosis, such as modulating the metabolism of fatty acids in the liver, have been hypothesized [63].

Sphingolipids are an important type of fat found in milk and other dairy foods. Long-term feeding (two generations) of sphingolipids (1%) to laboratory rats significantly decreased total blood cholesterol levels by about 30% [74]. Sphingomyelin (the most abundant sphingolipid in milk) has been demonstrated to inhibit the absorption of cholesterol, fat, and other lipids in laboratory rats [75]. The potential roles of CLA and sphingolipids in cardiovascular health warrant additional study.

In summary, findings of studies of the effects of individual fatty acids on blood lipid levels indicate that three fatty acids in milk fat (i.e., the long-chain SFAs — palmitic, myristic, and lauric acids) raise blood cholesterol levels, whereas other bovine milk fats do not [35,37,76]. The latter includes the long-chain SFA stearic acid; short- and medium-chain SFAs; MUFAS; PUFAs; and possibly CLA and sphingolipids.

2.3.1.2 Dietary Fat Quantity

The relationship between total fat intake and CHD is of lesser importance than the type or quality of fat consumed [8,11,28,40]. Findings from a number of prospective epidemiological studies, controlled feeding trials, and limited randomized clinical trials have suggested relationships between specific types of fat and CHD, but not with total fat [35,44,59,77–80]. For example, the Nurses' Health Study found no association between total fat intake and risk of CHD over a 14-year period after adjusting for CHD risk factors [78]. However, there was a nonsignificant trend toward a positive association between SFA intake and CHD and an inverse association between MUFA intake and PUFA intake and risk of CHD [78]. When this follow-up study, among more than 78,000 women initially free of heart disease, was extended to 20 years, no statistically-significant associations were found between intakes of total fat, saturated fat, or monounsaturated fat and CHD in multivariate analyses [80]. However, intake of PUFA, at least up to approximately 7% of energy, was associated with reduced risk of CHD, particularly among women who were younger or overweight. Additionally, a high intake of *trans* fat increased the risk of CHD, particularly for younger women [80].

Some studies have shown that reducing total fat intake has beneficial effects on the incidence of cardiovascular events when SFA and cholesterol are also low [28]. However, a low-fat diet can potentially have adverse effects on CHD risk factors, evidenced by the decrease in HDL cholesterol and increase in triglyceride and lipoprotein (a) levels [5,8,11,28,81]. Compared to higher fat intakes, low-fat/high-carbohydrate diets can induce a lipoprotein pattern called the atherogenic lipoprotein phenotype, which is associated with increased risk of CHD [11,20,82]. This phenotype is minimally expressed in physically-active, lean populations, while it is developed in sedentary, overweight/obese populations [11]. In addition to this, individuals differ in their blood lipoprotein response to a low-fat diet [20,82–84]. When normolipidemic male subjects with initially low HDL cholesterol levels were fed a low-fat diet, there was a nonsignificant decrease in HDL cholesterol and a substantial decrease in LDL cholesterol, resulting in a significant improvement in the LDL/HDL cholesterol ratio [83]. However, in the men with normal HDL cholesterol levels, both LDL and HDL cholesterol levels decreased, resulting in an unchanged LDL/HDL cholesterol ratio. Another study found that persons who are overweight or insulin-resistant have a less favorable lipoprotein response (i.e., smaller reductions in LDL cholesterol) to diets low in total and saturated fat than do those who are not overweight or who are insulin-sensitive [84].

Evidence indicates that altering the quality or type of fat consumed (i.e., replacing SFAs with USFAs) is more effective in lowering the risk of CHD than previously appreciated [78,80,85,86]. Extremes in dietary fat intake should be avoided. High-fat diets (>35% of energy) increase the risk of CHD, while very low-fat diets (<20% of energy) may induce adverse metabolic changes (i.e., reduce HDL cholesterol and increase triglyceride levels), fail to maintain weight loss, and possibly lead to nutrient inadequacies [5,28,29]. Dietary guidelines advocate a diet moderate in total fat (20 to 35% of energy) for the majority of the population [4,5,11,13,14]. There is also growing support for tailoring fat intake to individuals to help reduce the risk of CHD [5,19,28].

2.3.1.3 Dietary Cholesterol

Studies show that as dietary cholesterol increases, there is an average increase in blood levels of total, LDL, and HDL cholesterol, although the magnitude of the response is less than that observed for saturated and *trans* fatty acid intake, and varies by individual [5,13,16]. A meta-analysis of 27 controlled metabolic feeding studies of added dietary cholesterol indicates that the change in total blood cholesterol is steeper in the range from zero to 300 to 400 mg/day of added dietary cholesterol than at cholesterol intakes above this level [87]. Additionally, the magnitude of the response to dietary cholesterol diminishes at higher baseline cholesterol intakes [87].

Equations based on data from numerous studies predict that 100 mg of added dietary cholesterol per day will increase blood cholesterol by 2 to 3 mg/dl on average, approximately 80% of which is the LDL fraction [11,17,18]. For an individual with a total blood cholesterol level of 200 mg/dl, a 2 to 3 mg increase represents an approximate 1% to 1.5% increase in blood cholesterol level (0.8% to 1.2% increase in LDL cholesterol), which is estimated to increase CHD risk by about 1%, although this may be offset in part by the increase in HDL cholesterol [11].

Individuals differ widely in their blood cholesterol response to dietary cholesterol intake [5,11,16–18,88,89]. The responsiveness to dietary cholesterol is reported to vary over a wider range than that found with other dietary variables [16]. According to a review by McNamara [89], 15% to 20% of the population is relatively sensitive to the effects of dietary cholesterol, whereas 80% to 85% is relatively insensitive. Reducing dietary cholesterol intake from 400 mg/day to 300 mg/day is estimated to lower plasma cholesterol levels by an average of 3.2 mg/dl in cholesterol-sensitive individuals (i.e., those who lack precise feedback control of endogenous cholesterol synthesis) [89]. At present, there is no biological marker to identify individuals who are more or less sensitive to dietary cholesterol. Individuals with hyperlipidemia may be more sensitive to dietary cholesterol [90]. In a study involving 21 subjects, an acute load of cholesterol (700 mg) with a meal did not produce a more atherogenic profile except in subjects with hypertriglyceridemia [90]. Insulin-resistant individuals have also been shown to have a reduced response to dietary cholesterol, as compared to insulin-sensitive individuals [91]. The variation in response to dietary cholesterol may be due to such factors as differences in intestinal cholesterol absorption, suppression of cholesterol synthesis in the liver by dietary cholesterol, and LDL catabolism, as well as genetics [11]. The AHA [5] summarizes the effects of dietary cholesterol on blood cholesterol levels as follows: "Dietary cholesterol can increase LDL cholesterol levels, although to a lesser extent than saturated fat. As is the case with saturated fat intake, this response varies widely among individuals."

2.3.1.4 Protein

A number of studies suggest that moderately replacing carbohydrate with protein, including animal protein, has a beneficial effect on the blood lipid profile and risk of heart disease [92–95]. In a crossover randomized controlled trial involving ten healthy normolipidemic adults in which fat intake was maintained at 35% of total energy, moderately replacing carbohydrate with animal protein reduced total, VLDL, and LDL cholesterol levels [92]. Unlike low-fat diets, this diet did not lower HDL cholesterol levels. Findings from the Nurses Health Study of 80,082 women between the ages of 34 and 59 years found that replacing carbohydrate with protein was weakly associated with lower risk of ischemic heart disease after controlling for major CHD risk factors [93]. In this prospective cohort study, both animal and vegetable proteins contributed to the lower risk, and the inverse association between protein intake and heart disease was similar in women with low- or high-fat diets. According to a recent review, exchanging protein (either animal or plant) for carbohydrate improves blood lipid profiles in clinical trials, and high protein intake is linked with low risk of CHD in epidemiological studies [95]. However, the author recommends more long-term studies to confirm this benefit of protein and to determine optimal amounts and sources of protein [95]. A recent investigation in overweight men found that a high-protein, moderately low-carbohydrate diet reduced the expression of a common genetically-influenced lipoprotein phenotype and had a favorable effect on atherogenic lipoprotein levels (e.g., total/HDL cholesterol) independent of saturated fat [96].

Some investigators have examined the role of dairy proteins, both casein and whey proteins, in cardiovascular health. Casein, the major protein in milk and dairy foods, has been shown to be moderately hypercholesterolemic when substituted for soy protein [97–105]. However, the effect of casein on blood cholesterol levels varies widely, and appears to depend on experimental conditions, including the amount of cholesterol in the diet; the percentage of protein and lipid in the diet; the species, age, and strain of the animal; duration of the study, the kind of casein; and the blood cholesterol level of the individual, among other factors [99,100,106].

Studies indicate that a hypercholesterolemic effect of casein compared to soy protein is dependent on a cholesterol-rich diet [97,98,103]. In a crossover study in which normolipidemic subjects consumed formula diets containing 500 mg cholesterol per day and 20% casein, blood LDL cholesterol levels increased by 10% and HDL cholesterol decreased by 10% [98]. When cholesterol intake was reduced to <100 mg/day, casein and soy protein had similar effects on blood lipoprotein levels.

In addition to dietary cholesterol, other dietary components, such as minerals, may influence the hypercholesterolemic response to casein. In a study involving rabbits, a reduction in dietary minerals enhanced casein-induced hypercholesterolemia [101]. In rabbits, casein is hypercholesterolemic and atherogenic compared to soy. However, when the casein:soy ratio is 1:1, blood cholesterol levels and atherosclerosis are similar to those observed when 100% soy is fed [102].

Most of the studies that have examined the effect of casein on blood cholesterol levels have been carried out in growing animals consuming a single source of protein [101]. Consequently, extrapolating the findings to adult humans consuming a mixed diet is questionable. Moreover, an individual's initial blood cholesterol level influences the response to proteins such as soybean [99,100]. Low-fat, low-cholesterol diets containing isolated soybean protein (25 or 50 g/day), as compared to casein, have been demonstrated to reduce blood cholesterol levels in men with elevated blood cholesterol, but not in those with lower initial blood cholesterol levels [99,100]. A study in normolipidemic men fed liquid formula diets containing either casein or soy protein found that the casein diet lowered lipoprotein(a), a risk factor for CHD, whereas soy protein had a lipoprotein(a)-raising effect [107]. According to an AHA science advisory, studies conducted over the last 10 years do not confirm the benefits of soy protein when compared to other proteins for cardiovascular health [108].

It has been proposed that consumption of a casein variant in cow's milk, specifically beta-casein A1, represents a risk factor for CHD [109–111]. Milk and dairy products contain a mixture of A1 and A2 beta-casein proteins. A study in rabbits showed that intake of beta-casein A1 increased blood total cholesterol, LDL cholesterol, HDL cholesterol, and triglyceride levels, as well as aortic fatty streaks, compared to beta-casein A2 [109]. Between-country correlations have observed a link between estimated national average beta-casein A1 consumption and CHD mortality in developed countries [110,111]. However, critical reviews of the available science have led to the conclusion that evidence for an involvement of beta-casein A1 in CHD, if far from conclusive [112,113]. As one researcher states, "there is no convincing or even probable evidence that the A-1 B-casein of cow milk has any adverse effect in humans" [113]. In fact, this statement is supported by findings of the first study in individuals at high risk of developing heart disease which examined the effect of B-casein A1 vs. A2 on heart disease risk factors [114]. This double-blind crossover study in 15 Australian individuals at high risk of developing heart disease found no evidence that dietary supplementation with B-casein A1 had any disadvantage in terms of cardiovascular risk factors compared to casein A2 [114]. Subjects received a daily supplement of either casein A1 or A2 (25 g) for 12 weeks each. Both caseins significantly reduced blood cholesterol levels by a similar amount. In addition, the two casein supplements did not differ in their effect on other risk factors for heart disease (i.e., homocysteine, C-reactive protein, blood pressure) [114].

Whey-derived peptides may help reduce the risk of CHD by lowering blood pressure, inhibiting platelet aggregation, and reducing blood cholesterol levels. Whey peptides have been shown to inhibit the activity of angiotensin-converting enzyme, thereby lowering blood pressure [115] (see Chapter 3 on Dairy Foods and Hypertension). Some whey proteins may also affect blood coagulation [116]. *In vitro* and experimental animal studies indicate that peptides derived from glycomacropeptide and lactoferrin may inhibit platelet aggregation and thrombosis [116]. In addition, whey proteins may reduce blood cholesterol levels or have a favorable impact on blood lipid levels [117,118]. When mice fed a standard commercial diet were administered milk-derived lactoferrin, plasma and liver cholesterol and triglyceride levels were reduced and blood HDL cholesterol levels were increased [118]. However, bovine lactoferrin had no significant effects on lipid metabolism in mice fed a high-fat diet. Further study of the role of dairy proteins, both casein and whey proteins, in cardiovascular disease is warranted.

2.3.1.5 Calcium

A number of studies support a hypocholesterolemic effect of calcium [119–127]. This finding is of significance, considering that dairy foods contribute 72% of the calcium available in the U.S. food supply [38]. It is important to recognize that, while the presence of calcium in arteries may be a risk factor for heart disease [128], there is no good data to suggest that oral calcium intake adds to calcification in the arteries. The calcium present in arteries is a byproduct of cholesterol and plaque build-up.

In a randomized single blind study, 13 men aged 38 to 49 years with moderate hypercholesterolemia were fed a metabolic diet approximating the typical American diet (i.e., 34% of calories from fat, 13% from SFAs, and 240 mg cholesterol a day) and either 400 mg or 2200 mg calcium (as calcium citrate malate) per day for 10 days [121]. When compared to the low-calcium diet, the high-calcium diet lowered total cholesterol by 6%, LDL cholesterol by 11%, and apoB levels by 7% (Table 2.2). No significant differences in HDL cholesterol levels were observed [121]. The excretion of SFAs doubled during the high-calcium diet, suggesting that calcium's beneficial effect may be explained by the formation of calcium–SFA complexes in the intestine. The findings of this study led the authors to conclude that increasing the calcium intake of a typical American diet "may be mildly effective in lowering total and LDL cholesterol concentrations, perhaps by its action on increasing SFA excretion" [121]. A complementary approach to the traditional recommendation to reduce SFA intake might be to decrease the absorption of this lipid by increasing calcium intake. From the results of this study, it can be anticipated that the hypercholesterolemic effect of SFAs in a food such as whole milk may be ameliorated, at least in part, by the presence of calcium in the same food.

In a randomized, double-blind, placebo-controlled crossover study involving 56 patients with mild to moderate hypercholesterolemia treated with a low-fat, low-cholesterol diet, increasing intake of calcium (as the carbonate) by 400 mg for 6 weeks reduced LDL cholesterol levels by 4.4% and increased HDL cholesterol by 4.1% [122]. The calcium in the carbonate treatment significantly decreased the ratio of LDL to HDL cholesterol by 6.5% [122]. Another randomized controlled trial in 223 healthy postmenopausal women found that supplementation with 1000 mg of calcium (as calcium citrate) per day for 1 year significantly increased HDL cholesterol by 7.3% and decreased LDL cholesterol by 6% (Figure 2.6) [124]. Reid [125] predicted that the resultant 16.4% increase in the HDL to LDL cholesterol ratio would reduce cardiovascular events by 20% to 30%.

Jacqmain et al. [126] reported that, compared to a low calcium intake (<600 mg/day), a high calcium intake (>1000 mg/day) has a beneficial effect on the blood lipoprotein-lipid profile, predictive of a lower risk of CHD. In this study of nearly 500 adults participating in Phase 2 of the Quebec Family Study, daily calcium intake was inversely associated with total cholesterol, LDL cholesterol, and the total:HDL cholesterol ratio in both women and men after adjusting for variations in body fat mass and waist circumference. According to 3-day diet records, the majority of calcium intake for men and women participating in this study came from dairy foods, including milk, cheese, and yogurt [126].

TABLE 2.2
Serum Lipid, Lipoprotein, and Apolipoprotein Concentrations in Humans Fed a Low or High Calcium Diet

Item	Low Ca	High Ca
Cholesterol (mmol/L)	5.99±0.62	5.66±0.57[a]
Triglycerides (mmol/L)	1.74±0.82	1.89±0.90[b]
LDL cholesterol (mmol/L)	4.13±0.54	3.67±0.49[a]
HDL cholesterol (mmol/L)	1.06±0.23	1.11±0.34
Apolipoprotein B (g/L)	10.4±1.7	9.7±1.5[a]
Apolipoprotein Al (g/L)	12.1±1.8	12.3±1.7

[a] Indicates significantly different from low Ca diet at $P<0.05$.

[b] Mean of both periods assumes residual effect observed in Period 1 attributed to baseline difference. With permission.

Source: Values are mean±SD, $n=3$. Samples from each subject were assayed in triplicate. From Denke, M. A. et al., *J. Nutr.*, 123, 1047, 1993.

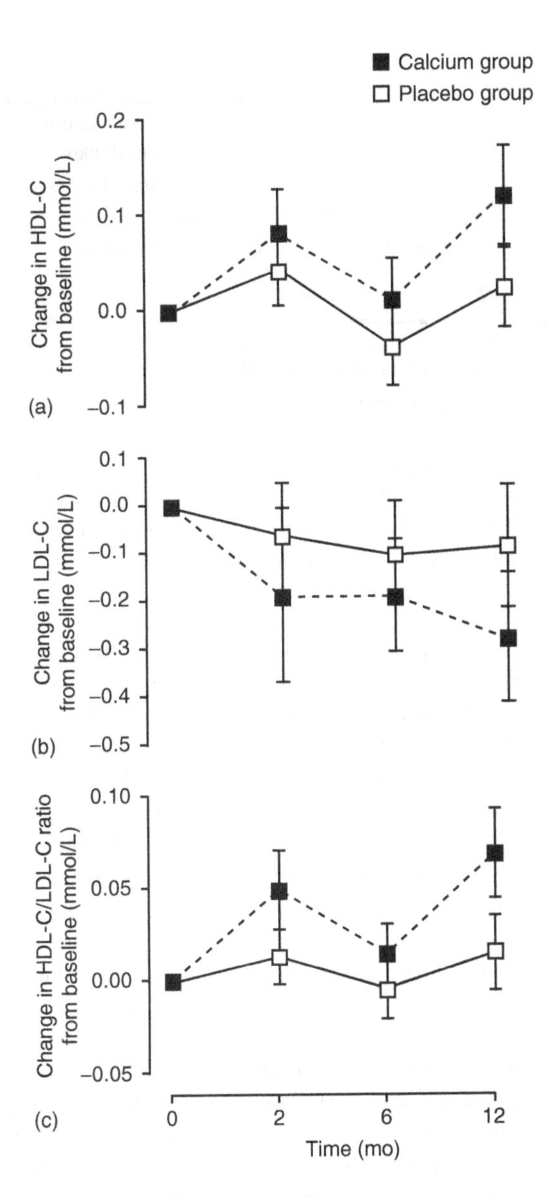

FIGURE 2.6 Effect of calcium citrate or placebo on (a) high-density lipoprotein-cholesterol (HDL-C), (b) low-density lipoprotein-cholesterol (LDL-C), and (c) their ratio in healthy late postmenopausal women. Data are changes from baseline and are shown as mean with standard errors. The between-groups differences in changes from baseline were significant, mo = months. (From Reid, I. R., *Drugs Aging*, 21, 7, 2004.)

Calcium's hypolipidemic effect may be explained by its interaction with fatty acids in the gut to reduce fatty acid absorption and by its ability to decrease the intestinal concentration of bile acids that facilitate fat absorption, as well as calcium's promotion of fat breakdown and decrease in fat formation within the fat cell [125,127]. In addition to calcium's favorable effect on blood lipids, this mineral may protect against CHD by lowering blood pressure (see Chapter 3 on Dairy Foods and Hypertension).

In addition to calcium, other minerals in dairy foods — such as magnesium and potassium — may have beneficial effects on cardiovascular health by influencing blood lipids and hypertension

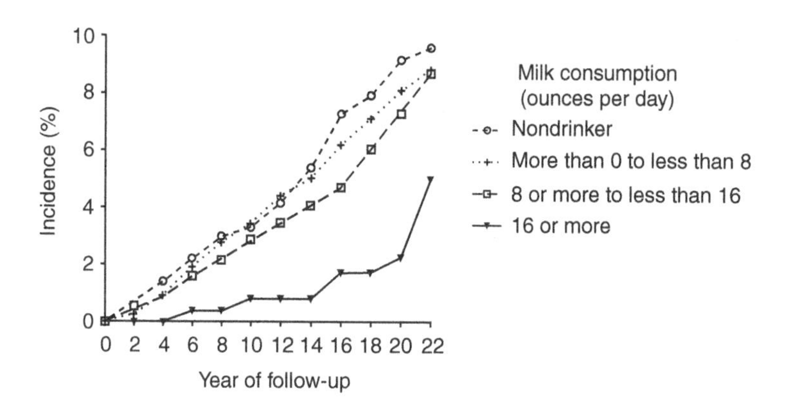

FIGURE 2.7 Cumulative incidence of thromboembolic stroke by year of follow-up and amount of milk consumed in men aged 55 to 68 years. All men were free of known coronary artery disease and stroke at the time of study enrollment. Follow-up began at the time of study enrollment (1965 to 1968) and lasted 22 years. (From Abbott, R. D. et al., *Stroke*, 27, 813, 1996. With permission.)

[127,129,130]. Moreover, calcium, particularly in combination with potassium and magnesium, has been linked to decreased risk of stroke [131–135].

In a cohort of 3150 older middle-aged (55 to 68 years) Japanese men enrolled in the Honolulu Heart Program and followed for 22 years, intake of calcium from milk, but not from nondairy sources, was associated with reduced risk of stroke [131]. Men who consumed 16 ounces per day or more of milk experienced half the rate of stroke (3.7 vs. 7.9 per 100, respectively) of men who did not drink milk (Figure 2.7). Although the rate of stroke decreased with increasing milk intake, the decline in stroke was modest for men who consumed less than 16 ounces per day. The finding that calcium intake from dairy sources, but not from nondairy sources, reduced risk of stroke indicates that other constituents in milk or concomitant health behaviors related to milk intake may be protective. The researchers concluded that, when combined with a balanced diet, weight control, and physical activity, drinking milk may help to decrease the risk of stroke [131].

High intakes of dietary calcium, especially dairy calcium, have been linked to a lower risk of ischemic stroke in the Nurses' Health Study of more than 85,000 U.S. women ages 34 to 59 years [132]. A prospective study of more than 53,000 Japanese men and women aged 40 to 79 years who were followed for 9.6 years found that total calcium intake and calcium from dairy products (milk, yogurt, cheese) were associated with a reduced risk of mortality from stroke [134].

In addition to calcium, higher intakes of potassium and magnesium are linked to decreased risk of stroke, presumably in large part due to lower blood pressure [132,133,135,136]. The FDA has approved a health claim for foods that are good sources of potassium and the reduction of high blood pressure and stroke [137]. Foods making this claim must contain at least 350 mg of potassium per serving, have no more than 140 mg of sodium per serving, and be low in fat, saturated fat, and cholesterol [137]. Nonfat milk qualifies to make this claim.

2.3.2 Genetics

Although efforts to prevent CHD have primarily focused on dietary and drug modifications of blood total cholesterol and lipoprotein cholesterol levels, accumulating scientific findings indicate that genetics has an important effect on blood lipid levels and CHD risk [5,19,20,138–140]. In fact, family history is considered to be a major risk factor for early onset CHD.

Studies clearly indicate that individuals differ in their blood lipid responses to diet, notably with regard to dietary intake of fat and cholesterol [24,25,42,43,87,141–143]. A large variability in blood

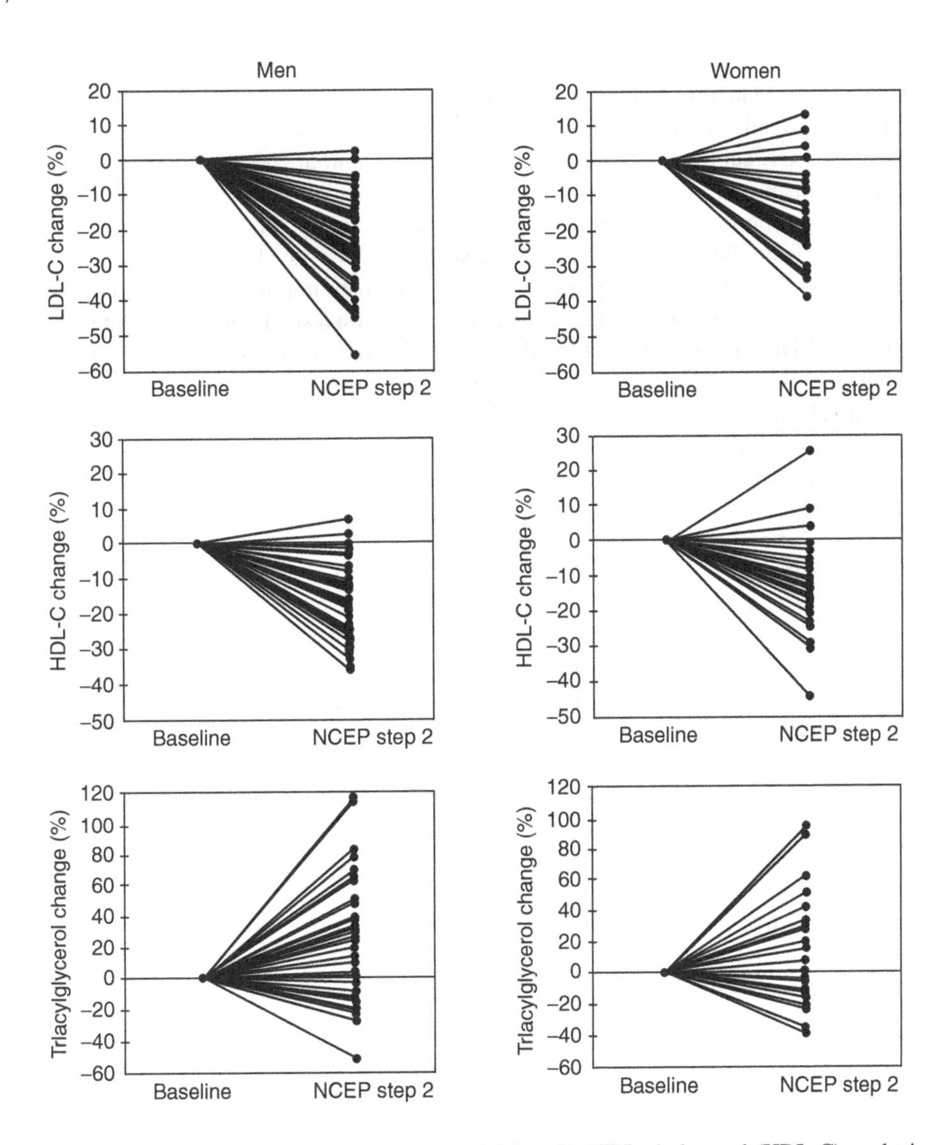

FIGURE 2.8 Individual variability in LDL-cholesterol (LDL-C), HDL-cholesterol (HDL-C), and triacygly-cerol concentrations in response to a National Cholesterol Education Program (NCEP) Step 2 diet in men and women. (From Schaefer, E. J. et. al., *Am. J. Clin. Nutr.*, 65, 823, 1997. With permission.)

lipid responses among individuals following the NCEP's Step 2 diet (i.e., 30% or less of calories from total fat, less than 7% of calories from saturated fat, and less than 200 mg cholesterol/day) has been reported (Figure 2.8) [42]. Changes in blood LDL cholesterol levels ranged from +3 to −55% in men and +13 and −39% in women [42]. The range of individual responses to the same dietary intervention has been attributed to multiple genes, each with a relatively small effect [5,19,42,138]. This variability in response supports individualized dietary and lifestyle recommendations to prevent and treat CHD [5]. The identification of genes that influence an individual's risk for CHD may ultimately result in tests to identify individuals most likely to benefit from specific dietary or other lifestyle interventions and allow for individualized dietary recommendations [19].

During the past few decades, considerable progress has been made in identifying genes influencing major risk factors for CHD, such as total blood cholesterol, lipoproteins (HDL and LDL cholesterol), and apolipoproteins (apo B, A-I, A-II, A-IV, E) [42,138,139,144–148]. Genetic defects in lipoprotein metabolism have increased understanding of how specific lipoproteins influence premature CHD [149,150]. Several genes have been shown to affect blood HDL cholesterol levels and consequently CHD risk [42,148,151].

Several investigations have demonstrated an influence of genetics on blood levels of LDL cholesterol and LDL subfraction patterns [19,152,153]. Familial forms of hypercholesterolemia, which are present in one in 500 persons in the general population, may result from deficient or defective LDL receptors [154]. A mutation in the gene coding for the LDL receptor prevents removal of LDL from the blood and results in a significant rise in LDL cholesterol and increased risk of CHD [154]. Genetic polymorphisms in apoE, which are important in the receptor-mediated uptake of small VLDL and intermediate-density LDL, explain a small but significant proportion of the variation in LDL cholesterol [19,42,140,146,148]. Variations in the apoE genotype have been shown to interact with the quantity and quality of dietary fat to modify blood total, LDL, or HDL cholesterol levels, as well as LDL subclasses [16,19,148,155]. Evidence indicates that the apoE4 allele is associated with a more atherogenic lipoprotein profile than apoE2 or apoE3 and that apoE4 carriers (found in approximately 14% of the population) are more responsive to changes in dietary fat and cholesterol than carriers of apoE2 or apoE3 alleles [16,19,148,155].

Researchers have identified defects in genes controlling LDL subclasses which could explain much of the familial clustering of lipid and lipoprotein levels in certain families and their increased risk of premature CHD [149,156–158]. In a community-based study of 301 subjects from 61 nuclear families, two distinct LDL subclasses were described [149]. Phenotype A is characterized by a predominance of large, buoyant LDL particles, and phenotype B consists mostly of small, dense LDL particles [19,159]. To date, seven different LDL subclasses and five different HDL subclasses based on their particle size and density have been identified [159].

LDL subclass pattern B is found in approximately 30% to 35% of adult males, in 5% to 10% of males <20 years of age, and in 5% to 10% of premenopausal women [19]. The majority of the population has the less-atherogenic LDL subclass pattern A. Individuals with LDL pattern B tend to have low HDL cholesterol, high triglyceride levels, high blood sugar levels, high blood pressure, and obesity — a constellation of disorders known as metabolic syndrome, and a profile associated with a two-to-three fold increase in CHD risk [19,150,152,156,160]. In the Quebec Cardiovascular Study which followed 2443 men for 5 years, small dense LDLs increased CHD risk independently of other risk factors, such as LDL cholesterol levels, body mass index, diabetes, blood pressure, age, alcohol intake, smoking, and a family history of heart disease [161]. The higher risk of heart disease in individuals with phenotype B may be explained by the increased susceptibility to oxidation of the smaller, denser LDL particles [19,160,162,163]. In addition, compared to its larger counterparts, small dense LDL binds less well to LDL receptors, is cleared more slowly from circulation, and may enter and bind to the arterial wall more readily [19,164,165]. Increased cholesterol deposition in the arterial wall increases the risk of atherosclerotic lesions. Studies indicate that risk of CHD is lower in subjects with higher levels of larger HDL2 subfractions as compared with the smaller, denser HDL3 subfractions [159,166].

Susceptibility to phenotype B appears to be inherited in most affected families as a major gene trait. Scientists have identified one possible genetic locus for this trait, designated atherosclerosis susceptibility (ATHS) on chromosome 19 [150]. This and other genes underlie predisposition to the atherogenic lipoprotein phenotype (ALP), a common heritable trait shared by up to 30% of the population [144]. The trait is characterized by an atherogenic lipoprotein profile, including LDL subclass pattern B. The effects of ATHS generally do not become apparent until after age 20 in men and after menopause in women [152]. The interaction of ATHS with other genetic or environmental factors, such as diet, may be responsible for a large proportion of the familial predisposition to CHD in the general population [150].

The same genetic factors that determine an individual's plasma lipoprotein subclass profile and CHD risk also may affect the response to diet [19,156–158]. Diet–gene interactions affecting LDL subclass patterns may contribute substantially to the variability among individuals in the effect of low-fat diets on CHD risk [19]. Adult males with LDL subclass pattern B have been found to differ

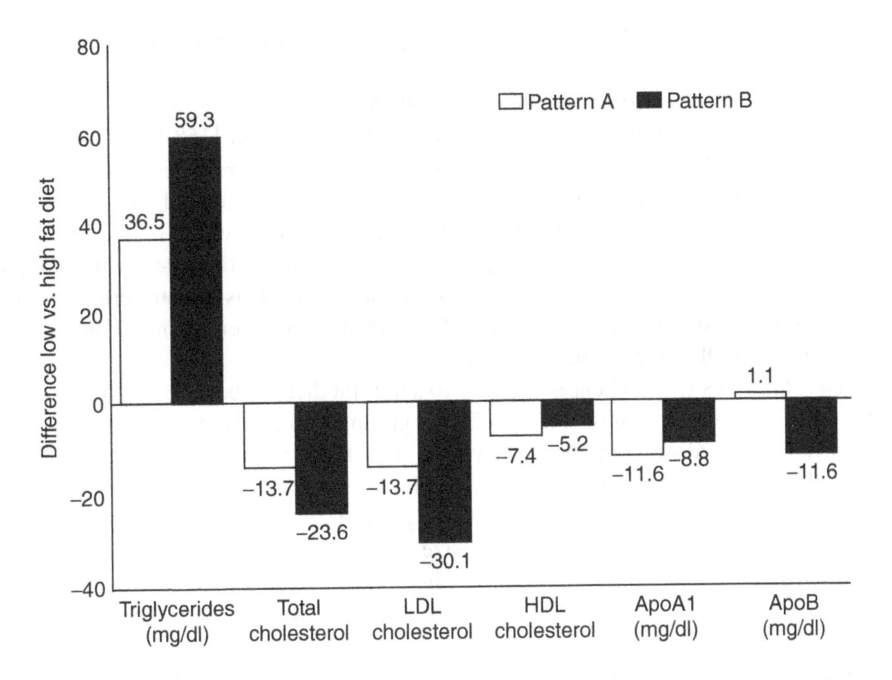

FIGURE 2.9 Differences between adults with genetically-determined LDL subclass pattern A and B in their blood lipid, lipoprotein cholesterol, and apolipoprotein responses to a change from a high-to-low-fat diet. (Adapted from Dreon, D. M. et al., *FASEB J.*, 8, 121, 1994. With permission.)

from men with LDL subclass pattern A in their lipoprotein response to a low-fat diet [156]. In a randomized crossover investigation, 105 healthy, middle-aged men consumed either a high-fat (46% of calories from fat, 34% from carbohydrates) or low-fat (24% of calories from fat, 56% from carbohydrates) diet for 6 weeks. Following the low-fat diet, pattern B subjects ($n = 18$) exhibited twice the decrease in LDL cholesterol as did pattern A subjects and plasma apoB levels decreased significantly, indicating a reduction in the total number of LDL particles and an expected lowering of CHD risk (Figure 2.9) [156]. Thus, the genetically-influenced LDL subclass pattern (A or B) is a significant factor contributing to the variation of LDL cholesterol response to a low-fat, high-carbohydrate diet. The benefits of a reduced-fat diet in terms of lipoprotein predictors of CHD risk, including LDL cholesterol, the ratio of LDL to HDL, and plasma apoB, were greatest in the minority of men who possessed LDL subclass pattern B [156]. This study also revealed that while the low-fat diet was especially beneficial for the pattern B men, it led to a more atherogenic lipoprotein response in some pattern A subjects [156]. Of the 87 men with pattern A on the high fat diet, 41% converted to the atherogenic pattern B profile with minimal change in particle number while consuming the low-fat diet [156]. In these men, the decrease in LDL cholesterol largely represents a reduction in the cholesterol content of LDL and, therefore, would not be expected to lead to a decrease in CHD risk [19].

The finding that a low-fat diet potentially may have adverse effects on CHD by switching some individuals' LDL subclass from A to a more atherogenic B subclass has been demonstrated in other studies in men [19,157,167]. Moreover, an increasing number of subjects with pattern A convert to the pattern B phenotype with progressive reduction in dietary fat (i.e., to 10% of calories from fat) and isocaloric substitution of carbohydrate [167]. These observations illustrate the complex interaction between diet and genetics. Genetically-determined LDL subclass pattern influences the blood lipid response to diet; conversely, diet influences changes in subclass pattern. Thus, both genetic and environmental factors, by influencing LDL subclass distributions, may contribute to differences in individuals' plasma lipoprotein response to a low-fat diet and subsequent risk of CHD [19,156,157,167].

A genetic predisposition to LDL pattern A or B may influence the blood lipid response to a reduced-fat diet even if individuals themselves do not have this trait [158,168]. When 72 premenopausal women ages 25 through 44 years were switched from a 35% fat diet to a 20% fat diet for eight weeks, changes in LDL cholesterol levels were related to the number of parents expressing the pattern B phenotype. Specifically, LDL cholesterol reduction on a low-fat, high-carbohydrate diet was greatest in daughters of two pattern B parents, intermediate in daughters with one pattern B parent, and least in daughters with no pattern B parents [158]. This genetic effect on the blood cholesterol response to diet was independent of the women's body weight, initial blood cholesterol levels, or their own LDL subclass pattern [158].

Likewise, children's LDL subclass response to a low-fat diet has been shown to be predicted by their parents' LDL subclass patterns [168]. When a group of 50 children, mean age 14, were fed a very-low-fat (10% of calories), high-carbohydrate diet, those with two pattern B parents had a greater prevalence of pattern B and higher LDL cholesterol and triglyceride levels compared to children of two pattern A parents [168]. Additionally, children of two pattern B parents were more likely to have diet-induced reductions in LDL size and to shift from pattern A to pattern B when consuming a very-low-fat, high-carbohydrate diet. These findings suggest that parents' LDL subclass pattern may help predict whether or not children would benefit from a low-fat, high-carbohydrate diet [168].

Additional support for a diet–gene interaction is provided by Lopez-Miranda and colleagues [169,170]. When young men with a mutation in the gene responsible for apoA-1 and previously normal cholesterol levels were fed a high-fat diet (40% of calories) rich in monounsaturated fat, total and LDL blood cholesterol levels increased. These results were surprising, given that the effect of monounsaturated fat on blood lipids is generally similar to that of a diet low in total and saturated fat. The authors conclude that for the 20% of the Caucasian population with this genetic mutation, reducing dietary fat successfully reduces plasma LDL cholesterol levels [169]. Genetic variations at the apoC3 gene locus appear to influence the LDL cholesterol response to dietary MUFAs [170]. Based on these findings, an individual's genetic make-up not only influences the size and shape of LDL particles, but may also influence the metabolic response to dietary fat.

An understanding of how diet and genetics interact to influence CHD risk is becoming much clearer. Identification of genetic polymorphisms that affect lipoproteins and CHD responses to specific dietary recommendations will eventually enable identification of individuals most likely to benefit from specific dietary modifications. It is clear that the same dietary pattern has unique effects in different individuals, and that reduced-fat diets may not be beneficial or equally beneficial for everyone [19].

Age and gender are other factors that can influence the extent to which individuals handle dietary fat [80,171–173]. Oxidation of the SFA, palmitic acid, in healthy children aged 5 to 10 years was almost twice that found in adults. Also, the metabolic disposal of palmitic acid was greater in men than in women [171]. Oh et al. [80] reported that the associations between PUFA intake and CHD and *trans* fat intake and CHD were stronger among younger than older women. Other researchers report that men and women may differ in their blood lipid responses and risk of CHD to dietary changes [172,173]. Low-density lipoprotein is a stronger predictor of CHD in men, whereas non-LDL lipid variables, such as HDL cholesterol abnormalities and triglyceride levels, are stronger predictors of CHD risk in women [25,172]. As mentioned previously, factors such as body fat, body mass index, and insulin sensitivity may influence an individual's blood lipid responses to diets reduced in total and saturated fat [84].

The complicating factor of genetic diversity and differences among individuals in their ability to handle dietary fat because of age, gender, body mass index, insulin levels, and possibly lifestyle factors supports dietary recommendations tailored to individuals. The AHA [5] recognizes the importance of genetics in influencing individuals' responses to diet and their ultimate risk for

CHD. In the future, based on individual genetically-based nutrition profiles, people may be able to map out a personal strategy of what to eat to minimize the risk of CHD. New technologies for gene analysis may eventually lead to greater individualization of dietary recommendations to reduce CHD, both for major subgroups of the population (e.g., children) and for individuals [174].

2.3.3 Dairy Foods

Studies of the effects of single nutrients, such as specific fats, in dairy foods on blood lipid levels are important for identifying mechanisms underlying observed responses, but are of little practical relevance. In whole foods, complex interactions occur among nutrients, which can modify the impact of a single nutrient on blood lipid levels. As reviewed below, studies employing dairy foods indicate that when these foods are consumed in usual amounts, they do not appear to adversely affect blood lipid levels or increase the risk of CHD. It is important to appreciate that the impact of a single food on risk of CHD also is influenced by the composition of the rest of the diet, as well as other lifestyle (e.g., physical activity, cigarette smoking) and genetic factors. Although there is a tendency to indict specific foods or food components, risk of CHD is associated with the total diet and other risk factors over time.

2.3.3.1 Milk and Culture-Containing Dairy Foods

Some researchers have hypothesized that certain dairy foods contain a blood cholesterol-lowering "milk factor" [175–183]. Interest in this possibility arose from the observation that Maasai tribesmen of East Africa, who consume large quantities (4 to 5 liter per person per day) of fermented whole milk, have low blood cholesterol levels and a low incidence of CHD [180].

Subsequent studies have examined the effect of a variety of dairy products on blood cholesterol levels. Several of these studies reveal that milk, yogurt, or *Lactobacillus acidophilus*-containing dairy foods are hypocholesterolemic in humans [176,178,179,182,184]. Howard and Marks [176] reported that humans exhibited a 5% to 15% decrease in blood cholesterol levels 1 week following intake of 2 quarts of whole and fat-free milk a day, respectively. Likewise, Hepner et al. [179] found that supplementing ordinary diets with three cups of pasteurized and unpasteurized yogurt a day for 1 week reduced blood cholesterol levels by 5% to 10%. In a study of men with high blood cholesterol levels, consumption of about 1 cup of yogurt containing *L. acidophilus* a day decreased blood cholesterol levels by about 3% [182]. This finding led the researchers to suggest that regular intake of yogurt with *L. acidophilus* could potentially reduce CHD by 6% to 10% [182].

In a well-controlled 8-week clinical trial, daily consumption of yogurt fermented with *Symbiobacterium thermophilus* and *Enterococcus faecium* reduced LDL cholesterol by 8.4% [185]. However, in a crossover, controlled feeding study in 29 women, intake of a symbiotic yogurt enriched with probiotics (*L. acidophilus* and *Bifidobacterium longum*) and a prebiotic (oligofructose) significantly increased HDL cholesterol and improved the LDL/HDL cholesterol ratio, but had no effect on blood total cholesterol, LDL cholesterol, or triglycerides over a period of 21 weeks [186].

Buonopane et al. [184] investigated the effect of consuming one quart of skim milk a day for eight weeks on blood cholesterol levels of 82 free-living adults. Blood cholesterol levels dropped 6.6% within 4 weeks in adults who consumed fat-free milk and whose initial blood cholesterol levels were elevated (217 to 233 mg/dl). The hypocholesterolemic effect of fat-free milk was greater in individuals with higher rather than lower baseline cholesterol levels [184]. A similar cholesterol-lowering effect of fat-free milk (400 mL/day or about two glasses) was observed in postmenopausal Japanese women [187]. The reduction in blood cholesterol levels with fat-free milk observed in these studies is in agreement with findings from some earlier investigations [188,189].

Experimental animal studies also indicate a hypocholesterolemic effect of several dairy products [190–193]. Kritchevsky et al. [190] demonstrated that either whole or fat-free milk fed to rats reduced blood cholesterol levels. When the effects of yogurt and acidophilus yogurt on blood lipids were examined in mice, blood total and LDL cholesterol significantly decreased in the animals fed acidophilus yogurt [191]. In contrast, yogurt or acidophilus yogurt did not affect blood HDL cholesterol and triglyceride levels [191]. In another study, total and LDL cholesterol levels decreased in laboratory rats fed yogurt containing either lactose-hydrolyzed condensed whey or bifidobacteria, whereas whole milk and standard yogurt had no hypocholesterolemic effect [192]. Zommara et al. [193] reported that whey from fat-free milk fermented with bifidobacteria and lactic acid bacteria reduced blood total and LDL cholesterol levels, increased the activity of antioxidant enzymes, and increased the resistance of LDL cholesterol to oxidation in laboratory rats. In this study, the nonfermented whey diet was less effective than whey from cultured milk in reducing blood cholesterol and oxidative stress [193].

A review of findings from experimental animal and human studies led Canadian researchers to conclude that intake of fermented dairy products moderately lowers blood cholesterol levels [183]. Although all the animal studies examined pointed to a cholesterol-lowering effect of fermented milk products, findings from studies in humans were less consistent [183]. The researchers suggest that fermented milk increases gut bacteria that ferment indigestible carbohydrates, which in turn produce short-chain fatty acids. The latter then decrease blood cholesterol concentrations, either by inhibiting cholesterol synthesis in the liver or by redistributing cholesterol from the blood to the liver [183]. More research is needed to document a hypocholesterolemic effect of nonfermented and fermented milk products and to identify the "milk factor." As discussed above, calcium is a possible candidate.

Regardless of whether or not milk and milk products have a hypocholesterolemic effect, there is growing evidence to suggest that consumption of milk and milk products does not adversely affect blood lipid levels or risk of CHD [119,178,189,194–196]. Thompson et al. [189] observed no significant change in blood cholesterol levels following intake of 1-liter supplements of various milk products fed daily for 3 weeks to human subjects. Likewise, McNamara et al. [194] found that 16 ounces of yogurt or a nonfermented dairy product (16 ounces low-fat milk, plus 10% milk solids) had no effect on plasma total, LDL, and HDL cholesterol levels when consumed by 18 normolipidemic males for 4 weeks. In an intervention study involving over 300 adults and in which calcium intake was increased to 1500 mg/day using mostly dairy foods (milk, cheese, yogurt) for 12 weeks, there was no effect on blood lipid levels despite the increased consumption of dairy foods [119].

A multicenter, randomized controlled trial of 204 healthy adults aged 55 to 85 years found no change in blood total and LDL cholesterol levels or the ratio of total cholesterol to HDL cholesterol in those who increased their intake of milk (skim or 1% reduced-fat) by 3 cups/day for 12 weeks [195]. A study of 70-year old Finnish men found an inverse association between intake of milk products and certain cardiovascular disease (CVD) risk factors, such as body mass index, waist circumference, and the LDL/HDL cholesterol ratio [196]. In this study, intake of milk products was positively associated with HDL cholesterol and apoA-1 levels [196]. Consumption of milk products may have a beneficial effect on LDL particle size [197]. In a study of nearly 300 healthy older men, Swedish researchers found that reported intakes of fat from dairy products and individual fatty acids typically found in milk products were associated with significantly fewer small dense LDL particles and a more favorable LDL profile [197].

Studies have shown that a healthy eating plan including dairy products reduces risk factors for CVD [198–202]. A low-fat (27% of calories) eating plan rich in low-fat dairy products (3 servings/day) and fruits and vegetables (8 to 10 servings/day) — known as the Dietary Approaches to Stop Hypertension (DASH) — has been demonstrated to have a beneficial effect on blood lipid levels [199]. A randomized controlled outpatient feeding trial in 436 participants of the DASH trial found a significant reduction in total cholesterol (−13.7 mg/dl), LDL cholesterol (−10.7 mg/dl), and

HDL cholesterol (−3.7 mg/dl) levels, with no change in triglyceride levels, in those who consumed the DASH diet compared to the control diet (i.e., typical American diet) [200]. These changes represent net reductions of 7.3, 9.0, and 7.5% in average concentrations of total, LDL, and HDL cholesterol, respectively. Although HDL cholesterol (i.e., the "good" cholesterol) was reduced along with LDL cholesterol, there were no significant changes in the ratio of total cholesterol to HDL cholesterol or the ratio of LDL to HDL cholesterol, which are considered to be better indicators of CVD risk [200]. Using the Framingham risk equation, the researchers estimated that consuming the DASH diet reduced the 10-year risk of developing CVD by 12.1%, whereas consuming the control diet increased the risk of CVD by 0.9% [200].

Harsha et al. [202] reported that the beneficial effects of the DASH trial on blood lipid levels are evident regardless of the level of sodium intake. Intake of the DASH diet at three different sodium levels (1500 mg, 2400 mg, and 3300 mg/day) for 30 days each in 390 adults resulted in lower levels of total cholesterol, LDL cholesterol, and HDL cholesterol in those consuming the DASH diet at each sodium level, compared to those consuming the typical American diet [202]. The DASH diet also lowers blood levels of homocysteine, an amino acid associated with increased risk of CVD [199]. An increased intake of milk and yogurt has been shown to be associated with lower blood levels of homocysteine [203]. When the relationship between food consumption frequencies and dietary intakes of B vitamins and blood levels of homocysteine were examined in the United States using data from the third National Health and Examination Survey (1988 to 1994), blood levels of homocysteine were approximately 15% higher in subjects who never consumed milk than in those who consumed milk at least once a day. Blood homocysteine levels were about 6.4% higher in those who never consumed yogurt than in those who consumed yogurt more than 15 times per month [203].

Consumption of milk and other dairy products may reduce the risk of CVD by their beneficial effect on blood pressure (see Chapter 7) and on body weight regulation (see Chapter 6). Reusser et al. [201] reviewed how dietary patterns that include an adequate intake of dairy products have a beneficial effect on several CVD risk factors, including hypertension, the metabolic syndrome, and obesity in the African American population. A multicenter prospective study, called the Coronary Artery Risk Development in Young Adults (CARDIA) study, conducted among 3157 African American and Caucasian young adults over a 10-year period, found that overweight participants who consumed the most dairy products (5 or more servings/day) had an approximately 70% lower incidence of the metabolic syndrome (also called insulin resistance syndrome) than those who consumed few dairy products (1.5 servings/day or fewer) [204]. All types of dairy products, both reduced-fat and full-fat versions, were associated with this benefit (Table 2.3). Other recent epidemiological studies link intake of dairy products with low risk of metabolic syndrome or risk factors associated with metabolic syndrome [205–207]. When researchers examined the association between dietary calcium, vitamin D, and the prevalence of the metabolic syndrome in more than 10,000 middle-aged and older women participating in the Women's Health Study, they found that intakes of calcium and dairy products were associated with a lower prevalence of the metabolic syndrome in this population [207].

Interestingly, a study in Sweden demonstrated that estimated intake of milk fat is negatively associated with "metabolic" risk factors for heart disease (insulin, body mass index, leptin, blood clotting factors, etc.) [208]. In this prospective case-control study involving 78 cases (who had a first heart attack) and 156 control subjects (who had not had a heart attack), a higher intake of fat from dairy products, as estimated by two milk fat biomarkers (i.e., pentadecanoic and heptadecanoic fatty acids in blood lipid esters), was associated with a reduced risk of developing a first-ever acute myocardial infarction [208]. The researchers recommend that further studies be conducted to verify these findings and to identify the mechanism responsible for the potentially beneficial relationship between milk fat and metabolic risk factors for heart disease.

Additional studies provide evidence that consumption of milk or dairy products is associated with no increase or a reduction in risk of CHD [209–213]. Ness et al. [209] reported results for CHD

TABLE 2.3
Odds Ratios for Components of Insulin Resistance Syndrome (IRS) per Daily Eating Occasion of Specific Types of Dairy Products among Individuals Who Were Overweight at Baseline

	Odds Ratio (95% Confidence Interval)				
Variables	Obesity	Abnormal Glucose Homeostasis	Elevated Blood Pressure	Dyslipldemia	IRS
All dairy products	0.82 (0.72 to 0.93)	0.83 (0.73 to 0.95)	0.81 (0.71 to 0.93)	0.92 (0.82 to 1.04)	0.79 (0.72 to 0.88)
Reduced-fat	0.81 (0.70 to 1.02)	0.95 (079 to 1.14)	0.79 (0.64 to 0.98)	0.95 (0.80 to 1.13)	0.78 (0.65 to 0.93)
High fat	0.84 (0.73 to 0.97)	0.77 (0.65 to 0.91)	0.84 (0.71 to 0.99)	0.91 (0.79 to 1.05)	0.82 (0.71 to 0.94)
Milk and milk drinks	0.83 (0.68 to 1.00)	0.84 (0.70 to 1.03)	0.80 (0.64 to 0.99)	0.91 (0.76 to 1.08)	074 (0.62 to 0.89)
Cheese and sour cream	0.82 (0.55 to 1.22)	0.96 (0.65 to 1.42)	0.67 (0.43 to 1.06)	1.23 (0.85 to 1.77)	0.64 (0.43 to 0.94)
Butter and cream	0.85 (0.72 to 1.02)	0.84 (0.69 to 1.03)	0.86 (0.70 to 1.05)	0.91 (0.76 to 1.08)	0.90 (0.76 to 1.05)
Dairy-based desserts	0.63 (0.24 to 1.64)	0.26 (0.09 to 0.80)	0.37 (0.12 to 1.13)	0.68 (0.26 to 1.79)	0.32 (0.13 to 0.83)
Yogurt	0.47 (0.16 to 1.43)	0.44 (0.12 to 1.62)	0.78 (0.22 to 2.72)	0.51 (0.15 to 1.72)	0.58 (0.20 to 1.66)

Source: From Pereira, M. A. et al., *JAMA*, 287, 2081, 2002. With permission.

and all causes mortality in a 25-year follow-up cohort of 5765 men ages 36 to 64 years living in Scotland. Between 1970 and 1973, the researchers interviewed the men to determine how much milk they drank and collected other detailed information on health habits and lifestyles. After 25 years of follow-up, men who drank between 2/3 and 2 to 2/3 cups of milk per day were 8% less likely to die of CHD or any cause than those who drank less than 2/3 cup. These results were statistically significant after adjusting for several variables such as socioeconomic position, health status, and health behaviors such as smoking [209]. Although the type of milk was not determined, the researchers speculate that the men probably drank mostly whole milk, as that was the type of milk mainly available in Scotland at that time. Ness et al. [209] referred to seven prospective studies that examined the association between milk consumption and heart disease or all causes of mortality. In none of these studies was milk consumption associated with increased CHD or total mortality [209].

Elwood et al. [210,211], in two studies — a cohort study and an analysis pooling the findings of ten cohort studies — concluded that milk drinking is associated with a reduction in heart disease and stroke risk. The Caerphilly Cohort Study followed a group of 2403 men aged 45 to 59 years in South Wales for 20 to 24 years to test the hypothesis that milk drinking increases the risk of ischaemic heart disease and ischaemic stroke. Contrary to the popular hypothesis, results showed that, after adjusting for other risk factors, men who drank the most milk (2 cups or more/day) vs. no milk had a 36% reduced risk of either heart disease or stroke (vascular disease). Among men with evidence of vascular disease at baseline, milk intake was associated with a 63% reduced risk [210]. No association was found between milk drinking and any cause of death (all-cause mortality). The same researchers pooled the results of ten prospective cohort studies that evaluated the relationship between milk consumption, or intake of calcium from dairy sources, and incidence of vascular disease [211]. All but one of the studies individually showed that a high intake of milk was associated with a reduced risk of heart disease and stroke. When the results were pooled, the highest vs. the lowest milk consumption was associated with a 13% reduced risk of heart disease, a 17% reduced risk of stroke, and a 16% reduced risk of any vascular event. The authors concluded that "the studies, taken together, suggest that milk drinking may be associated with a small but worthwhile reduction in heart disease and stroke risk." The cohort studies were carried out at a time when the availability of reduced-fat milks was limited [211]. Milk intake in the Caerphilly Cohort Study was estimated by using a semi-quantitative frequency questionnaire which may have overestimated food intake. When a more accurate method of diet assessment (i.e., 7-day weighed food records) was used in a subsequent study, similar observations were found [213].

2.3.3.2 Butter and Cheese

Intake of butter generally causes blood total and LDL cholesterol levels to increase, more so when consumed by individuals with elevated blood cholesterol levels [214–216]. When moderately hypercholesterolemic subjects consumed a diet containing 36% of calories from fat, half of which was obtained from butter, blood total and LDL cholesterol levels increased [215]. Similarly, in an investigation in which normocholesterolemic young men were fed diets containing 37% of calories from fat, 81% of which was provided by cocoa butter, olive oil, soybean oil, or dairy butter, butter was hypercholesterolemic [214].

Of interest are the findings of an investigation which examined the effects of five different fats, including butter, for 6 weeks on blood lipid and lipoprotein levels in 38 healthy, normolipidemic free-living men aged 30 to 60 years [217]. In this study, consuming butter at a level of about 19% of total calories (i.e., 60% of total fat intake or at least 20 times more than usually consumed) produced only a small (5%), although statistically significant, rise in total and LDL cholesterol levels [217]. Thus, under free-living conditions, intake of butter appears to have a relatively small influence on blood cholesterol levels [217]. No link between intake of butter and CHD was found in a prospective study examining the effect of margarine (a source of *trans* fatty acids) intake on the development of CHD among over 800 middle-aged men followed for 21 years [218]. The researchers caution, however, that conclusions may be premature, because this study used a single 24-hour dietary recall which may not accurately reflect dietary intake. However, their findings are supported by an earlier prospective study of more than 85,000 women participating in the Nurses' Health Study, in which intake of butter was not significantly associated with CHD risk [58].

When the effects of butter and cheese on blood lipoprotein levels, haemostatic variables, and homocysteine were examined in 22 adults participating in a randomized crossover study, cheese intake was found to be less cholesterol-raising than butter at equal fat content [219]. In another randomized crossover feeding study, in which the effects of milk, cheese, and butter on blood lipids were examined in 14 healthy young men, cheese intake did not significantly increase LDL cholesterol levels [220]. The diets provided 35% of calories from fat (20% from dairy fat, as whole milk, butter, or hard cheese), 17% from protein, and 48% from carbohydrate. The researchers speculate that cheese may not raise blood cholesterol levels due to its calcium content or because fermentation may have a cholesterol-lowering effect [220]. In a similar study in middle-aged men and women with mildly elevated blood cholesterol levels, dairy fat in cheese raised LDL cholesterol 6% less on average than that of butter at comparable intakes of total and saturated fat [221]. This finding of the lower cholesterol-raising effect of cheese than butter led the researchers to suggest that the "inclusion of moderate amounts of cheese in the diet may need to be reevaluated even for subjects with elevated plasma cholesterol" [221]. A study in laboratory rats fed cheese demonstrated that plasma total cholesterol and non-HDL cholesterol levels were lower than in rats fed beef meat (tallow) diets [222]. Moreover, the cheese-fed rats had a healthier fatty acid composition of liver triglycerides [222].

A review of findings from observational and intervention trials of dairy products and cardiovascular disease led Tholstrup [223] to conclude that "there is no strong evidence that dairy products increase the risk of CHD in healthy men of all ages or young and middle-aged healthy women." This investigator called for more research, especially well-designed clinical trials in humans, to elucidate the role of milk and milk products in the risk of heart disease [223].

2.4 EFFICACY AND SAFETY OF LOW-FAT, LOW-SATURATED FAT DIETS

A number of questions have arisen regarding the efficacy (i.e., in reducing CHD and improving life expectancy) and safety (i.e., nutritional adequacy) of following low-fat, low-saturated fat diets [24,35,224,225]. This is particularly true for very-low-fat diets [29]. It is evident that the potential gain accrued by dietary interventions to reduce fat intake is unique to each individual. Consequently, there is increasing support for tailoring dietary fat/saturated fat recommendations to individuals to reduce the risk of CHD [5,19,20,28].

2.4.1 EFFICACY

Meta-analyses using data from both metabolic ward studies and studies in free-living populations indicate that lowering total dietary fat from 37% of calories and cholesterol from 385 mg/day to the NCEP Step 1 diet (i.e., 30% of calories as fat and 300 mg cholesterol/day) reduces blood total and LDL cholesterol by an average of 5% [17,18]. In addition, a large degree of individual variability in response to this dietary intervention is reported. In a review of 16 published trials of six months or longer of the Step 1 diet, Ramsay et al. [226] found little effect on blood cholesterol levels in free-living individuals. However, in high-risk subjects, reductions in blood cholesterol levels averaged about 2% over 6 months to 6 years, equivalent to an estimated reduction in coronary events of 3% [226].

In the first study to evaluate the effectiveness of the NCEP's Step 2 diet (30% or less of total calories from fat, <7% of total calories from SFA, <200 mg cholesterol) on blood cholesterol levels in nearly 100 asymptomatic free-living adults with mild hypercholesterolemia, diet had only a small effect on blood cholesterol levels [227]. The low-fat diet reduced total and LDL blood cholesterol levels each by 5%, but was accompanied by a 5% decrease in HDL cholesterol. The effect of the low-fat diet on blood cholesterol levels in this study was only one-third the level predicted by the NCEP Expert Panel. Although Schaefer et al. [42] reported more significant decreases in blood total and LDL cholesterol levels in 72 men and 48 women following the NCEP Step 2 diet, a wide variation in blood lipid responses was observed. Moreover, HDL cholesterol decreased and triglyceride levels rose [42].

According to the Women's Health Initiative Dietary Modification Trial, which was an 8-year, randomized, controlled trial conducted in more than 48,000 healthy postmenopausal women recruited from 40 clinical centers across the United States, a low-fat dietary pattern had no significant effect on the incidence of CHD, stroke, or cardiovascular disease [228]. Moreover, the low-fat diet had only modest beneficial effects on heart disease risk factors (e.g., LDL cholesterol, blood pressure, a clotting factor). The findings of this trial led the researchers to conclude that "more focused diet and lifestyle interventions may be needed to improve risk factors and reduce CVD risk" [228].

The ratio of total cholesterol to HDL cholesterol is a better predictor of CHD risk than either one alone [229]. A low-fat diet may result in no or even a slightly negative change in the total cholesterol/HDL ratio. Researchers have found that low-fat, high-carbohydrate diets can lead to changes in lipoprotein metabolism associated with increased risk of CHD, such as a decrease in HDL cholesterol and ApoA1 (the major transport protein for HDL) and increases in triglyceride and small dense LDL (subclass pattern B) levels [18,28,35,79,81,229–235]. A study in eight healthy adults who consumed either a low-fat (25% of energy), high-carbohydrate (60% of energy) diet or a high-fat (45% of energy), low-carbohydrate (40% of energy) diet in random order for two weeks found that those on the low-fat, high-carbohydrate diet had lower blood HDL cholesterol levels, higher triglyceride levels, and a persistent increase in remnant lipoproteins [234].

Research findings also demonstrate that a low-fat diet increases blood Lp(a) levels and leads to detrimental changes in LDL particle size [236,237]. In a double-blind multicenter study called the Delta study, reducing total and SFA intake in healthy adults decreased blood total, LDL, and HDL cholesterol levels, and increased blood Lp(a) levels [236]. The researchers suggest that the potentially atherogenic changes (i.e., reduction in HDL cholesterol and increase in Lp(a) levels) in response to decreasing total and saturated fat intake must be weighed against the benefit of reducing LDL cholesterol levels [236].

Diets high in saturated fat are also associated with an increase in larger, less atherogenic LDL particles [237]. In a crossover diet study involving 103 healthy men, a low-fat diet (24% vs. 46% of calories as fat) was associated with increased levels of the more atherogenic small LDL particles [237]. This study found that an increase in SFAs, particularly myristic and palmitic acids, was positively associated with larger LDL particles and negatively associated with small (more atherogenic) LDL particles, whereas dietary stearic acid had no effect [237]. Saturated fat intake was also inversely related to the activity of hepatic lipase, an enzyme involved in the formation of small, dense LDL cholesterol [237]. Dietary total and saturated fat intake can also influence HDL particle size and density [238]. Reducing total and saturated fat intake has been shown to result in a pronounced decrease in the larger size HDL2 subfractions compared with the smaller-sized HDL3 subfractions (i.e., a more atherogenic profile) [238].

A 3-year investigational study which examined the effects of dietary macronutrients on atherosclerotic progression in 235 postmenopausal women who had at least one coronary stenosis (>30% reduction in luminal diameter) found that a higher intake of saturated fat was associated with a more favorable lipoprotein profile (i.e., higher HDL, higher apoA-1, lower triglycerides, and a lower ratio of total cholesterol to HDL cholesterol) and less progression of coronary atherosclerosis [172]. Saturated fat intake was associated with significantly less narrowing (stenosis) of the arteries. In the highest quartile of saturated fat intake, there was no increase in stenosis, compared to an 8% increase in the lowest quartile, and 3.6% increase in the second quartile. With respect to specific SFAs, each 1% increase in calorie intake from stearic acid was associated with a 0.11-mm smaller decline in luminal diameter, whereas each 1% increase in calorie intake from lauric, myristic, or palmitic acid was associated with a 0.05-mm smaller decline in luminal diameter [172]. The beneficial effect of saturated fat on progression of atherosclerosis was especially pronounced in postmenopausal women whose intake of monounsaturated fat was low or whose intake of carbohydrate was high [172]. Monounsaturated fat, total fat, and protein intakes were not associated with the progression of atherosclerosis in these postmenopausal women. In an accompanying editorial, the researchers note that the women participating in the study had risk factors associated with the metabolic syndrome, and that triglyceride and HDL cholesterol abnormalities are stronger predictors of coronary artery disease in women, whereas LDL concentration is a stronger predictor in men [25].

These findings indicate that SFAs may not be as detrimental to the lipoprotein profile or heart disease risk for some individuals as once believed. Researchers suggest that the increase in HDL cholesterol from a diet high in saturated fat compensates for the adverse effects of SFAs on LDL [239].

Studies in children and adolescents have examined the effects of fat intake on blood lipid levels. In an investigation of 110 preschool children in Spain, those who consumed diets containing 13% or more of calories from SFA had higher HDL cholesterol levels and better HDL cholesterol/LDL cholesterol ratios than did children whose saturated fat intake was less than 13% of calories [240]. When relationships between specific fatty acids and blood levels of cholesterol, ApoB (which aids transport of LDL cholesterol), and insulin were examined in 94 adolescents in Sweden, higher intakes of SFAs derived from milk fat were associated with lower blood levels of cholesterol and ApoB [241]. The findings led the researchers to suggest that "milk fat contains or is associated with some component of the diet, or some other characteristics of food intake, which counterbalances the expected positive relationships between saturated fat intake and lipid levels" [241].

When more than 600 children initially aged 8 to 10 years with elevated LDL cholesterol levels participated in the Dietary Intervention Study in Children (DISC), diets reduced in fat, saturated fat, and cholesterol significantly lowered LDL cholesterol at 1 and 3 years, but at 5 years and at the end of the 7-year study, the low-fat diet intervention had no significant effect on LDL cholesterol levels [242]. In this multicenter, controlled trial, children were randomly assigned either to a diet intervention group instructed to follow a Step 2 NCEP diet (28% fat, <8% saturated fat, <75 mg cholesterol per 1000 calories) or a usual care group who were given educational material on heart-healthy eating with an examination once a year. Average fat and saturated fat intakes for all the children at the beginning of the study were 33% to 34% and 12.5%, respectively. As a result of the intervention, children reduced their total fat and saturated fat intakes to an average of 28.5 and 10.2% of calories, respectively. Participants in the usual care group reduced their fat and saturated fat intakes as well, to roughly 31% and 11% of calories, respectively [242]. The researchers suggest that the lack of difference in blood LDL cholesterol levels could be due to the decline in compliance in the intervention group, evidenced by higher total fat, saturated fat, and cholesterol intake over time [242]. The study provided no data on nutrient intakes, so it is unknown how the 7-year intervention impacted nutrient intakes. However, an earlier study reporting results of the DISC study at 3 years indicated that children following a low-fat diet had lower intakes of several nutrients, including calcium [243].

Consuming a fat-reduced diet appears to have an overall modest effect on blood cholesterol levels [17,18]. Moreover, individuals vary greatly in their blood lipid response to changes in dietary total and saturated fat [5,19,20,35,42,148]. In addition, very low-fat diets may have undesirable effects on blood lipids, thereby potentially increasing some individuals' risk of developing CHD. For this reason, as well as the risk of nutrient deficiencies and unresolved questions regarding the effectiveness of very-low-fat diets (i.e., <20% of total calories from fat), the AHA does not recommend the use of these diets [29]. In particular, very-low-fat diets could lead to health problems in young children, older adults, pregnant women, and individuals with hypertriglyceridemia or insulin-dependent diabetes mellitus [29].

Epidemiological and clinical trials of the impact of dietary interventions on CHD and total mortality are inconsistent [35,85,225,244–246]. In general, the benefits of following a cholesterol-lowering diet on life expectancy are greater for people at higher risk of CHD [245]. When the relationship between dietary variables and CHD mortality over 12 years was examined in 4546 adults participating in the Lipid Research Clinics Prevalence Follow-up Study, none of the dietary components examined (e.g., cholesterol, total fat, saturated fat) was linked to total deaths [246]. Although epidemiologic studies often indicate a relationship between reduced dietary fat and lower CHD risk, findings from clinical studies are less impressive [85]. A review of six primary prevention trials in high-risk, but otherwise healthy, people demonstrated no significant reduction in either CHD or all-cause mortality in most of the trials [85]. Similar findings were observed in the only two controlled secondary prevention trials in which diets low in saturated fat and cholesterol were fed to CHD patients [85]. In contrast, in five out of six studies in which the type of fat fed was altered, a more beneficial effect on CHD mortality and, to a lesser extent, all-cause mortality was observed [85]. The author of this review concluded that diets high in polyunsaturated fat and low in saturated fat are preferable to diets low in total fat in reducing CHD risk. Similar findings are reported from the Nurses' Health Study [78]. In this 14-year prospective study of over 80,000 women, substituting MUFAs and PUFAs for SFAs and *trans* USFAs was more effective in preventing CHD than reducing total fat intake [78]. No statistically-significant associations were found between intakes of total fat, animal fat, or saturated fat and CHD risk after adjusting for confounding variables [78]. Likewise, when this study was extended to 20 years, intakes of total fat intake as a percentage of energy, saturated fat, and monounsaturated fat were not statistically associated with CHD risk after adjusting for confounding risk factors [80]. Pietinen et al. [59] reported a statistically-significant inverse association between risk of CHD mortality and intake of SFAs in a cohort of 21,930 Finnish men participating in the Alpha-Tocopherol, Beta-Carotene Cancer Prevention Study.

According to a recent review of randomized clinical trials of diet interventions (i.e., reductions in total fat, saturated fat, and cholesterol intakes) and CHD outcome, there is little conclusive evidence that dietary intervention reduces total or CHD mortality [35]. The large number of studies that have examined the effect of combinations of lifestyle changes with diet on CHD outcome and total mortality yield conflicting findings [35,225]. Taubes [27], following an analysis of the history and politics behind the diet-heart hypothesis, concluded that, after 50 years of research, evidence fails to prove that consuming a low-fat diet prolongs life.

At very low levels of blood cholesterol (<160 mg/dl), the possibility that mortality increases due to some cancers, cerebral hemorrhage, respiratory disease, alcoholism, depression, suicide, and violence has been reported [247–251]. A prospective study of 2277 older adults found that low blood cholesterol was a strong predictor of all-cause mortality and could be an indicator of frailty or subclinical disease [251]. However, a causal relationship between low blood cholesterol and the above conditions remains to be established [252,253]. A meta-analysis of 19 randomized clinical trials of cholesterol-lowering interventions with diet modification or drug treatment found that low blood cholesterol levels did not increase the odds of dying from suicide, accidents, and violence [253]. However, a nonstatistically significant trend toward increased deaths from suicide and violence was observed in trials of dietary interventions and nonstatin drugs. These findings led the researchers to suggest that, although nonillness mortality was not significantly increased by cholesterol-lowering treatments, the possibility of adverse effects on psychological well-being and quality of life cannot be ruled out [253]. Clearly, additional research is needed to clarify the association between low blood cholesterol levels and mortality.

Although reducing dietary fat is a worthwhile goal for some individuals, it is not a "magic bullet" or simple solution to complex health problems like CHD. Additionally, not everyone benefits or benefits equally from reducing dietary total and saturated fat. Dietary fat may be more likely to have effects on lipoproteins and CHD risk in men vs. women, in individuals with metabolic syndrome vs. those without this disorder, and in individuals with genetically-influenced lipoprotein profiles [25,91,172,173]. Age may also influence the blood cholesterol response to dietary fat reduction. In an investigation in The Netherlands that involved 724 adults 85 years and older, high blood cholesterol levels were associated with reduced risk of death from all causes [254]. This study raises questions about the benefits of cholesterol lowering, at least in the "oldest old."

2.4.2 Safety

Although reducing fat intake as recommended is considered to be safe [5,14], some studies indicate that children and adults who consume low-fat diets may not meet their needs for specific nutrients. Depending on the fat-reduction strategy used, the overall nutritional adequacy of the diet may be compromised. In a study in Bogalusa, Louisiana, in which more than 800 children with an average age of 10 years were grouped according to fat intake, a higher percentage of children consuming a low-fat diet (<30% energy) failed to meet recommendations for vitamins B_6, B_{12}, E, thiamin, riboflavin, niacin, calcium, phosphorus, magnesium, and iron compared to those with a higher fat intake (30% to >40% of energy) [255]. Further, children following self-selected low-fat diets consumed 20% more sugar, mainly in the form of candy, sweetened beverages, and desserts than children who consumed higher-fat diets [255]. Intakes of calcium and phosphorus were significantly decreased in healthy, predominately-Hispanic preschool children in New York City who reduced their fat intake to $\leq$30% kcal (Figure 2.10) [256]. Ballew et al. [257], using reported dietary intake from the CSFII, 1994 to 1996, found that young children who consumed between

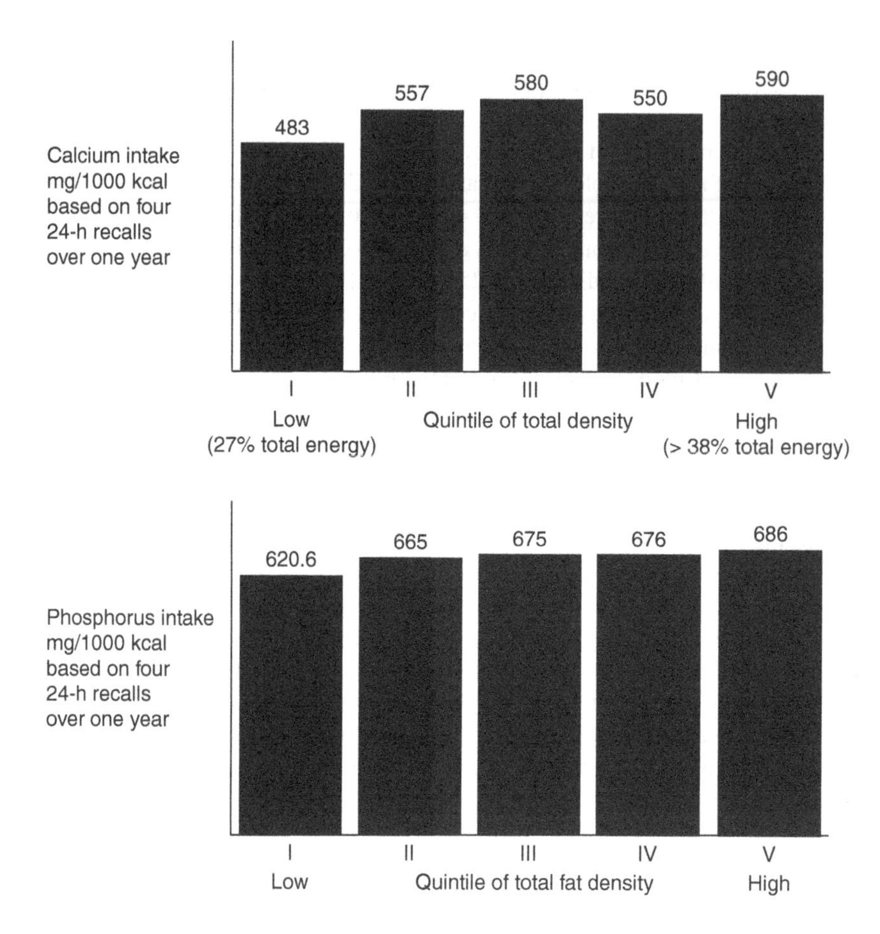

FIGURE 2.10 Intakes of calcium and phosphorus according to quintiles of total fat density in children. (Adapted from Shea, S. et al., *Pediatrics*, 92, 579, 1993. With permission.)

29% and 31.9% of calories from fat were at greater risk of inadequate intakes of vitamin E, calcium, and zinc than children with higher fat intakes.

However, children who consume a low-fat diet can meet their nutrient needs by appropriate selections of low-fat foods [11,14]. The nutrient adequacy of fat-reduced diets depends on the strategies used to decrease fat intake [11,258]. If the message to "eat less fat" is misconstrued to mean "drink less milk," children's intake of calcium, as well as some other essential nutrients, may be compromised [258]. Emphasizing fat-modified diets, while encouraging intake of low-fat and nonfat dairy products, fruits, vegetables, and grains, can help ensure that children's diets are adequate in nutrients [14,258]. Parents should receive dietary counseling on how to reduce their children's fat intake without compromising the nutritional quality of their diets [259]. Parental role modeling also is important to help children make healthful food choices [14].

Similar to children, adults who consume low-fat ($\leq$30% kcal) diets may be at risk of deficiencies of nutrients if healthful food choices are not made. According to an analysis of the diets of over 6000 middle-aged men participating in the Multiple Risk Factor Intervention Trial (MRFIT), men at risk of CHD who switched to a low-fat diet often decreased their intakes of calcium, vitamin D, iron, and zinc [260]. Similar findings were reported in another investigation of the nutrient intakes of 409 adults following the NCEP Step I and II diets for 6 months [261]. Women who followed the low-fat diet advice significantly reduced their intakes of calcium and other nutrients, such as vitamins D and E, which were already low in their diets [261]. Men following these diets had low intakes of vitamin E and zinc. Women's low intakes of calcium and vitamin D were attributed to their low intake of milk. The findings of this study led the authors to recommend that "assessment and counseling for cholesterol-lowering diets should include attention to low-fat sources of calcium and zinc in women, and zinc in men" [261].

By selecting a combination of regular and low-fat foods, including cheeses, yogurt, salad dressings, and snacks, adults and children can reduce their fat intake without compromising nutrient intake, according to a study of individuals participating in the 1994 to 1996 CSFII [262]. Eliminating certain fat-containing foods from the diet to lower the risk of CHD can lead to nutrient shortcomings and increase the risk of other diseases [262]. These researchers conclude that their findings support the paradigm that "all foods can fit" [262]. A case-control study of postmenopausal women in Italy found that those who inappropriately avoided or severely limited calcium-rich dairy products from their diet in an attempt to lower their high blood cholesterol levels had a significantly higher prevalence of osteoporosis and forearm fractures after 27 months than women in the control group who had a high intake of dairy products [263]. The researchers recommend that dietary advice to lower blood cholesterol should also focus on maintaining an adequate calcium intake by providing calcium from sources such as low-fat dairy products.

2.4.3 Dietary Compliance

A major problem with following low-fat (≤30% of energy) diets, especially among free-living populations, is long-term adherence to such diets [85,235,264,265]. Prolonged compliance to diets reduced in fat and cholesterol is difficult even for individuals who receive intensive training and follow the diet initially [264]. In a 12-week study which followed over 100 patients with high blood cholesterol levels, compliance (as determined by changes in blood lipid and lipoprotein levels and from dietary records) to a low-fat (≤30% of energy), low-cholesterol (≤300 mg/day) diet was sustained in only 30% of the patients, even after an initial 3 months of intensive diet training [264]. In another study, women participating in the Women's Health Trial were more likely to maintain a low-fat diet if they switched to low-fat versions of foods they normally consumed (except for cheese) and used low-fat cooking methods [265]. In contrast, compliance to a low-fat diet was more problematic if the women consistently avoided certain foods (e.g., meat, ice cream) and fats normally used as flavoring (e.g., butter) [265]. Men participating in the MRFIT were more likely to adhere to a low-fat diet if they were older, did not drink alcohol or smoke, did not frequently eat away from home, had high blood cholesterol and blood pressure levels, and experienced fewer stressful life events [266]. A multicenter intervention trial involving 560 adults at risk of CHD who received either prepackaged foods or nutrition guidance on low-fat diets found that compliance was better in individuals receiving the prepackaged foods (47%) than in those who self-selected low-fat diets (8%) [267]. Adults receiving the prepackaged foods also consumed twice as much calcium and higher intakes of other nutrients than those who self-selected low-fat diets [267]. In general, the more restrictive the diet is, the poorer the compliance [85].

2.4.4 The Role of Various Dairy Foods in Meeting Dietary Guidelines for Fat Intake

A nationwide public opinion survey of 700 adults conducted for the American Dietetic Association found that 57% of those interviewed believed that they had to give up certain foods to have a healthful diet [268]. However, studies indicate that all foods can be included in a healthful diet [13,262]. According to a computer analysis, individuals can choose from a variety of fat-reducing methods tailored to their tastes, lifestyles, and family's food choices [269]. This analysis indicates that individuals can meet recommended dietary goals for fat and cholesterol by making a variety of relatively simple dietary changes without reducing the amount of or eliminating foods like whole milk or substituting low-fat for whole milk. Consequently, individuals who prefer the taste of whole milk over lower-fat (2%, 1%, or fat-free) milk can still meet their total fat goal by making other selections by, for example, choosing only lean meats and reduced-fat salad dressings [269].

According to an analysis of the usage and impact of fat-modified products, adults who used two or three fat reduction strategies (e.g., fat-free milk, lean meats, fat-modified products) achieved diets containing 30% or less of fat from calories, less than 10% of calories from saturated fat, reduced in total calories, and high in vitamins and minerals [270]. The author states that energy and nutrient needs vary among individuals and that "all foods can fit into the boundaries of both micro- and macronutrient needs" [270]. When eight healthy male volunteers aged 20 to 36 years consumed diets meeting the AHA recommendations, plus one cup of whole or fat-free milk per 1000 kcal of diet for 6 weeks, both of the milk diets provided a substantial reduction in fat intake compared to the subjects' usual diet [178]. Plasma total and LDL cholesterol levels were decreased on both milk diets compared with the baseline diet, although the reductions in blood total and LDL cholesterol were greater when the fat-free milk was consumed [178]. Similar findings related to the inclusion of fast foods in a low-fat diet were reported by Davidson et al. [271]. These investigators concluded that "familiar foods with a higher fat content in the context of a well-counseled balanced diet do not need to be sacrificed to comply with the goals of the NCEP" [271].

2.5 SUMMARY

Scientific evidence fails to support the notion that intake of dairy foods in moderation contributes to increased CHD risk. In fact, several components in dairy foods may have effects that could reduce the risk of CHD. The misperception that dairy may have a negative impact on CHD risk stems from the total and saturated fat content of some products such as whole milk, cheese, and ice cream. Yet national food availability data indicate that dairy foods make a relatively small contribution to total fat, contributing far less than that provided by fats, oils, meat, poultry, and fish [38]. Moreover, individual fats in dairy foods have unique effects on blood lipid levels. Some dairy food fats (e.g., SFAs such as palmitic, myristic, and lauric acids, and cholesterol) are hypercholesterolemic, whereas others (e.g., MUFAs, PUFAs, the SFA stearic acid, low and medium chain SFAs) may have a modest hypocholesterolemic or no effect in comparison with longer-chain SFAs. Additionally, some components in dairy fats, such as CLA and sphingolipids, as well as other nutrients, such as whey peptides and calcium, in dairy products may have cardioprotective effects.

The influence of any single nutrient on blood lipid levels is highly individualized, in large part because of genetic variability. In addition, the effects of single nutrients may be different when delivered in the complex matrix of food and the overall diet. There is little evidence from scientific studies which have examined foods, rather than specific nutrients, that dairy foods contribute to an atherogenic blood profile or CHD when consumed in recommended amounts. In studies in which various milks or culture-containing dairy products such as yogurt are consumed in moderate amounts, blood lipid levels generally do not increase.

According to an analysis, if Americans increased their dairy food intake to 3 to 4 servings per day, the incidence of CHD and stroke would be reduced by 10 and 20%, respectively, beginning in 3 years, and would result in 5-year cost savings of $16.5 billion and 20 billion, respectively [272]. A consensus report from the National Medical Association recommends that the American public in general and African Americans in particular consume 3 to 4 servings a day of low-fat milk, cheese, and/or yogurt to reduce the risk of chronic diseases, including CHD, as well as CHD risk factors such as obesity/overweight and hypertension [273].

Much remains to be learned about the relationship between dietary fat intake and CHD and, in particular, how other factors (e.g., nutrients, genetics) may interact to increase or decrease CHD risk in populations or individuals. Some studies report that low-fat diets are ineffective in reducing CHD and in improving life expectancy, and may lead to potential health risks (e.g., nutritional inadequacies). In addition, only a proportion of the U.S. population responds significantly to the fat content of the diet with a change in blood lipids, and an even smaller portion is significantly responsive to the cholesterol content of their diets. Scientists are identifying genes that influence blood lipid and lipoprotein levels and individuals' responses to specific dietary interventions. This genetic information one day may allow identification of individuals most likely to benefit from consuming a low-fat diet (or other intervention). These considerations, along with the difficulty experienced by many in adhering to fat-restricted diets, are resulting in increased emphasis on an individualized approach to identifying and treating CHD. Improved identification of individuals at high risk of CHD and of those who will benefit most from specific interventions can be expected to improve health, reduce mortality, and decrease health care costs.

Recognition that very-low-fat diets ($<20\%$ of calories) may lead to nutrient shortcomings and potentially be harmful to cardiovascular health (e.g., by decreasing HDL cholesterol and increasing blood triglyceride levels) has led to less-restrictive dietary fat recommendations in recent years. Nevertheless, an overzealous attempt to reduce total and saturated fat may lead some individuals to eliminate nutrient-dense foods containing these nutrients from their diet. Omitting specific foods or food groups from the diet can lead to shortcomings of essential nutrients. Individuals who prefer higher-fat milks may switch to less-nutritious beverages, thereby jeopardizing their intake of many essential nutrients in dairy foods. Studies reveal that intake of dairy foods in recommended amounts is associated with improved intakes of essential nutrients without an adverse effect on dietary fat or cholesterol intake.

Individuals who need to follow a low-fat diet can choose from a variety of fat-reducing strategies, which can include all dairy foods. Most dietary fat recommendations encourage intake of low-fat and nonfat milk products to help keep saturated fat and cholesterol low and to maintain caloric balance. There are no "good" foods or "bad" foods relative to blood cholesterol levels or CHD risk. If an individual consumes favorite foods (e.g., whole milk, ice cream) in moderation and reduces fat intake by making other personal food choices (e.g., choosing low-fat salad dressings, fewer snack foods like potato chips), compliance to a fat-reduced diet can improve.

For a healthy vigorous existence for as long as possible, it is important to consume a variety of foods from each of the major food groups in moderation. Also important in the prevention and treatment of CHD is consideration of the individual's total risk profile (i.e., body weight, physical activity, cigarette smoking, etc.). Recognition of the variety of genetic and environmental (dietary and nondietary) factors involved in the development of CHD is leading health professionals to move away from "one-size-fits-all" dietary recommendations to more individualized guidance. Better targeting of dietary interventions to reduce CHD can improve their effectiveness and lower costs. A narrow focus on a single food, food group, or diet can be counterproductive and may, in fact, be deleterious to health.

REFERENCES

1. American Heart Association, *Heart Disease and Stroke Statistics — 2005 Update*, American Heart Association, Dallas, TX, 2005.
2. Thom, T. et al., Heart disease and stroke statistics — 2006 Update, A report from the American Heart Association Statistics Committee and Stroke Statistics Subcommittee, *Circulation*, 113, 85, 2006.
3. U.S. Department of Health and Human Services, *Healthy People 2010* (Conference Edition, in Two Volumes), Washington, D.C., January 2000.
4. Expert Panel on Detection, Evaluation, and Treatment of High Blood Cholesterol in Adults, Executive Summary of the Third Report of the National Cholesterol Education Program (NCEP) Expert Panel on Detection, Evaluation, and Treatment of High Blood Cholesterol in Adults (Adult Treatment Panel III), *JAMA*, 285, 2486, 2001.
5. Krauss, R. M. et al., AHA dietary guidelines. Revision 2000: A statement for healthcare professionals from the Nutrition Committee of the American Heart Association, *Circulation*, 102, 2284, 2000.

6. Joint WHO/FAO Expert Consultation on Diet, Nutrition and the Prevention of Chronic Diseases, WHO Technical Report Series 916, World Health Organization, Geneva, 2003.
7. Grundy, S. M. et al., Diagnosis and management of the metabolic syndrome, An American Heart Association/National Heart, Lung, and Blood Institute scientific statement, *Circulation*, 112, 2735, 2005.
8. McNamara, D. J., Dietary fatty acids, lipoproteins, and cardiovascular disease, *Adv. Food Nutr. Res.*, 36, 253, 1992.
9. Kris-Etherton, P. M. and Yu, S., Individual fatty acid effects on plasma lipids and lipoproteins: human studies, *Am. J. Clin. Nutr.*, 65 (suppl.), 1628s, 1997.
10. Grundy, S. M., What is the desirable ratio of saturated, polyunsaturated, and monounsaturated fatty acids in the diet? *Am. J. Clin. Nutr.*, 66 (suppl.), 988s, 1997.
11. Institute of Medicine of the National Academies, *Dietary Reference Intakes for Energy, Carbohydrate, Fiber, Fat, Fatty Acids, Cholesterol, and Amino Acids*, The National Academies Press, Washington, D.C., 2002.
12. Kavey, R.-E.W. et al., American Heart Association guidelines for primary prevention of atherosclerotic cardiovascular disease beginning in childhood, *Circulation*, 107, 1562, 2003.
13. U.S. Department of Health and Human Services and U.S. Department of Agriculture, Dietary Guidelines for Americans, 2005, 6th ed., U.S. Government Printing Office, Washington, D.C., 2005, www.healthierus.gov/dietaryguidelines.
14. Gidding, S. S. et al., Dietary recommendations for children and adolescents, a guide for practitioners, Consensus statement from the American Heart Association, endorsed by the American Academy of Pediatrics, *Circulation*, 112, 2061, 2005.
15. Freedman, D. S. et al., Relation of lipoprotein subclasses as measured by proton nuclear magnetic resonance spectroscopy to coronary artery disease, *Arterioscler. Thromb. Vasc. Biol.*, 18, 1046, 1998.
16. Schaefer, E. J., Lipoproteins, nutrition, and heart disease, *Am, J. Clin. Nutr.*, 75, 191, 2002.
17. Howell, W. H. et al., Plasma lipid and lipoprotein responses to dietary fat and cholesterol: a meta-analysis, *Am. J. Clin. Nutr.*, 65, 1747, 1997.
18. Clarke, R. et al., Dietary lipids and blood cholesterol: quantitative meta-analysis of metabolic ward studies, *Br. Med. J.*, 314, 112, 1997.
19. Krauss, R. M., Dietary and genetic effects on low-density lipoprotein heterogeneity, *Annu. Rev. Nutr.*, 21, 283, 2001.
20. Krauss, R. M., Dietary and genetic probes of atherogenic dyslipidemia, *Arterioscler. Thromb. Vasc. Biol.*, 25, 2265, 2005.
21. Hegsted, D. M. et al., Quantitative effects of dietary fat on serum cholesterol in man, *Am. J. Clin. Nutr.*, 17, 281, 1965.
22. Yu, S. et al., Plasma cholesterol predictive equations demonstrate that stearic acid is neutral and monounsaturated fatty acids are hypocholesterolemic, *Am. J. Clin. Nutr.*, 61, 1129, 1995.
23. Mensink, R. P. and Katan, M. B., Effect of dietary fatty acids on serum lipids and lipoproteins in a meta-analysis of 27 trials, *Arterioscler. Thromb.*, 12, 911, 1992.
24. German, J. B. and Dillard, C. J., Saturated fats: what dietary intake? *Am. J. Clin. Nutr.*, 80, 550, 2004.
25. Knopp, R. H. and Retzlaff, B. M., Saturated fat prevents coronary artery disease? An American paradox, *Am. J. Clin. Nutr.*, 80, 1102, 2004.
26. Katan, M. B., Grundy, S. M., and Willett, W. C., Should a low-fat, high-carbohydrate diet be recommended for everyone? Beyond low-fat diets, *N. Engl. J. Med.*, 337, 563, 1997.
27. Taubes, G., The soft science of dietary fat, *Science*, 291, 2535, 2001.
28. Kris-Etherton, P. M. et al., Dietary fat: assessing the evidence in support of a moderate-fat diet; the benchmark based on lipoprotein metabolism, *Proc. Nutr. Soc.*, 61, 287, 2002.
29. Lichtenstein, A. H., Van Horn, L., and for the Nutrition Committee, Very low-fat diets, *Circulation*, 98, 935, 1998.
30. American Academy of Pediatrics, Committee on Nutrition, Cholesterol in children, *Pediatrics*, 101, 141, 1998.
31. Zlotkin, S. H., A review of the Canadian "Nutrition Recommendations Update: Dietary Fat and Children," *J. Nutr.*, 126, 1022s, 1996.

32. Briefel, R. R. and Johnson, C. L., Secular trends in dietary intake in the United States, *Annu. Rev. Nutr.*, 24, 401, 2004.
33. Department of Health and Human Services, Food and Drug Administration, Food labeling: health claims and label statements; dietary saturated fat and cholesterol and coronary heart disease, *Fed. Reg.*, 58 (3), 2739, 1993.
34. U.S. Department of Agriculture, Agricultural Research Service, USDA Nutrient Database for Standard Reference, Release 18, 2005, Nutrient Data Laboratory Home Page www.ars.usda.gov/ba/bhnrc/ndl.
35. Parodi, P. W., Milk fat in human nutrition, *Austr. J. Dairy Technol.*, 59, 3, 2004.
36. Pfeuffer, M. and Schrezenmeir, J., Bioactive substances in milk with properties decreasing risk of cardiovascular diseases, *Br. J. Nutr.*, 84 (suppl. 1), 155s, 2000.
37. German, J. B. and Dillard, C. J., Composition, structure and absorption of milk lipids: a source of energy, fat-soluble nutrients and bioactive molecules, *Crit. Rev. Food Sci. Nutr.*, 46, 57, 2006.
38. Gerrior, S., Bente, L. and Hiza, H., *Nutrient Content of the U.S. Food Supply, 1909–2000*, Home Economics Research Report No. 56, U.S. Department of Agriculture, Center for Nutrition Policy and Promotion, 2004.
39. Weinberg, L. G., Berner, L. A., and Graves, J. E., Nutrient contributions of dairy foods in the United States, Continuing Survey of Food Intakes by Individuals, 1994–1996, *J. Am. Diet. Assoc.*, 104, 895, 2004.
40. Woodside, J. V. and Kromhout, D., Fatty acids and CHD, *Proc. Nutr. Soc.*, 64, 554, 2005.
41. Institute of Medicine, Food and Drug Administration, Letter Report on Dietary Reference Intakes for *Trans* Fatty Acids. Drawn from the Report on Dietary Reference Intakes for Energy, Carbohydrate, Fiber, Fat, Fatty Acids, Cholesterol, Protein, and Amino Acids, A Report of the Panel on Macronutrients, Subcommittees on Upper Reference Levels of Nutrients and on Interpretation and Uses of Dietary Reference Intakes, and the Standing Committee on the Scientific Evaluation of Dietary Reference Intakes, July 2002.
42. Schaefer, E. J. et al., Individual variability in lipoprotein cholesterol response to National Cholesterol Education Program Step 2 diets, *Am. J. Clin. Nutr.*, 65, 823, 1997.
43. Denke, M. A., Review of human studies evaluating individual dietary responsiveness in patients with hypercholesterolemia, *Am. J. Clin. Nutr.*, 62 (suppl.), 471s, 1995.
44. Mensink, R. P. et al., Effects of dietary fatty acids and carbohydrates on the ratio of serum total to HDL cholesterol and on serum lipids and apolipoproteins: a meta-analysis of 60 controlled trials, *Am. J. Clin. Nutr.*, 77, 1146, 2003.
45. Tholstrup, T. et al., Fat high in stearic acid favorably affects blood lipids and factor VII coagulant activity in comparison with fats high in palmitic acid or high in myristic and lauric acids, *Am. J. Clin. Nutr.*, 59, 371, 1994.
46. Denke, M. A. and Grundy, S. M., Comparison of effects of lauric and palmitic acid on plasma lipids and lipoproteins, *Am. J. Clin. Nutr.*, 56, 895, 1992.
47. Tholstrup, T., Vessby, B., and Sandstrom, B., Difference in effect of myristic and stearic acid on plasma HDL cholesterol within 24 hours in young men, *Eur. J. Clin. Nutr.*, 57, 735, 2003.
48. Temme, E. H., Mensink, R. P., and Hornstra, G., Comparison of the effects of diets enriched in lauric, palmitic, or oleic acids on serum lipids and lipoproteins in healthy women and men, *Am. J. Clin. Nutr.*, 63, 897, 1996.
49. Grundy, S. M., Influence of stearic acid on cholesterol metabolism relative to other long-chain fatty acids, *Am. J. Clin. Nutr.*, 60 (suppl.), 986, 1994.
50. Kritchevsky, D., Stearic acid metabolism and atherogenesis: history, *Am. J. Clin. Nutr.*, 60 (suppl.), 997, 1994.
51. Kris-Etherton, P. et al., AHA scientific statement: summary of the scientific conference on dietary fatty acids and cardiovascular health, *J. Nutr.*, 131, 1322, 2001.
52. Rudel, L. L., Parks, J. S., and Sawyer, J. K., Compared with dietary monounsaturated and saturated fat, polyunsaturated fat protects African green monkeys from coronary artery atherosclerosis, Arterioscler, *Thromb. Vasc. Biol.*, 15, 2101, 1995.
53. Rudel, L. L., Hepatic origin of cholesteryl oleate in coronary artery atherosclerosis in African green monkeys: enrichment of dietary monounsaturated fat, *J. Clin. Investig.*, 100, 74, 1997.

54. Vogel, R. A., Brachial artery ultrasound: a noninvasive tool in the assessment of triglyceride-rich lipoproteins, *Clin. Cardiol.*, 22, 6, (suppl.), 1134, 1999.
55. Lock, A. L., Parodi, P. W., and Bauman, D. E., The biology of trans fatty acids: implications for human health and the dairy industry, *Aust. J. Dairy Technol.*, 60, 134, 2005.
56. Hunter, J. E., Dietary levels of trans fatty acids: basis for health concerns and industry efforts to limit use, *Nutr. Res.*, 25, 499, 2005.
57. Food and Drug Administration, Department of Health and Human Services, Food labeling; *trans* fatty acids in nutrition labeling; consumer research to consider nutrient content and health claims and possible footnote or disclosure statements; final rule and proposed rule, *Fed. Reg.*, 68 (133), 41434, 2003.
58. Willett, W. C. et al., Intake of *trans* fatty acids and risk of coronary heart disease among women, *Lancet*, 341, 581, 1993.
59. Pietinen, P. et al., Intake of fatty acids and risk of coronary heart disease in a cohort of Finnish men: the Alpha Tocopherol, Beta-Carotene Cancer Prevention Study, *Am. J. Epidemiol.*, 145, 876, 1997.
60. Lee, K. N., Kritchevsky, D., and Pariza, M. W., Conjugated linoleic acid and atherosclerosis in rabbits, *Atherosclerosis*, 108, 19, 1994.
61. Nicolosi, R. J. et al., Dietary conjugated linoleic acid reduces plasma lipoproteins and early aortic atherosclerosis in hypercholesterolemic hamsters, *Artery*, 22 (5), 266, 1997.
62. Belury, M. A., Dietary conjugated linoleic acid in health: physiological effects and mechanisms of action, *Annu. Rev. Nutr.*, 22, 505, 2002.
63. McLeod, R. S. et al., Conjugated linoleic acids, atherosclerosis, and hepatic very-low-density lipoprotein metabolism, *Am. J. Clin. Nutr.*, 79 (suppl.), 1169s, 2004.
64. Wahle, K. W. J., Heys, S. D., and Rotondo, D., Conjugated linoleic acids: are they beneficial or detrimental to health? *Prog. Lipid Res.*, 43, 553, 2004.
65. Kritchevsky, D. et al., Influence of graded levels of conjugated linoleic acid (CLA) on experimental atherosclerosis in rabbits, *Nutr. Res.*, 22, 1275, 2002.
66. Kritchevsky, D. et al., Conjugated linoleic acid isomer effects in atherosclerosis: growth and regression of lesions, *Lipids*, 39, 611, 2004.
67. Toomey, S. et al., Regression of pre-established atherosclerosis in the apoE mouse by conjugated linoleic acid, *Biochem. Soc. Trans.*, 31, 1075, 2003.
68. Lock, A. L. et al., Butter naturally enriched in conjugated linoleic acid and vaccenic acid alters tissue fatty acids and improves the plasma lipoprotein profile in cholesterol-fed hamsters, *J. Nutr.*, 135, 2005, 1934.
69. Arbones-Mainar, J. M. et al., *Trans*-10, *cis*-12 and *cis*-9, *trans*-11-conjugated linoleic acid isomers selectively modify HDL-apolipoprotein composition in apolipoprotein E knockout mice, *J. Nutr.*, 136, 353, 2006.
70. Burdge, G. et al., Incorporation of *cis*-9, *trans*-11 conjugated linoleic acid and vaccenic acid (trans-11 18:1) into plasma and leucocyte lipids in healthy men consuming dairy products naturally enriched in these fatty acids, *Br. J. Nutr.*, 94, 237, 2005.
71. Tricon, S. et al., Opposing effects of *cis*-9, *trans*-11 and *trans*- 10, *cis*-12 conjugated linoleic acid on blood lipids in healthy humans, Am, *J. Clin. Nutr.*, 80, 614, 2004.
72. Terpstra, A. H. M., Effect of conjugated linoleic acid on body composition and plasma lipids in humans: an overview of the literature, *Am. J. Clin. Nutr.*, 79, 352, 2004.
73. Desroches, S. et al., Lack of effect of dietary conjugated linoleic acids naturally incorporated into butter on the lipid profile and body composition of overweight and obese men, *Am. J. Clin. Nutr.*, 82, 309, 2005.
74. Kobayaski, T. et al., A long-term feeding of sphingolipids affected the levels of plasma cholesterol and hepatic tricyglycerol but not tissue phospholipids and sphingolipids, *Nutr. Res.*, 17 (1), 111, 1997.
75. Noh, S. K. and Koo, S. I., Milk sphingomyelin is more effective than egg sphingomyelin in inhibiting intestinal absorption of cholesterol and fat in rats, *J. Nutr.*, 134, 2611, 2004.
76. Bernier, L. A., Roundtable discussion on milk fat, dairy foods, and coronary heart disease risk, *J. Nutr.*, 123, 1175, 1993.
77. Ascherio, A. et al., Dietary fat and risk of coronary heart disease in men: cohort follow up study in the United States, *Br. Med. J.*, 313, 84, 1996.

78. Hu, F. B. et al., Dietary fat intake and the risk of coronary heart disease in women, *N. Engl. J. Med.*, 337, 1491, 1997.
79. Sacks, F. M. and Katan, M., Randomized clinical trials on the effects of dietary fat and carbohydrate on plasma lipoproteins and cardiovascular disease, *Am. J. Med.*, 113 (suppl. 9B), 13s, 2002.
80. Oh, K. et al., Dietary fat intake and risk of coronary heart disease in women: 20 years of follow-up of the Nurses' Health Study, *Am. J. Epidemiol.*, 161, 672, 2005.
81. Katan, M. B., Effect of low-fat diets on plasma high-density lipoprotein concentrations, *Am. J. Clin. Nutr.*, 67 (suppl.), 573s, 1998.
82. Krauss, R. M., Atherogenic lipoprotein phenotype and diet–gene interactions, *J. Nutr.*, 131, 340s, 2001.
83. Asztalos, B. et al., Differential response to low-fat diet between low and normal HDL-cholesterol subjects, *J. Lipid Res.*, 41, 321, 2000.
84. Lefevre, M. et al., Individual variability in cardiovascular disease risk factor responses to low-fat and low-saturated-fat diets in men: body mass index, adiposity, and insulin resistance predict changes in LDL cholesterol, *Am. J. Clin. Nutr.*, 82, 957, 2005.
85. Oliver, M. F., It is more important to increase the intake of unsaturated fats than to decrease the intake of saturated fats: evidence from clinical trials relating to ischemic heart disease, *Am. J. Clin. Nutr.*, 66 (suppl.), 980s, 1997.
86. Morgan, S. A., O'Dea, K., and Sinclair, A. J., A low-fat diet supplemented with monounsaturated fat results in less HDL-C lowering than a very-low-fat diet, *J. Am. Diet. Assoc.*, 97, 151, 1997.
87. Hopkins, P. N., Effects of dietary cholesterol on serum cholesterol: a meta-analysis and review, *Am. J. Clin. Nutr.*, 55, 1060, 1992.
88. Ginsberg, H. N. et al., Increases in dietary cholesterol are associated with modest increases in both LDL and HDL cholesterol in healthy young women, *Arterioscler. Thromb. Vasc. Biol.*, 15, 169, 1995.
89. McNamara, D. J., Cholesterol intake and plasma cholesterol: an update, *J. Am. Coll. Nutr.*, 16 (6), 530, 1997.
90. Clifton, P. M. and Nestel, P. J., Effect of dietary cholesterol on postprandial lipoproteins in three phenotypic groups, *Am. J. Clin. Nutr.*, 64, 361, 1996.
91. Knopp, R. H. et al., Effects of insulin resistance and obesity on lipoproteins and sensitivity to egg feeding, *Arterioscler. Thromb. Vasc. Biol.*, 23, 1437, 2003.
92. Wolfe, B. M. and Piche, L. A., Replacement of carbohydrate by protein in a conventional-fat diet reduces cholesterol and triglyceride concentrations in healthy normolipidemic subjects, *Clin. Investig. Med.*, 22, 140, 1999.
93. Hu, F. B. et al., Dietary protein and risk of ischemic heart disease in women, *Am. J. Clin. Nutr.*, 70, 221, 1999.
94. Wolfe, B. M., Potential role of raising dietary protein intake for reducing the risk of atherosclerosis, *Can. J. Cardiol.*, 11 (suppl.), 127G, 1995.
95. Hu, F. B., Protein, body weight, and cardioavascular health, *Am. J. Clin. Nutr.*, 82 (suppl.), 242s, 2005.
96. Krauss, R. M., Genetic and dietary probes of atherogenic lipoprotein metabolism, presented at the American Heart Association, Robert Levy Memorial Lecture, New Orleans, LA, November 9, 2004.
97. Anonymous, Casein versus soy protein: further elucidation of their differential effect on serum cholesterol in rabbits, *Nutr. Rev.*, 49, 121, 1991.
98. Meinertz, H., Nilausen, K., and Faergeman, O., Soy protein and casein in cholesterol-enriched diets: effects on plasma lipoproteins in normolipidemic subjects, *Am. J. Clin. Nutr.*, 50, 786, 1989.
99. Potter, S. M. et al., Depression of plasma cholesterol in men by consumption of baked products containing soy protein, *Am. J. Clin. Nutr.*, 58, 501, 1993.
100. Bakhit, R. M. et al., Intake of 25 g of soybean protein with or without soybean fiber alters plasma lipids in men with elevated cholesterol concentrations, *J. Nutr.*, 124, 213, 1994.
101. Samman, S., Khosla, P., and Carroll, K. K., Influence of dietary minerals on apolipoprotein B metabolism in rabbits fed semipurified diets containing casein, *Atherosclerosis*, 82, 69, 1990.
102. Kritchevsky, D. et al., Experimental atherosclerosis in rabbits fed cholesterol-free diets, 9. Beef protein and textured vegetable protein, *Atherosclerosis*, 39, 169, 1981.

103. Sakono, M. et al., Comparison between dietary soybean protein and casein of the inhibitory effect on atherogenesis in the thoracic aorta of hypercholesterolemic (ExHc) rats treated with experimental hypervitamin D, *Biosci. Biotechnol. Biochem., (Japan)*, 61, 514, 1997.
104. Nicolosi, R. J. and Wilson, T. A., The anti-atherogenic effect of dietary soybean protein concentrate in hamsters, *Nutr. Res.*, 17 (9), 1457, 1997.
105. Lu, Y.-F. and Jian, M.-R., Effects of soy protein and casein on lipid metabolism in mature and suckling rats, *Nutr. Res.*, 17, 1341, 1997.
106. Kritchevsky, D., Dietary protein, cholesterol and atherosclerosis: a review of early history, *J. Nutr.*, 125, 589s, 1995.
107. Nilausen, K. and Meinertz, H., Lipoprotein(a) and dietary proteins: casein lowers lipoprotein(a) concentrations as compared with soy protein, *Am. J. Clin. Nutr.*, 69, 419, 1999.
108. Sacks, F. M. et al. and for the American Heart Association Nutrition Committee, Soy protein, isoflavones, and cardiovascular health, *Circulation*, 113, 1034, 2006.
109. Tailford, K. A. et al., A casein variant in cow's milk is atherogenic, *Atherosclerosis*, 170, 13, 2003.
110. McLachlan, C. N. S., B-casein A, ischemic heart disease mortality, and other illnesses, *Med. Hypotheses*, 56, 262, 2001.
111. Laugesen, M. and Elliott, R., Ischaemic heart disease, Type 1 diabetes, and cow milk A1 beta-casein, *N.Z. Med. J.*, 116, U295, 2003.
112. Mann, J. and Skeaff, M., Beta-casein variants and atherosclerosis-claims are premature (Editorial), *Atherosclerosis*, 170, 11, 2003.
113. Truswell, A. S., The A2 milk case: a critical review, *Eur. J. Clin. Nutr.*, 59, 623, 2005.
114. Chin-Dusting, J. et al., Effect of dietary supplementation with B-casein A1 or A2 on markers of disease development in individuals at high risk of cardiovascular disease, *Br. J. Nutr.*, 95, 136, 2006.
115. FitzGerald, R. J., Murray, B. A., and Walsh, D. J., Hypotensive peptides from milk proteins, *J. Nutr.*, 134, 980s, 2004.
116. Rutherford, K. J. and Gill, H. S., Peptides affecting coagulation, *Br. J. Nutr.*, 84 (suppl. 1), 99s, 2000.
117. Walzem, R. L., Dillard, C. J., and German, J. B., Whey components: millennia of evolution create functionalities for mammalian nutrition: what we know and what we may be overlooking, *Crit. Rev. Food Sci. Nutr.*, 42, 353, 2002.
118. Takeuchi, T. et al., Bovine lactoferrin reduces plasma triacyglycerol and NEFA accompanied by deceased hepatic cholesterol and triacylglycerol contents in rodents, *Br. J. Nutr.*, 91, 533, 2004.
119. Karanja, N. et al., Impact of increasing calcium in the diet on nutrient consumption, plasma lipids, and lipoproteins in humans, *Am. J. Clin. Nutr.*, 59, 900, 1994.
120. Karanja, N. et al., Plasma lipids and hypertension: response to calcium supplementation, *Am. J. Clin. Nutr.*, 45, 60, 1987.
121. Denke, M. A., Fox, M. M., and Schulte, M. C., Short-term dietary calcium fortification increases fecal saturated fat content and reduces serum lipids in men, *J. Nutr.*, 123, 1047, 1993.
122. Bell, L. et al., Cholesterol-lowering effects of calcium carbonate in patients with mild to moderate hypercholesterolemia, *Arch. Intern. Med.*, 152, 2441, 1992.
123. Bostick, R. M. et al., Relation of calcium, vitamin D, and dairy food intake to ischemic heart disease mortality among postmenopausal women, *Am. J. Epidemiol.*, 149, 151, 1999.
124. Reid, I. R. et al., Effects of calcium supplementation on serum lipid concentrations in normal older women: a randomized controlled trial, *Am. J. Med.*, 112, 343, 2002.
125. Reid, I. R., Effects of calcium supplementation on circulating lipids, *Drugs Aging*, 21, 7, 2004.
126. Jacqmain, M. et al., Calcium intake, body composition, and lipoprotein-lipid concentrations in adults, *Am. J. Clin. Nutr.*, 77, 1448, 2003.
127. Vaskonen, T., Dietary minerals and modification of cardiovascular risk factors, *J. Nutr. Biochem.*, 14, 492, 2003.
128. Greenland, P. et al., Coronary artery calcium score combined with Framingham Score for risk prediction in asymptomatic individuals, *JAMA*, 291, 210, 2004.
129. Al-Delaimy, W. K. et al., Magnesium intake and risk of coronary heart disease among men, *J. Am. Coll. Nutr.*, 23, 63, 2004.
130. McCarron, D. A. and Reusser, M. E., Are low intakes of calcium and potassium important causes of cardiovascular disease? *Am. J. Hypertens.*, 14, 206s, 2001.

131. Abbott, R. D. et al., Effect of dietary calcium and milk consumption on risk of thromboembolic stroke in older middle-aged men. The Honolulu Heart Program, *Stroke*, 27, 813, 1996.
132. Iso, H. et al., Prospective study of calcium, potassium, and magnesium intake and risk of stroke in women, *Stroke*, 30, 1772, 1999.
133. Massey, L. K., Dairy food consumption, blood pressure and stroke, *J. Nutr.*, 131, 2001, 1875.
134. Umesawa, M. et al., Dietary intake of calcium in relation to mortality from cardiovascular disease, the JACC study, *Stroke*, 37, 20, 2006.
135. Ascherio, A. et al., Intake of potassium, magnesium, calcium, and fiber and risk of stroke among U.S. men, *Circulation*, 98, 1198, 1998.
136. Bazzano, L. A. et al., Dietary potassium intake and risk of stroke in U.S. men and women. National Health and Nutrition Examination Survey. I. Epidemiological follow-up study, *Stroke*, 32, 1473, 2001.
137. U.S. Food and Drug Administration, Health claim notification for potassium containing foods, October 31, 2000 (http://vm.cfsan.fda.gov/~dms/hclm-k.html).
138. Krauss, R. M., Genetic influences on lipoprotein response to dietary fat and cholesterol: an overview, *Am. J. Clin. Nutr.*, 62, 457s, 1995.
139. Berdanier, C., Nutrient–gene interactions, *Nutr. Today*, 35, 8, 2000.
140. Dreon, D. M. and Krauss, R. M., Diet–gene interactions in human lipoprotein metabolism, *J. Am. Coll. Nutr.*, 16, 313, 1997.
141. Katan, M. B., Beynen, A. C., and de Vries, J. H. M., Existence of consistent hypo- and hyperresponders to dietary cholesterol in man, *Am. J. Epidemiol.*, 123, 221, 1986.
142. Quivers, E. S. et al., Variability in response to a low-fat, low-cholesterol diet in children with elevated low-density lipoprotein cholesterol levels, *Pediatrics*, 89, 925, 1992.
143. Denke, M. A. and Grundy, S. M., Individual responses to a cholesterol-lowering diet in 50 men with moderate hypercholesterolemia, *Arch. Intern. Med.*, 154 (3), 317, 1994.
144. Carmena-Ramon, R. et al., Genetic variation at the ApoA-IV gene locus and response to diet in familial hypercholesterolemia, *Artherioscler. Thromb. Vasc. Biol.*, 18, 1266, 1998.
145. Ordovas, J. M. et al., Gene–diet interaction in determining plasma lipid response to dietary intervention, *Atherosclerosis*, 118 (suppl.), 11s, 1995.
146. Gylling, H. et al., Polymorphisms of the genes encoding apoproteins A-1, B, C-III, and E and LDL receptor, and cholesterol and LDL metabolism during increased cholesterol intake. Common alleles of the apoprotein E gene show the greatest regulatory impact, *Arterioscler. Thromb. Vasc. Biol.*, 17, 38, 1997.
147. Breslow, J. L. et al., Genetic susceptibility to atherosclerosis, *Circulation*, 80, 724, 1989.
148. Masson, L. F., McNeill, G., and Avenell, A., Genetic variation and the lipid response to dietary intervention: a systematic review, *Am. J. Clin. Nutr.*, 77, 1098, 2003.
149. Austin, M. A. et al., Atherogenic lipoprotein phenotype: a proposed genetic marker for coronary heart disease risk, *Circulation*, 82, 495, 1990.
150. Nishina, P. M. et al., Linkage of atherogenic lipoprotein phenotype to the low density lipoprotein receptor locus on the short arm of chromosome 19, *Proc. Natl Acad. Sci. U.S.A.*, 89, 708, 1992.
151. Cohen, J. C. et al., Multiple rare alleles contribute to low plasma levels of HDL cholesterol, *Science*, 305, 869, 2004.
152. Austin, M. A. et al., Inheritance of low-density lipoprotein subclass patterns: results of complex segregation analysis, *Am. J. Hum. Genet.*, 43, 838, 1988.
153. De Graaf, J. et al., Both inherited susceptibility and environmental exposure determine the low-density lipoprotein-subfraction pattern distribution in healthy Dutch families, *Am. J. Hum. Genet.*, 51, 1295, 1992.
154. Brown, M. S. and Goldstein, J. L., Teaching old dogmas new tricks, *Nature*, 330, 113, 1987.
155. Dreon, D. M. et al., Apolipoprotein E isoform phenotype and LDL subclass response to a reduced fat diet, *Arterioscler. Thromb. Vasc. Biol.*, 15, 105, 1995.
156. Dreon, D. M. et al., Low-density lipoprotein subclass patterns and lipoprotein response to a reduced fat diet in men, *FASEB J.*, 8, 121, 1994.
157. Krauss, R. M. and Dreon, D. M., Low-density-lipoprotein subclasses and response to a low-fat diet in healthy men, *Am. J. Clin. Nutr.*, 62, 478s, 1995.

158. Dreon, D. M. et al., LDL subclass patterns and lipoprotein response to a low-fat, high-carbohydrate diet in women, *Arterioscler. Thromb. Vasc. Biol.*, 17, 707, 1997.
159. Williams, P. T. and Smallest, L. D. L. et al., particles are most strongly related to coronary disease progression in men, *Arterioscler. Thromb. Vasc. Biol.*, 23, 314, 2003.
160. Berneis, K. K. and Krauss, R. M., Metabolic origins and clinical significance of LDL heterogeneity, *J. Lipid Res.*, 43, 1363, 2002.
161. Lamarche, B. et al., Small, dense low-density lipoprotein particles as a predictor of the risk of ischemic heart disease in men, *Circulation*, 95, 69, 1997.
162. De Graaf, J. et al., Enhanced susceptibility to *in vitro* oxidation of the dense low density lipoprotein subfraction in healthy subjects, *Atherosclerosis*, 11 (2), 298, 1991.
163. Tribble, D. L. et al., Variations in oxidative susceptibility among six low density lipoprotein subfactions of differing density and particle size, *Atherosclerosis*, 93, 189, 1992.
164. Packard, C. J. and Shepard, J., Lipoprotein heterogeneity and apolipoprotein B metabolism, *Arterioscler. Thromb. Vasc. Biol.*, 17, 3542, 1997.
165. Bjornheden, T. et al., Accumulation of lipoprotein fractions and subfractions in the arterial wall, determined in an *in vitro* perfusion system, *Atherosclerosis*, 123, 43, 1996.
166. Barzilai, N. et al., Unique lipoprotein phenotype and genotype associated with exceptional longevity, *JAMA*, 290, 2030, 2003.
167. Dreon, D. M. et al., A very-low-fat diet is not associated with improved lipoprotein profiles in men with a predominance of large, low-density lipoproteins, *Am. J. Clin. Nutr.*, 69, 411, 1999.
168. Dreon, D. M., Reduced, L. D. L. et al., particle size in children consuming a very-low-fat diet is related to parental LDL-subclass patterns, *Am. J. Clin. Nutr.*, 71, 1611, 2000.
169. Lopez-Miranda, J. et al., Influence of mutation in human apolipoprotein A-1 gene promoter on plasma LDL cholesterol response to dietary fat, *Lancet*, 343, 1246, 1994.
170. Lopez-Miranda, J., Jansen, S., and Ordovas, J. M., Influence of the Sst1 polymorphism at the apolipoprotein C-III gene locus on the plasma low-density-lipoprotein-cholesterol response to dietary monounsaturated fat, *Am. J. Clin. Nutr.*, 66, 97, 1997.
171. Jones, A. E. et al., The effect of age and gender on the metabolic disposal of [1–13C] palmitic acid, *Eur. J. Clin. Nutr.*, 52, 22, 1998.
172. Mozaffarian, D., Rimm, E. B., and Herrington, D. M., Dietary fats, carbohydrate, and progression of coronary atherosclerosis in postmenopausal women, *Am. J. Clin. Nutr.*, 80, 1175, 2004.
173. Li, Z. et al., Men and women differ in lipoprotein response to dietary saturated fat and cholesterol restriction, *J. Nutr.*, 133, 3428, 2003.
174. Krauss, R. M., Genetic recipes for heart-healthy diets, *Am. J. Clin. Nutr.*, 71, 668, 2000.
175. Richardson, T., The hypocholesterolemic effect of milk — a review, *J. Food Protect.*, 41, 226, 1978.
176. Howard, N. A. and Marks, J., Hypocholesterolemic effect of milk, *Lancet*, 2, 255, 1977.
177. Hitchins, A. D. and McDonough, F. E., Prophylactic and therapeutic aspects of fermented milk, *Am. J. Clin. Nutr.*, 49, 675, 1989.
178. Steinmetz, K. A. et al., Effect of consumption of whole milk and skim milk on blood lipid profiles in healthy men, *Am. J. Clin. Nutr.*, 59, 612, 1994.
179. Hepner, G. et al., Hypocholesterolemic effect of yogurt and milk, *Am. J. Clin. Nutr.*, 32, 19, 1979.
180. Mann, G. V. and Spoerry, A., Studies of a surfactant and cholesteremia in the Masai, *Am. J. Clin. Nutr.*, 27, 464, 1974.
181. Mann, G. V., A factor in yogurt which lowers cholesteremia in man, *Atherosclerosis*, 26, 335, 1977.
182. Anderson, J. W. and Gilliland, S. E., Effect of fermented milk (yogurt) containing *Lactobacillus acidophilus* LI on serum cholesterol in hypercholesterolemic humans, *J. Am. Coll. Nutr.*, 18, 43, 1999.
183. St. Onge, M.-P., Farnworth, E. R., and Jones, P. J. H., Consumption of fermented and nonfermented dairy products: effects on cholesterol concentrations and metabolism, *Am. J. Clin. Nutr.*, 71, 674, 2000.
184. Buonopane, G. J. et al., Effect of skim milk supplementation on blood cholesterol concentration, blood pressure, and triglycerides in a free-living human population, *J. Am. Coll. Nutr.*, 11 (1), 56, 1992.
185. Agerholm-Larsen, L. et al., Effect of 8 week intake of probiotic milk products on risk factors for cardiovascular diseases, *Eur. J. Clin. Nutr.*, 54, 288, 2000.

186. Kiebling, G., Schneider, J., and Jahreis, G., Long-term consumption of fermented dairy products over 6 months increases HDL cholesterol, *Eur. J. Clin. Nutr.*, 56, 843, 2002.
187. Maruyama, C. et al., The effect of milk and skim milk intake on serum lipids and apoproteins in postmenopausal females, *J. Nutr. Sci. Vitaminol.*, 38, 203, 1992.
188. Rossouw, J. E. et al., The effect of skim milk, yogurt, and full cream milk on human serum lipids, *Am. J. Clin. Nutr.*, 34, 351, 1982.
189. Thompson, L. U. et al., The effect of fermented and unfermented milks on serum cholesterol, *Am. J. Clin. Nutr.*, 36, 1106, 1982.
190. Kritchevsky, D. et al., Influence of whole or skim milk on cholesterol metabolism in rats, *Am. J. Clin. Nutr.*, 32, 597, 1979.
191. Akalin, A. S., Gonc, S., and Duzel, S., Influence of yogurt and acidophilus yogurt on serum cholesterol levels in mice, *J. Dairy Sci.*, 80, 2721, 1997.
192. Beena, A. and Prasad, V., Effect of yogurt and bifidus yogurt fortified with skim milk powder, condensed whey and lactose-hydrolysed condensed whey on serum cholesterol and triacylglycerol levels in rats, *J. Dairy Sci.*, 64, 453, 1997.
193. Zommara, M. et al., Whey from cultured skim milk decreases serum cholesterol and increases antioxidant enzymes in liver and red blood cells in rats, *Nutr. Res.*, 16 (2), 293, 1996.
194. McNamara, D. J., Lowell, A. E., and Sabb, J. E., Effect of yogurt intake on plasma lipid and lipoprotein levels in normolipidemic males, *Atherosclerosis*, 79, 167, 1989.
195. Barr, S. I. et al., Effects of increased consumption of fluid milk on energy and nutrient intake, body weight, and cardiovascular risk factors in healthy older adults, *J. Am. Diet. Assoc.*, 100, 810, 2000.
196. Smedman, A. E. M. et al., Pentadecanoic acid in serum as a marker for intake of milk fat: relations between intake of milk fat and metabolic risk factors, *Am. J. Clin. Nutr.*, 69, 22, 1999.
197. Sjogren, P. et al., Milk-derived fatty acids are associated with a more favorable LDL particle size distribution in healthy men, *J. Nutr.*, 134, 1729, 2004.
198. McCarron, D. A. and Reusser, M., Reducing cardiovascular disease risk with diet, *Obes. Res.*, 9 (suppl. 5), 335s, 2001.
199. Appel, L. J. et al., Effect of dietary patterns on serum homocysteine. Results of a randomized, controlled feeding trial, *Circulation*, 102, 852, 2000.
200. Obarzanek, E. et al., Effects on blood lipids of a blood pressure-lowering diet: the Dietary Approaches to Stop Hypertension (DASH) Trial, *Am. J. Clin. Nutr.*, 74, 80, 2001.
201. Reusser, M. et al., Adequate nutrient intake can reduce cardiovascular disease risk in African Americans, *J. Natl Med. Assoc.*, 95, 188, 2003.
202. Harsha, D. W. et al., Effect of dietary sodium intake on blood lipids. Results from the DASH-Sodium Trial, *Hypertension*, 43 (part 2), 393, 2004.
203. Ganji, V. and Kafai, M. R., Frequent consumption of milk, yogurt, cold breakfast cereals, peppers, and cruciferous vegetables and intakes of dietary folate and riboflavin but not vitamins B-12 and B-6 are inversely associated with serum total homocysteine concentrations in the U.S. population, *Am. J. Clin. Nutr.*, 80, 1500, 2004.
204. Pereira, M. A. et al., Dairy consumption, obesity, and the insulin resistance syndrome in young adults, The CARDIA study, *JAMA*, 287, 2081, 2002.
205. Azadbakht, L. et al., Dairy consumption is inversely associated with the prevalence of the metabolic syndrome in Tehranian adults, *Am. J. Clin. Nutr.*, 82, 523, 2005.
206. Yoo, S. et al., Comparison of dietary intakes associated with metabolic syndrome risk factors in young adults: the Bogalusa Heart Study, *Am. J. Clin. Nutr.*, 80, 841, 2004.
207. Liu, S. et al., Dietary calcium, vitamin D, and the prevalence of metabolic syndrome in middle-aged and older U.S. women, *Diab. Care*, 28, 2926, 2005.
208. Warensjo, E. et al., Estimated intake of milk fat is negatively associated with cardiovascular risk factors and does not increase the risk of a first acute myocardial infarction. A prospective case-control study, *Br. J. Nutr.*, 91, 635, 2004.
209. Ness, A. R., Smith, G. D., and Hart, C., Milk, coronary heart disease, and mortality, *J. Epidemiol. Community Health*, 55, 379, 2001.
210. Elwood, P. C. et al., Milk drinking, ischaemic heart disease, and ischaemic stroke. I. Evidence from the Caerphilly cohort, *Eur. J. Clin. Nutr.*, 58, 711, 2004.

211. Elwood, P. C. et al., Milk drinking, ischaemic heart disease, and ischaemic stroke. II. Evidence from cohort studies, *Eur. J. Clin. Nutr.*, 58, 718, 2004.
212. Elwood, P. C., Milk and cardiovascular disease: a review of the epidemiological evidence, *Aust. J. Dairy Technol.*, 60, 58, 2005.
213. Elwood, P. C. et al., Milk consumption, stroke, and heart disease risk: evidence from the Caerphilly cohort of older men, *J. Epidemiol. Community Health*, 59, 502, 2005.
214. Kris-Etherton, P. M. et al., The role of fatty acid saturation on plasma lipids, lipoproteins, and apolipoproteins. I. Effects of whole food diets high in cocoa butter, olive oil, soybean oil, dairy butter, and milk chocolate on the plasma lipids of young men, *Metabolism*, 42 (1), 121, 1993.
215. Cox, C. et al., Effects of coconut oil, butter and safflower oil on lipids and lipoproteins in persons with moderately elevated cholesterol levels, *J. Lipid Res.*, 36, 1787, 1995.
216. Chisholm, A. et al., Effect on lipoprotein profile of replacing butter with margarine in a lowfat diet: randomised crossover study with hypercholesterolemic subjects, *Br. Med. J.*, 312, 931, 1996.
217. Wood, R. et al., Effect of butter, mono- and polyunsaturated fatty acid-enriched butter, trans fatty acid margarine, and zero trans fatty acid margarine on serum lipids and lipoproteins in healthy men, *J. Lipid Res.*, 34 (1), 1, 1993.
218. Gillman, M. W. et al., Margarine intake and subsequent coronary heart disease in men, *Epidemiology*, 8, 144, 1997.
219. Biong, A. S. et al., A comparison of the effects of cheese and butter on serum lipids, haemostatic variables and homocysteine, *Br. J. Nutr.*, 92, 791, 2004.
220. Tholstrup, T. et al., Does fat in milk, butter and cheese affect blood lipids and cholesterol differently? *J. Am. Coll. Nutr.*, 23, 169, 2004.
221. Nestel, P. J., Chronopulos, A., and Cehun, M., Dairy fat in cheese raises LDL cholesterol less than that in butter in mildly hypercholesterolemic subjects, *Eur. J. Clin. Nutr.*, 59, 1059, 2005.
222. Roupas, P. et al., The impact of cheese consumption on markers of cardiovascular risk in rats, *Int. Dairy J.*, 16, 243, 2006.
223. Tholstrup, T., Dairy products and cardiovascular disease, *Curr. Opin. Lipidol.*, 17, 1, 2006.
224. Ravnskov, U., The questionable role of saturated and polyunsaturated fatty acids in cardiovascular disease, *J. Clin. Epidemiol.*, 51, 443, 1998.
225. Hooper, L. et al., Dietary fat intake and prevention of cardiovascular disease: systematic review, *Br. Med. J.*, 322, 757, 2001.
226. Ramsay, L. E., Yeo, W. W., and Jackson, P. R., Dietary reduction of serum cholesterol: time to think again, *Br. Med. J.*, 303, 953, 1991.
227. Hunninghake, D. B. et al., The efficacy of intensive dietary therapy alone or combined with Lovastatin in outpatients with hypercholesterolemia, *N. Engl. J. Med.*, 328, 1213, 1993.
228. Howard, B. V. et al., Low-fat dietary pattern and risk of cardiovascular disease: the Women's Health Initiative Randomized Controlled Dietary Modification Trial, *JAMA*, 295, 655, 2006.
229. Kinosian, B., Glick, H., and Garland, G., Cholesterol and coronary heart disease: predicting risks by levels and ratios, *Ann. Intern. Med.*, 121, 641, 1996.
230. Knopp, R. H. et al., Long-term cholesterol-lowering effects of 4 fat-restricted diets in hypercholesterolemic and combined hyperlipidemic men, *JAMA*, 278, 1509, 1997.
231. Jeppersen, J. et al., Effects of low-fat, high-carbohydrate diets on risk factors for ischaemic heart disease in postmenopausal women, *Am. J. Clin. Nutr.*, 65, 1027, 1997.
232. Walden, C. E. et al., Lipoprotein lipid response to the National Cholesterol Education Program Step II diet by hypercholesterolemic and combined hyperlipidemic women and men, *Arterioscler. Thromb. Vasc. Biol.*, 17, 375, 1997.
233. Cheung, M. C., Lichtenstein, A. H., and Schaefer, E. J., Effects of a diet restricted in saturated fatty acids and cholesterol on the composition of apolipoprotein A-1-containing lipoprotein particles in the fasting and fed states, *Am. J. Clin. Nutr.*, 60, 911, 1994.
234. Abbasi, F. et al., High carbohydrate diets, triglyceride-rich lipoproteins, and coronary heart disease risk, *Am. J. Cardiol.*, 85, 45, 2000.
235. Meksawan, K. et al., Effect of low and high fat diets on nutrient intakes and selected cardiovascular risk factors in sedentary men and women, *J. Am. Coll. Nutr.*, 23, 131, 2004.

236. Ginsberg, H. N., for the DELTA Research Group et al., Effects of reducing dietary saturated fatty acids on plasma lipids and lipoproteins in healthy subjects, The Delta Study, Protocol 1, *Arterioscler. Thromb. Vasc. Biol.*, 18, 441, 1998.
237. Dreon, D. M. et al., Change in dietary saturated fat intake is associated with change in mass of large low-density-lipoprotein particles in men, *Am. J. Clin. Nutr.*, 67, 828, 1998.
238. Berglund, L. et al., HDL-subpopulation patterns in response to reductions in dietary total and saturated fat intakes in healthy subjects, *Am. J. Clin. Nutr.*, 70, 992, 1999.
239. Hu, F. B. and Willett, W. C., Reply to OH Holmquist: protein, fat and ischemic heart disease, *Am. J. Clin. Nutr.*, 71, 848, 2000.
240. Ortega, R. M. et al., Effect of saturated fatty acid consumption on energy and nutrient intake and blood lipid levels in preschool children, *Ann. Nutr. Metab.*, 45, 121, 2001.
241. Samuelson, G. et al., Dietary fat intake in healthy adolescents: inverse relationships between the estimated intake of saturated fatty acids and serum cholesterol, *Br. J. Nutr.*, 85, 333, 2001.
242. Obarzanek, E. et al., Long-term safety and efficacy of a cholesterol-lowering diet in children with elevated low-density lipoprotein cholesterol: seven-year results of dietary intervention study in children (DISC), *Pediatrics*, 107, 256, 2001.
243. Obarzanek, E. et al., Safety of a fat-reduced diet: the dietary intervention study in children (DISC), *Pediatrics*, 100, 51, 1997.
244. Ravnskov, U. et al., Studies of dietary fat and heart disease, *Science*, 295, 1464, 2002.
245. Smith, G. D., Song, F., and Sheldon, T. A., Cholesterol lowering and mortality: the importance of considering initial level of risk, *Br. Med. J.*, 306, 1367, 1993.
246. Esrey, K. L., Joseph, L., and Grover, S. A., Relationship between dietary intake and coronary heart disease mortality: Lipid Research Clinics Prevalence Follow-up Study, *J. Clin. Epidemiol.*, 49, 211, 1996.
247. Zureik, M., Courbon, D., and Ducimetiere, P., Decline in serum total cholesterol and the risk of death from cancer, *Epidemiology*, 8, 137, 1997.
248. Raiha, I. et al., Effect of serum lipids, lipoproteins, and apolipoproteins on vascular and nonvascular mortality in the elderly, *Arterioscler. Thromb. Vasc. Biol.*, 17, 1224, 1997.
249. Zureik, M., Courbon, D., and Ducimetiere, P., Serum cholesterol concentration and death from suicide in men: Paris prospective study, *Br. Med. J.*, 313, 649, 1996.
250. Golumb, B. A., Cholesterol and violence: is there a connection? *Ann. Intern. Med.*, 128, 478, 1998.
251. Schupf, N. et al., Relationship between plasma lipids and all-cause mortality in nondemented elderly, *J. Am. Geriatr. Soc.*, 53, 219, 2005.
252. Wardle, J. et al., Randomized trial of the effects of cholesterol-lowering dietary treatment on psychological function, *Am. J. Med.*, 108, 547, 2000.
253. Muldoon, M. F. et al., Cholesterol reduction and non-illness mortality: meta-analysis of randomized clinical trials, *Br. Med. J.*, 322, 11, 2001.
254. Weverling-Rijnsburger, A. W. E. et al., Total cholesterol and risk of mortality in the oldest old, *Lancet*, 350, 1119, 1997.
255. Nicklas, T. A. et al., Nutrient adequacy of lowfat intakes for children: the Bogalusa Heart Study, *Pediatrics*, 89, 221, 1992.
256. Shea, S. et al., Is there a relationship between dietary fat and stature or growth in children three to five years of age? *Pediatrics*, 92, 579, 1993.
257. Ballew, C. et al., Nutrient intakes and dietary patterns of young children by dietary fat intakes, *J. Pediatr.*, 136, 181, 2000.
258. Johnson, R. K., Can children follow a fat-modified diet and have adequate nutrient intakes essential for optimal growth and development? *J. Pediatr.*, 136, 143, 2000.
259. Kaistha, A. et al., Overrestriction of dietary fat intake before formal nutritional counseling in children with hyperlipidemia, *Arch. Pediatr. Adolesc. Med.*, 155, 1225, 2001.
260. Dolecek, T. A. et al., Nutritional adequacy of diets reported at baseline and during trial years 1–6 by the special intervention and usual care groups in the Multiple Risk Factor Intervention Trial, *Am. J. Clin. Nutr.*, 65 (1), 305s, 1997.
261. Retzlaff, B. M. et al., Nutritional intake of women and men on the NCEP Step I and Step II diets, *J. Am. Coll. Nutr.*, 16 (1), 52, 1997.

262. Sigman-Grant, M., Warland, R., and Hsieh, G., Selected lower-fat foods positively impact nutrient quality in diets of free-living Americans, *J. Am. Diet. Assoc.*, 103, 570, 2003.
263. Varenna, M. et al., Unbalanced diet to lower serum cholesterol level is a risk factor for postmenopausal osteoporosis and distal forearm fracture, *Osteop. Int.*, 12, 296, 2001.
264. Henkin, Y. et al., Saturated fats, cholesterol, and dietary compliance, *Arch. Intern. Med.*, 152, 1167, 1992.
265. Kristal, A. R. et al., Long-term maintenance of a low-fat diet: durability of fat-related dietary habits in the women's health trial, *J. Am. Diet. Assoc.*, 92, 553, 1992.
266. Van Horn, L. V. et al., Adherence to dietary recommendations in the special intervention group in the Multiple Risk Factor Intervention Trial, *Am. J. Clin. Nutr.*, 65 (1), 289s, 1997.
267. McCarron, D. A. et al., Nutritional management of cardiovascular risk factors, *Arch. Intern. Med.*, 157, 169, 1997.
268. The American Dietetic Association, *Nutrition and You, Trends 2000*, The American Dietetic Association, Chicago, IL, 2002.
269. Smith-Schneider, L. M., Sigman-Grant, M. J., and Kris-Etherton, P. M., Dietary fat reduction strategies, *J. Am. Diet. Assoc.*, 92, 34, 1992.
270. Sigman-Grant, M., Can you have your low-fat cake and eat it too? The role of fat-modified products, *J. Am. Diet. Assoc.*, 97 (suppl.), 76s, 1997.
271. Davidson, M. H. et al., Efficacy of the National Cholesterol Education Program Step 1 Diet, *Arch. Intern. Med.*, 156, 305, 1996.
272. McCarron, D. A. and Heaney, R. P., Estimated healthcare savings associated with adequate dairy food intake, *Am. J. Hypertens.*, 17, 88, 2004.
273. Wooten, W. J. and Price, W., Consensus Report of the National Medical Association. The role of dairy and dairy nutrients in the diet of African Americans, *J. Natl Med. Assoc.*, 96 (Dec. suppl.), 1s, 2004.

3 Dairy Foods and Hypertension

3.1 INTRODUCTION

At least 65 million adults — or nearly one-third (31.3%) of the U.S. adult population — have hypertension, according to 1999 to 2000 data from the National Health and Nutrition Examination Survey (NHANES) [1]. This number represents a 30% increase in the past decade [1]. Hypertension is defined as a blood pressure equal to or greater than 140 mm Hg systolic (contracting), or 90 mm Hg diastolic (resting), or use of antihypertensive medications, or a medical history of hypertension [1]. In addition, an estimated 45 million Americans are considered to be prehypertensive [2]. Prehypertension is defined as a systolic blood pressure of 120 to 139 mm Hg or a diastolic blood pressure of 80 to 89 mm Hg (Table 3.1) [2]. Individuals with pre-hypertension are at high risk of developing hypertension and are advised to adopt lifestyle changes that lower their blood pressure [2]. Blood pressure has also risen among children and adolescents over the past decade, in part because of the increased prevalence of overweight in this population [3]. Children whose blood pressure falls into the 95th percentile or higher for size and age are considered hypertensive [4]. Those in the 90th to 95th percentiles are now called prehypertensive. Similar to the adult guidelines, the threshold for prehypertension in adolescents is 120/80 [4].

The increase in obesity and an aging and growing population underlie the increased burden of hypertension in the United States [1,3]. The age-related increase in systolic blood pressure is primarily responsible for the increase in hypertension with advancing age [2]. The prevalence of hypertension is higher for African Americans than for Mexican Americans or non-Hispanic whites (Table 3.2) [1,2]. High blood pressure is nearly 40% higher in African Americans, and they develop it earlier in life and with greater consequences than Caucasians [5]. Until age 55, men are at greater risk of high blood pressure than women, whereas after age 55, the percentage of women with high blood pressure is higher [6]. Hypertension can also result as a complication of pregnancy [2].

Uncontrolled high blood pressure increases the risk for cardiovascular disease, stroke, heart failure, and kidney disease [2]. For every 20 mm Hg systolic or 10 mm Hg diastolic increase in blood pressure, mortality from ischemic heart disease and stroke doubles [2]. Control of blood pressure, particularly systolic blood pressure, can reduce morbidity and mortality from stroke, heart disease, and renal failure. Researchers estimate that a 5 mm Hg reduction in systolic blood pressure in the population would reduce mortality due to stroke by 14%, mortality due to heart disease by 9%, and all-cause mortality by 7% [2]. Not only is hypertension in children, adolescents, and adults on the rise, but more than 40% of adult hypertensives are not being treated, and two-thirds of adult hypertensives are not reaching the goal of blood pressure levels of <140/90 mm Hg (Table 3.3) [2]. For 2006, the estimated cost of hypertension is $63.5 billion in direct medical (e.g., cost of physicians, medications) and indirect (e.g., lost wages, lowered productivity) expenditures [6].

Given the high prevalence, serious health consequences, and staggering economic burden of hypertension, the U.S. Department of Health and Human Services' National Health Promotion and Disease Prevention Objectives for the year 2010 call for reducing uncontrolled high blood pressure [5]. A specific goal is to increase blood pressure control (i.e., from an estimated 18% to 50%)

TABLE 3.1
Classification of Blood Pressure for Adults

BP Classification	SBP (mm Hg)	DBP (mm Hg)
Normal	<120	And <80
Prehypertension	120 to 139	Or 80 to 69
Stage 1 hypertension	140 to 159	Or 90 to 99
Stage 2 hypertension	≥ 160	Or ≥ 100

Source: From Chobanian, A. V. et al., *Hypertension*, 42, 1206, 2003. With permission.

in people with high blood pressure [5]. Modestly reducing the general population's blood pressure level can have a major positive impact on health [2].

Both genetic and environmental factors influence the risk of hypertension [2,7]. Because of the high cost of and potential adverse side effects associated with pharmacological therapy for this disease, individuals are encouraged to adopt lifestyle modifications to treat or reduce their risk of high blood pressure (Table 3.4) [2,4]. These lifestyle modifications include weight reduction, if overweight; adoption of the Dietary Approaches to Stop Hypertension (DASH) eating plan, which is a low-fat diet rich in fruits and vegetables and low-fat dairy products; dietary sodium reduction

TABLE 3.2
Trend of Age-Adjusted Rates for U.S. Adults with Hypertension by Sex, Race, and Ethnicity

	Age-Adjusted Hypertension Prevalence			
	1988 to 1994		1999 to 2000	
Sex, Race, and Ethnicity	Percent	SE	Percent	SE
Both sexes	24.5	0.6	28.4[a]	1.1
Non-Hispanic white	23.4	0.7	27.2	1.3
Non-Hispanic black	36.2	0.9	38.8	1.5
Mexican American	25.4	0.8	28.7	1.3
Other	20.3	1.7	29.8	2.8
Male	25.4	0.9	28.3	1.5
Non-Hispanic white	24.6	1.0	27.4	1.7
Non-Hispanic black	35.7	1.2	37.5	2.1
Mexican American	25.9	1.1	28.7	2.2
Other	20.7	2.5	26.5	3.8
Female	23.3	0.6	28.7	1.2
Non-Hispanic white	21.9	0.7	26.6	1.4
Non-Hispanic black	36.3	0.9	39.5	2.0
Mexican American	24.5	0.8	28.0	2.1
Other	19.6	1.8	31.1	3.0

Age-adjusted to year 2000 standard; hypertension defined by NHANES BP readings (systolic ≥ 140 mm Hg or diastolic ≥ 90 mm Hg) or use of antihypertensive medication,

[a] Value computed using crude age-specific and sex-specific rates and copulation numbers.

Source: From Fields, L. E. et al., *Hypertension*, 44, 1, 2004. With permission.

TABLE 3.3
Trends in Awareness, Treatment, and Control of High Blood Pressure: 1976 to 2000

	National Health and Nutrition Examination Survey, %			
	1976 to 1980 [257]	**1988 to 1991 [257]**	**1991 to 1994 [4]**	**1999 to 2005 [5]**
Awareness	51	73	68	70
Treatment	31	55	54	59
Control[a]	10	29	27	34

Percentage of adults aged 18 to 74 years with systolic blood pressure (SBP) of 140 mm Hg or greater, diastolic blood pressure (DBP) of 90 mm Hg or greater, or taking antihypertensive medication.

[a] SBP below 140 mm Hg and DBP below 90 mm Hg and on antihypertensive medication.

Source: From Chobanian, A. V. et al., *Hypertension*, 42, 1206, 2003. With permission.

(no more than 2.4 g sodium or 6 g sodium chloride for adults); regular physical activity; and, for adults, moderation in alcohol consumption [2,4]. Historically, sodium restriction has been the focus of hypertension prevention and treatment; however, the National Heart, Lung and Blood Institute (NHLBI), in its lifestyle modifications for adults, ranks the DASH diet ahead of sodium restriction as the most effective nutritional intervention to control blood pressure [2].

This chapter reviews scientific evidence supporting the beneficial role of a dietary pattern, including dairy foods in the prevention and treatment of hypertension, and how dairy food nutrients (e.g., calcium, potassium, magnesium, protein) contribute to this beneficial effect. It is important to recognize that nutrients are not consumed in isolation, but as interactive components of the total

TABLE 3.4
Life-Style Modifications to Prevent and Manage Hypertension

Modification	Recommendation	Approximate SBP Reduction (Range)[a]
Weight reduction	Maintain normal body weight (body mass index 18.5 to 24.9 kg/m^2)	5 to 20 mm Hg/10 kg [92,93]
Adopt DASH eating plan	Consume a diet rich in fruits, vegetables, and low-fat dairy products with a reduced content of saturated and total fat	8 to 14 mm Hg [94,95]
Dietary sodium reduction	Reduce dietary sodium intake to no more than 100 mmol per day (2.4 g sodium or 6 g sodium chloride)	2 to 8 mm Kg [94–96]
Physical activity	Engage in regular aerobic physical activity such as brisk walking (at least 30 minutes per day, most days of the week)	4 to 9 mm Hg [97,98]
Moderation of alcohol consumption	Limit consumption to no more than two drinks (e.g., 24 oz beer, 10 oz wine, or 3 oz 80-proof whiskey) per day in most men and to no more than 1 drink per day in women and lighter-weight persons	2 to 4 mm Hg [99]

DASH indicates dietary approaches to stop hypertension. For overall cardiovascular risk reduction, stop smoking.

[a] The effects of implementing these modifications are dose- and time-dependent and could be greater for some individuals.

Source: From Chobanian, A. V. et al., *Hypertension*, 42, 1206, 2003. With permission.

diet [8]. The high degree of intercorrelation among dietary factors may account for some of the heterogeneity in blood pressure response to variations in intake of individual nutrients [8]. Moreover, findings from a single intervention (i.e., a specific nutrient) may underestimate the effects achieved with combined interventions. Studies indicate that dietary patterns yielding nutrients as they occur together in foods significantly lower blood pressure [9–11]. Other lifestyle modifications to prevent or treat hypertension, such as weight reduction and dietary sodium reduction, are also discussed, as well as the effect of a combination of lifestyle interventions.

3.2 DIETARY PATTERNS INCLUDING DAIRY FOODS AND BLOOD PRESSURE

Twenty years ago, changes in the overall dietary pattern to include more dairy foods, fruits, and vegetables were associated with lower blood pressure [12]. Support for this approach to blood pressure control has more recently been provided by U.S. government-sponsored controlled-feeding intervention trials, called DASH [9,11].

The first multicenter DASH trial sponsored by the NHLBI included 459 adults with systolic blood pressures of less than 160 mm Hg and diastolic pressures of 80 to 95 mm Hg (i.e., high-normal blood pressure) [9]. About half of the participants were women and nearly 60% were African Americans. For 8 weeks, participants were randomly assigned to one of the following three dietary plans: a "control" diet similar to what many Americans consume (low in fruits, vegetables, and dairy products, and containing 36% of calories from fat); a "fruits and vegetables" diet (higher in fiber, potassium, and magnesium than in the control diet, but similar in fat); or a "combination" diet (the so-called DASH diet) high in low-fat dairy foods, fruits, and vegetables and reduced in total fat (26% of calories), saturated fat, and cholesterol (i.e., higher in fiber, protein, potassium, magnesium, and calcium than the control diet). The DASH combination diet also included whole grains, poultry, fish, and nuts and small amounts of red meat, sweets, and sugar-containing beverages [9]. Sodium intake (approximately 3 g/day), body weight, and physical activity remained constant throughout the study. An in-depth description of the DASH feeding trial can be found in a supplement to the Journal of the American Dietetic Association [13].

The DASH combination diet, which included low-fat dairy foods, fruits, and vegetables, produced the largest reductions in blood pressures (Figure 3.1) [9]. Overall, this diet reduced systolic blood pressure by 5.5 mm Hg and diastolic blood pressure by 3.0 mm Hg compared to the control diet. The fruits and vegetables diet also reduced systolic and diastolic blood pressures (i.e., by 2.8 mm Hg and 1.1 mm Hg, respectively), although by about half that achieved with the DASH combination diet (Table 3.5). For participants with hypertension, the blood pressure-lowering effect of the DASH combination diet was even more impressive, with average reductions of 11.4 mm Hg for systolic and 5.5 mm Hg for diastolic blood pressures compared to the control diet (Table 3.5) [9]. The reduction in blood pressure on the DASH combination diet occurred quickly (within 2 weeks), remained lower as long as the participants stayed on the diet, and rivaled that achieved with typical single-drug therapy [9]. Participants following the DASH diet (at the 2000 calorie level) consumed about 3 servings/day of dairy foods and 8 to 10 servings/day of fruits and vegetables. The blood pressure-lowering effect of the DASH diet was independent of body weight, sodium intake, or alcohol intake [9].

The potential savings in health care costs attributed to the DASH diet are likely substantial, considering that after 8 weeks of consuming the DASH diet, 70% of participants with an initially high blood pressure had a normal blood pressure and would no longer need pharmacological management of their hypertension [14]. The DASH researchers estimate that if Americans eating a typical Western diet adopt the DASH dietary pattern, heart disease could be reduced by 15% and stroke by 27% [9].

A second DASH study, DASH-Sodium, was conducted to examine the blood pressure effects of the DASH diet in combination with various levels of sodium intake [11]. This multicenter, randomized controlled trial included 412 adults (41% hypertensives, 40% Caucasians, and 57% African

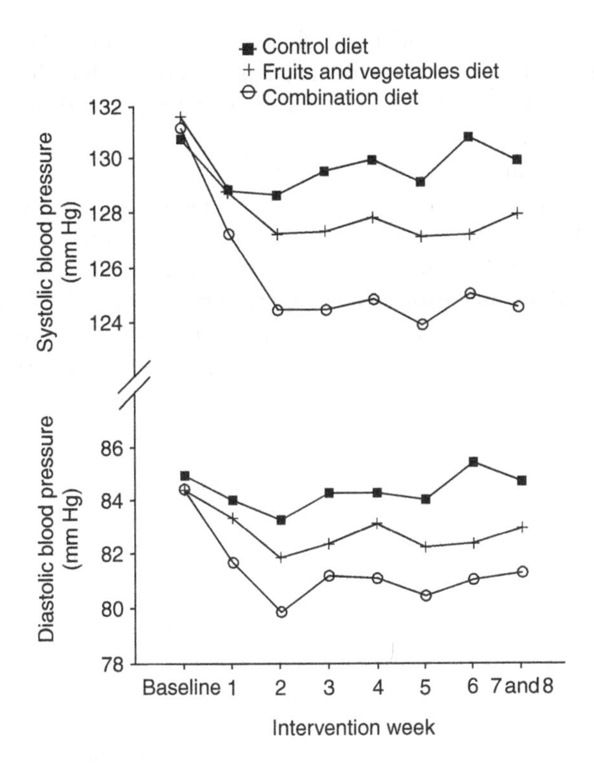

FIGURE 3.1. Mean systolic and diastolic blood pressures at baseline and during each intervention week, according to diet, for 379 subjects with complete sets of weekly blood pressure measurements. (From Appel, L. J. et al., *N. Engl. J. Med.*, 336, 1117, 1997.)

TABLE 3.5
Mean Changes in Blood Pressure in the Intervention Diets Compared to the Control Diet in the DASH Study

Category	Combination Group (97.5% CI)	P value	Fruits and Vegetables Group (97.5% CI)	P value
Systolic blood pressure (mm Hg)				
All subjects ($n = 459$)	−5.5(−7.4 to −3.7)	<0.001	−2.8(−4.7 to −0.9)	<0.001
Hypertensive ($n = 133$)[a]	−11.4(−15.9 to −6.9)	<0.0001	7.2(−11.4 to −3.0)	<0.001
Nonhypertensive ($n = 326$)	−3.5(−5.3 to −1.6)	<0.001	−0.8(−2.7 to 1.1)	0.33
Diastolic blood pressure (mm Hg)				
All subjects ($n = 459$)	−3.0(−4.3 to −1.6)	<0.001	−1.1(−2.4 to 0.3)	0.07
Hypertensive ($n = 133$)	−5.5(−8.2 to −2.7)	<0.001	−2.8(−5.4 to −0.3)	0.01
Nonhypertensive ($n = 326$)	−2.1(−3.6 to −0.5)	0.003	−0.3(−1.9 to 1.3)	0.71

CI, Confidence interval; DASH, Dietary approaches to stop hypertension.

[a] Hypertension was defined as a baseline systolic blood pressure ≥140 mm Hg or a dlastolic blood pressure ≥90 mm Hg.

Source: From McCarron, D. A. and Reusser, M. E., *Am. J. Hypertens.*, 14, 206s, 2001. With permission.

Americans) [11]. Participants were randomly assigned to either a typical American diet (control) or the DASH diet. Within each of these diets, participants ate foods with high (~3.5 g or 150 mmol), intermediate (~2.3 g or 100 mmol), or low (~1.2 g or 50 mmol) targeted levels of sodium for 30 days each in random order.

The DASH diet significantly lowered systolic blood pressure, regardless of the level of sodium consumed [11]. This finding confirms and extends the findings of the previous DASH trial [9], which demonstrated that the first step in blood pressure control is improving the overall diet by increasing intake of low-fat dairy foods, fruits, and vegetables. With both the control and the DASH diet, reducing sodium intake lowered blood pressure in a step-wise fashion [11]. The DASH diet at the highest sodium level reduced systolic blood pressure by 5.9 mm Hg compared to the control diet at the same sodium level. For participants consuming the DASH diet, reducing sodium intake to the intermediate level lowered systolic blood pressure by an additional 1.3 mm Hg, and reducing sodium to the lowest level resulted in an additional 1.7 mm Hg drop in systolic blood pressure [11].

Because blood pressure data (i.e., means and standard deviations) on the effect of the DASH-Sodium diet in normotensive subjects has not been reported and a study by Bray et al. [15] shows that the "delta" did not change in this group once on the DASH diet, it remains unproven whether the entire population would benefit by any degree of sodium reduction once on the DASH diet [16]. With the exception of older African American adults with established hypertension, consuming the DASH diet alone provided the most significant reduction in blood pressure for the majority of participants [16]. The findings of the DASH-Sodium diet, like the DASH diet, demonstrate that intake of a diet that meets currently recommended nutrient levels is the most effective nutritional approach for managing blood pressure. If the nutrient quality of the diet is adequate, sodium intake may have little effect on blood pressure control in the majority of individuals [16].

Although the blood pressure-lowering effect of the DASH diet is applicable to most people, both normotensives and hypertensives, some individuals benefit more than others. The DASH diet has been shown to lower blood pressure more in persons with hypertension than in those without hypertension [9,11,17,18]. In persons without hypertension, the DASH combination diet lowered systolic and diastolic blood pressures by 3.5 and 2.2 mm Hg, respectively, compared to the control diet [17]. However, in hypertensive subjects, systolic and diastolic blood pressures were reduced by 11.6 and 5.3 mm Hg, respectively, compared to the control diet [17]. A subgroup analysis of 133 hypertensive participants in the DASH trial supports the benefits of this dietary pattern for individuals with hypertension [14]. The DASH diet was found to be an effective treatment for adults with stage 1 isolated systolic hypertension, evidenced by a reduction in systolic blood pressure comparable to that achieved with a typical antihypertensive drug [19]. Moreover, the DASH diet enhances the effectiveness of antihypertensive medication [20]. The beneficial effect of the DASH eating pattern for hypertensives was also observed in the DASH-Sodium trial [11,18].

The DASH dietary pattern is particularly effective for minorities, such as African Americans, who are at higher risk of developing hypertension and its complications than are their white counterparts [11,21–24]. According to a subgroup analysis of the DASH trial, the DASH combination diet lowered systolic blood pressure significantly more in African Americans (6.8 mm Hg) than in whites (3.3 mm Hg) [17]. Similar beneficial findings for African Americans are reported in the DASH-Sodium trial [11]. The increased effectiveness of the DASH combination diet for African Americans supports other findings suggesting racial differences in blood pressure responses to diet [22]. African Americans' high risk for hypertension may be explained in part by deficiencies of multiple nutrients [24]. A study of 180 minority adolescents at risk of developing high blood pressure found that blood pressure was lower in adolescents who had higher intakes of potassium, calcium, magnesium, and vitamins [24]. The researchers suggest "diets rich in combination of nutrients derived from fruits, vegetables, and low-fat dairy products could contribute to primary prevention of hypertension when instituted at an early age" [24].

The beneficial effect of a dietary pattern similar to the DASH diet has been demonstrated in other studies [10,12,25–28]. Nowson and colleagues in Australia compared the effectiveness of a modified DASH diet containing 4 daily servings of fruit, 4 daily servings of vegetables, 3 daily servings of nonfat dairy products, and fish three times a week with that of a conventional low-fat diet, both in promoting weight loss and in reducing blood pressure [26]. This 12-week clinical trial included 54 overweight/obese middle-aged men with higher-than-normal blood pressure. In addition to defined diets, each subject was instructed to exercise moderately for at least 30 minutes on all or most days of the week. Both diet groups lost approximately 11 pounds over the 12-week study period. However, the reduction in systolic and diastolic blood pressures was much greater in the group consuming the modified DASH diet [26]. There were no differences between the groups in fruit or vegetable intakes, whereas the group consuming the modified DASH diet had a significantly higher dairy food intake than the other group. The researchers speculate that a combination of factors, including lower sodium with increased potassium, calcium, and magnesium intakes, may account for the greater reduction in blood pressure achieved with the modified DASH diet than with the low-fat diet [26].

Similar to the DASH diet, OmniHeart diets reduced in saturated fat and cholesterol and rich in fruit, vegetables, fiber, potassium, and other minerals have been shown to reduce systolic blood pressure [25]. The OmniHeart randomized trial compared the effects on blood pressure of three healthy dietary patterns in 164 adults with prehypertension or stage 1 hypertension. One diet was rich in carbohydrate (58% of total calories); a second was rich in protein (approximately half from plant sources); and another was rich in unsaturated fat, predominately monounsaturated fat [25]. Each diet lowered systolic blood pressure, but the blood pressure-lowering effect was greater in those who consumed the diets in which some of the carbohydrate was substituted with either protein or monounsaturated fat [25].

Findings of a large, multicenter prospective study of more than 4300 young black and white adults (aged 18 to 30 years) enrolled in the Coronary Artery Risk Development in Young Adults (CARDIA) Study support the benefits of an overall dietary pattern high in plant foods and milk in protecting against the development of high blood pressure and hypertension [27]. In this 15-year study, consumption of plant foods (i.e., whole grains, fruit, nuts) and milk was associated with a reduced incidence of elevated blood pressure. The researchers suggest that the beneficial effect of these foods on blood pressure may be explained by their rich array of nutrients and constituents (fiber, magnesium, potassium, calcium, and other food components) [27].

In a study involving 560 adults with hypertension, dyslipidemia, or diabetes at ten different medical centers in the U.S. participants were randomized to receive either prepackaged meals meeting individual nutrient requirements, or they self-selected an American Heart Association Step 1 or Step 2 diet under a nutritionist's guidance for 10 weeks [10]. Although blood pressure improved on both nutrition plans, the prepackaged meal plan resulted in a greater decrease in blood pressures (6.4 and 4.2 mm Hg for systolic and diastolic blood pressures, respectively) than the self-selected diets (4.6 and 3.0 mm Hg for systolic and diastolic blood pressures, respectively) [10]. The beneficial effects on blood pressure with the prepackaged meal plan were accompanied by improvements in dietary levels of calcium, potassium, and magnesium, approximating intakes achieved in the DASH study, and correlated with improvements in biochemical markers modified by those minerals [10]. The researchers concluded that consuming nutritionally-balanced meals that meet the recommendations of national health organizations can improve cardiovascular risk factors such as blood pressure [10].

Findings of a recent study suggest that a DASH-like dietary pattern characterized by higher intakes of fruits, vegetables, and dairy products (whether full-fat or reduced fat) has beneficial effects on blood pressure throughout childhood [28]. The independent and combined effects of intakes of fruits and vegetables (4 or more servings/day) and dairy products (2 or more servings/day) on blood pressure changes over a period of 8 years were examined in 95 children initially aged 3 to 6 years. By early adolescence, children who consumed a DASH-like diet higher in fruits and vegetables and dairy products had a lower systolic blood pressure (106 mm Hg) than those with lower intakes of these food groups (113 mm Hg) [28]. Children who consumed a higher intake of fruits and vegetables alone or dairy foods alone had intermediate levels of systolic blood pressure in adolescence. Although a similar trend was shown for both systolic and diastolic blood pressure, the effects were stronger for systolic blood pressure [28]. These findings lend support to the blood pressure guidelines which suggest that the DASH diet may help prevent and treat hypertension in children and adolescents [4].

Further support for the importance of the overall diet on blood pressure is provided by an analysis of regional variations in blood pressure and dietary intakes in the United States using data from the National Health and Nutrition Examination Survey III (NHANES III) in over 17,500 individuals [29]. This analysis found that participants living in the southern part of the United States had the highest systolic and diastolic blood pressures and reported the highest consumption of polyunsaturated and monounsaturated fats, cholesterol, and sodium, and the lowest amounts of fiber, potassium, calcium, phosphorus, magnesium, copper, riboflavin, niacin, iron, and vitamins A, C, and B_6. The findings suggest that this nutritional pattern may explain in part the higher prevalence of hypertension in the south [29].

Since publication of the DASH study in 1997 [9], the DASH combination diet has been acknowledged or incorporated into a number of dietary recommendations issued by health professional organizations and health advisory groups [2,4,30–33]. As indicated by the NHLBI in its most recent report of the Joint National Committee on Prevention, Detection, Evaluation, and Treatment of High Blood Pressure (JNC 7) for adults, the DASH diet is more effective than the long-standing recommendation to reduce sodium intake [2]. The 2005 edition of the *Dietary Guidelines for Americans* [32] refers to the DASH eating plan as an example of an eating pattern that exemplifies the recommendations in the Guidelines. In addition, the American Heart Association, in its recent scientific statement on dietary approaches to prevent and treat hypertension, supports consumption of the DASH dietary pattern for all Americans to both reduce and prevent elevated blood pressure [30]. Miller et al. [33] have identified other health professional groups that support the DASH diet.

3.3 DAIRY FOOD NUTRIENTS AND BLOOD PRESSURE

Although the DASH trial [9] was not designed to evaluate the effects of specific nutrients on blood pressure, the DASH diet is rich in calcium, potassium, and magnesium (~75th percentile of U.S. intake compared to ~25th percentile of U.S. intake for the control diet) [13]. Dairy products in the DASH diet are among the major contributors of calcium, potassium and magnesium, nutrients shown to lower blood pressure [33–35]. In fact, dairy products (e.g., fluid milk, yogurt) are the best food source for providing all three nutrients simultaneously in meaningful amounts [36]. In 2000, dairy foods contributed 72% of the calcium, 18% of the potassium, and 15% of the magnesium available in the nation's food supply [36]. As indicated in Table 3.6, dairy foods provide an appreciable percentage of the current dietary recommendations for calcium, potassium, and magnesium [31,37,38]. Numerous studies have demonstrated a blood pressure-lowering effect of these nutrients [33,35,39,40]. The association between inadequate mineral consumption (calcium, potassium, magnesium) and high blood pressure has persisted for over two decades, according to data from NHANES I (1984), NHANES III (1989 to 1991 and 1991 to 1994), and NHANES IV (1999 to 2000) [12,40]. Compared to the dramatic effects of the DASH diet, which likely resulted from the combined impact of several nutrients, the blood pressure response of a single nutrient is typically modest and heterogeneous. Nevertheless, even a modest population-wide reduction in blood pressure can lead to substantial reductions in cardiovascular disease [2].

TABLE 3.6
Calcium, Potassium, and Magnesium Content of Selected Dairy Products

Dairy Product	Calcium		Potassium		Magnesium	
	Mg	(%AI)[a]	Mg	(%AI)[b]	Mg	(%RDA)[c]
Whole milk, 1 cup	276	(23)	349	(7)	24	(8)
Reduced fat milk, 2%, 1 cup	285	(24)	366	(8)	27	(8)
Nonfat milk, 1 cup	306	(26)	382	(8)	27	(8)
Low-fat (1%) chocolate milk, 1 cup	288	(24)	425	(9)	32	(10)
Buttermilk, cultured, 1 cup	284	(24)	370	(8)	27	(8)
Yogurt, plain low-fat, 8 fl. ounces	448	(37)	573	(12)	42	(13)
Yogurt, plain skim milk, 8 fl. ounces	488	(41)	625	(13)	47	(15)

[a] 1200 Mg calcium.
[b] 4700 Mg potassium.
[c] 320 Mg magnesium (Institute of Medicine 1997; 2004).

Source: Institute of Medicine 1997; 2004.

3.3.1. Calcium, Dairy Foods, and Blood Pressure

Since the early 1980s, a considerable body of scientific evidence has accumulated from investigations in experimental animals, epidemiological studies, and clinical intervention trials in humans to support a beneficial role for calcium or calcium-rich foods such as milk and other dairy foods in blood pressure control [8,33,35,39,41,42]. Findings from a large body of scientific data indicate that increasing calcium intake to 1000 to 1500 mg/day, equivalent to the amount in 3 to 4 servings of milk, cheese, or yogurt, reduces the risk of hypertension [33,35].

3.3.1.1 Experimental Animal Studies

A blood pressure-lowering effect of calcium has been demonstrated in several models of genetically-hypertensive rats, including spontaneous hypertensive rats (SHR), salt-sensitive Dahl rats, (DOC)-salt rats, and Lyon genetically hypertensive rats [8,41,43–47], as well as in normotensive Wistar-Kyoto (WKY) rats [48]. A low calcium intake increases the hypertensive effect of a high-sodium chloride diet, while a high calcium intake lowers sodium chloride-induced blood pressure or attenuates the development of hypertension in these animals. More calcium is needed to reduce blood pressure in genetic hypertensive rats than in normotensive animals [49].

Abnormalities in calcium metabolism (e.g., reduced serum ionized calcium, increased parathyroid hormone, enhanced urinary calcium excretion) have been described in virtually all animal models of hypertension [47,50–55]. Blakeborough et al. [56] reported that less calcium is absorbed in SHR rats than in normotensive WKY rats.

Several studies demonstrate that the hypotensive effect of calcium in experimental animals requires a normal or high normal intake of sodium chloride [50,51,54,57–59]. Oshima et al. [57] found that a high-calcium diet lowered blood pressure in SHR rats only when intake of sodium chloride was high. These findings indicate that increased calcium helps to prevent dietary sodium chloride-induced hypertension. Oparil et al. [54] observed that dietary calcium supplementation prevented salt-sensitive hypertension in SHR rats by increasing diuretic and natriuretic responses to acute volume loading and by activating central nervous system pathways (i.e., neuronal mechanisms). Wyss et al. [58] likewise concluded that neuronal mechanisms underlie the blood pressure-lowering effect of dietary calcium in salt-sensitive SHR rats. Specifically, the addition of calcium to a high-sodium chloride diet may prevent a rise in blood pressure by preventing the sodium chloride-induced decrease in anterior hypothalamic norepinephrine [58].

In DOC-salt rats (a low-renin model of experimental hypertension which is particularly sensitive to the hypotensive effects of calcium), a high-calcium diet was demonstrated to attenuate the rise in renal vascular resistance, which accompanies DOC-salt hypertension [51,60]. DiPette et al. [60] reported that this effect of calcium was associated with a suppression of 1,25-dihydroxyvitamin D3. Calcium regulatory hormones, namely parathyroid hormone and 1,25-dihydroxyvitamin D3, have been demonstrated to have properties that can increase peripheral vascular resistance [61–63]. Enhanced vascular relaxation may be a mechanism whereby calcium supplementation reduces blood pressure in sodium-volume-dependent hypertension [51].

Increased dietary calcium has been reported to reduce smooth muscle reactivity in SHR rats. Porsti et al. [64] investigated the effects of oral calcium supplementation on blood pressure and intracellular free calcium concentration in SHR (hypertensive) and WKY (normotensive) rats. They also measured associated changes in vascular smooth muscle reactions. Calcium supplementation altered vascular smooth muscle responses and significantly attenuated the rise in systolic blood pressure and reduced intracellular free calcium in the hypertensive, but not normotensive, animals (Figure 3.2).

Experimental animal studies have demonstrated that increased calcium intake not only protects against salt-induced increases in blood pressure, but also modifies the effects of specific fats on blood pressure. Karanja et al. [65] observed that supplemental calcium reduced the severity of hypertension associated with a corn oil-rich diet in SHR rats. Further, a high-calcium/butterfat diet was as effective as fish oil in lowering blood pressure (Figure 3.3).

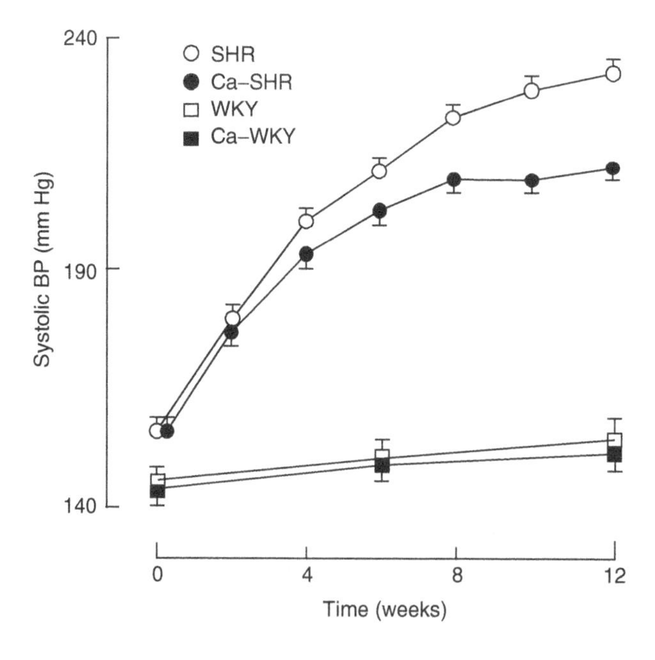

FIGURE 3.2. Line graphs show the effect of high calcium (Ca) diet on systolic blood pressure (BP) in the spontaneously hypertensive rates (SHR) and Wistar-Kyoto rats (WKY) during the 12-week study, development of hypertension was attenuated in the Ca–SHR group ($P < 0.0001$) ($n = 16$ for SHR and Ca–SHR, and $n = 9$ for WKY and Ca–WKY groups). (From Porsti, I., Arvola, P., Wuorela, H., and Vapaatalo, H., *Hypertension*, 19, 85, 1992. With permission.)

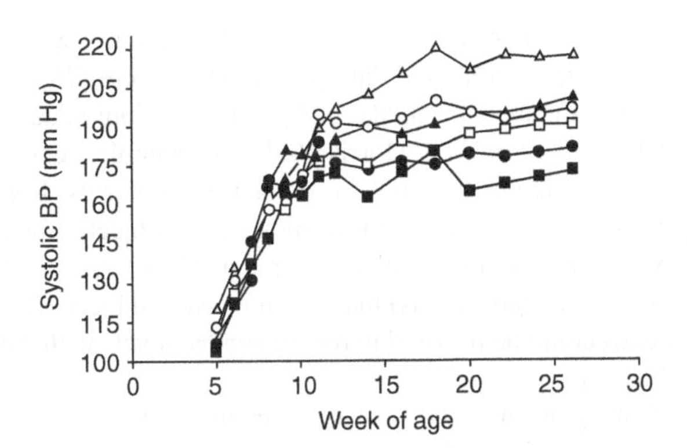

FIGURE 3.3 Line graph showing time course of blood pressure (BP) development for each of the six diets, △, CO/0.25% Ca^{2+}; ○, BF/0.25% Ca^{2+}; □, FO/0.25% Ca^{2+}; ▲, CO/2.0% Ca^{2+}; ●, BF/2.0% Ca^{2+}; ■, FO/2.0% Ca^{2+}., CO, corn oil; BF, butterfat; FO, fish oil. (From Karanja, N., Phanouvong, T., and McCarron, D. A., *Hypertension*, 14, 674, 1989. With permission.)

3.3.1.2 Epidemiological Studies

Numerous epidemiological studies support an inverse relationship between dietary calcium and blood pressure, with the strongest association between low intakes of calcium and higher blood pressure (Figure 3.4) [8,12,35,39–42,49,66–75]. A 1984 analysis of the first NHANES I, comprising dietary data from more than 10,000 American adults, identified an inverse association between dietary calcium and blood pressure levels [12]. Dietary calcium intake of >1000 mg/day was associated with a 40 to 50% reduction in the prevalence of hypertension [12]. Of the 17 nutrients assessed in the study, including sodium and potassium, calcium was the only nutrient that differed significantly in intake between persons with and without hypertension. In an analysis

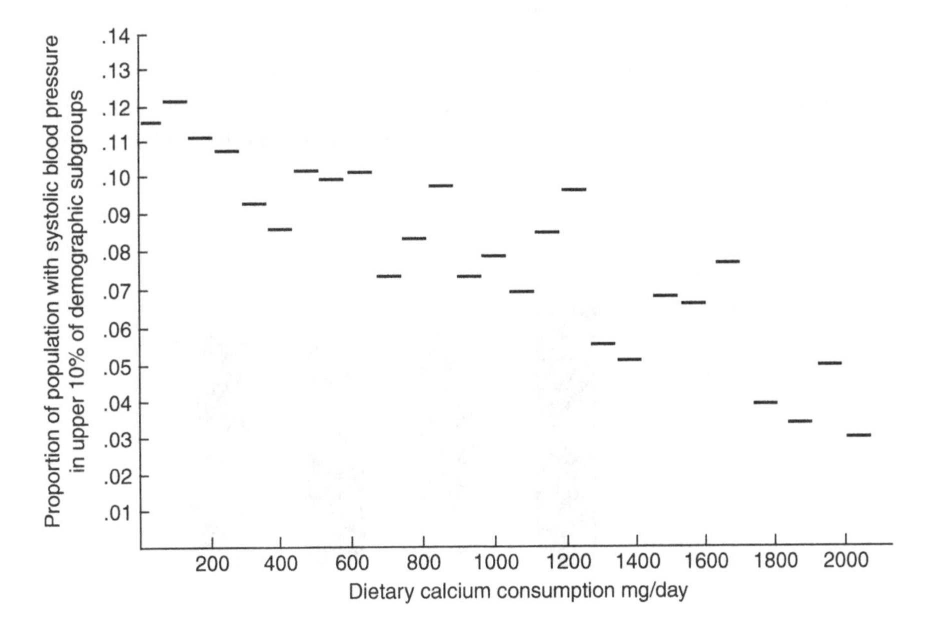

FIGURE 3.4 Percentage of individuals at risk of developing or having hypertension on the basis of daily calcium intake as reported in the National Health and Nutrition Examination Survey (NHANES) I. (From McCarron, D. A. et al., *Am. J. Clin. Nutr.*, 54, 215s, 1991. With permission.)

of data from NHANES III, a higher calcium intake (>1200 mg/day) was associated with lower rates of age-related increases in systolic and diastolic blood pressure [76].

Studies demonstrate that the calcium intake of hypertensive individuals is lower than that of normotensive individuals. McCarron and Morris [66], for example, reported that hypertensive women consumed 21% less calcium than their normotensive controls. Karanja et al. [77], in a cross-sectional study of 326 hypertensive and normotensive subjects, found that hypertensives consumed significantly lower amounts of calcium, magnesium, and potassium (i.e., nutrients found in substantial quantities in dairy foods) than normotensive subjects. They also demonstrated that intake of these minerals could be restored to recommended levels with dairy foods and without impacting blood lipid levels [77].

An inverse association has been found between calcium intake and hypertensive disorders of pregnancy (gestational hypertension and preeclampsia) [42,75]. Similarly, an inverse association between calcium intake and blood pressure has been observed in children [78,79]. In a study involving 80 preschoolers, systolic blood pressure dropped by 2.0 mm Hg for each 100 mg calcium per 1000 Kcal/day consumed [78]. Simons-Morton et al. [79] reported an inverse association between calcium intake and diastolic blood pressure, based on data analyzed from 662 children participating in the Dietary Intervention Study in Children (DISC). This 3-year study, which provided dietary advice to lower fat intake for 8-year-old children with elevated low-density lipoprotein cholesterol levels, also found that higher intakes of magnesium, potassium, protein, and carbohydrate were associated with lower blood pressure [79]. The blood pressure-lowering effect of calcium in children is supported by an intervention trial involving 101 school-aged children (11 years at baseline) [80]. Increasing calcium intake by 600 mg a day for 12 weeks reduced systolic blood pressure, especially in children whose calcium intake was initially low [80]. Ensuring adequate calcium intake during childhood may be one way to lower the risk of developing hypertension later in life. There is some evidence supporting the concept that essential hypertension has its roots in childhood, and high blood pressure represents a significant clinical problem in children and adolescents [3,4,81]. Approximately one-half of children with high blood pressure have hypertension as adults, according to the Bogalusa Heart Study, which followed 1505 children for 15 years [81].

Several prospective studies support a blood pressure-lowering effect of calcium. Findings from the first 4 years of follow-up of the Nurses Health Study involving nearly 60,000 females in the United States demonstrated a 23% reduction in the relative risk for developing hypertension with a

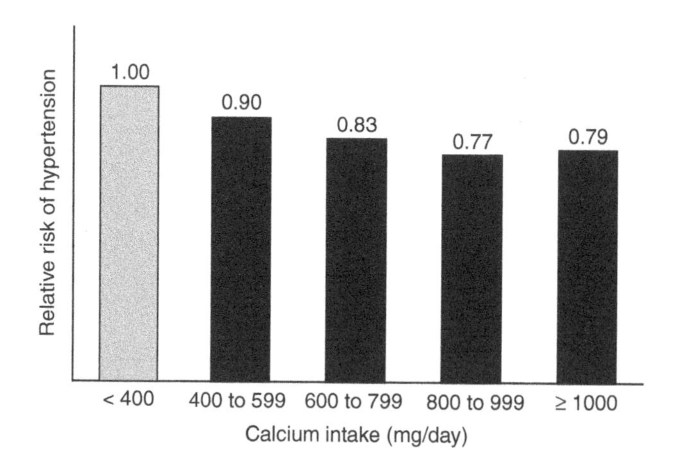

FIGURE 3.5 Relative risk of hypertension by level of energy-adjusted daily intake of calcium by U.S. female nurses. (Adapted from Witteman, J. C. M. et al., *Circulation*, 80, 1320, 1989. With permission.)

dietary calcium intake of at least 800 mg/day, compared with an intake of less than 400 mg/day (Figure 3.5) [68]. The lower risk of hypertension was independently associated with calcium from both dairy and nondairy sources. Calcium intake has also been demonstrated to have a strong independent inverse association with risk of hypertension in men, according to a 4-year prospective study which examined the relationship between various nutritional factors and blood pressure in 30,681 predominantly white U.S. male health professionals, 40 to 75 years of age, without diagnosed hypertension [82]. High blood pressure was associated with calcium intakes below 500 mg/day. In a 10-year epidemiological follow-up study of NHANES I involving more than 6600 adults, those who reported higher calcium intakes were less likely to develop hypertension 10 years later than subjects who reported lower calcium intakes [71].

When Burkett [72] reanalyzed a meta-analysis of 23 published epidemiological studies that examined the relation between dietary calcium intake and blood pressure [83], calcium was found to have a greater beneficial effect on blood pressure than originally reported. Several methodological errors were identified in the original meta-analysis that led to an underestimation of the relationship between calcium and blood pressure.

Calcium from dairy foods specifically has been associated with a decrease in blood pressure in numerous epidemiological studies. Garcia-Palmieri et al. [84], in a report from the Puerto Rico Heart Study, found that milk intake was inversely associated with both systolic and diastolic blood pressure in men and that this correlation was independent of coffee and alcohol intake, weight, education, cigarette smoking, and other dietary variables. Systolic blood pressure was reduced by 2 mm Hg for every 2 cups of milk (730 mg calcium) consumed per day. No association was observed between nondairy calcium intake and blood pressure. Reed et al. [85], in a study of diet and blood pressure among 800 Japanese men in Hawaii, observed that calcium from dairy foods, but not from nondairy foods, was inversely associated with blood pressure. The authors attributed this finding to the fact that dairy foods contain not only calcium, but also other nutrients (for example, potassium) that influence blood pressure.

In a cross-sectional study of calcium intake and blood pressure of 1790 adults in Erie County, New York, Freudenheim et al. [86] found that the calcium intake of normotensives tended to be higher than that of hypertensives, and that calcium from milk and yogurt (but not cheese) was inversely associated with diastolic blood pressure in Caucasian females. These findings are in agreement with those of a previous study demonstrating that milk, but not cheese, protected against hypertension [87].

A study reported by Iso et al. [69] involving more than 1900 Japanese men ages 40 to 69 years found that systolic blood pressure was higher among men whose daily calcium intake, particularly from dairy foods, was low (449 to 695 mg). The authors suggest that increasing total calcium intake by 300 mg (i.e., the amount in an 8-ounce glass of milk) corresponds to a 1.6 mm Hg decrease in systolic blood pressure. Recognizing that dairy calcium intake is typically low among the Japanese, Iso and coworkers [69] recommend that this population group increase their calcium intake, primarily by consuming more milk and milk products.

When the effect of calcium intake from dairy products was investigated in more than 7500 men and 8000 women in Norway, a significant linear decrease in systolic and diastolic blood pressures with increasing dairy calcium was found in both sexes [88]. Individuals with the highest dairy calcium intake had blood pressures equal to or lower than 1 to 3 mm Hg than those with the lowest dairy calcium intake [88].

A high calcium intake (1575 mg/day) from dairy products during the first 20 weeks of pregnancy was associated with a low risk of gestational hypertension in a case-control study in Quebec, Canada [89]. The association was independent of body mass index, exercise, maternal age, education, and cigarette smoking. In a study of pregnant women from the Child Health and Development Study, women who drank two glasses of milk a day were at the lowest risk for preeclampsia [90].

In the CARDIA Trial, a multicenter population-based prospective observational study of 3157 young adults aged 18 to 30 years followed for a 10-year period, a consistent reduction in the incidence of hypertension and other components of insulin resistance syndrome was observed with higher consumption of dairy foods (including low- and full-fat varieties) in overweight individuals [91]. The 10-year cumulative incidence of hypertension with the lowest dairy consumption (<10 times/week or <1.5 servings/day) was 22.9%, compared to 8.7% in those with the highest dairy consumption (35 or more times per week or 5 or more servings per day). The odds of elevated blood pressure were considerably lower with both low-fat (OR 0.79) and full-fat (OR 0.84) dairy [91]. For each daily eating occasion of dairy products, the odds of elevated blood pressure were lower by nearly 20%.

A prospective (27-month) study of 5880 university graduates (average age of 37 years) in Spain found that those who reported the highest intakes of low-fat dairy foods (mostly low-fat and nonfat milk) were 54% less likely to develop high blood pressure than those with the lowest intakes [92]. No significant association was observed between whole-fat dairy consumption and blood pressure. Additionally, calcium from low-fat dairy products, but not total calcium intake or calcium intake from whole fat dairy foods, was associated with a lower risk of high blood pressure [92]. According to the researchers, calcium only partly explains the inverse association between low-fat dairy foods and blood pressure found in this study. Adjusting the data for other dietary components of dairy foods, such as potassium, magnesium, phosphorus, protein, and total fat, did not alter the results [92]. The researchers speculate that interactions between dietary components of dairy foods may have contributed to the beneficial results [92].

3.3.1.3 Clinical Studies

Clinical intervention trials using different biochemical indices and sources of calcium (i.e., supplements or calcium from foods such as dairy products) indicate a beneficial, although variable, blood pressure-lowering effect of calcium [8,39,41,42,66,70,74,75,93–95].

When McCarron and Morris [66] compared the blood pressure response of 48 hypertensive and 32 normotensive individuals to 1000 mg of calcium salt (as the carbonate or citrate) per day for 8 weeks, the blood pressure response of the hypertensive patients was greater than that of the normotensives. However, there was considerable individual variation for both groups [66]. Likewise, a meta-analysis of 22 randomized clinical trials of the effect of calcium supplementation (1000 mg a day) on blood pressure in 1231 persons revealed that calcium lowered systolic blood pressure more in hypertensive persons (1.68 mm Hg) than in normotensive persons (0.53 mm Hg) [93]. Calcium supplementation was associated with a statistically-significant decrease in systolic blood pressure of 1 to 2 mm Hg both in the overall sample and in hypertensive individuals. In this meta-analysis, calcium significantly reduced systolic blood pressure, but not diastolic blood pressure [93]. Calcium supplementation also had the largest blood pressure-lowering effect in older persons and women.

Bucher et al. [96] suggest that the findings reported above [93], which demonstrated a greater blood pressure-lowering effect in hypertensive than in normotensive individuals, may be explained by the cut-off used to define normotensive and hypertensive individuals or failure to do a regression analysis on the effect of increased calcium based on baseline blood pressure levels. In their meta-analysis of 33 randomized controlled clinical trials involving 2412 individuals, both normotensive and hypertensive, Bucher et al. [94] examined the relation between baseline blood pressure and calcium supplementation by using regression analysis. In this meta-analysis, increasing calcium intake by 1000 to 2000 mg a day was associated with a small, but statistically-significant reduction in systolic blood pressure (1.27 mm Hg), but not diastolic blood pressure (0.24 mm Hg) for the study group as a whole. The researchers hypothesized that the marked heterogeneity in the blood pressure response to increased calcium observed in their meta-analysis may be explained by several factors, including baseline calcium intake [94]. That is, calcium's hypotensive effect may be greater in individuals consuming low levels of dietary calcium intake than in individuals whose calcium intake is adequate. They also speculated that, because of nutrient interactions, increasing calcium intake from food sources might have a greater blood pressure-lowering effect than calcium supplements. In addition, these researchers noted that increasing calcium intake might have a stronger beneficial effect in groups at high risk for hypertension, such as African Americans, salt-sensitive individuals, and pregnant women [94]. In an update of the meta-analysis, the researchers addressed the possibility that the source of calcium — dietary vs. nondietary — may explain the marked differences in blood pressure responses [97]. This analysis demonstrated that the blood pressure-lowering effect of calcium derived from foods, primarily dairy products, was consistent, whereas the response to supplements was heterogenous. This finding indicates that, in many studies, calcium may serve as a marker for dairy foods, and that observed blood pressure benefits are not derived solely from calcium, but from the full nutritional profile of dairy foods, which include multiple minerals, vitamins, protein, and essential fatty acids.

In essential hypertensive patients, Resnick et al. [98] observed that patients with a serum profile of lower renin, lower ionized calcium, and elevated 1,25-dihydroxyvitamin D levels experienced a significantly greater reduction in blood pressure in response to calcium supplementation (2 g/day) than hypertensive patients with the opposite profile. Similarly, Grobbee and Hofman [99] observed that calcium supplementation (1 g/day) lowered diastolic blood pressure in mildly-hypertensive adults aged 16 to 29 years, especially in subjects with high plasma parathyroid hormone levels and/or low serum total calcium. Strazzullo et al. [100], in a long-term (15-week) double-blind trial of calcium supplementation (1 g/day) in 18 patients with mild hypertension, also found that hypertensive patients with abnormal calcium metabolism (e.g., hypercalciuria) were most likely to respond to increased calcium with a reduction in blood pressure.

Additional findings by Resnick et al. [101], similar to those from experimental animal studies (see above), indicated that calcium supplementation was effective in offsetting the pressure-elevating effect of salt in salt sensitive individuals. Zemel et al. [102], on the basis of their studies in salt-sensitive African Americans, also concluded that — salt sensitive hypertensives are more likely to demonstrate blood pressure reductions in response to calcium supplementation than individuals who are not salt-sensitive. Vaughan et al. [103] found that systolic and diastolic blood pressure decreased (9% and 8%, respectively) in mildly-hypertensive men who consumed a high-calcium (1400 mg/day), moderate-sodium (3300 mg/day) diet for 6 weeks compared to men who consumed a low-calcium (400 mg/day), moderate-sodium diet. Sodium excretion increased 13 to 21% in the men who consumed the high-calcium diet [103].

Increasing calcium also helps to maintain normal blood pressure during pregnancy and reduce the risk of preeclampsia [41,75,104–109]. Pregnancy-induced hypertension occurs in 10% to 20% of all pregnancies. Women pregnant for the first time or pregnant with twins or triplets are at the highest risk of pregnancy-induced hypertension. Preeclampsia, a severe complication of pregnancy that develops in previously-normotensive women, is characterized by hypertension, retention of fluid, and proteinuria. It usually presents between the 20th week of gestation and term. The condition occurs in 2% to 8% of all pregnancies, or a higher percentage in high-risk pregnancies, and can endanger the health of both the mother and child [104].

Belizan et al. [107], in a multicenter, double-blind, randomized clinical trial involving 1194 Argentinean women in their first pregnancies, found that risk of hypertensive disorders of pregnancy was significantly lower in women who received 2000 mg of elemental calcium (as the carbonate) than in those who received a placebo (9.8% vs. 14.8%). The protective effect of calcium was more evident after the 28th week of pregnancy than at earlier stages (Figure 3.6). Individuals with low calcium levels and low plasma renin levels were most likely to benefit from increased calcium intake [107]. A beneficial effect of increased calcium during pregnancy was also demonstrated in teenagers enrolled in the Johns Hopkins Hospital Adolescent Pregnancy Program [109]. The pregnant teens who received an additional 2000 mg of calcium a day not only had lower blood pressures, but also were less likely to deliver premature infants than the pregnant teens who

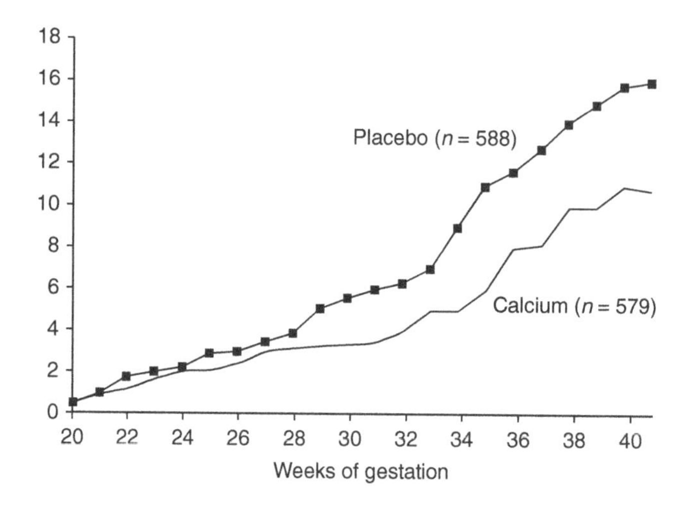

FIGURE 3.6 Percentage of women in the calcium and placebo groups in whom hypertensive disorders of pregnancy (gestational hypertension and preeclampsia) developed according to the week of gestation. (From Belizan, J. M. J. et al., *N. Engl. J. Med.*, 325, 1402, 1991. With permission.)

did not receive increased calcium [109]. Knight and Keith [108] reported that calcium supplementation (1 g/day for 20 weeks) significantly lowered diastolic blood pressure in hypertensive, but not normotensive, pregnant women.

A meta-analysis of 14 randomized trials involving 2459 pregnant women found that increasing calcium intake by 1500 to 2000 mg a day during pregnancy lowered systolic and diastolic blood pressure by 5.40 and 3.44 mm Hg, respectively (Figure 3.7) [104]. This meta-analysis also found that increasing calcium intake reduced the incidence of pregnancy-induced hypertension by 70% and preeclampsia by 62% [104].

In contrast to these positive results, the Calcium for Preeclampsia Prevention (CPEP) trial, conducted among over 4500 healthy pregnant women at five U.S. medical centers, found a slight, but nonsignificant, beneficial effect of 2000 mg of supplemental calcium on risk of preeclampsia, pregnancy-associated hypertension, or other adverse outcomes of pregnancy [110]. The failure to find a significant beneficial effect of calcium on pregnancy outcome in this study may be explained

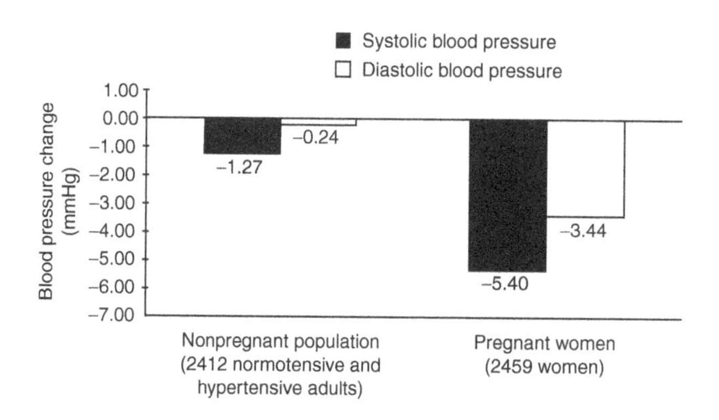

FIGURE 3.7 Blood pressure-lowering effect of calcium in a nonpregnant population and in pregnant women, according to meta-analyses. (Adapted from Bucher, H. C. et. al., *JAMA*, 275, April 10, 1016, 1996, Copyright 1996, American Medical Association. With permission.)

by the women's already relatively high calcium intake of 1100 mg a day and low risk status such as age [75]. Moreover, this study did not evaluate the effect of a dairy source of calcium. Because calcium-rich foods such as dairy foods contain other nutrients, including potassium and magnesium, which are associated with lowering blood pressure, the benefits could be even greater if calcium were obtained from foods rather than supplements [104]. A Cochrane review of ten studies involving more than 6000 women found that increasing calcium intake modestly reduced high blood pressure and risk of preeclampsia [111]. These effects were greatest for women at high risk of hypertension and those with initially low calcium intakes [111]. A recent randomized, double-blind, placebo-controlled trial conducted at four clinics in two developing countries (Bangladesh and Colombia) found that calcium (600 mg/day) plus conjugated linoleic acid (450 mg/day) supplementation significantly reduced the incidence of pregnancy-induced hypertension [112]. The 48 women in this study were at either end of the most common reproductive years (<19 years or >35 years) and were at high risk for pregnancy-induced hypertension because of a family history of this condition.

Meeting calcium needs during pregnancy may not only lower the risk of hypertensive disorders during pregnancy and its adverse outcomes, but may also have a beneficial effect on the offsprings' blood pressure [113–115]. An inverse association has been reported between maternal calcium intake and the blood pressure of breast-fed infants at 1, 6, and 12 months of age [114]. In a follow-up study, systolic blood pressure was significantly lower in 7-year-old children whose mothers received 2000 mg of supplemental calcium during pregnancy than in children whose mothers did not receive extra calcium [113]. Similarly, a more recent study found that increasing calcium intake (2000 mg/day) of pregnant women resulted in lower blood pressure in their 2-year-old offspring [115]. Researchers speculate that a high calcium intake during pregnancy may influence or program mechanisms in utero to regulate blood pressure of the offspring [113,115].

Clinical trials utilizing dairy foods as a source of calcium have shown a blood pressure-lowering effect [116–121]. A small hypotensive effect of milk intake was related to its mineral content in a 6-week double-blind trial examining regular milk vs. a "mineral-poor" milk (Figure 3.8) [117]. In this study of young normotensive women, the decrease in systolic blood pressure was significantly greater in the group supplemented with the regular milk (4.1%) than in

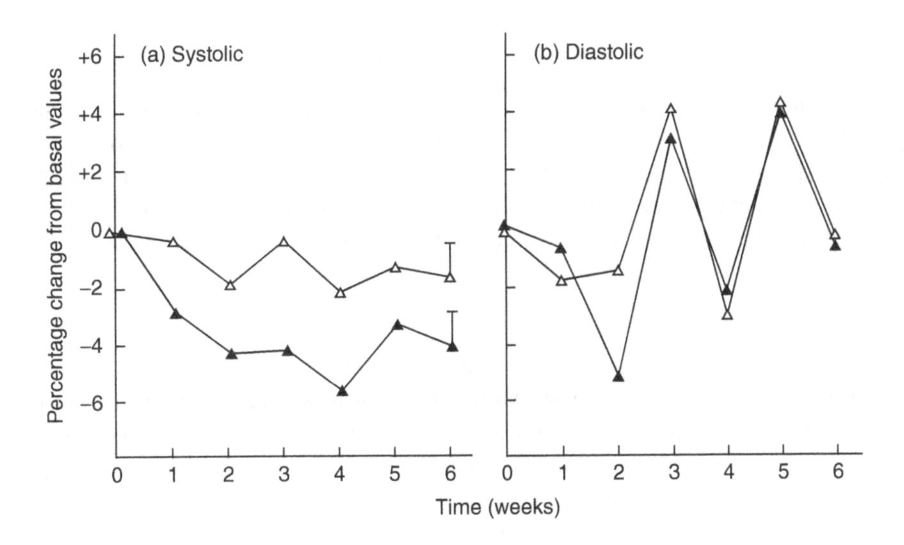

FIGURE 3.8 Mean percentage changes in systolic and diastolic blood pressure from basal values vs. time. Bar represents 1 SEM. (▲) = normal milk group; (△) = "mineral-poor" milk group. Significance level between groups: $*P<0.05$. (From Van Beresteijn, E. C. H., Van Schaik, M., and Schaafsma, G., *J. Intern. Med.*, 228, 477, 1990. With permission.)

the women given the mineral-poor milk (1.3%). No effect on diastolic blood pressure was observed. When the researchers compared their findings with those of trials of calcium supplements alone, they found that the effect of milk on blood pressure was greater and more rapid than that of calcium alone [117]. Thus, the combination or interaction of nutrients in milk may be more hypotensive than the blood pressure-lowering effect of individual nutrients. Another study in normotensive subjects reported by Bierenbaum et al. [116] found that dairy products as a source of calcium (1150 mg/day) significantly reduced systolic blood pressure by an average of 5 mm Hg. Other researchers have reported that increasing milk intake lowers blood pressure [119,120]. In older adults, especially hypertensive older adults, blood pressure decreased when their milk consumption increased from <1.5 to 2.9 servings/day [120]. Zemel et al. [118] reported that calcium (600 mg/day) in the form of yogurt was more effective than calcium carbonate supplements in reducing systolic blood pressure and intracellular calcium in African American noninsulin dependent diabetic hypertensives.

Increasing calcium intake through foods such as dairy products appears to have a greater and more consistent blood pressure-lowering effect than calcium supplements [97,118]. In a meta-analysis of 42 randomized controlled trials of calcium supplementation on blood pressure, systolic blood pressure decreased by 2.10 mm Hg in the dietary calcium studies, compared to 1.09 mm Hg in the calcium supplement studies [97]. The difference in the effect of dietary vs. nondietary calcium on diastolic blood pressure was smaller (1.09 vs. 0.87 mm Hg) than that for systolic blood pressure. Particularly noteworthy was the observation that dietary calcium had a more consistent blood pressure-lowering effect than did calcium supplements [97].

As reviewed by McCarron and Reusser [35], a large body of epidemiological and clinical research findings supports a blood pressure-lowering effect of adequate calcium intake (1000 to 1500 mg/day). However, a variety of factors, as discussed below, impact calcium's effect on blood pressure. Findings from clinical intervention studies using different indices demonstrate that increased calcium intake is most effective in lowering blood pressure in the face of a calcium deficit as found in pregnancy, in older age, among African American and diabetic subjects, and in individuals with lower renin activity, lower circulating calcium levels, higher urinary calcium excretion, secondary hyperparathyroidism, and elevated vitamin D hormone.

3.3.1.4 Determinants of a Hypotensive Response to Calcium

Heterogeneity in the blood pressure response to calcium alone is not surprising, given interactions among nutrients in the diet and food and the fact that hypertension is the expression of a variety of disorders with different mechanisms which, singly or in combination, result in increased vascular tone and total peripheral resistance [8,39–42,73]. A number of factors related to the study design, the individual, and the composition of the diet can influence the effect of calcium on blood pressure.

3.3.1.4.1 Study Design

The duration of the intervention and the dose and source of calcium can influence blood pressure response [42]. According to McCarron and Morris [66], at least 8 weeks of intervention is necessary for the antihypertensive effect of calcium to be expressed. Thus, the failure of some calcium intervention trials to find an effect, such as those reported by van Beresteyn et al. [122] and Kynast-Gales and Massey [123] may be explained in part by their short duration (<8 weeks).

"Negative" findings for a hypotensive role of calcium may also be due to an insufficient amount of supplemental calcium or to a high level of calcium intake prior to supplementation. Inaccurate determination of blood pressure and dietary calcium intake, inconsistent screening of subjects for factors such as salt intake, and a small sample size also may contribute to the failure of some studies to demonstrate an inverse association between calcium and blood pressure [40]. In addition, the source of calcium may influence the findings: a stronger hypotensive effect is found with food sources of calcium than with calcium supplements [9,33,35,97].

3.3.1.4.2 Individual Characteristics

In general, older persons appear to be particularly responsive to the blood pressure-lowering effect of increased calcium intake [93,124,125]. This may be explained by the lower initial calcium intake and reduced ability to absorb calcium in older adults. Studies indicate that individuals with low initial calcium intakes (e.g., African Americans, the elderly) are more responsive to the blood pressure-lowering effects of calcium than are calcium-replete individuals [53,63,69,95,126]. In a randomized, double-blind clinical trial of 116 African American adolescents, calcium supplementation (1.5 g/day) reduced diastolic blood pressure more in adolescents with lower dietary calcium intakes than in those with higher calcium intakes [95]. An antihypertensive effect of calcium cannot be expected from a population whose calcium intake already meets or exceeds recommended intakes. The failure of some studies to demonstrate a significant blood pressure-lowering effect of calcium may be explained by the participants' already-high calcium intake [110,126,127].

Several researchers suggest that there is a threshold of calcium, beyond which there is an attenuated relationship between calcium intake and blood pressure [41,49,63,94,126,128]. According to McCarron et al. [49], the "set point" of this threshold is 700 to 800 mg calcium per day (i.e., risk of hypertension increases at calcium intakes below this level), although many factors such as other dietary components and genetics can influence this "set point."

An individual's initial blood pressure status also may influence the blood pressure response to calcium supplementation. Individuals with a higher initial blood pressure may be more likely to respond to increased calcium or dairy intake with a reduction in blood pressure than individuals with a lower initial blood pressure [66,70,93,94,119,120]. In a study of 204 older adults who increased their milk consumption from <1.5 to 2.9 servings/day, blood pressure was reduced more in the hypertensive individuals than in those with normal blood pressure [120]. Systolic blood pressure also appears to be affected more than diastolic pressure by increased calcium intake [40,53,66,69,70,93,94]. An analysis of data from NHANES III and IV found that low mineral intake (calcium, potassium, magnesium) was most pronounced in participants with only high systolic blood pressure [40].

Body weight may determine the blood pressure response to calcium intake [74]. There is a strong and consistent relationship between body weight and blood pressure. Overweight increases risk of hypertension while weight loss reduces blood pressure [2,30,129–135]. Failure of increased calcium to lower blood pressure in some overweight individuals may be explained by the overriding influence of excess weight compared to a low calcium intake [68,82].

"Salt sensitivity" is a potential predictor of blood pressure response to calcium [41,53,61,63,98,99,106,136,137]. Salt-sensitive, low-renin individuals exhibit disturbances in calcium metabolism, such as low serum ionized calcium, increased calciuresis, and elevated levels of calcium regulatory hormones (i.e., parathyroid hormone and 1,25 dihydroxyvitamin D) (Figure 3.9). Individuals with characteristics of salt sensitivity have been observed to be more likely to respond to dietary calcium with a decrease in blood pressure — at least when sodium intake is not restricted — than nonsalt-sensitive individuals. The protective effect of calcium in salt-sensitive individuals appears to be most pronounced in the presence of a high sodium intake [62,138–141]. A low salt intake may preclude a blood pressure-lowering response to calcium supplementation, as calcium serves to attenuate the hypertensive response to high salt diets. Zemel et al. [141] found that hypertensive, salt-sensitive African American adults consuming a high-sodium (4000 mg)/low-calcium (356 mg) diet exhibited a decrease in blood pressure in response to increased calcium intake (956 mg/day), whereas adding calcium to a low-sodium (1000 mg) diet had no effect on blood pressure.

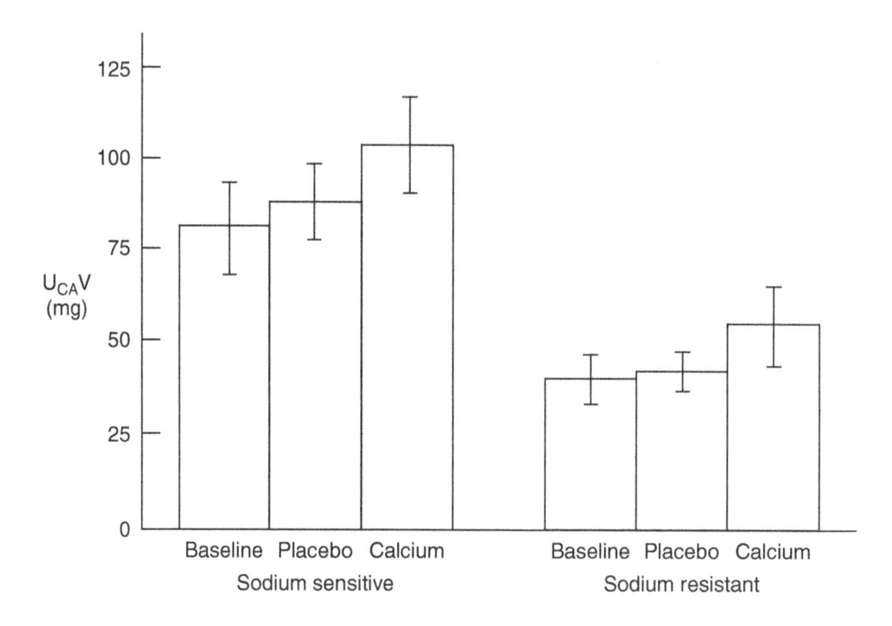

FIGURE 3.9 Mean ± standard deviation for urinary calcium excretion in sodium sensitive (left panel) and sodium resistant (right panel) subjects at baseline, during placebo, and during calcium supplementation. Sodium-sensitive subjects had significantly ($P < 0.001$) greater calcium excretion during all three periods. (From Weinberger, M. H., Wagner, U. L., and Fineberg, N. S., *Am. J. Hypertens.*, 6, 799, 1993. With permission.)

3.3.1.4.3 Other Dietary Components

Interactions among calcium and other nutrients or dietary components may contribute to inconsistent effects of calcium on blood pressure [8,73,142]. As studies indicate, calcium's effect on blood pressure is influenced by salt intake. Other dietary components, such as potassium, magnesium, and alcohol intake, also may influence the antihypertensive effect of calcium [8,41,49,68,71,73,85,125,138,142–144]. Calcium's protective effect on blood pressure is diminished in the presence of high intakes of alcohol [68,144]. This means that calcium in amounts higher than recommended intakes may be necessary to reduce elevated blood pressure in individuals who consume high alcohol intakes (>20 g/day or more than two drinks/day). Hamet et al. [138] suggest that high intakes of calcium (800 mg/1000 kcal) may help protect against sodium-induced as well as alcohol-induced hypertension. In contrast, less calcium may be needed to lower blood pressure in individuals consuming a high intake of potassium [144]. The effect of a single nutrient on blood pressure may be too small to detect, whereas several antihypertensive nutrients consumed together in a diet such as the DASH diet appear to have a more significant effect [9,40]. Clearly, nutrients interact in their effect on blood pressure regulation [8].

3.3.1.4.4 Who Is Most Likely to Respond?

There is no absolute predictor of the blood pressure response to increased calcium intake. However, the groups indicated in Table 3.7 are considered to be the most likely to respond to increased calcium intake with a decrease in blood pressure [49,63,145]. Additionally, specific clinical characteristics described in Table 3.7 predict individuals likely to have a blood pressure reduction in response to increased calcium intake [63].

TABLE 3.7
Groups and Clinical Characteristics Associated with an Antihypertensive Effect of Calcium

Groups	Clinical Characteristics
Blacks	Salt-sensitive
Southeast Asians (Japanese)	Elevated parathyroid hormone
Alcoholics	Elevated 1,25-dihydroxyvitamin D
Diabetics	Low ionized calcium
Salt-sensitive subjects	Hypercalciuria
Pregnant women	Low rennin activity
Elderly people	
Individuals consuming low calcium diets	

Source: Adapted from McCarron et al., *Am. J. Clin. Nutr.*, 54 (Suppl. 1), 215, 1991; Sowers, J. R. et al., *Am. J. Hypertens.*, 4, 557, 1991.

3.3.2 Potassium and Blood Pressure

Experimental animal studies, epidemiological investigations, and clinical trials in humans indicate that an adequate potassium intake may protect against hypertension [8,12,30,35,38,39,146–149]. Overall findings also indicate that dietary potassium (e.g., in foods such as fruits, vegetables, and dairy foods) may have a major role as a nonpharmacological agent in the control of high blood pressure [38]. Not only may potassium protect against hypertension and its associated vascular diseases including stroke, but it may also reduce the need for antihypertensive medication [8]. Increasing potassium intake blunts the effect of sodium chloride on blood pressure and mitigates salt sensitivity [38]. Based on evidence demonstrating that diets rich in potassium (and low in sodium) reduce blood pressure and stroke risk, the food and drug administration has approved a health claim for qualifying foods that are good sources of potassium [150]. Nonfat milk qualifies for this claim.

3.3.2.1 Experimental Animal Studies

In several animal models of hypertension, increasing potassium intake reduces blood pressure, often by attenuating a salt-induced rise in blood pressure [8,147,148,151,152]. In a study involving Dahl salt-sensitive and salt-resistant rats, low potassium intake was not only associated with increased blood pressure in both strains, but it also increased the hypertensive effects of a high-salt diet, even in previously salt-resistant rats [152]. In another experiment involving hypertensive rats, a high potassium diet markedly influenced salt sensitivity, evidenced by the reduction in blood pressure and mortality in the rats fed a high-potassium, high-sodium diet compared to those fed a normal-potassium, high-sodium diet [148].

3.3.2.2 Epidemiological Studies

Numerous epidemiological investigations indicate an inverse association between potassium intake or urinary potassium excretion (a proxy of intake) and blood pressure, although the findings are not entirely consistent [38]. Higher intake of potassium was associated with lower mean systolic blood pressure and lower risk of hypertension in a study of 10,372 individuals aged 18 to 74 years who participated in NHANES I [12]. Likewise, in NHANES III, potassium intake was associated with lower systolic and diastolic blood pressures [153]. Increasing potassium intake was also associated with a decrease in the age-related rise in blood pressure [153]. In the INTERSALT study (a study investigating the relationships between electrolytes and blood pressure in over 10,000 adults in 52 population centers around the world), potassium intake or serum, urine, or total body potassium was inversely associated with blood pressure [154,155]. According to analyses of INTERSALT data, an increase in urinary potassium excretion of 60 mmol/day is associated with a 2.7 mm Hg reduction in systolic blood pressure [154]. The INTERSALT data also demonstrated a drop in systolic blood pressure by 3.4 mm Hg, with a decrease in the 24-hour urinary sodium-potassium ratio from 3.1 (170 mmol of sodium/55 mmol potassium) to 1.0 (70 mmol of sodium /70 mmol potassium) [155].

When the relationship between electrolytes (sodium, potassium, calcium, and magnesium) and blood pressure was investigated in over 400 Yi farmers in the People's Republic of China, dietary, serum, and urinary potassium levels were inversely associated with systolic and diastolic blood pressures [143]. An increase in potassium intake of 100 mmol/day (7.5 g) corresponded to a decrease of 8.3 and 5.7 mm Hg in systolic and diastolic blood pressures, respectively [143].

In 615 older men of Japanese ancestry participating in the Honolulu Heart Study, total potassium intake (i.e., from food and supplements) was significantly and inversely associated with both systolic and diastolic blood pressures [156]. Potassium from food was associated with a decrease in both systolic and diastolic blood pressures, while supplemental potassium was associated only with a decrease in diastolic blood pressure. Moreover, when potassium intake from dairy and nondairy sources was examined, dairy potassium was inversely associated with systolic and diastolic blood pressures, while nondairy potassium showed only a borderline inverse association with systolic blood pressure [156]. This epidemiological study indicates that potassium from dairy foods has a stronger relationship to blood pressure than potassium from nondairy foods.

Prospective studies support a beneficial role for dietary potassium in blood pressure regulation [82,129,132]. When 30,681 predominantly white American male health professionals aged 40 to 75 years without diagnosed hypertension increased their dietary potassium intake, risk of hypertension was significantly lower after adjusting for age, relative weight, and alcohol and energy intake (Figure 3.10) [82]. In men participating in the Multiple Risk Factor Intervention Trial (MRFIT), dietary potassium intake was inversely associated with both systolic and diastolic blood pressure [129]. During the 6 years of the trial, potassium had a greater blood pressure-lowering effect on systolic than diastolic blood pressure. In the Nurses Health Study II, an epidemiological cohort study of 300 women with normal blood pressure and habitually low intakes of potassium, increasing potassium intake to 102 mmol/day for 16 weeks significantly lowered systolic and diastolic blood pressures by 2.0 and 1.7 mm Hg, respectively [149].

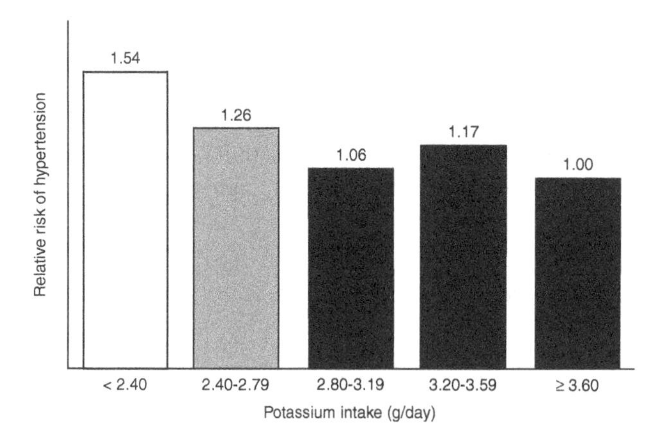

FIGURE 3.10 Relative risk of hypertension in U.S. male health professionals by level of energy-adjusted daily intake of potassium. (Adapted from Ascherio, A. et al., *Circulation*, 86, 1475, 1992. With permission.)

Findings of a longitudinal study in The Netherlands involving 233 children aged 5 to 17 years suggest that a sufficient intake of potassium (especially from food) or a reduction in the dietary sodium to potassium ratio may be beneficial in the early prevention of hypertension [157]. Children with a high dietary intake of potassium had a smaller yearly increase in systolic blood pressure than children with a low potassium intake. The sodium-to-potassium ratio also had an inverse relationship with blood pressure, although there was no clear effect for sodium alone. According to a 3-year study of potassium supplementation (or sodium reduction), increased dietary potassium reduced blood pressure within the first two decades of life in adolescent girls [158].

Similar to findings from experimental animal studies, some epidemiological studies in humans suggest that potassium's effect on the development of arterial disease may be independent of changes in blood pressure [159,160]. In a 12-year prospective study, a high intake of potassium from food sources reduced risk of stroke without a marked lowering of blood pressure [159]. When the relationship between urinary cations obtained from the INTERSALT study and cerebrovascular mortality was examined, 24-hour urinary potassium excretion was inversely associated with cerebrovascular disease mortality in women with no change in systolic and diastolic blood pressures [160].

3.3.2.3 Clinical Studies

Clinical trials in normotensive and, in particular, hypertensive individuals point to a blood pressure-lowering effect of increased potassium intake [161–166]. In a randomized, crossover trial in the United Kingdom, systolic blood pressure decreased by an average of 15 points in eight hypertensive patients over 68 years old who increased their intake of potassium by 60 mmol a day for 1 month and 48 mmol for four additional months [163]. In an investigation of African Americans who consumed a low-potassium diet (32 to 35 mmol/day), those receiving a potassium supplement (80 mmol/day) for 3 weeks experienced a decrease in systolic and diastolic blood pressure of 6.9 and 2.5 mm Hg, respectively [162]. In a randomized, double-blind, placebo-controlled trial of 150 Chinese adults with mild hypertension or high-normal blood pressure, increasing potassium intake by 60 mmol/day for 12 weeks significantly reduced systolic blood pressure by 5 mm Hg [164].

Available evidence from meta-analyses supports a blood pressure-lowering effect of potassium [161,165]. In a meta-analysis of 33 randomized, controlled clinical trials involving over 2600 participants (age range 18 to 79 years), potassium supplementation was associated with a significant reduction in mean systolic (3.11 mm Hg) and diastolic (1.97 mm Hg) blood pressure (Figure 3.11). Compared to normotensive subjects, greater reductions in blood pressure were observed in hypertensive subjects. Potassium supplements reduced blood pressure by 1.8/1.0 in normotensive subjects and 4.4/2.5 mm Hg in hypertensive subjects (Figure 3.11) [161]. In addition, the blood pressure-lowering effect of potassium appeared to be more pronounced in subjects consuming a high sodium intake. These findings led the authors of this meta-analysis to suggest that increasing potassium intake may be beneficial for the prevention and treatment of hypertension, especially in individuals who have difficulty lowering their sodium intake [161]. In another meta-analysis of 27 potassium trials in adults over a minimum duration of 2 weeks, increasing potassium intake (44 mmol/day or 1.8 g/day) reduced systolic blood pressure by 2.42 mm Hg and diastolic blood pressure by 1.57 mm Hg [165]. The blood pressure response to increased potassium intake was greater in hypertensives than in normotensives [165].

Increasing dietary potassium intake from foods (e.g., fruits, vegetables, milk) appears to be as beneficial as potassium supplements in lowering blood pressure [167]. This was demonstrated in a study in which 28 hypertensive patients undergoing drug (antihypertensive) therapy increased their dietary potassium intake by an average of 50% (from 2.76 to 4.35 g/day), while another 26 participants maintained their usual diets [167]. The participants consuming the high-potassium diets needed less medication (i.e., 36% reduction in drug use) than the control group to keep their blood pressure below 165/95 mm Hg. When the blood pressure-lowering effect of potassium

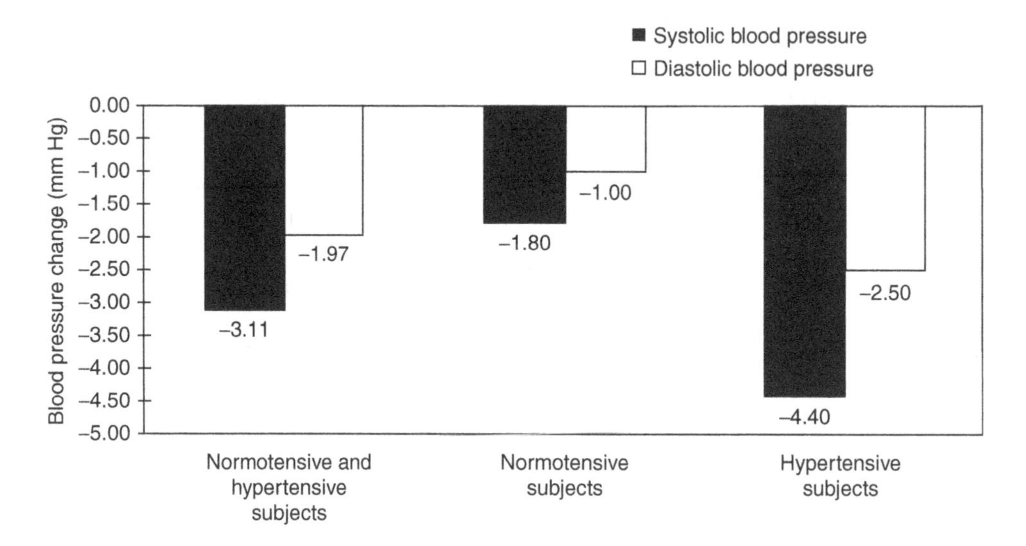

FIGURE 3.11 Effect of potassium supplementation on blood pressure in normotensive and hypertensive subjects. (Adapted from Whelton, P. K. et al., *JAMA*, 277, May 28, 1624, 1997. Copyright 1997, American Medical Association. With permission.)

chloride was compared to potassium citrate in a randomized crossover trial in 14 hypertensive adults, potassium citrate (as found in some food sources of potassium) had a similar effect on blood pressure as potassium chloride [166]. Based on these findings, the researchers concluded that "increasing the consumption of foods high in potassium is likely to have the same effect on blood pressure as potassium chloride" [166]. They add that increasing potassium intake from foods may be preferable, as many foods may have beneficial health effects independent of their potassium content.

In general, the hypotensive effect of potassium is more pronounced in hypertensive than in normotensive individuals [39,161,165]. African Americans and others whose potassium intake is habitually low appear to benefit more from increased potassium intake than do whites or other groups consuming higher amounts of potassium [30,161,162,168]. African Americans usually consume and excrete less potassium and their blood pressure tends to be higher than Caucasians [168]. African Americans also have lower plasma renin sensitivity than Caucasians. A 10-week trial of the effect of an 80-mEq potassium chloride supplement a day on blood pressure showed that plasma renin activity in African Americans increased to the same level as in Caucasians after potassium supplementation [168]. This finding suggests that the low plasma renin activity in African Americans is due in part to low potassium intake. Increasing dietary intake of food sources of potassium may be particularly beneficial for African Americans and others whose prevalence or risk of hypertension is high [38].

The effects of potassium on blood pressure are also influenced by other nutrients, such as sodium, calcium, and magnesium [121,149,169,170]. Most studies that have demonstrated an antihypertensive effect of potassium have involved subjects consuming a high-sodium (salt) diet rather than a low-sodium diet [161,164,169]. A major mechanism by which increased potassium intake lowers blood pressure appears to be related to natriuresis (sodium excretion). Thus, individuals on high-sodium diets need to maintain an adequate potassium intake to reduce their risk for hypertension. Increased potassium intake also reduces urinary losses of calcium and magnesium, nutrients demonstrated to have a protective effect on blood pressure [8]. Ensuring an adequate intake (AI) of potassium (120 mmol/day or 4.7 g/day), preferentially from foods, such as vegetables, fruits, and dairy foods (milk, yogurt) is recommended to help reduce the risk of hypertension [30,38]. Unfortunately, many population groups in the United States have low potassium intakes [38].

The U.S. Food and Drug Administration (FDA) has approved a health claim that "Diets containing foods that are good sources of potassium and low in sodium may reduce the risk of high blood pressure and stroke" [150]. Qualifying foods must contain at least 350 mg of potassium per serving and no more than 140 mg sodium. They must also be low in fat, saturated fat, and cholesterol. Nonfat milk qualifies for this claim. The 6th Edition (2005) of the *Dietary Guidelines for Americans* [32] recommends that Americans consume potassium-rich foods (e.g., fruits, vegetables, dairy products such as milk and yogurt) to reduce their risk of hypertension. Meeting the potassium recommendation (4.7 g/day) with food is especially important for individuals with hypertension, blacks, and middle-aged and older adults [32]. Likewise, the American Heart Association encourages increasing potassium intake from foods as foods are accompanied by a variety of other nutrients [30].

3.3.3 Magnesium and Blood Pressure

Magnesium has been observed to directly and indirectly affect cardiac and vascular smooth muscle [171]. Because magnesium promotes vascular smooth-muscle relaxation, it is reasonable to suggest that this mineral may play a role in blood pressure regulation. Experimental animal, human epidemiological, and clinical studies have examined the relationship between dietary magnesium intake and blood pressure; however, the evidence is less conclusive than that for calcium or potassium [8,30,171].

3.3.3.1 Experimental Animal Studies

Lower levels of magnesium in the plasma, kidney, heart, lung, and tibia and lower erythrocyte intracellular free magnesium have been found in the SHR (hypertensive) strain of rats compared to normotensive WKY rats [172,173]. In several different experimental rat models of hypertension, alterations in urinary magnesium excretion are reported [55]. In addition, diets that increase or decrease intracellular free magnesium also lower or raise blood pressure, respectively [171]. Experimental animals fed a magnesium-deficient diet have been shown to exhibit an increase in blood pressure, and high-magnesium diets attenuate the development of hypertension [174–176]. When the effect of dietary magnesium supplementation (10 g/kg diet) on blood pressure of Sprague–Dawley normotensive and mineralocorticoid-salt (DOCA-salt) hypertensive rats was investigated, magnesium supplementation significantly reduced blood pressure in the hypertensive, but not normotensive, rats [177].

3.3.3.2 Epidemiological Studies

In a review of epidemiological studies of magnesium and blood pressure (mostly cross-sectional), Whelton and Klag [178] reported inconsistent findings. According to these authors, methodological shortcomings in the studies — including their brief duration, use of a single 24-hour dietary recall to measure magnesium intake, and the complicating presence of antihypertensive medication — preclude definitive conclusions regarding the effects of magnesium on blood pressure. Interactions among nutrients also influence the findings [49,85]. Reed and colleagues [85], in their analysis of data from the Honolulu Heart Project, were unable to isolate the beneficial effects of magnesium from those of potassium and calcium.

Three studies reviewed by Whelton and Klag [178], however, deserve mention, the first two because of their strong designs and the third because of a possible added explanation for the inconsistent findings. Magnesium was examined in a cross-sectional study of 61 dietary variables and blood pressure in 615 men participating in the Honolulu Heart Study, a community-based study of coronary heart disease and stroke in a cohort of elderly Japanese men living in Oahua, Hawaii.

Magnesium intake had the strongest inverse association with both systolic and diastolic blood pressures (Figure 3.12) [156]. Systolic and diastolic blood pressures were found to be 6.4 and 3.1 mm Hg lower, respectively, in the highest vs. the lowest quintile of magnesium intake [156]. In a hospital-based study in Detroit, dietary magnesium (determined by 4-day food records) was higher in Caucasian normotensive subjects than in either African American normotensives or Caucasian or African American hypertensives [141]. When serum magnesium levels and blood pressure were examined, Resnick et al. [179] found no difference in serum magnesium levels between hypertensive and control patients. However, when these investigators separated the hypertensive patients according to their renin status, those with high renin hypertension had the lowest serum magnesium levels [179]. These studies provide some evidence for a role for magnesium in regulating blood pressure.

Some prospective studies support a protective role for magnesium in the regulation of blood pressure [68,82,132]. Dietary magnesium had an independent and significant inverse association with hypertension in the first 4 years of follow-up (1980 to 1984) of the Nurses Health Study [68]. This prospective study examined the relationship of various nutritional factors to hypertension in over 58,000 predominantly Caucasian U.S. female registered nurses, aged 34 to 59 years [68]. The nurses who consumed at least 280 mg of magnesium a day had a one-third lower chance of developing hypertension than those who consumed lower intakes of magnesium (<200 mg/day). The main contributors to magnesium intake in this study were fruits and vegetables (27%), cereals (17%), and dairy products (13%). The nurses who consumed at least recommended intakes for magnesium and calcium experienced a lower risk of developing hypertension compared to the nurses with low intakes of both nutrients [68]. In the second 4 years of follow-up (1984 to 1988) of 41,541 U.S. females participating in the Nurses Health Study [132], magnesium intake was inversely associated with systolic and diastolic blood pressures, but not with the incidence of hypertension.

A beneficial role for magnesium in blood pressure regulation has also been reported in a prospective study involving nearly 31,000 predominantly Caucasian U.S. male health professionals, after adjusting for age, relative weight, and alcohol and energy intake (Figure 3.13) [82]. Another study of over 15,000 subjects found an inverse association between dietary and blood levels of magnesium with systolic and diastolic blood pressures [180]. In older adults participating in a study in The Netherlands, increasing magnesium intake by 100 mg a day from foods was associated with a decrease in systolic and diastolic blood pressure of 1.2 and 1.1 mm Hg,

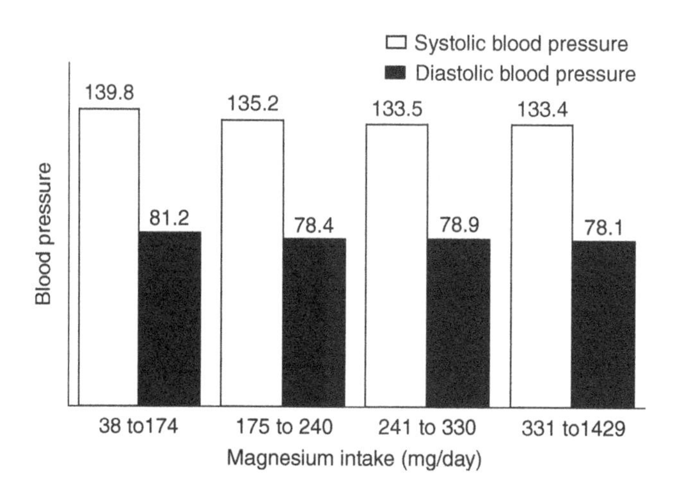

FIGURE 3.12 Inverse association between total magnesium intake and systolic and diastolic blood pressure in Japanese men. (Adapted from Joffres, M. R. et al., *Am. J. Clin. Nutr.*, 45, 469, 1987. With permission.)

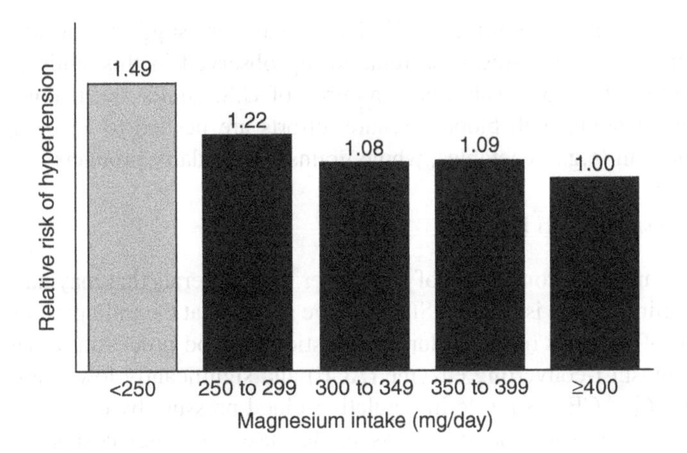

FIGURE 3.13 Relative risk of hypertension by level of energy-adjusted daily intake of magnesium in U.S. male health professionals. (Adapted from Ascherio, A. et al., *Circulation*, 86, 1475, 1992. With permission.)

respectively [170]. In this study, the blood pressure lowering effect of magnesium was greater in men than in women. A pooled analysis of 29 observational studies pointed to a negative association between dietary magnesium intake and blood pressure [181].

3.3.3.3 Clinical Studies

Clinical studies of the influence of magnesium on blood pressure have yielded inconsistent findings, thus neither proving nor refuting an antihypertensive effect of this mineral. In phase I of the Trials of Hypertension Prevention [127], no difference in blood pressure was observed between 227 subjects who received magnesium supplements (360 mg/day) for 6 months vs. 234 who received a placebo. However, the possibility of low magnesium absorption and low compliance, as well as the decrease in blood pressure in the placebo group, may have contributed to the lack of a blood pressure-lowering effect of magnesium in this trial. The hypotensive effect of magnesium may be restricted to magnesium-deficient individuals [182]. According to a 3-month study of 13 patients with mild hypertension, oral supplements of magnesium lowered blood pressure only in patients identified as magnesium deficient based on blood magnesium levels [182]. However, in the Nurses Health Study II, increasing magnesium intake to 585 mg/day for 16 weeks in normotensive women whose usual dietary intake of magnesium was low had no effect on blood pressure [149]. Other methodological variables, such as the use of antihypertensive medication and the length of follow-up, may contribute to the inconsistent findings.

In the Multiple Risk Factor Intervention Trial, dietary magnesium was inversely related to systolic and diastolic blood pressures with the greater effect for men not receiving antihypertensive medication [129]. Additionally, in a double-blind, placebo-controlled study involving 91 women with mild to moderate hypertension, increasing magnesium intake by 485 mg (20 mm) a day had no significant effect on blood pressure after 3 months of magnesium supplementation [183]. However, after 6 months, magnesium modestly but significantly reduced diastolic blood pressure (3.4 mm Hg). The decrease in systolic blood pressure (2.7 mm Hg) was not statistically significant [183]. Possible interactions of magnesium with other nutrients also may explain the inconsistent effects of magnesium on blood pressure [171].

A meta-analysis of 20 randomized clinical trials of the effects of magnesium on blood pressure found that, overall, magnesium supplementation (10 to 40 mmol/day) resulted in only a small reduction in blood pressure, 0.6 mm Hg systolic and 0.8 mm Hg diastolic [184]. However, the researchers detected a dose-response effect. For each 10 mmol/day (240-mg) increase in magnesium, systolic blood pressure was significantly reduced by 4.3 mm Hg and diastolic blood pressure was reduced by 2.3 mm Hg [184]. The researchers suggest that additional studies be conducted to confirm the dose-response relationship observed in this study [184]. Considering the low magnesium intake of a substantial number of U.S. adults and magnesium's potentially beneficial role in reducing high blood pressure, efforts are needed to encourage intake of food sources of magnesium (e.g., vegetables, whole grains, fruits, dairy products) [185].

3.3.4 Protein and Blood Pressure

Protein is one example of a constituent of milk other than minerals that may have vascular effects, although current clinical data is limited. Studies have shown that the milk proteins casein and whey are a rich source of peptides (derived during digestion or food processing) that inhibit the vasoconstrictor angiotensin-I-converting enzyme (ACE) and significantly lower systolic and diastolic blood pressure [186]. ACE has a role in regulating blood pressure by converting angiotensin I to angiotensin II, which constricts the blood vessels. Because of the high cost and various side effects associated with ACE-inhibitory drugs, attention has focused on milk peptides as potential natural hypotensive agents.

In spontaneously hypertensive rats (SHRs), individual caseins (casokinins) and whey proteins (lactokinins) with ACE-inhibitory peptides significantly reduce blood pressure [186]. Additionally, a limited number of human studies associate different milk protein hydrolysates and fermented dairy products, which have been shown *in vitro* to contain ACE-inhibitory peptides, with significant decreases in systolic and diastolic blood pressures [186–190]. In a double-blind, placebo-controlled study of 30 older adults, the majority of whom were taking antihypertensive medication, both systolic and diastolic blood pressures were significantly reduced following intake of a fermented sour milk drink containing peptides for 8 weeks [187]. In a longer-term (5-month) double-blind, placebo-controlled trial involving 39 hypertensive subjects, intake of a fermented milk with bioactive peptides reduced systolic and diastolic blood pressure [188]. The researchers suggested that, in addition to the ACE-inhibitory effect of the peptides in fermented milk, the higher calcium intake might also have contributed to this dairy product's blood pressure-lowering effect [188]. Another randomized, placebo-controlled, double-blind study found that intake of powdered *Lactobacillus helveticus* fermented milk tablets containing bioactive peptides for 2 weeks reduced blood pressure in subjects with high-normal blood pressure or mild hypertension [190]. In a pilot study described by FitzGerald et al. [186], intake of a whey protein hydrolysate by 30 borderline hypertensive adults for 6 weeks significantly reduced systolic and diastolic blood pressure. The reduction in blood pressure occurred within 1 week after consumption of the whey protein hydrolysate and was maintained for the remaining 5 weeks of the study. In a single-blind, placebo-controlled study in Japanese adults with high-normal blood pressure or mild hypertension, systolic blood pressure decreased in those given a daily casein hydrolysate containing bioactive peptides for 6 weeks [189]. The decrease in systolic blood pressure was dose-dependent and the antihypertensive effect was greatest in subjects with mild hypertension [189].

To date, specific milk protein hydrolysates and fermented dairy products have been demonstrated to reduce blood pressure in SHRs and hypertensive subjects, with no effect on the blood pressure in normotensive laboratory rats or humans [186]. Although findings of a hypotensive effect of milk-derived peptides are promising, additional research is needed to confirm these findings and to determine the mechanism(s) involved.

3.4 OTHER LIFESTYLE MODIFICATIONS

3.4.1 Weight Reduction

The recent increase in the prevalence of high blood pressure among children, adolescents, and adults in the United States is attributed in part to the rise in obesity between 1988 and 2000 [1–4].

Excess body weight, especially central or abdominal obesity, increases risk of hypertension, and weight reduction in individuals who are at least 10% above ideal weight may reduce blood pressure [2,30,130–134,191]. In a study of more than 5000 children aged 10 to 19 years, overweight was associated with high blood pressure, especially in minorities [192]. A meta-analysis of 25 randomized controlled trials involving 4874 participants found that a weight loss of 5.1 kg (11 pounds) reduced systolic blood pressure by 4.44 mm Hg and diastolic blood pressure by 3.57 mm Hg [191]. Weight loss may also reduce or eliminate the need for antihypertensive medication [2,130].

Increasing intake of dairy foods not only reduces blood pressure, but may also help to prevent and treat obesity, a risk factor for hypertension. Emerging scientific evidence indicates a beneficial role for calcium and dairy products in adult weight management when combined with an energy-reduced diet [189] (see Chapter 7). High dairy diets have been demonstrated to reduce lipid accumulation in fat cells and increase fat breakdown during caloric restriction [193]. Dairy sources of calcium reduce weight and fat gain to a greater extent than do supplemental sources of calcium. Based on findings from epidemiological studies and recent clinical trials, consuming diets that include three or more servings/day of dairy products significantly reduces adipose tissue mass in overweight adults not on calorie-reduced diets (and not consuming excessive calories) and markedly accelerates weight and body fat loss secondary to calorie restriction compared with diets low in dairy products [193].

Regular aerobic physical activity, such as brisk walking at least for 30 minutes a day on most days of the week, also can lower blood pressure in many previously sedentary hypertensive patients [2,194]. A meta-analysis of 54 randomized controlled trials (2419 participants) found that aerobic exercise reduced blood pressure in both hypertensive and normotensive individuals [194]. A combined program of physical activity and weight loss is recommended for managing overweight individuals with high blood pressure [135].

3.4.2 Dietary Sodium Reduction

Dietary sodium has traditionally been the nutrient most often associated with blood pressure control. However, despite extensive research, whether or not there should be a universal recommendation to reduce dietary sodium continues to be debated [16,195–198]. While some researchers cite evidence demonstrating that sodium intake is positively associated with blood pressure, others are of the opinion that the link between sodium intake and blood pressure is unproven, particularly in individuals with normal blood pressure [198]. While a reduction in sodium intake, on average, lowers blood pressure, there is considerable heterogeneity in individual blood pressure responses to changes in sodium or salt [38,199]. Meta-analyses have found that reducing sodium intake lowers blood pressure more in hypertensive than in normotensive individuals [200,201]. Moreover, sodium intake may have unique effects on blood pressure categories [40]. An analysis of mineral intakes and blood pressure using data from NHANES III and IV found that sodium intake was significantly lower in those with isolated systolic hypertension (i.e., those most at risk for cardiovascular disease) compared to those with normal blood pressure [40]. In contrast, persons with elevated diastolic hypertension tended to be overweight and to have a higher sodium intake.

Much of the controversy surrounding sodium is related to "salt sensitivity." Salt-sensitive individuals are generally considered to be those whose blood pressure increases with salt loading and decreases with salt restriction, although there is no precise definition [38]. For the majority of the population that is salt-resistant, sodium intake has little or no effect on blood pressure [38,197,202]. At present, there is no diagnostic test to differentiate salt-sensitive from salt-resistant individuals [38]. The difficulty in identifying individuals as salt-sensitive or salt-resistant is due in part to the considerable variation in changes in blood pressure within individuals, even when sodium, weight, and diet are held constant [199]. However, certain population groups — including hypertensive individuals, African Americans, overweight persons, patients with chronic kidney disease, individuals with a family history of hypertension, older adults, and people with low plasma renin levels — are more likely to be salt-sensitive than others [200,202]. Genetic as well as non-genetic factors (e.g., diet) contribute to salt sensitivity [16,38,202]. Diet can modify salt sensitivity, as evidenced by the DASH-Sodium study [11]. This low-fat diet adequate in nutrients, including the mineral profile available through dairy products (calcium, potassium, magnesium), reduced the negative effects of high salt intake on blood pressure in salt-sensitive individuals. That is, dietary salt increases blood pressure in certain individuals (e.g., minorities, those with hypertension) if they consume a nutrient-poor diet. However, if the quality of the diet is adequate, salt intake has little effect on the blood pressure of the vast majority of individuals [15,16,23,38].

Many federal, professional, and health organizations recommend that sodium intake be reduced to no more than 2.3 or 2.4 g /day (100 mmol sodium/day or approximately 1 tsp of salt) [2,30,32]. The Institute of Medicine (IOM) recently lowered the dietary sodium recommendations even further — to 1.5 g/day for all healthy 19- to 50-year olds, 1.3 g/day for those over 50 years, and 1.2 g/day for people older than 70 years [38]. The IOM has set a tolerable upper intake level (UL) of 2.3 g sodium/day for healthy adults through age 50 years, and recommends that older adults, African Americans, and individuals with chronic diseases such as hypertension, diabetes, and chronic kidney disease consume less than this upper limit of sodium [38]. Similar recommendations are provided in the 6th Edition of the 2005 *Dietary Guidelines for Americans* [32]. Critics of the IOM's sodium recommendations cite the lack of evidence to support the recommendations [16,198]. The IOM's sodium recommendations were based largely on findings from the DASH-Sodium trial (11), which was biased toward subjects with mild hypertension, African Americans, and slightly overweight individuals. Researchers argue that this study failed to provide evidence that reducing sodium intake influences hypertension risk in individuals with normal blood pressure levels [16,198]. In fact, according to recommendations for the management of hypertension for Canadians, a reduction in sodium intake is not advised for individuals with normal blood pressure [203].

The safety and efficacy of low-sodium diets are of concern [198,204,205]. Diets reduced in sodium are potentially low in several essential nutrients, such as calcium, potassium, and magnesium, which have been demonstrated to be beneficial in blood pressure regulation [202,206,207]. Other potential problems associated with low sodium intake include hydration and insulin resistance [198]. In addition, there is no evidence that restricting sodium is associated with a reduction in cardiovascular disease or all-cause mortality [204,205,208]. An analysis of 11 long-term ($>$6 months to 7 years) interventions to reduce sodium intake in more than 3500 adults found only minimal reductions in blood pressure and an unclear effect on mortality and cardiovascular disease [208]. The researchers concluded that lowering sodium intake may lessen the need for medication in hypertensive individuals, but has little effect on overall health [208]. While reducing sodium intake appears to be beneficial for persons at risk for hypertension, scientific evidence indicates that the focus of national nutrition policy directed at hypertension should be on the overall nutritional quality of the diet [9,15,16].

3.5 COMPREHENSIVE LIFESTYLE MODIFICATIONS AND BLOOD PRESSURE: PUTTING IT ALL TOGETHER

Comprehensive lifestyle modifications have been demonstrated to have a beneficial effect on blood pressure [209,210]. The effectiveness of implementing several lifestyle interventions simultaneously (e.g., the DASH diet, sodium reduction, weight loss, aerobic exercise) was investigated in a 9-week randomized clinical trial (diet, exercise, and weight loss intervention Trial or DEW-IT) involving 44 hypertensive, overweight adults taking blood pressure-lowering medication [209]. Participants were randomly assigned to the lifestyle group or the control group (i.e., no nutrition or lifestyle counseling). The results showed that by the end of the 9 weeks, blood pressure was substantially reduced in the lifestyle group and the improvement in blood pressure control was similar in magnitude to that achieved with drug therapy. Compared to the control group, average 24-hour systolic and diastolic blood pressures in the lifestyle group were significantly reduced by 9.5/5.3 mm Hg [209].

Results of the PREMIER trial, a randomized clinical trial which assessed the effects of simultaneous lifestyle modifications to improve blood pressure, demonstrated that free-living individuals could make multiple lifestyle changes, including increased intake of dairy products, at one time that lower blood pressure [210]. In this study, 810 free-living adults (62% women, 34% African Americans) with above-optimal blood pressure, including stage 1 hypertension, were randomized to one of three intervention groups for 6 months; i) an "advice-only" group; ii) an "established" group, which received behavioral interventions to implement weight loss, sodium reduction, increased physical activity, and limited alcohol consumption; and iii) an "established plus DASH" group which, in addition to the above, received instruction and counseling on the DASH diet. Consumption of dairy products increased significantly more in the "established plus DASH" group (0.5 servings), with almost 60% of participants in this group consuming 2 or more dairy servings/day, than in the other two groups [210]. Likewise, fruit and vegetable intake increased in "established plus DASH" group compared to the other two groups. The blood pressure reduction in the "established plus DASH" group was consistently greater than the corresponding blood pressure reduction in the "established" group; however, the difference was not statistically significant. The researchers suggest that this may be because participants did not fully reach the goals of the DASH diet or because the combined effect of several blood pressure-reducing interventions is not additive. Based on the findings, the researchers suggest that widespread implementation of the PREMIER behavioral interventions, particularly the "established plus DASH" intervention, should reduce blood pressure or increase blood pressure control [210].

3.6 SUMMARY

Hypertension affects more than 65 million American adults (i.e., about one-third of the adult population), and an additional 45 million adults are considered to be pre-hypertensive or at high risk of hypertension [1,2]. This disease is also detectable in an increasing number of children and young adults [3,4]. Hypertension, which increases the risk for cardiovascular disease, stroke, heart failure, and kidney disease, is estimated to cost the nation $63.5 billion a year [2,6]. Because of its high prevalence, serious health consequences, and economic burden, lifestyle modifications, including dietary interventions, are recommended to help prevent and treat hypertension [2,4].

Traditionally, changes in single nutrients (e.g., reducing excess sodium intake) were the primary focus of dietary interventions to prevent and treat hypertension. However, scientific evidence accumulated over the past 20 years indicates that the overall diet, specifically a dietary pattern that increases intake of multiple nutrients, is more important in blood pressure regulation than modifications in any single dietary component. This change in focus is exemplified in the National Heart, Lung and Blood Institute's most recent lifestyle modifications for hypertension prevention and treatment in adults [2]. For the first time, these lifestyle recommendations rank adoption of the DASH (Dietary Approaches to Stop Hypertension) eating plan, which is a low-fat diet rich in fruits, vegetables, and low-fat dairy products, as more important than sodium reduction to control blood pressure [2]. In addition, the National High Blood Pressure Education Program Working Group on High Blood Pressure in Children and Adolescents, in its guidelines, recommends lifestyle modifications for children and adolescents with hypertension or prehypertension [4]. These include weight reduction if overweight, regular physical activity, dietary modification, and family-based interventions [4]. Although firm evidence regarding the efficacy of dietary interventions to control blood pressure in children is lacking, intake of the DASH diet is encouraged [4].

The DASH trial demonstrated that a low-fat dietary pattern high in fruits and vegetables (8 to 9 servings/day) and dairy products (~3 servings/day) — i.e., DASH diet — produces significant reductions in systolic and diastolic blood pressures in adults [9]. The blood pressure-lowering effect of the DASH diet is particularly beneficial for hypertensives and African Americans who are at high risk for hypertension [9,17,18]. A follow-up study, called the DASH-Sodium trial, has confirmed the blood pressure-lowering effect of the DASH diet [11]. Reducing sodium intake in combination with the DASH diet lowered blood pressure even further. However, with the exception of older adults with hypertension, consuming the DASH diet alone provided the most significant reduction in blood pressure for the majority of participants [11].

Data from the DASH trials support a blood pressure-lowering effect of dairy products and provide strong support for recommending at least 3 servings/day of dairy foods as part of an overall healthy diet [9,11,33]. Although the DASH diet was not designed to evaluate the effects of specific nutrients on blood pressure, dairy products are major sources of calcium, potassium, magnesium, and protein, nutrients demonstrated to lower blood pressure [33–36].

A large body of scientific evidence supports a blood pressure-lowering effect of dietary calcium [33,35]. However, the findings are not as dramatic or as consistent as in the DASH trial. A variety of factors can affect the blood pressure–calcium relationship (e.g., baseline calcium intake, calcium source, study design, etc.). Despite the heterogeneity in the blood pressure response to increasing calcium intake, consuming recommended dietary intakes of calcium is encouraged to help prevent or treat hypertension [33,35]. Dairy products are recognized as being more effective than calcium supplements in reducing blood pressure [9,33,35,41,97]. Food sources of calcium such as dairy foods (milk, cheese, and yogurt) are recommended because, in addition to calcium, they provide other nutrients, such as potassium and magnesium, which may protect against hypertension [33,77,123,211]. One researcher stated, "a diet devoid of dairy products will often be a poor diet not just in respect to calcium, but for many other nutrients as well" [212]. Milk and other dairy foods make a significant contribution to the nation's supply of nutrients [36]. Diets low in dairy foods compromise the nutritional quality of the diet [77,212–216]. Studies in both adults [77,120,213] and children [215–220] indicate that consuming dairy foods improves the overall nutrient adequacy of the diet. Moreover, increasing calcium intake to 1500 to 1600 mg/day (i.e., an amount greater than the 1000 to 1300 mg currently recommended for adults [31]) from dairy foods (e.g., yogurt, skim, and low-fat milk) does not raise plasma lipids, lipoproteins, or body weight (i.e., other risk factors for coronary heart disease) [77], a finding supported by other investigators [120,213,215,216,218]. In fact, emerging research indicates that consuming 3 servings of dairy foods a day as part of a calorie-reduced diet has a beneficial effect on body weight [193] (see Chapter 7), which is of significance considering that overweight is a risk factor for hypertension. In addition, consuming calcium-rich foods like dairy products is likely to be associated with fewer compliance problems than associated with salt-restricted diets [63]. Consuming calcium-rich foods such as dairy foods is also advantageous, considering that sodium-restricted diets are often limited in other essential nutrients, such as calcium, iron, magnesium, and vitamin B6 [206].

Experimental animal, epidemiological investigations, and clinical trials in humans indicate that an adequate intake of potassium (120 mmol/day or 4.7 g/day), preferably from foods such as vegetables, fruits, and dairy products (milk and yogurt, for example), protects against hypertension [8,12,30,35,38,146–149]. Dairy foods, because of their potassium content, may be especially beneficial for African Americans, the elderly, and others at high risk for hypertension; for hypertensive individuals on drugs (dairy foods may reduce their need for medication); and for young people, to lower their later risk of this disease. The FDA has approved a health claim that "Diets containing foods that are good sources of potassium and low in sodium may reduce the risk of high blood pressure and stroke" [150]. Nonfat milk qualifies for this claim. The 6th Edition of the 2005 *Dietary Guidelines for Americans* [32] recommends that Americans consume potassium-rich foods (e.g., fruit, vegetables, dairy products such as milk and yogurt). Meeting the potassium recommendation (4.7 g/day) with food is especially important for individuals with hypertension, blacks, and middle-aged and older adults [32].

Compared to calcium or potassium, the evidence supporting a hypotensive effect of magnesium is less conclusive. However, considering the low magnesium intake of a substantial proportion of Americans and magnesium's potentially beneficial role in reducing high blood pressure, efforts are needed to encourage intake of food sources of magnesium (e.g., vegetables, whole grains, fruits, dairy products) [185].

Emerging findings in hypertensive animals and humans indicate that milk peptides derived from casein and whey may have a hypotensive effect [186].

In addition to the DASH diet, other lifestyle modifications to prevent and treat hypertension include weight reduction if overweight, dietary sodium reduction (no more than 100 mmol/day or 2.4 g/day), physical activity, and moderation in alcohol intake [2,30]. The results of the PREMIER trial, a randomized clinical trial which assessed the effects of simultaneous lifestyle modifications to improve blood pressure, demonstrates that free-living individuals can make multiple lifestyle changes, including increased intake of dairy foods, at one time to lower their blood pressure [210].

Considering the high costs associated with hypertension and the U.S. government's goal of reducing the nation's health care expenditures, prevention of hypertension by consuming a nutritionally adequate diet containing recommended servings of dairy foods is essential. Based on collective observations from a variety of studies, including the DASH trial, McCarron and Heaney [221] estimate that consuming a healthful diet containing 3 to 4 servings of dairy foods/day would lead to a 40% reduction in the prevalence of mild to moderate hypertension and result in first year health care cost savings of $14 billion with cumulative savings of $70 billion at 5 years.

REFERENCES

1. Fields, L. E. et al., The burden of adult hypertension in the United States 1999 to 2000. A rising tide, *Hypertension*, 44, 1, 2004.
2. Chobanian, A. V. et al., The National High Blood Pressure Education Program Coordinating Committee, 7th Report of the Joint National Committee on Prevention, Detection, Evaluation, and Treatment of High Blood Pressure, *Hypertension*, 42, 1206, 2003.
3. Munter, P. et al., Trends in blood pressure among children and adolescents, *JAMA*, 291, 2107, 2004.
4. National High Blood Pressure Education Program Working Group on High Blood Pressure in Children and Adolescents, The 4th report on the diagnosis, evaluation, and treatment of high blood pressure in children and adolescents, *Pediatrics*, 114, 555, 2004.
5. Department of Health and Human Services, Public Health Service, *Healthy People 2010*, Vol. I, U.S. Government Printing Office, Washington, D.C., December, 2000.
6. Thom, T. et al., Heart disease and stroke statistics — 2006 update: a report from the American Heart Association Statistics Committee and Stroke Statistics Subcommittee, *Circulation*, 113, 85, 2006.
7. Preuss, H. G., Diet, genetics, and hypertension, *J. Am. Coll. Nutr.*, 16, 296, 1997.
8. Reusser, M. E. and McCarron, D. A., Micronutrient effects on blood pressure regulation, *Nutr. Rev.*, 52, 367, 1994.
9. Appel, L. J. et al., For the DASH Collaborative Research Group, a clinical trial of the effects of dietary patterns on blood pressure, *N. Engl. J. Med.*, 336, 1117, 1997.
10. McCarron, D. A. et al., Nutritional management of cardiovascular risk factors, *Arch. Intern. Med.*, 157, 169, 1997.
11. Sacks, F. M. et al., Effects on blood pressure of reduced sodium and the Dietary Approaches to Stop Hypertension (DASH) diet, *N. Engl. J. Med.*, 322, 3, 2001.
12. McCarron, D. A. et al., Blood pressure and nutrient intake in the United States, *Science*, 224, 1392, 1984.
13. Obarzanek, E. and Moore, T. J., Eds., The Dietary Approaches to Stop Hypertension (DASH) Trial, *J. Am. Diet. Assoc.*, 99 (suppl.), 9s, 1999.

14. Conlin, P. R. et al., For the DASH research group, The effect of dietary patterns on blood pressure control in hypertensive patients: results from the Dietary Approaches to Stop Hypertension (DASH) trial, *Am. J. Hypertens.*, 13, 949, 2000.
15. Bray, G. A. et al., A further subgroup analysis of the effects of the DASH diet and three dietary sodium levels on blood pressure: results of the DASH-Sodium trial, *Am. J. Cardiol.*, 94, 222, 2004.
16. McCarron, D. A., DASH-Sodium trial: where are the data? *Am. J. Hypertens.*, 16, 92, 2003.
17. Svetkey, L. P. et al., Effects of dietary patterns on blood pressure. Subgroup analysis of the dietary approaches to stop, *Arch. Intern. Med.*, 159, 285, 1999.
18. Vollmer, W. M. et al., Effects of diet and sodium intake on blood pressure: subgroup analysis of the DASH-Sodium trial, *Ann. Intern. Med.*, 135, 1019, 2001.
19. Moore, T. J. et al., DASH (Dietary Approaches to Stop Hypertension) diet is effective treatment for stage 1 isolated systolic hypertension, *Hypertension*, 38, 155, 2001.
20. Conlin, P. R. et al., The DASH diet enhances the blood pressure response to Losartan in hypertensive patients, *Am. J. Hypertens.*, 16, 337, 2003.
21. McCarron, D. A., Metz, J. A., and Hatten, D. C., Mineral intake and blood pressure in African Americans, *Am. J. Clin. Nutr.*, 68, 517, 1998.
22. Tucker, K., Dietary Patterns and blood pressure in African Americans, *Nutr. Rev.*, 57, 11, 1999.
23. Reusser, M. E. et al., Adequate nutrient intake can reduce cardiovascular disease risk in African Americans, *J. Natl. Med. Assoc.*, 95, 188, 2003.
24. Falkner, B. et al., Dietary nutrients and blood pressure in urban minority adolescents at risk for hypertension, *Arch. Pediatr. Adolesc. Med.*, 154, 918, 2000.
25. Appel, L. J. et al., Effects of protein, monounsaturated fat, and carbohydrate intake on blood pressure and serum lipids, Results of the OmniHeart Randomized Trial, *JAMA*, 294, 2455, 2005.
26. Nowson, C. A. et al., Blood pressure change with weight loss is affected by diet type in men, *Am. J. Clin. Nutr.*, 81, 983, 2005.
27. Steffen, L. M. et al., Associations of plant food, dairy product, and meat intakes with 15-y incidence of elevated blood pressure in young black and white adults: the Coronary Artery Risk Development in Young Adults (CARDIA) Study, *Am. J. Clin. Nutr.*, 82, 1169, 2005.
28. Moore, L. et al., Intake of fruits, vegetables, and dairy products in early childhood and subsequent blood pressure change, *Epidemiology*, 16, 4, 2005.
29. Hajjar, I. and Kotchen, T., Regional variations of blood pressure in the United States are associated with regional variations in dietary intakes: the NHANES-III data, *J. Nutr.*, 133, 211, 2003.
30. Appel, L. J. et al., Dietary approaches to prevent and treat hypertension, a scientific statement from the American Heart Association, *Hypertension*, 47, 296, 2006.
31. IOM (Institute of Medicine), *Dietary Reference Intakes for Calcium, Phosphorus, Magnesium, Vitamin D, and Fluoride, Standing Committee on the Scientific Evaluation of Dietary Reference Intakes, Food and Nutrition Board*, National Academies Press, Washington, D.C., 1997.
32. U.S. Department of Health and Human Services, U.S. Department of Agriculture. *Dietary Guidelines for Americans, 2005*, 6th ed, Washington, D.C., U.S. Government Printing Office, January 2005, www.healthierus.gov/dietaryguidelines.
33. Miller, G. D. et al., Benefits of dairy product consumption on blood pressure in humans: a summary of the biomedical literature, *J. Am. Coll. Nutr.*, 19, 147s, 2000.
34. Lin, P.-H. et al., Food group sources of nutrients in the dietary patterns of the DASH-Sodium trial, *J. Am. Diet. Assoc.*, 103, 488, 2003.
35. McCarron, D. A. and Reusser, M. E., Finding consensus in the dietary calcium–blood pressure debate, *J. Am. Coll. Nutr.*, 18, 398s, 1999.
36. Gerrior, S., Bente, L., and Hiza, H., Nutrient Content of the U.S. Food Supply, 1909 to 2000, U.S. Department of Agriculture, Center for Nutrition Policy and Promotion, Home Economics Research Report No. 55, 2004.
37. U.S. Department of Agriculture, Agricultural Research Service, U.S.D.A National Nutrient Database for Standard Reference, Release 18. Nutrient Data Laboratory Home Page, www.ars.usda.gov/ba/bhnrc/ndl.
38. Institute of Medicine of the National Academies, Dietary Reference Intakes for Water, Potassium, Sodium, Chloride, and Sulfate, The National Academies Press, Washington, D.C., 2004.

39. McCarron, D. A. and Reusser, M. E., Are low intakes of calcium and potassium important causes of cardiovascular disease? *Am. J. Hypertens.*, 14, 206s, 2001.
40. Townsend, M. S. et al., Low mineral intake is associated with high systolic blood pressure in the Third and Fourth National Health and Nutrition Examination Surveys, *Am. J. Hypertens.*, 18, 261, 2005.
41. Hamet, P., The evaluation of the scientific evidence for a relationship between calcium and hypertension, *J. Nutr.*, 125 (suppl.), 311s, 1995.
42. Osborne, C. G. et al., Evidence for the relationship of calcium to blood pressure, *Nutr. Rev.*, 54, 365, 1996.
43. Hatton, D. C. and McCarron, D. A., Dietary calcium and blood pressure in experimental models of hypertension. A review, *Hypertension*, 23 (4), 513, 1994.
44. McCarron, D. A. et al., Blood pressure development of the spontaneously hypertensive rat after concurrent manipulations of dietary Ca^{2+} and Na^{+}: relation to intestinal Ca^{2+} fluxes, *Clin. J. Invest.*, 76, 1147, 1985.
45. Ayachi, S., Increased dietary calcium lowers blood pressure in the spontaneously hypertensive rat, *Metabolism*, 28, 1234, 1979.
46. Pernot, F. et al., Dietary calcium, vascular reactivity, and genetic hypertension in the Lyon rat strain, *Am. J. Hypertens.*, 3, 846, 1990.
47. Schleiffer, R. and Gairard, A., Blood pressure effects of calcium intake in experimental models of hypertension, *Semin. Nephrol.*, 15, 526, 1995.
48. McCarron, D. A., Blood pressure and calcium balance in the Wistar-Kyoto rat, *Life Sci.*, 30, 683, 1982.
49. McCarron, D. A. et al., Dietary calcium and blood pressure: modifying factors in specific populations, *Am. J. Clin. Nutr.*, 54 (suppl. I), 215s, 1991.
50. Porsti, I. and Makynen, H., Dietary calcium intake: effects on central blood pressure control, *Semin. Nephrol.*, 15, 550, 1995.
51. Makynen, H. et al., Endothelial function in deoxycorticosterone–NaCl hypertension. Effect of calcium supplementation, *Circulation*, 93, 1000, 1996.
52. Hamet, P. et al., Calcium levels and platelet responsiveness in spontaneously hypertensive rats on high-calcium diet (Abst.), *J. Hypertens.*, 4 (suppl. 6), 716s, 1986.
53. Sowers, J. R. et al., Calcium and hypertension, *J. Lab. Clin. Med.*, 114, 338, 1989.
54. Oparil, S. et al., Dietary Ca^{2+} prevents NaCl-sensitive hypertension in spontaneously hypertensive rats via sympatholytic and renal effects, *Am. J. Clin. Nutr.*, 54 (suppl.), 227s, 1991.
55. Young, E. W., Bukoski, R. D., and McCarron, D. A., Calcium metabolism in experimental hypertension, *Proc. Soc. Exp. Biol. Med.*, 187, 123, 1988.
56. Blakeborough, P., Neville, S. G., and Rolls, B. A., The effect of diets adequate and deficient in calcium on blood pressures and the activities of intestinal and kidney plasma membrane enzymes in normotensive and spontaneously hypertensive rats, *Br. J. Nutr.*, 63, 65, 1990.
57. Oshima, T. et al., Modification of platelet and lymphocyte calcium handling and blood pressure by dietary sodium and calcium in genetically hypertensive rats, *J. Lab. Clin. Med.*, 119, 151, 1992.
58. Wyss, J. M. et al., Dietary Ca^{2+} prevents NaCl-induced exacerbation of hypertension and increases hypothalamic norepinephrine turnover in spontaneously hypertensive rats, *J. Hypertens.*, 7, 711, 1989.
59. Wuorela, H., The effect of high calcium intake on intracellular free $[Ca^{2+}]$ and Na^{+}–H^{+} exchange in DOC–NaCl-hypertensive rats, *Pharmacol. Toxicol.*, 71, 376, 1992.
60. DiPette, D. J. et al., Effect of dietary calcium supplementation on blood pressure and calcitropic hormones in mineralocorticoid-salt hypertension, *J. Hypertens.*, 8, 515, 1990.
61. Resnick, L. M., Calcium calcitropic hormones in human and experimental hypertension, in *Endocrine Metabolism in Hypertension*, Laragh, J. H., Brenner, B., and Kaplan, N. M., Eds., Raven Press, New York, p. 265, 1989.
62. Resnick, L. M., Muller, F. B., and Laragh, J. H., Calcium regulating hormones in essential hypertension, relation to plasma renin activity and sodium metabolism, *Ann. Intern. Med.*, 105, 649, 1986.
63. Sowers, J. R. et al., Calcium metabolism and dietary calcium in salt sensitive hypertension, *Am. J. Hypertens.*, 4, 557, 1991.

64. Porsti, I. et al., High calcium diet augments vascular potassium relaxation in hypertensive rats, *Hypertension*, 19, 85, 1992.
65. Karanja, N., Phanouvong, T., and McCarron, D. A., Blood pressure in spontaneously hypertensive rats fed butterfat, corn oil, or fish oil, *Hypertension*, 14, 674, 1989.
66. McCarron, D. A. and Morris, C. D., Blood pressure response to oral calcium in persons with mild to moderate hypertension, *Ann. Intern. Med.*, 103, 825, 1985.
67. McCarron, D. A., Calcium metabolism and hypertension, *Kidney Int.*, 35, 717, 1989.
68. Witteman, J. C. M. et al., A prospective study of nutritional factors and hypertension among U.S. women, *Circulation*, 80, 1320, 1989.
69. Iso, H. et al., Calcium intake and blood pressure in seven Japanese populations, *Am. J. Epidemiol.*, 133, 776, 1991.
70. Grobbee, D. E. and Waal-Manning, H. J., The role of calcium supplementation in the treatment of hypertension, current evidence, *Drugs*, 39 (1), 7, 1990.
71. Dwyer, J. H. et al., Dietary calcium, alcohol, and incidence of treated hypertension in the NHANES I epidemiologic follow-up study, *Am. J. Epidemiol.*, 144, 828, 1996.
72. Birkett, N. J., Comments on a meta-analysis on the relationship between dietary calcium intake and blood pressure, *Am. J. Epidemiol.*, 148, 223, 1998.
73. Morris, C. D. and Reusser, M. E., Calcium intake and blood pressure: epidemiology revisited, *Sem. Nephrol.*, 15, 490, 1995.
74. Geleijnse, J. M. and Grobbee, D. E., Calcium intake and blood pressure: an update, *J. Cardiovasc. Risk*, 7, 23, 2000.
75. Ritchie, L. D. and King, J. C., Dietary calcium and pregnancy-induced hypertension: is there a relation? *Am. J. Clin. Nutr.*, 71, 1371s, 2000.
76. Hajjar, I. M., Grim, C. E., and Kotchen, T. A., Dietary calcium lowers the age-related rise in blood pressure in the United States: The NHANES III Survey, *J. Clin. Hypertens.*, 5, 122, 2003.
77. Karanja, N. et al., Impact of increasing calcium in the diet on nutrient consumption, plasma lipids, and lipoproteins in humans, *Am. J. Clin. Nutr.*, 59, 900, 1994.
78. Gillman, M. W. et al., Inverse association of dietary calcium with systolic blood pressure in young children, *JAMA*, 267, 2340, 1992.
79. Simons-Morton, D. G. et al., Nutrient intake and blood pressure in the Dietary Intervention Study in Children, *Hypertension*, 29, 930, 1997.
80. Gillman, M. W. et al., Effect of calcium supplementation on blood pressure in children, *J. Pediatr.*, 127, 186, 1995.
81. Bao, W. et al., Essential hypertension predicted by tracking of elevated blood pressure from childhood to adulthood: the Bogalusa Heart Study, *Am. J. Hypertens.*, 8, 657, 1995.
82. Ascherio, A. et al., A prospective study of nutritional factors and hypertension among U.S. men, *Circulation*, 86, 1475, 1992.
83. Cappuccio, F. P. et al., Epidemiologic association between dietary calcium intake and blood pressure: a meta-analysis of published data, *Am. J. Epidemiol.*, 142, 935, 1995.
84. Garcia-Palmieri, M. R. et al., Milk consumption, calcium intake, and decreased hypertension in Puerto Rico: Puerto Rico Heart Health Program Study, *Hypertension*, 6, 322, 1984.
85. Reed, D. et al., Diet, blood pressure, and multicollinearity, *Hypertension*, 7, 405, 1985.
86. Freudenheim, J. L. et al., Calcium intake and blood pressure in blacks and whites, *Ethnicity Dis.*, 1, 114, 1991.
87. Trevisan, M. et al., Calcium-rich foods and blood pressure: findings from the Italian National Research Council Study (The Nine Communities Study), *Am. J. Epidemiol.*, 127, 1155, 1988.
88. Jorde, R. and Bonaa, K. H., Calcium from dairy products, vitamin D intake, and blood pressure: the Tromso study, *Am. J. Clin. Nutr.*, 71, 1530, 2000.
89. Marcoux, S., Brisson, J., and Fabia, J., Calcium intake from dairy products and supplements and the risks of preeclampsia and gestational hypertension, *Am. J. Epidemiol.*, 133, 1266, 1991.
90. Richardson, B. E. and Baird, D. D., A study of milk and calcium supplement intake and subsequent preeclampsia in a cohort of pregnant women, *Am. J. Epidemiol.*, 141, 667, 1995.
91. Pereira, M. A. et al., Dairy consumption, obesity, and the insulin resistance syndrome in young adults: the CARDIA study, *JAMA*, 287, 2081, 2002.

92. Alonso, A. et al., Low-fat dairy consumption and reduced risk of hypertension: the Sequimiento Universidad de Navarra (SUN) cohort, *Am. J. Clin. Nutr.*, 82, 972, 2005.
93. Allender, P. S. et al., Dietary calcium and blood pressure: a meta-analysis of randomized clinical trials, *Ann. Intern. Med.*, 124, 825, 1996.
94. Bucher, H. C. et al., Effects of dietary calcium supplementation on blood pressure: a meta-analysis of randomized controlled trials, *JAMA*, 275, 1016, 1996.
95. Dwyer, J. H. et al., Dietary calcium, calcium supplementation, and blood pressure in African American adolescents, *Am. J. Clin. Nutr.*, 68, 648, 1998.
96. Bucher, H. C., Guyatt, G. H., and Cook, R. J., Dietary calcium and blood pressure, *Ann. Intern. Med.*, 126, 492, 1997.
97. Griffith, L. E. et al., The influence of dietary and nondietary calcium supplementation on blood pressure. An updated meta-analysis of randomized controlled trials, *J. Hypertens.*, 12, 84, 1999.
98. Resnick, L. M., Nicholson, J. P., and Laragh, J. H., Calcium metabolism in essential hypertension: relationship to altered renin system activity, *Fed. Proc.*, 45, 2739, 1986.
99. Grobbee, D. E. and Hofman, A., Effect of calcium supplementation on diastolic blood pressure in young people with mild hypertension, *Lancet*, 2, 703, 1986.
100. Strazzullo, P. et al., Controlled trial of long-term oral calcium supplementation in essential hypertension, *Hypertension*, 8, 1084, 1986.
101. Resnick, L. et al., Dietary calcium modifies the pressor effects of dietary salt intake in essential hypertension, *J. Hypertens.*, 4 (suppl. 6), 679s, 1986.
102. Zemel, M. B., Gualdoni, S. M., and Sowers, J. R., Reductions in total and extracellular water associated with calcium-induced natriuresis and the antihypertensive effect of calcium in blacks, *Am. J. Hypertens.*, 1, 70, 1988.
103. Vaughan, L. A. et al., Blood pressure responses of mild hypertensive Caucasian males to a metabolic diet with moderate sodium and two levels of dietary calcium, *Nutr. Res.*, 17, 215, 1997.
104. Bucher, H. C. et al., Effect of calcium supplementation on pregnancy-induced hypertension and preeclampsia, *JAMA*, 275, 1113, 1996.
105. Hojo, M. and August, P., Calcium metabolism in normal and hypertensive pregnancy, *Semin. Nephrol.*, 15, 504, 1995.
106. Repke, J. T. and Villar, J., Pregnancy-induced hypertension and low birth weight: the role of calcium, *Am. J. Clin. Nutr.*, 54 (suppl.), 237s, 1991.
107. Belizan, J. M. et al., Calcium supplementation to prevent hypertensive disorders of pregnancy, *N. Engl. J. Med.*, 325, 1399, 1991.
108. Knight, K. B. and Keith, R. E., Calcium supplementation on normotensive and hypertensive pregnant women, *Am. J. Clin. Nutr.*, 55, 891, 1992.
109. Villar, J. and Repke, J. T., Calcium supplementation during pregnancy may reduce preterm delivery in high-risk populations, *J. Obstet. Gynecol.*, 163, 1124, 1990.
110. Levine, R. J. et al., Trial of calcium for prevention of preeclampsia, *N. Engl. J. Med.*, 337, 69, 1997.
111. Atallah, A. N., Hofmeyr, G. J., and Duley, L., Calcium supplementation during pregnancy for preventing hypertensive disorders and related problems, *Cochrane Database Syst. Rev.*, 1, CD001059, 2002.
112. Herrera, J. A. et al., Calcium plus linoleic acid therapy for pregnancy-induced hypertension, *Int. J. Gynecol. Obstet.*, 91, 221, 2005.
113. Belizan, J. M. et al., Long term effect of calcium supplementation during pregnancy on the blood pressure of offspring: follow up of a randomised controlled trial, *Br. Med. J.*, 315, 281, 1997.
114. McGarvey, S. T. et al., Maternal prenatal dietary potassium, calcium, magnesium, and infant blood pressure, *Hypertension*, 17, 218, 1991.
115. Hatton, D. C. et al., Gestational calcium supplementation and blood pressure in the offspring, *Am. J. Hypertens.*, 16, 801, 2003.
116. Bierenbaum, M. L. et al., Dietary calcium: a method of lowering blood pressure, *Am. J. Hypertens.*, 1 (suppl.), 149s, 1988.
117. Van Beresteijn, E. C. H., Van Schaik, M., and Schaafsma, G., Milk: does it affect blood pressure? A controlled intervention study, *J. Intern. Med.*, 228, 477, 1990.
118. Zemel, M. B. et al., Altered cation transport in non-insulin-dependent diabetic hypertension: effects of dietary calcium, *J. Hypertens.*, 6 (suppl. 4), 228s, 1988.

119. Green, J. H. et al., Blood pressure responses to high-calcium skim milk and potassium-enriched high-calcium skim milk, *J. Hypertens.*, 18, 1331, 2000.
120. Barr, S. I. et al., Effects of increased consumption of fluid milk on energy and nutrient factors, body weight and cardiovascular risk factors in healthy older adults, *J. Am. Diet. Assoc.*, 100, 810, 2000.
121. Massey, L. K., Dairy food consumption, blood pressure and stroke, *J. Nutr.*, 131, 2001, 1875.
122. Van Beresteyn, E. C. H., Schaafsma, G., and de Waard, H., Oral calcium and blood pressure: a controlled intervention trial, *Am. J. Clin. Nutr.*, 44, 883, 1986.
123. Kynast-Gales, S. A. and Massey, L. K., Effects of dietary calcium from dairy products on ambulatory blood pressure in hypertensive men, *J. Am. Diet. Assoc.*, 92, 1497, 1992.
124. Takagi, Y. et al., Calcium treatment of essential hypertension in elderly patients evaluated by 24H monitoring, *Am. J. Hypertens.*, 4, 836, 1991.
125. McCarron, D. A., A consensus approach to electrolytes and blood pressure Could we all be right? *Hypertension*, 17 (suppl. I), 170s, 1991.
126. Orwoll, E. S. and Oviatt, S., Relationship of mineral metabolism and long-term calcium and cholecalciferol supplementation to blood pressure in normotensive men, *Am. J. Clin. Nutr.*, 52, 717, 1990.
127. The Trials of Hypertension Prevention Collaborative Research Group, The effects of nonpharmacologic interventions on blood pressure of persons with high normal levels: results of the Trials of Hypertension Prevention, Phase 1, *JAMA*, 267, 1213, 1992.
128. Gruchow, H. W., Sobocinski, K. A., and Barboriak, J. J., Calcium intake and the relationship of dietary sodium and potassium to blood pressure, *Am. J. Clin. Nutr.*, 48, 1463, 1988.
129. Stamler, J., Caggiula, A. W., and Grandits, G. A., Relation of body mass and alcohol, nutrient, fiber, and caffeine intakes to blood pressure in the special intervention and usual care groups in the Multiple Risk Factor Intervention Trial, *Am. J. Clin. Nutr.*, 65 (suppl.), 338s, 1997.
130. McCarron, D. A. and Reusser, M. E., Body weight and blood pressure regulation, *Am. J. Clin. Nutr.*, 63 (suppl.), 423s, 1996.
131. Pickering, T. G., Lessons from the Trials of Hypertension Prevention, Phase II, energy intake is more important than dietary sodium in the prevention of hypertension, *Arch. Intern. Med.*, 157, 596, 1997.
132. Ascherio, A. et al., Prospective study of nutritional factors, blood pressure, and hypertension among U.S. women, *Hypertension*, 27, 1065, 1996.
133. Whelton, P. K. et al., for the Trials of Hypertension Prevention Collaborative Research Group, efficacy of nonpharmacologic interventions in adults with high-normal blood pressure: results from phase I of the Trials of Hypertension Prevention, *Am. J. Clin. Nutr.*, 65 (suppl.), 652s, 1997.
134. Stevens, V. J. et al., Long-term weight loss and changes in blood pressure: results from the Trials of Hypertension Prevention, Phase II, *Ann. Intern. Med.*, 134, 1, 2001.
135. Blumenthal, J. A. et al., Exercise and weight loss reduce blood pressure in men and women with mild hypertension, *Arch. Intern. Med.*, 160, 2000, 1947.
136. Weinberger, M. H., Wagner, U. L., and Fineberg, N. S., The blood pressure effects of calcium supplementation in humans of known sodium responsiveness, *Am. J. Hypertens.*, 6, 799, 1993.
137. Zemel, M. B. et al., Effects of sodium and calcium on calcium metabolism and blood pressure regulation in hypertensive black adults, *J. Hypertens.*, 4 (suppl.), 364s, 1986.
138. Hamet, P. et al., Interactions among calcium, sodium, and alcohol intake as determinants of blood pressure, *Hypertension*, 17 (suppl. I), 150s, 1991.
139. Hamet, P. et al., Epidemiological evidence of an interaction between calcium and sodium intake impacting on blood pressure, a Montreal study, *Am. J. Hypertens.*, 5, 378, 1992.
140. Saito, K. et al., Effect of oral calcium on blood pressure response in salt-loaded borderline hypertensive patients, *Hypertension*, 13, 219, 1989.
141. Zemel, P., Gualdoni, S., and Sowers, J. R., Racial differences in mineral intake in ambulatory normotensives and hypertensives, *Am. J. Hypertens.*, 1, 1465, 1988.
142. Oparil, S. Ed., Conference on Dietary Sodium and Health, *Am. J. Clin. Nutr.*, 65 (suppl. 2), 583s, 1997.
143. He, J. et al., Relation of electrolytes to blood pressure in men, The Yi people study, *Hypertension*, 17, 378, 1991.
144. Criqui, M. H., Langer, R. D., and Reed, D. M., Dietary alcohol, calcium, and potassium: independent and combined effects on blood pressure, *Circulation*, 80, 609, 1989.
145. Resnick, L. M., Dietary calcium and hypertension, *J. Nutr.*, 117, 1806, 1987.

146. Linas, S. L., The role of potassium in the pathogenesis and treatment of hypertension, *Kidney Int.*, 39, 771, 1991.
147. Haddy, F. J., Roles of sodium, potassium, calcium, and natriuretic factors in hypertension, *Hypertension*, 18 (suppl. III), 179s, 1991.
148. Tobian, L., Dietary sodium chloride and potassium have effects on the pathophysiology of hypertension in humans and animals, *Am. J. Clin. Nutr.*, 65 (s), 606s, 1997.
149. Sacks, F. M. et al., Effect on blood pressure of potassium, calcium, and magnesium in women with low habitual intake, *Hypertension*, 31 (Part 1), 131, 1998.
150. U.S. Food and Drug Administration, Health claim notification for potassium containing foods, October 31, 2000, http://vm.cfsan.fda.gov/~dms/hclm-k.html.
151. Barden, A., Beilin, L. J., and Vandongen, R., Effect of potassium supplementation on blood pressure and vasodilator mechanisms in spontaneously hypertensive rats, *Clin. Sci.*, 75, 527, 1988.
152. Wu, X., Ackermann, U., and Sonnenberg, H., Potassium depletion and salt-sensitive hypertension in Dahl rats: effect on calcium, magnesium, and phosphate excretions, *Clin. Exp. Hypertens.*, 17, 989, 1995.
153. Hajjar, I. M. et al., Impact of diet on blood pressure and age-related changes in blood pressure in the U.S. population, *Arch. Intern. Med.*, 161, 589, 2001.
154. Intersalt Cooperative Research Group, Intersalt: an international study of electrolyte excretion and blood pressure: results for 24 h urinary sodium and potassium excretion, *Br. Med. J.*, 297, 319, 1988.
155. Stamler, R., Implications of the INTERSALT Study, *Hypertension*, 17 (suppl. 1), 16s, 1991.
156. Joffres, M. R., Reed, D. M., and Yano, K., Relationship of magnesium intake and other dietary factors to blood pressure: the Honolulu heart study, *Am. J. Clin. Nutr.*, 45, 469, 1987.
157. Geleijnse, J. M., Grobbee, D. E., and Hofman, A., Sodium and potassium intake and blood pressure change in childhood, *Br. Med. J.*, 300, 899, 1990.
158. Sinaiko, A. R., Gomez-Marin, O., and Prineas, R. J., Effect of low sodium diet or potassium supplementation on adolescent blood pressure, *Hypertension*, 21, 989, 1993.
159. Khaw, K. T. and Barrett-Connor, E., Dietary potassium and stroke-associated mortality: a 12-year prospective population study, *N. Engl. J. Med.*, 316, 235, 1987.
160. Xie, J. X. et al., The relationship between urinary cations obtained from the INTERSALT study and cerebrovascular mortality, *J. Hum. Hypertens.*, 6, 17, 1992.
161. Whelton, P. K. et al., Effects of oral potassium on blood pressure: meta-analysis of randomized controlled clinical trials, *JAMA*, 277, 1624, 1997.
162. Brancati, F. L. et al., Effect of potassium supplementation on blood pressure in African Americans on a low-potassium diet, *Arch. Intern. Med.*, 156, 61, 1996.
163. Fotherby, M. D. and Potter, J. F., Long-term potassium supplementation lowers blood pressure in elderly hypertensive subjects, *Int. J. Clin. Practice*, 51, 219, 1997.
164. Gu, D. et al., Effect of potassium supplementation on blood pressure in Chinese: a randomized, placebo-controlled trial, *J. Hypertens.*, 19, 1325, 2001.
165. Geleijnse, J. M., Kok, F. J., and Grobbee, D. E., Blood pressure response to changes in sodium and potassium intake: a metaregression analysis of randomised trials, *J. Hum. Hypertens.*, 17, 471, 2003.
166. He, F. J. et al., Effect of short-term supplementation of potassium chloride and potassium citrate on blood pressure in hypertensives, *Hypertension*, 45, 571, 2005.
167. Siani, A. et al., Increasing the dietary potassium intake reduces the need for antihypertensive medication, *Ann. Intern. Med.*, 115, 753, 1991.
168. Langford, H. G., Cushman, W. C., and Hsu, H., Chronic affect of KCl on black–white differences in plasma renin activity, aldosterone, and urinary electrolytes, *Am. J. Hypertens.*, 4, 399, 1991.
169. Grimm, R. H. Jr. et al., The influence of oral potassium chloride on blood pressure in hypertensive men on a low-sodium diet, *N. Engl. J. Med.*, 322, 569, 1990.
170. Geleijnse, J. M. et al., Dietary electrolyte intake and blood pressure in older subjects: the Rotterdam Study, *J. Hypertens.*, 14, 737, 1996.
171. Paolisso, G. and Barbagallo, M., Hypertension, diabetes mellitus, and insulin resistance. The role of intracellular magnesium, *Am. J. Hypertens.*, 10, 346, 1997.
172. Berthelot, A. et al., Disturbances of magnesium metabolism in the spontaneously hypertensive rat, *J. Am. Coll. Nutr.*, 6, 329, 1987.

173. Matuura, T. et al., Decreased intracellular free magnesium in erythrocytes of spontaneously hypertensive rats, *Biochem. Biophys. Res. Commun.*, 143, 1012, 1987.
174. Berthelot, A. and Esposito, J., Effects of dietary magnesium on the development of hypertension in the spontaneously hypertensive rat, *J. Am. Coll. Nutr.*, 4, 343, 1983.
175. Wolf, P. et al., Blood pressure and plasma renin activity after magnesium supplementation in the spontaneously hypertensive rat: a study during developing and established hypertension, *Magnesium*, 6, 243, 1987.
176. Laurant, P. et al., Effect of magnesium deficiency on blood pressure and mechanical properties of rat carotid artery, *Hypertension*, 33, 1105, 1999.
177. Laurant, P., Kantelip, J.-P., and Berthelot, A., Dietary magnesium supplementation modifies blood pressure and cardiovascular function in mineralocorticoid-salt hypertensive rats but not in normotensive rats, *J. Nutr.*, 125, 830, 1995.
178. Whelton, P. K. and Klag, M. J., Magnesium and blood pressure: review of the epidemiologic and clinical trial experience, *Am. J. Cardiol.*, 63 (suppl. G), 26s, 1989.
179. Resnick, L. M. et al., Divalent cations in essential hypertension, relations between serum ionized calcium, magnesium and plasma renin activity, *N. Engl. J. Med.*, 309, 888, 1983.
180. Ma, J. et al., Associations of serum and dietary magnesium with cardiovascular disease, hypertension, diabetes, insulin, and carotid arterial wall thickness: the ARIC study, *J. Clin. Epidemiol.*, 48, 927, 1995.
181. Mizushima, S. et al., Dietary magnesium intake and blood pressure: a qualitative overview of the observational studies, *J. Hum. Hypertens.*, 12, 447, 1998.
182. Zemel, P. C. et al., Metabolic and hemodynamic effects of magnesium supplementation in patients with essential hypertension, *Am. J. Clin. Nutr.*, 51, 665, 1990.
183. Witteman, J. C. M. et al., Reduction of blood pressure with oral magnesium supplementation in women with mild to moderate hypertension, *Am. J. Clin. Nutr.*, 60, 129, 1994.
184. Jee, S. H. et al., The effect of magnesium supplementation on blood pressure: a meta-analysis of randomized clinical trials, *Am. J. Hypertens.*, 15, 691, 2002.
185. Ford, E. S. and Mokdad, A. H., Dietary magnesium intake in a national sample of U.S. adults, *J. Nutr.*, 133, 2879, 2003.
186. FitzGerald, R. J., Murray, B. A., and Walsh, D. J., Hypotensive peptides from milk proteins, *J. Nutr.*, 134, 980s, 2004.
187. Hata, Y. et al., A placebo-controlled study of the effect of sour milk on blood pressure in hypertensive subjects, *Am. J. Clin. Nutr.*, 64, 767, 1996.
188. Seppo, L. et al., A fermented milk high in bioactive peptides has a blood pressure-lowering effect in hypertensive subjects, *Am. J. Clin. Nutr.*, 77, 326, 2003.
189. Mizuno, S. et al., Antihypertensive effect of casein hydrolysate in a placebo-controlled study in subjects with high-normal blood pressure and mild hypertension, *Br. J. Nutr.*, 94, 84, 2005.
190. Aihara, K. et al., Effect of powdered fermented milk with *Lactobacillus helveticus* on subjects with high-normal blood pressure or mild hypertension, *J. Am. Coll. Nutr.*, 24, 257, 2005.
191. Neter, J. E., Influence of weight reduction on blood pressure: a meta-analysis of randomized controlled trials, *Hypertension*, 42, 878, 2003.
192. Sorof, J. M. et al., Overweight, ethnicity, and the prevalence of hypertension in school-aged children, *Pediatrics*, 113, 475, 2004.
193. Zemel, M. B., Role of calcium and dairy products in energy partitioning and weight management, *Am. J. Clin. Nutr.*, 79, 907s, 2004.
194. Whelton, S. P. et al., Effect of aerobic exercise on blood pressure: a meta-analysis of randomized, controlled trials, *Ann. Intern. Med.*, 136, 493, 2002.
195. Kaplan, N. M., The dietary guideline for sodium: should we shake it up? No, *Am. J. Clin. Nutr.*, 71, 1020, 2000.
196. McCarron, D. A., The dietary guideline for sodium: should we shake it up? Yes! *Am. J. Clin. Nutr.*, 71, 1013, 2000.
197. Taubes, G., The (political) science of salt, *Science*, 281, 898, 1998.
198. Mitka, M., Dash of dissent on salt intake advice, *JAMA*, 291, 1686, 2004.
199. Obarzanek, E. et al., Individual blood pressure responses to changes in salt intake. Results from the DASH-Sodium Trial, *Hypertension*, 42, 459, 2003.

200. Graudal, N. A., Galloe, A. M., and Garred, P., Effects of sodium restriction on blood pressure, renin, aldosterone, catecholamines, cholesterols, and triglyceride. A meta-analysis, *JAMA*, 279, 1383, 1998.
201. He, F. J. and MacGregor, G. A., Effects of modest salt reduction on blood pressure: a meta-analysis of randomized trials. Implications for public health, *J. Hum. Hypertens.*, 16, 761, 2002.
202. Oparil, S., Blood pressure and metabolic responses to moderate sodium restriction in Isradipine-treated hypertensive patients, *Am. J. Hypertens.*, 10, 68, 1997.
203. Touyz, R. M. et al., The Canadian recommendations for the management of hypertension: Part III — lifestyle modifications to prevent and control hypertension, *Can. J. Cardiol.*, 20, 55, 2004.
204. Alderman, M. H., Cohen, H., and Madhavan, S., Dietary sodium intake and mortality: The National Health and Nutrition Examination Survey (NHANES I), *Lancet*, 351, 781, 1998.
205. Alderman, M. H., Salt, blood pressure, and human health, *Hypertension*, 36, 890, 2000.
206. Morris, C. D., Effect of dietary sodium restriction on overall nutrient intake, *Am. J. Clin. Nutr.*, 65 (suppl.), 687s, 1997.
207. McCarron, D. A. et al., Blood pressure and metabolic responses to moderate sodium restriction in Isradipine-treated hypertensive patients, *Am. J. Hypertens.*, 10, 68, 1997.
208. Hooper, L. et al., Systematic review of long term effects of advice to reduce dietary salt in adults, *Br. Med. J.*, 325, 628, 2002.
209. Miller, E. R. III et al., Results of the Diet, Exercise and Weight Loss Intervention Trial (DEW-IT), *Hypertension*, 40, 612, 2002.
210. Writing Group of the PREMIER Collaborative Research Group, effects of comprehensive lifestyle modifications on blood pressure control, *JAMA*, 289, 2083, 2003.
211. Miller, G. D., Jarvis, J. K., and McBean, L. D., The importance of meeting calcium needs with foods, *J. Am. Coll. Nutr.*, 20, 168s, 2001.
212. Heaney, R. P., Calcium, dairy products and osteoporosis, *J. Am. Coll. Nutr.*, 19, 83s, 2000.
213. Devine, A., Prince, R. L., and Bell, R., Nutritional effect of calcium supplementation by skim milk powder or calcium tablets on total nutrient intake in postmenopausal women, *Am. J. Clin. Nutr.*, 64, 731, 1996.
214. Barger-Lux, M. J. et al., Nutritional correlates of low calcium intake, *Clin. Appl. Nutr.*, 2 (4), 39, 1992.
215. Chan, G. M., Hoffman, K., and McMurray, M., Effects of dairy products on bone and body composition in pubertal girls, *J. Pediatr.*, 126, 551, 1995.
216. Cadogan, J. et al., Milk intake and bone mineral acquisition in adolescent girls: randomized, controlled intervention trial, *Br. Med. J.*, 315, 1255, 1997.
217. Ballew, C., Kuester, S., and Gillespie, C., Beverage choices affect adequacy of children's nutrient intakes, *Arch. Pediatr. Adolesc. Med.*, 154, 1148, 2000.
218. Bowman, S. A., Beverage choices of young females: changes and impact on nutrient intakes, *J. Am. Diet. Assoc.*, 102, 1234, 2002.
219. Johnson, R. K., Frary, C., and Wang, M. Q., The nutritional consequences of flavored-milk consumption by school-aged children and adolescents in the United States, *J. Am. Diet. Assoc.*, 102, 853, 2002.
220. Frary, C. D., Johnson, R. K., and Wang, M. Q., Children and adolescents' choices of foods and beverages high in added sugars are associated with intakes of key nutrients and food groups, *J. Adol. Health*, 34, 56, 2004.
221. McCarron, D. A. and Heaney, R. P., Estimated healthcare savings associated with adequate dairy food intake, *Am. J. Hypertens.*, 17, 88, 2004.

4 Dairy Foods and Cancer

4.1 INTRODUCTION

Cancer is the second leading cause of death in the United States (after heart disease), responsible for one out of every four deaths [1]. Both genetic and environmental factors contribute to this disease [1,2]. Heredity accounts for approximately 5% to 10% of all cancers [1]. Among environmental factors, about one-third of cancer deaths are estimated to be related to poor nutrition and physical inactivity, including obesity [1].

Although some dietary factors such as fat are suspected of contributing to specific cancers, other dietary factors may be protective [2]. Several components in dairy foods, specifically calcium and vitamin D, bacterial cultures (for example, *Lactobacillus acidophilus*), a class of fatty acids known as conjugated dienoic derivatives of linoleic acid (CLA), sphingolipids, butyric acid, and milk proteins may protect against cancer [3–10].

This chapter reviews research on the role of dairy foods and dairy food nutrients in three common cancers: colon or colorectal cancer, breast cancer, and prostate cancer. By far, most of the research has focused on the potentially beneficial effect of dairy foods/dairy food nutrients on colorectal cancer risk.

4.1.1 Dietary Fat and Cancer Risk

High intake of dietary fat has been implicated in the development of some cancers, including those of the colon, breast, and prostate gland [11]. Early support for this theory comes from experimental animal and some cross-cultural studies (for example, international food disappearance data, migrant, and time trend studies) [11]. However, findings from more recent epidemiological studies and clinical trials weaken this theory [11–14].

4.1.1.1 Dietary Fat and Colon Cancer

With respect to colon cancer, experimental animal studies support the suggestion that total fat increases the risk of this cancer. Colon cancer has been shown to develop more readily in animals fed a high-fat diet than in those fed a low-fat diet, especially when carcinogens are administered concurrently [15–17]. As reviewed by Reddy [15], carcinogen-induced colon tumor incidence was greater in rats fed high fat (23% by weight) semipurified diets containing either corn oil, safflower oil, lard, or beef tallow than in animals fed low fat (5% by weight) versions of these diets. High-fat diets containing coconut oil, olive oil, or *trans* fatty acids had no colon-tumor enhancing effect. When fat intake is low (less than 4% to 5%), polyunsaturated fatty acids are more effective than saturated fats in enhancing tumorigenesis, apparently because of the requirement for the essential fatty acid — linoleic acid [18]. When this requirement is satisfied, the total amount of dietary fat, not the type of fat, appears to be more important in tumorigenesis. Dietary fat appears to promote, rather than initiate, carcinogenesis [15]. In a review of fat and colon cancer in experimental animals, Klurfeld and Bull [19] suggest that total dietary fat generally increases colon tumorigenesis; however, other confounding factors such as total energy intake and the interaction of fat with other nutrients influence this relationship. No one specific type of fat appears to promote colon cancer in experimental animals except linoleic acid when dietary fat intake is low.

Experimental animal studies suggest mechanisms by which fat may affect colon cancer risk [15]. Dietary fat intake increases free fatty acids and bile acid secretion, which subsequently leads to a rise in the concentration of potentially toxic secondary bile acids (for example, deoxycholic acid and lithocholic acid) in the colonic lumen [20]. Free fatty acids and secondary bile acids can induce mucosal cell damage, increase epithelial cell proliferation rates, and enhance carcinogenesis by acting as tumor promoters in experimental animals [20].

Findings from recent epidemiological studies indicate little or no association between dietary fat intake and colon cancer risk. In a pooled analysis of 13 case-control studies of colorectal cancer, Howe et al. [21] found no association between dietary fat intake and risk of this cancer after adjusting for total energy intake. Several prospective studies have failed to find an association between total fat intake and colorectal cancer risk [22–24]. Neither total fat, different types of fat, nor major fatty acids were associated with risk of colorectal cancer in a prospective study of more than 37,000 female health professionals participating in the Women's Health Study [24]. However, intake of fried foods eaten away from home was significantly related to increased risk of colon cancer [24]. Based on a review of 40 case-control and cohort studies, Giovannucci and Goldin [25] conclude that total fat intake is not associated with colon cancer risk.

Inconsistencies in the relationship between total fat and colon cancer risk in epidemiological studies may be explained in part by the difficulty in separating the effects of fat from those of calories [25–27]. Excess calories may be more important than total fat in the pathogenesis of colon cancer [26]. According to a case-control study involving more than 4400 U.S. adults, consuming an extra 500 calories per day increased colon cancer risk by 15% in men and by 11% in women after controlling for physical activity and body weight [28]. Individual sources of energy (that is, dietary fat, protein, carbohydrate) did not affect colon cancer risk beyond the risk associated with energy intake. Also, failure to demonstrate an association between fat intake and colon cancer in some epidemiological studies may be explained by a narrow range of fat intake and/or protective factors in the diet. Consumption of a low-fat diet did not reduce the risk of colorectal cancer in the Women's Health Initiative Dietary Modification Trial, an 8-year, randomized, controlled clinical trial conducted in more than 48,000 healthy U.S. postmenopausal women [13].

4.1.1.2 Dietary Fat and Breast Cancer

High dietary fat is hypothesized to increase fat secretion into the small ducts of the mammary gland where the fat can be partly metabolized to free fatty acids [29]. Free fatty acids can be highly cytotoxic to local epithelial cells, leading to cell damage and necrosis followed by increased cell proliferation [29]. Although some evidence from experimental animal studies indicates that dietary fat enhances mammary carcinogenesis [30,31], findings from epidemiological studies of fat intake and breast cancer risk are weak and inconsistent [12,31–35]. In a pooled analysis of several prospective studies of more than 350,000 women, dietary fat intake was not associated with cancer risk [32]. In contrast, a prospective study of more than 90,000 women found that fat and animal fat intake, in particular, was associated with increased risk of breast cancer [35]. However, the researchers state that "intake of dairy fat *per se* was not statistically significantly associated with breast cancer risk" [35]. In a recent comprehensive review of dairy products and risk of breast cancer, Moorman and Terry [31] report that epidemiological studies fail to show that dietary fat or the fat content of dairy products increases breast cancer risk. Inconsistencies in findings from epidemiological studies examining the association between dietary fat intake and breast cancer may be related to several confounding factors such as intake of energy and other nutrients, as well as differences in methodologies used to assess fat intake [36]. In the Women's Health Initiative Dietary Modification Trial, which is a randomized, controlled clinical trial, intake of a low-fat diet did not reduce the risk of breast cancer [14].

4.1.1.3 Dietary Fat and Prostate Cancer

Although some epidemiological studies report that high dietary fat intake is linked to increased risk of advanced prostate cancer [37,38], other epidemiological studies do not support this finding [39,40]. A recent review of prospective cohort and intervention studies of potential dietary risk factors for prostate cancer found an inconsistent association between total fat or individual fatty acids and prostate cancer [41].

4.2 DAIRY FOODS, CALCIUM, VITAMIN D, AND PREVENTION OF COLON CANCER

Colorectal cancer is the third leading cause of cancer morbidity and mortality for both men and women in the United States [1]. In 2005, it was estimated that 145,290 Americans would develop this disease and 56,290 were expected to die from it [1]. An equal number of men and women are affected by colorectal cancer. Because the cause(s) of cancers of the colon and rectum is presumably the same, these cancers will be treated as one in this chapter. Epidemiological, experimental animal, *in vitro*, and clinical studies in humans have investigated a potential protective role for dairy foods, and particularly dairy food nutrients such as calcium and vitamin D, against colon cancer [9,10,42–49].

4.2.1 Epidemiological Studies

More than 25 years ago, Garland and Garland [50] proposed that calcium and vitamin D could reduce the risk of colon cancer. Since that time, many epidemiological studies have examined this hypothesis [48,51,52]. Calcium intake has been demonstrated to be inversely associated with colon cancer incidence and mortality in human population studies conducted both within the United States and among different countries (Figure 4.1) [46,53,54]. Similar types of studies demonstrate an inverse relationship between vitamin D (which increases calcium absorption) and colon cancer [10,46,55]. Vitamin D is obtained through synthesis in the body from exposure to sunlight and by consuming vitamin D-containing foods such as vitamin D-fortified milk. In ecologic studies, geographic variations in colon cancer mortality rates are associated with differences in latitudes and exposure to sunlight [50,56].

A number of case-control epidemiological studies suggest a protective effect for calcium and/or vitamin D against colon cancer [53,55,57–64]. In a case-control study in Utah in which male and female subjects were interviewed 2 years prior to the onset of cancer, Slattery et al. [53] found that a moderate intake of dietary calcium (i.e., greater than 800 mg daily) was associated with reduced risk of colon cancer, particularly in males. Findings from a large case-control study (746 matched pairs) in Los Angeles County, California demonstrated that increased calcium intake, and to a lesser extent vitamin D, are significantly associated with reduced risk of colon cancer after adjusting for total calories [59]. In another case-control study involving over 4000 adults in California, Utah, and Minnesota (1993 colon cancer cases and 2410 controls), risk of colon cancer was lower in both men and women who consumed diets higher in calcium [62]. In this study, consumption of total low-fat dairy products and calcium supplements, but not dietary vitamin D or sunshine exposure, was statistically associated with a decreased risk of colon cancer. Likewise, case-control studies of adults in Sweden [60] and Montreal, Quebec [58] support a protective effect of calcium against colon cancer.

Adenomas (benign noncancerous tumors) are an early stage of cancer development. Calcium intake was associated with a significant decrease in colorectal cancer risk in a case-control study in Uruguay involving 282 patients with adenocarcinomas of the colon and rectum and 564 hospitalized controls [61]. Higher intakes of vitamin D were also associated with reduced risk of colorectal cancer. Martinez et al. [65] reported that a calcium intake of nearly 1400 mg/day was protective

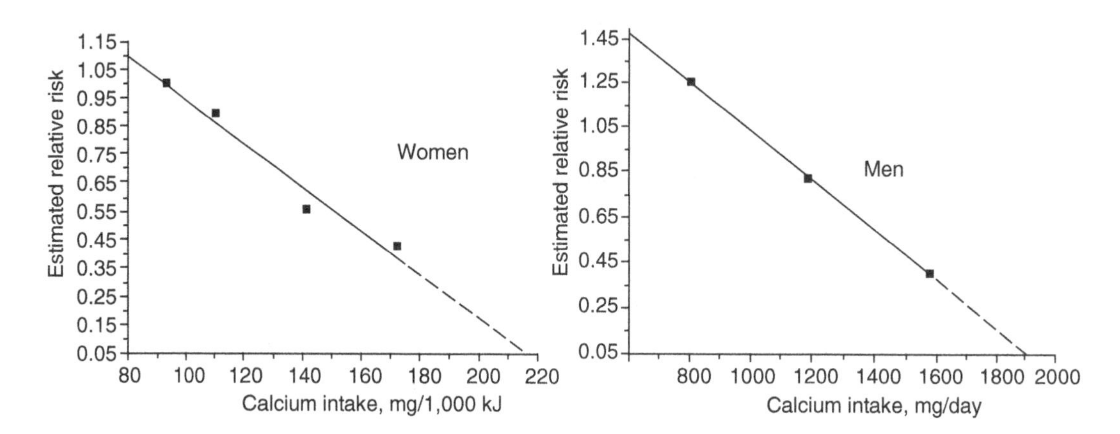

FIGURE 4.1 Estimated relative risk of colon cancer according to calcium intake per 1000 Kj in adults aged 40 to 79 years, Utah, 1979–1982. (From Slattery, M. L., Sorenson, A. W., and Ford, M. H., *Am. J. Epidemiol.*, 128, 504, 1988. With permission.)

against adenomatous polyps. The results of a case-control study of dietary intakes and other lifestyle factors for hyperplastic polyps in more than 500 adults indicate that high intakes of calcium (greater than 1000 mg/day) may be protective [66]. Hyperplastic polyps may be markers for the subsequent development of adenomas or carcinomas. Peters et al. [64], in a recent case-control study, evaluated the effect of calcium intake on colorectal adenoma in 3696 adults with adenoma of the distal colon and in 34,817 adults who did not have an adenoma. Calcium intake was determined using a food frequency questionnaire plus additional questions about calcium supplement use. Results showed that participants with the highest total calcium intake (greater than 1767 mg/day) had a 12% lower risk of colorectal adenoma than those with the lowest calcium intake (less than 731 mg/day), after adjusting for known risk factors (Figure 4.2). Participants taking more than 1200 mg/day of supplemental calcium had a 27% lower risk of colorectal adenoma than did those who did not use calcium supplements. Although this study found that high calcium intake, particularly from supplements, was associated with reduced risk of colorectal adenoma, other studies have found calcium-rich dairy foods, particularly milk, to be the most protective [48]. In another case-control study conducted by Peters et al. [57], a 73% reduction in risk of advanced colorectal adenomas was found in women in the highest quintile of serum 25(OH) D levels compared to those in the lowest quintile [57]. No association was found between serum 25(OH) D levels and adenoma risk in men.

Numerous prospective (cohort) epidemiological studies have examined the effect of calcium and/or vitamin D on colon cancer risk [23,52,55,56,67–81]. In an early 19-year prospective study of 1954 men working at the Western Union Electric Company in Chicago, the incidence of colorectal cancer was reduced by 75% in men who consumed 1200 mg or more of calcium a day and by 50% in those whose intake of vitamin D exceeded 3.75 μg (150 International Unit [IU]) a day [56]. Based on these early findings, Newmark and Lipkin [43] suggested that calcium intakes of more than 1800 and 1500 mg/day for men and women, respectively, are necessary to reduce the incidence of colon cancer. These amounts of calcium exceed current recommendations of 1000 to 1200 mg calcium per day for most adults [82]. In a 4-year prospective study of over 35,000 Iowa women aged 55 to 69 years without a history of cancer, calcium and vitamin D intakes were associated with a modest reduction in colon cancer risk [67].

The Antioxidant Polyp Prevention Study, a prospective study involving more than 700 adults, found that increased intake of dietary calcium, but not calcium supplements, was associated with a reduced risk of recurrent colorectal adenomas [68]. Adults who consumed more than 2 servings of

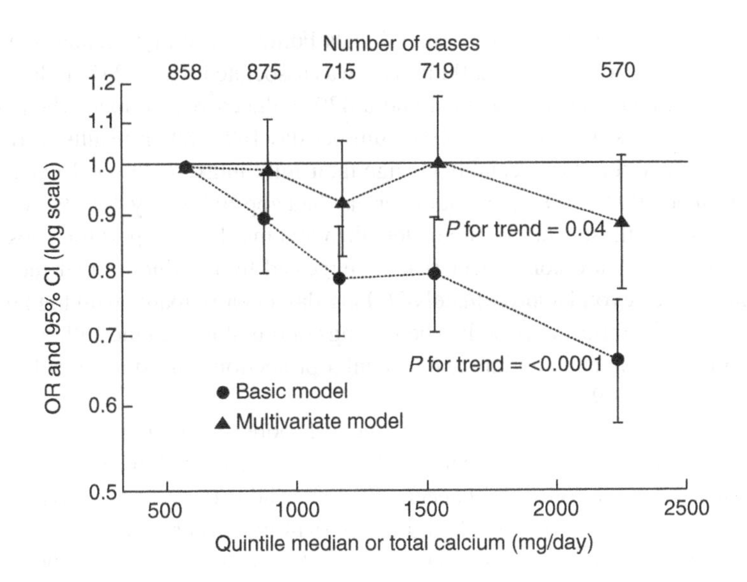

FIGURE 4.2 Association between total calcium intake and distal colorectal adenoma. Basic model adjusted for age, screening center, sex, and energy intake. Multivariate model adjusted for age, screening center, sex, energy intake, ethnic origin, educational attainment, tobacco use, alcohol intake, aspirin and ibuprofen use, physical activity, body mass index, and intakes of red meat, folate, and dietary fiber. (From Peters, U. et al., *Am. J. Clin. Nutr.*, 80, 1358, 2004.)

dairy foods a day had a slightly lower incidence of recurrent colon cancer than adults who consumed less than 1/2 a serving of dairy foods a day [68]. Dietary calcium appeared to have a more beneficial effect on colon cancer risk in individuals with a high-fat diet than those with a low-fat diet [68]. A more recent study of 1304 adults participating in the Wheat Bran Fiber Trial found that high dietary calcium (greater than 1068 mg/day) was associated with reduced risk of adenoma recurrence compared to those with dietary calcium intake below 698 mg/day, whereas calcium supplementation above 200 mg/day did not affect risk of recurrence [71].

Several other prospective studies published in the mid-1990s are less supportive of a protective effect of calcium against colon cancer. Findings from the Nurses' Health Study, a 6-year prospective study in the United States involving more than 89,000 women, revealed no consistent, significant association between calcium intake and risk of colon or rectal cancers [73]. However, a possible protective effect of vitamin D was observed, especially for rectal cancer. In the Health Professionals Follow-up Study Cohort, men who consumed higher intakes of calcium and vitamin D exhibited a slight, but statistically insignificant, reduction in risk of colon cancer compared to men who consumed lower intakes of these nutrients [74]. This study followed 47,935 male U.S. health professionals for 6 years, during which time 203 men developed colon cancer. Intake of milk and fermented milk products was not significantly associated with colon cancer risk [74].

A 1996 meta-analysis of 24 epidemiological studies (16 case-control and 8 prospective) of calcium and colon and/or rectal cancer or polyps failed to support the hypothesis that calcium protects against colorectal cancer [75]. The authors suggest that other dietary factors that affect calcium absorption and metabolism (for example, vitamin D, phosphate, and fiber) may influence the findings. Also, whether calcium has a protective effect only during a specific time of cancer development or at a specific subsite of the large bowel cannot be ruled out [79].

More recent prospective studies support a fairly consistent modest inverse association between calcium and/or vitamin D and colon cancer risk [52,69,70,76–78,80,81]. Wu et al. [69] combined the results from two large-scale, prospective studies in the United States, the Nurses' Health Study (almost 88,000 women) and the Health Professionals Follow-up Study (greater than 47,000 men). Higher calcium intake (greater than 1250 mg/day) was associated with a 27% reduced risk of distal (but not proximal) colon cancer in women and a 42% reduced risk in men when compared with those who consumed less than 500 mg of calcium per day [69]. When results were combined for men and women who did not appreciably change their milk intake over the 16 years of the study, those who consumed 700 to 800 mg calcium per day had approximately 40% to 50% lower risk of distal colon cancer than those who consumed less than 500 mg/day. Support for a possible threshold effect of calcium intake on colon cancer risk is suggested by the finding that increasing supplemental calcium intake beyond approximately 700 mg/day in participants with high dietary calcium appeared to have minimal further benefit. The findings of this study led the authors to conclude that "even a modest increase in calcium intake may confer protection against distal colon cancer among those with low intakes" [69].

In a large-scale observational prospective study of more than 61,000 women in Sweden who were followed for an average of 11 years, higher dietary calcium intake was associated with a moderately reduced risk of colorectal cancer [70]. After adjusting for other risk factors, women over 55 years of age with the highest calcium intake (914 mg/day) had a significant 28% and 55% lower risk of colorectal and distal colon cancer, respectively, than those with the lowest (486 mg/day) calcium intake. A prospective study of more than 45,000 Swedish men aged 45 to 79 years who were followed for 6.7 years found that the relative risk of colorectal cancer was 32% lower in those who consumed the highest quartile of total calcium (1445 mg/day or higher) compared to those in the lowest quartile (less than 956 mg calcium per day) [80].

In a 5-year observational prospective study of more than 60,000 men and more than 66,000 women participating in the Cancer Prevention Study II Nutrition Cohort (United States), those with the highest quintile of total calcium intake from diet and supplements had a 13% significantly lower risk of colorectal cancer than those in the lowest quintile of calcium intake [76]. The researchers suggest that their findings, along with those of Wu et al. [69] that also indicate a modest role for calcium in reducing colorectal cancer risk, call for more research to determine the optimal dose of calcium to reduce colorectal cancer risk. In their study, McCullough et al. [76] found that the association was strongest for calcium from supplements; dairy product intake was not related to overall colorectal risk. Total vitamin D intake from diet and multivitamins was associated with a lower risk of colorectal cancer, particularly among men [76].

A prospective study of more than 45,000 women without a history of colorectal cancer who were followed for an average of 8.5 years found that a difference of less than 400 to more than 800 mg calcium per day was associated with an approximately 25% decreased risk of colorectal cancer [78]. Moreover, simultaneously consuming high levels of calcium from both diet and supplements further reduced the risk (i.e., by approximately 45%). Although the risk of colorectal cancer was reduced regardless of the source of calcium, dietary calcium intakes greater than 400 mg/day resulted in a marked reduction in risk, whereas no association was observed for calcium supplements of less than 800 mg/day [78]. The researchers suggest that this discrepancy may be explained by differences in the bioavailability of calcium between diet and supplements. Based on their findings, the researchers suggest that a calcium intake of over 800 to 1200 mg/day may reduce the risk of colorectal cancer by 15% to 25% [78].

An investigation of approximately 73,000 French women ages 40 to 65 participating in the E3N-EPIC prospective study found that with increasing calcium intake there was a trend of decreasing risk of both adenoma and colorectal cancer [81]. Participants with the highest vs. lowest calcium intakes had a 20% lower risk of adenoma and a 28% lower risk of colorectal cancer. Higher phosphorus intake was associated with a 30% reduction in adenoma risk [81]. In addition, a protective effect of dairy products on adenoma (20% risk reduction) and of milk consumption on colorectal cancer (46% risk reduction) was observed, although the latter did not reach statistical significance [81]. In this study, dietary vitamin D did not appear to affect colorectal tumor risk.

The researchers conclude that their findings support the hypothesis that intakes of total dietary calcium and phosphorus reduce the risk of colorectal cancer [81].

Findings from a recent 10-year prospective study of more than 36,000 women participating in the U.S. Women's Health Study failed to support a protective role for calcium (from food or supplements) and vitamin D intakes against colorectal cancer incidence [79]. In this group of women, median intakes of total calcium and vitamin D were 882 mg/day and 271 IU/day, respectively. The researchers suggest that the lack of a protective effect of calcium against colorectal cancer in this study may be due to the relatively low intake of calcium consumed [79]. The failure to show a protective effect of vitamin D may be due to the lack of information on sun exposure as an additional source of vitamin D. The researchers concluded that, although their study did not support a protective effect of calcium and vitamin D against colorectal cancer incidences, given the strong evidence from both animal studies and *in vitro* studies, the benefits of these two nutrients cannot be ruled out [79].

Epidemiological studies that have investigated the effect of vitamin D *per se* on risk of colorectal cancer have yielded inconsistent findings [56,62,67,70,73,74,76,79,81]. In a prospective study of more than 1900 men in Chicago over a 19-year period, a significant inverse relation was observed between dietary intake of vitamin D and colon cancer [56]. In an 8-year prospective study in Maryland, Garland et al. [83] reported an inverse association between serum 25-hydroxyvitamin D and the incidence of colon cancer. In the Nurses' Health Study, a possible protective effect of vitamin D on rectal cancer was noted [73]. Likewise, in the 5-year observational prospective study of more than 126,000 adults in the Cancer Prevention Study II Nutrition Cohort, McCullough et al. [76] found an inverse association between vitamin D intake from diet and supplements and the risk of colorectal cancer, but the results were stronger for men than women. The researchers suggest that several factors, including gender and total dietary fat intake, may influence the effect of vitamin D on colon cancer risk [76]. A recent prospective, cross-sectional, multicenter study of more than 3000 asymptomatic adults over 50 years old who underwent screening colonoscopy exams found that diets high in vitamin D (greater than 645 IU/day) were associated with significantly reduced risk of advanced colorectal tumors [23]. In contrast, Terry et al. [70] found no effect of vitamin D on colon cancer risk in Swedish women. However, the vitamin D intake is this study was fairly low (approximately 130 IU/day) and generally uniform. Also, no effect of vitamin D on colorectal adenoma and cancer was found in a prospective study of French women [81]. A recent review of 20 epidemiological studies (case-control and cohort studies) of the relationship of vitamin D and colorectal cancer concluded that vitamin D from dietary sources may be sufficient to significantly reduce the risk of colorectal cancer, but the reduction is not large enough to consistently appear in all types of studies [55]. Most studies found that dietary and supplemental vitamin D combined is associated with a reduction in colon cancer risk [55].

A possible protective effect of dairy foods, the major source of calcium and vitamin D, against colon cancer has been demonstrated in epidemiological studies [52,58,59,62,67,68,80,81,84–86]. An early investigation in southern California, where milk is routinely fortified with vitamin D and where there is high exposure to sunlight, identified an inverse association between milk intake and risk of colon cancer [84]. This study of Seventh-Day Adventists who, on the average, have a low incidence of colorectal cancer, indicates a protective effect of vitamin D-fortified milk [84].

Findings from a large case-control study (746 matched pairs) in Los Angeles County, California found that when specific foods and cancer risk were examined, yogurt was protective against colon cancer, particularly in the distal colon, in men and women [59]. The effect of yogurt on colon cancer risk was independent of its calcium content and remained significant after adjustments for sources of calories and nondietary risk factors. This finding suggests that yogurt reduces the incidence of colon cancer by a factor other than just its calcium content. When calcium was omitted from the statistical model, milk was protective against colon cancer in both males and females [59].

In an early case-control study in Utah, Slattery et al. [53] observed an inverse association between risk of colon cancer in both men and women and intake of milk and other dairy foods. Another large case-control study of adults in California, Utah, and Minnesota found that intake of low-fat dairy products was associated with a statistically significant decrease in colon cancer risk [62]. A case-control study conducted among more than 14,000 men enrolled in the Physicians' Health Study found that intake of low-fat milk was associated with a lower risk of colorectal cancer, especially in those at highest risk as indicated by a high ratio of insulin-like growth factor to insulin-like growth factor binding protein (IGF-1/IGFBP-3) [63]. A protective effect of milk (and calcium) against colorectal cancer was found in a case-control study in Korea that compared the diets of 136 patients newly diagnosed with colorectal cancer or large bowel polyps and 134 control patients with no history of cancer or polyps [86].

Based on a review of 30 case-control or cohort studies of dairy foods and colorectal cancer using a meta-analytical approach, Norat and Riboli [48] concluded that "there is some epidemiological evidence that the consumption of total dairy products and in particular milk, may be associated to a modest reduction in colorectal cancer risk." An inverse association was found between milk intake and colorectal cancer in cohort studies, whereas case-control studies provided heterogeneous results [48]. No clear association was found between cheese or yogurt intake and colorectal cancer.

In a published pooled analysis of ten prospective cohort studies in North America and Europe that included 4992 incident colorectal cancer cases, increasing milk intake was associated with reduced risk of colorectal cancer [52]. The highest versus the lowest intake of milk was associated with a significant 27% and 20% reduction of cancers of the distal colon and rectum, respectively [52]. Compared to those who drank the least amount of milk (less than 1/3 cup per day), those who consumed one cup or more of milk per day had a 15% reduced risk of colorectal cancer. Each 16 ounce increase in milk consumption was associated with a 12% reduced risk of colorectal cancer [52]. For most other dairy products, the results were only suggestive of a protective effect against colorectal cancer. When the association between dairy foods and colorectal cancer risk was examined by cancer site, it was found that the inverse association was limited to cancers of the distal colon and rectum [52]. High intakes of dietary calcium (food source) and total calcium (from food and supplements) showed a reduction in colon cancer risk that was similar to that observed for milk. When compared to participants with the lowest calcium intake (less than 500 mg/day), those who consumed 900 to 1099 mg/day or more had a 26% reduction in colon cancer risk [52]. The relative risk for developing colon cancer was lowest for persons with the highest intakes of both calcium and vitamin D. The researchers state that "if individuals who consumed less than 1000 mg/day of calcium increased their intake to 1000 mg/day or more, 15 and 10% of the colorectal cancer cases in this study population would have been avoided for women and for men, respectively" [52]. When the association between dietary patterns and colorectal adenomas was investigated in 1341 Japanese men who had undergone a total colonoscopy, a dietary pattern including greater consumption of dairy products, fruits, and vegetables with low intake of local alcoholic beverages was associated with a reduced risk of colorectal adenomas [87].

In a prospective study of French women conducted by Kesse and coworkers [81], a significant protective effect of dairy products against adenoma was observed. Also, an inverse association between milk consumption and colorectal cancer was found, although it was not statistically significant [81]. Prospective studies in Swedish women and men support a protective effect of dairy products against colorectal cancer [80,85]. Intake of full-fat dairy products (that is, whole milk, full-fat cultured milk, cheese, cream, sour cream, and butter) and CLA were associated with a reduced risk of colorectal cancer in a study of more than 60,000 Swedish women aged 40 to 76 years who were followed for almost 15 years [85]. After adjusting for age and other potential confounding factors, intake of 4 or more servings of full-fat dairy foods a day was associated with a 41% reduced risk of colorectal cancer compared with the risk in women who consumed less than 1 serving per day [85]. Risk of colorectal cancer was also reduced with increased intake of CLA [85].

In a follow-up (6.7 years) study of Swedish men aged 45 to 79 years, increased consumption of total dairy foods was associated with reduced risk of colon cancer from all regions of the colon and rectum [80]. Dairy products' protective effect was mainly observed with intakes of more than 1.5 servings of milk a day (regardless of fat content). Also, the cancer-protective effect of milk calcium (approximately 1400 mg/day) was greatest for rectal cancer [80]. The researchers suggest that, in addition to calcium, other components in milk (for example, CLA, sphingolipids, and protein) may be protective [80].

A growing number of epidemiological studies support an inverse association between calcium, vitamin D, dairy food intake, and colon cancer. However, some inconsistencies occur as a result of factors such as the relative homogeneity of diets within populations, confounding dietary factors, and imprecise measurement of dietary intake in large population studies. Nevertheless, despite these limitations, epidemiological studies appear to be supportive of a modest protective effect of calcium, vitamin D, and dairy foods against colorectal cancer.

4.2.2 Animal Studies

A protective role for calcium and vitamin D in colon carcinogenesis is supported by many experimental animal studies [16,42,88–95]. In most of these studies, the effects of calcium and vitamin D on tumors induced in animals by chemical carcinogens (for example, injections of 1,2-dimethylhydrazine [DMH]) are examined.

Potential mechanisms underlying the protective effect of calcium against colon cancer are indicated from animal studies [44,93,96]. High-fat diets increase levels of bile acids and free fatty acids in the colonic lumen, resulting in damage to the colonic epithelium and increased epithelial proliferation. Increasing dietary calcium in rats fed high fat diets has been shown to reduce bile acid and free fatty acid excretion [20,93,94,96–99]. Intraluminal calcium chelates unconjugated bile acids, and/or free ionized fatty acids, especially in a basic pH environment, forming relatively insoluble (nontoxic) calcium complexes of fatty acids/bile acids. Binding of calcium to fatty acids in the small bowel prevents the reabsorption of fatty acids/bile acids and increases free fatty acid excretion. Calcium complexes of fatty acids are less toxic to the colorectal mucosa than are free fatty acids [93,96–98]. Therefore, increasing calcium may counteract any cancer-promoting effect of fat.

Direct evidence of this effect of calcium in experimental animals has been provided by Appleton et al. [97]. These investigators showed that the fecal content of bile acids decreased 33% and total fecal concentrations of free fatty acids increased 117% in laboratory rats fed a calcium-enriched diet. And when the effects of three different concentrations of calcium on organ cultures of rat colonic explants were examined, crypt cell production fell by 43% when calcium was doubled, and by an additional 43% when calcium was increased threefold (Figure 4.3) [97]. Skrypec [99] found that bile acid excretion increased and lower tumor incidence occurred in laboratory animals that were fed increased quantities of dietary calcium. Likewise, Lupton et al. [93] observed that when rats were fed a high-fat diet and a calcium intake equivalent to 1600 mg/day for humans, fecal excretion of bile acids and certain individual bile acids were reduced to a level found in the feces of rats fed a low-fat diet. However, the effect on indices of colonic proliferation was minimal (Figure 4.4) [93].

Hyperproliferation of colonic epithelial cells is a consistent and early marker of increased risk of colon cancer [43,100]. Increased calcium intake inhibits hyperproliferation of colon epithelial cells induced by carcinogens or high levels of fatty acids or bile acids present in the colon [20,89,101–104]. In a study in which rats were fed a high fat (40% of energy) diet supplemented with calcium phosphate, total fatty acid and bile acid concentration in the feces increased and proliferation of colonic epithelium decreased compared to control animals that did not receive calcium phosphate [92]. Van der Meer et al. [20] also found that, in experimental animals, the hyperproliferative effect of fat is inversely related to the amount of dietary calcium.

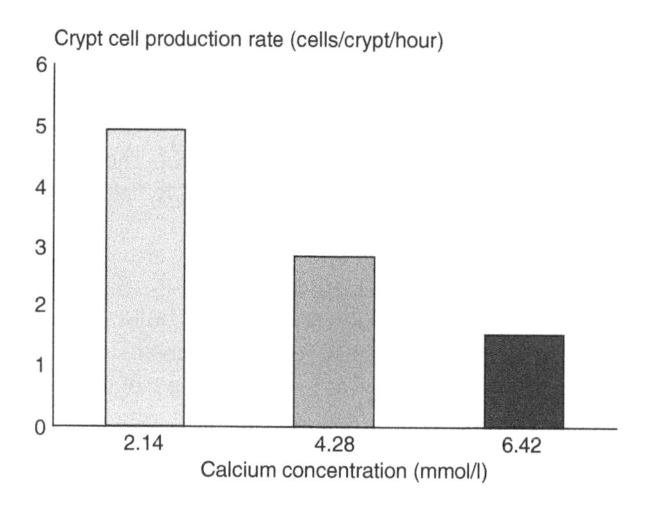

FIGURE 4.3 Doubling calcium concentrations reduced crypt cell production by 43%; trebling calcium concentrations caused an additional 43% fall in crypt cell production. (From Appleton, G. V. N. et al., *Gut*, 32, 1374, 1991. With permission.)

On a low-calcium diet, fat significantly increases colonic epithelial proliferation, whereas on a high-calcium diet the hyperproliferative effect of fat is dramatically reduced (Figure 4.5) [20]. The antiproliferative effect of dietary calcium phosphate has been demonstrated to be greater in the presence of saturated than polyunsaturated fat (Figure 4.6) [92].

Several investigators have shown that increasing dietary calcium and/or vitamin D reduces carcinogen-induced tumors in experimental animals [89,99,104–110]. Wargovich et al. [108] found that a calcium-enriched diet (equivalent to an intake of 2000 mg calcium by humans) suppressed azoxymethane-induced colon cancer at the promotional stage.

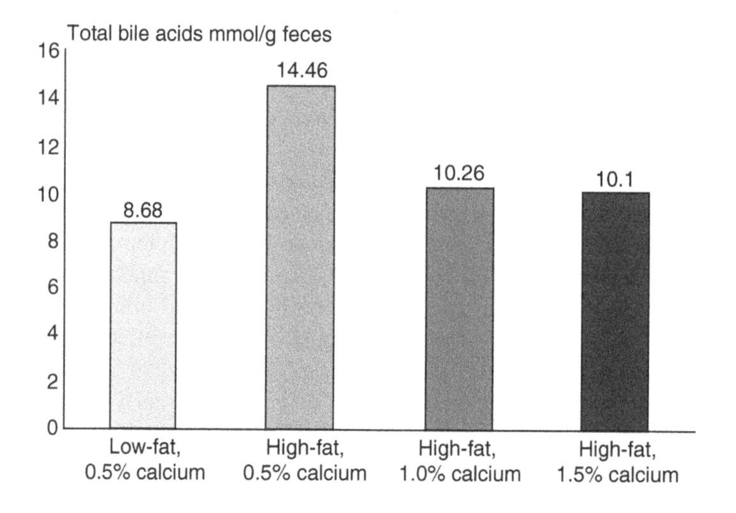

FIGURE 4.4 Effect of dietary calcium on fecal bile acid excretion in rats. Note that the high-fat, low-calcium diet resulted in the highest excretion of total fecal bile acids. As the amount of calcium increased in the high-fat diet, total bile acid excretion fell to a level approaching that in rats fed the low-fat diet. (Based on Lupton, J. R. et al., *J. Nutr.*, 124, 188, 1994. With permission.)

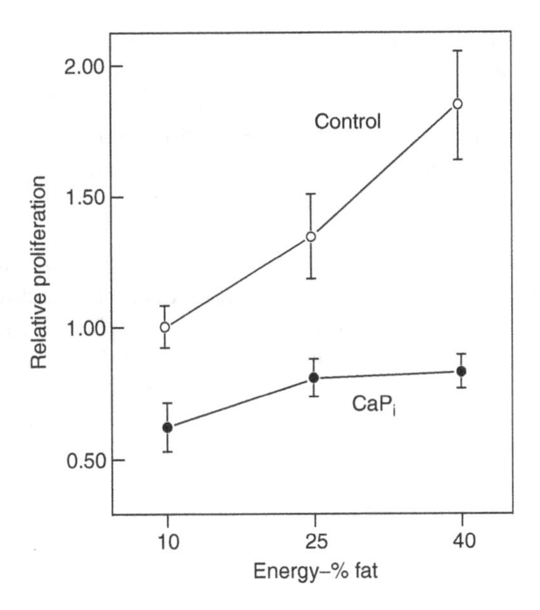

FIGURE 4.5 Effects of increasing amounts of fat and of calcium phosphate in purified diets of rats on colonic epithelial cell proliferation. The results are given relative to those for 10 Energy–% fat on the low-calcium control diet (mean $\pm$SE; $n = 6$). (Reprinted from Van der Meer, R. et al., *Cancer Lett.*, 114, 79, 1997. With permission from Elsevier Science.)

Colon tumor incidence decreased by 45% when laboratory rats injected with a single dose of DMH were fed a diet high in fat (20% corn oil), calcium, and vitamin D [105]. In this study, neither calcium nor vitamin D independently reduced tumor incidence. Both calcium and vitamin D were required for the anticarcinogenic effect, suggesting that these nutrients may act synergistically to

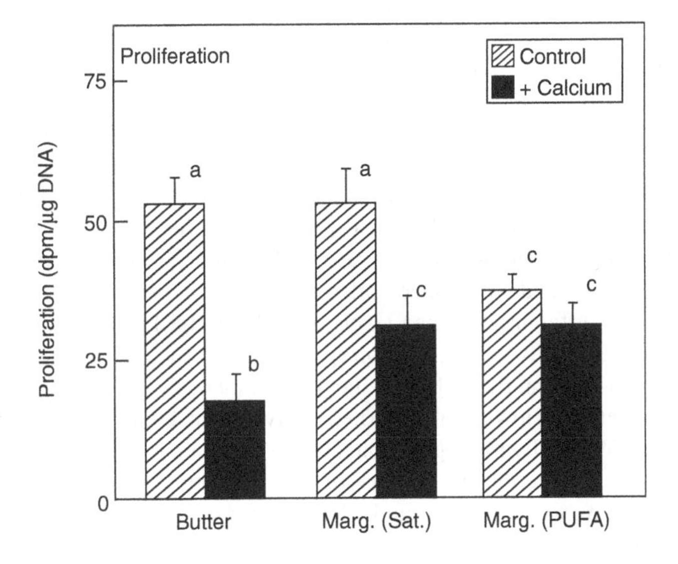

FIGURE 4.6 Colonic epithelial proliferation of rats fed diets differing in type of dietary fat and amount of $CaHPO_4$. Values are means of six rats $\pm$SEs. Bars not sharing the same superscript are significantly different: $P<0.05$. Control diets contain 25 µmol $CaHPO_4$/g diet, and diets with supplemental calcium contain 225 µmol $CaHPO_4$/g diet. (From Lapré, J. A. et al., *Cancer Res.*, 53, 784, 1993. With permission.)

protect against colon cancer [105]. The anticarcinogenic effect of calcium and vitamin D was most pronounced in the distal colon, as opposed to the entire or proximal colon, of the animals [105,110].

Sitrin et al. [109] examined the role of supplemental calcium alone or in combination with vitamin D on colonic tumorigenesis in rats receiving multiple injections of the carcinogen, DMH. Dietary calcium decreased the number and size of tumors, but only when adequate vitamin D was present in the diet [109]. Vitamin D deficiency abolished the protective effects of calcium on colon cancer.

In contrast to the above, Pence and Buddingh [89] found that the combination of calcium and vitamin D was less effective in reducing tumorigenesis than either nutrient alone. These investigators used a $2 \times 2 \times 2$ factorial design in rats to examine the effects of dietary fat, calcium, and vitamin D on colon tumors induced by multiple injections of DMH. Tumor incidence was reduced more in the animals fed a high-fat, low-vitamin D diet containing 1% calcium than in rats fed the same diet containing half as much calcium (0.5%). Calcium was not protective in rats fed low-fat or high-vitamin D diets [89]. The reason for the conflicting findings regarding the relationship between calcium and vitamin D and carcinogenesis is unknown. However, Pence and Buddingh [89], as well as other investigators [16,108,110], generally agree that the anticarcinogenic effect of calcium and/or vitamin D is most pronounced when animals are fed a high fat, rather than a low fat, diet. In a study investigating the effectiveness of two sources of calcium, elemental calcium (calcium carbonate) and dairy calcium (nonfat dried milk), in inhibiting chemically induced colon tumors in laboratory rats, the lowest incidence of cancer occurred when calcium was fed in conjunction with a high fat (20%) diet rather than a low fat (5%) diet [16]. Both sources of calcium were equally effective in reducing fecal bile acid concentrations and colon tumors. The researchers concluded that the ability of dietary calcium to protect against cancer depends in part on the fat content of the diet [16]. Vitamin D's ability to inhibit chemically induced colon cancer appears to depend on a certain minimum amount of calcium [105,111]. A recent review of studies of vitamin D and colon carcinogenesis in rodent models supports the efficacy of vitamin D, and especially vitamin D in combination with calcium, in colon cancer prevention [112].

Other researchers have provided evidence that colonic epithelial cell hyperproliferation is decreased in laboratory animals fed increased calcium and vitamin D [42,44,88–91,97,104,107,113]. As mentioned above, dietary lipids can accelerate colonic epithelial proliferation. Calcium appears to reduce the tumor-promoting effects of dietary fat in the colon by binding with cytotoxic bile acids and/or free fatty acids [44].

Appleton et al. [88,104] found that dietary calcium (calcium lactate) inhibited hyperproliferation of colonic epithelium in rats at high risk of colon cancer. Risk of colon cancer in these animals increased as a result of a surgical procedure (that is, removal of a portion of the small bowel) to impair the uptake and reabsorption of bile acids, or exposure to the chemical carcinogen, azoxymethane. Calcium has been demonstrated to restrict the tumor-promoting effects of dietary fat in the colon of rats or mice treated with ionized bile acids or free fatty acids such as deoxycholic acid or oleic acid, as well as different types and levels of fat [103,108,114]. It is the pattern of nutrient intake that confers susceptibility to or protection against colon cancer development. When mice and rats were fed a Western-style nutritional stress diet high in fat (40%) and phosphate (i.e., equivalent to 700 mg in human diets) and low in calcium (i.e., equivalent to 440 to 600 mg in human diets) and vitamin D (i.e., equivalent to slightly higher than 200 IU for human adults), colonic hyperplasia and hyperproliferation were induced in the absence of a carcinogen [90,91]. However, when calcium intake was increased (i.e., to an amount equivalent to 3000 mg in a 2400 kcal diet for humans), hyperproliferation of epithelial cells in colonic crypts was reduced to almost control levels [91]. Of interest in this experimental animal study was the observation that calcium's effects on epithelial cell proliferation were greater in the sigmoid than in the ascending colon (that is, the area of the colon where most human colon tumors occur) (Table 4.1) [91]. Risio et al. [94] reported that when mice were fed a Western-style diet high in fat and phosphate and low in calcium and vitamin D for 2

TABLE 4.1
High Calcium Intake Reduces Colonic Hyperproliferation Induced in Animals by a Western-Style Diet High in Fat and Phosphate and Low in Calcium and Vitamin D

	Control Diet	Stress Diet 1	Stress Diet 2	Control vs. Diet 1	Control vs. Diet 2	Diet 1 vs. Diet 2
Calcium (mg/kcal)	1.4	0.22	1.3			
Phosphorus (mg/kcal)	1.1	0.8	0.8			
Vitamin D (IU/kcal)	0.3	0.1	0.1			
Corn oil						
% kcal	12	40	40			
kcal/g	3.6	4.5	4.5			
			Sigmoid-Colon Results			
Rats						
Labeling index (%)	7.2±0.7[a,b]	9.9±0.7	8.6±0.4	$P<0.02$	NS	NS
Cells/crypt	36.9±0.9[b]	37.4±0.9	36.2±0.5	NS	NS	NS
Labeled cells/crypt	2.6±0.2[b]	3.7±0.3	3.1±0.1	$P<0.02$	NS	NS
Mice						
Labeling index (%)	4.1±0.3	6.1±0.4	4.3±0.4	$P<0.001$	NS	$P<0.01$
Cells/crypt	18.6±0.6	21.1±0.5	19.5±0.2	$P<0.01$	NS	$P<0.01$
Labeled cells/crypt	0.8±0.06	1.3±0.09	0.9±0.09	$P<0.001$	NS	$P<0.01$
			Ascending Colon Results			
Rats						
Labeling index (%)	8.0±0.5[b]	7.5±0.8	7.0±0.8	NS	NS	NS
Cells/crypt	30.1±2.0[b]	29.7±4.2	32.7±1.9	NS	NS	NS
Labeled cells/crypt	2.5±0.2[b]	2.3±0.6	2.3±0.2	NS	NS	NS
Mice						
Labeling index (%)	6.5±0.7	8.7±0.8	6.5±1.0	$P=0.05$	NS	$P<0.05$
Cells/crypt	15.9±1.8	18.2±1.9	1.6.6±1.0	NS	NS	NS
Labeled cells/crypt	1.0±0.1	1.6±0.1	1.1±0.1	$P=0.01$	NS	$P<0.02$

[a] 1±SEM; $n=6$ for rats and mice, except where indicated.
[b] $n=5$.
Source: From Newmark, H. L., Lipkin, M., and Maheshwari, N., *Am. J. Clin. Nutr.*, 54, 209s, 1991. With permission.

years, advanced dysplastic morphological changes in the colon related to tumor development and progression occurred. Specifically, this diet triggered and sustained the early phases of tumorigenesis in the colonic mucosa, inducing significant changes in cell renewal, apoptosis (programmed cell death), and genetic instability of the epithelium. The gross colonic lesions and other changes in the colon induced by the Western-style diet were similar to those produced by a chemical carcinogen [94]. An anticancer effect of vitamin D (1,25-dihydroxyvitamin D3) has been demonstrated in DMH-treated rats fed a stress diet (20% fat, high phosphorus, and low calcium) [95]. In the vitamin D-treated rats, proliferative indexes of colonic epithelium decreased, as well as tumor multiplicity [95].

Rafter et al. [98] showed that when the calcium content of a fluid containing bile acids was increased and perfused into rat colons, calcium inhibited the damaging effects of the bile acids. Calcium bound the bile acids, rendering them nontoxic to epithelial tissues. This protective effect of calcium on bile or fatty acid-induced hyperproliferation in animal models has been demonstrated by other investigators [115].

Reshef et al. [107] showed that calcium reduced colonic epithelial hyperproliferation in rats during the initiation (induction) phase of colon cancer induced by the carcinogen, *N*-methyl-*N*-nitro-*N*-nitrosoguanidine, even when the animals received a low-fat diet. This beneficial effect of calcium on colon carcinogenesis in the presence of low-fat diets suggests that the effect of calcium on tumorigenesis may include mechanisms other than binding fatty acids and bile acids. The source of calcium used (that is, calcium lactate or calcium carbonate) did not influence the results. A study in rats demonstrated that calcium precipitates cytotoxic surfactants (for example, bile acids, fatty acids, and phospholipids) in the colonic lumen, thereby resulting in decreased cytotoxicity of fecal water [116]. Calcium carbonate, calcium phosphate, and milk calcium elicited similar antiproliferative effects, indicating that calcium in milk is responsible for this effect.

4.2.3 *In Vitro* Studies

Cell proliferation, differentiation, and apoptosis are critical in tissue homeostasis and carcinogenesis. Substances inducing cell proliferation are considered to be tumor promoters, whereas many antitumor agents induce cell differentiation and apoptosis. The potential role of calcium in cell cycling and carcinogenesis has been investigated by *in vitro* studies [117]. *In vitro* studies of animal and human colonic mucosa cell cultures indicate that increasing dietary calcium intake decreases hyperproliferation of mucosal colonic epithelial cells and protects against the damaging effects of bile acids and fatty acids on colonic epithelial cells. However, when colonic epithelial cell proliferation is normal, calcium appears to have little, if any, effect on proliferation rates. *In vitro* studies also demonstrate that calcium phosphate precipitates hydrophobic bile acids and fatty acids in fecal water which decreases their concentrations and cytotoxicity, thus inhibiting epithelial cell damage and colonic proliferation [116].

In vitro studies indicate that early calcium intervention may be particularly effective in preventing colon cancer in individuals at high risk of this disease [97,102,118–120]. According to findings of an *in vitro* study conducted by Buset et al. [118], levels of extracellular calcium equivalent to those found in the blood of humans inhibited colonic epithelial cell proliferation, but not after the cells had progressed to adenomas (precursors of cancer) and carcinomas. The researchers hypothesized that sensitivity to calcium may be lost once colonic cells become malignant.

To determine if colonic cells lose their sensitivity to calcium once they progress to adenomas and carcinomas, Guo et al. [120] measured the direct effects of calcium on the growth of established colonic cancer cell lines *in vitro*. These researchers found that, in contrast to normal cells, colon cancer cell lines continued to grow in the presence of low concentrations of extracellular calcium, but that increasing the concentration of calcium specifically and directly inhibited growth of human and mouse colon cancer cells. Thus, increased intake of dietary calcium may reduce the risk of developing colon cancer by a direct inhibiting effect on the growth of colonic cancer cells. A potential role for calcium in apoptosis is under investigation. An increase in intracellular free calcium appears to trigger apoptosis induced by some agents [117,121]. Further, the role of calcium in the regulation of apoptosis may be dependent on dietary vitamin D3 [122].

4.2.4 Clinical Trials

Most clinical trials have indirectly assessed the effects of calcium intake on colorectal cancer. In general, clinical intervention trials in humans support a protective effect of calcium and vitamin D on several markers of colorectal cancer [43,46,101,102,119,123–132]. Calcium intake has been shown to reduce colonic epithelial hyperproliferation (that is, an intermediate biomarker of colon cancer risk) in individuals at risk of colon cancer. When Lipkin and Newmark [101] examined epithelial cell proliferation in the colonic mucosa of 10 patients from families with hereditary nonpolyposis colon cancer, those whose diets were supplemented with 1250 mg calcium (as carbonate) a day for 2 to 3 months experienced a significant reduction in colonic epithelial cell proliferation activity. Thus calcium reversed abnormal colonic epithelial cell proliferation known to be associated with increased risk of colon cancer [101]. These findings were later confirmed by the same investigators in a study employing a larger number of persons at high risk for colorectal cancer [102]. In this study, calcium (1300 to 1500 mg/day) given for several days decreased and normalized hyperproliferation of whole colonic crypts in individuals whose colonic proliferative activity was high, but not in those whose proliferative activity was close to normal [102].

Wargovich et al. [123] add further support that calcium regulates the proliferative behavior of colonic epithelium in individuals at high risk for colon cancer. In a placebo-controlled, single-blinded crossover study of the effect of calcium (2000 mg/day as carbonate) for 30 days on proliferation of rectal epithelium in subjects with sporadic adenomas, calcium markedly suppressed proliferation rates during the calcium phase of the study, but not during the placebo phase. These investigators also showed in two pilot clinical trials that 1500 mg supplemental calcium per day (in addition to about 700 mg dietary calcium for a total of 2200 mg) for 90 days failed to significantly reduce rectal epithelial cell proliferation in six subjects with sporadic adenoma, whereas 2000 mg supplemental calcium per day (i.e., total of 2700 mg) in another six patients was effective (Table 4.2) [123]. Likewise, O'Sullivan et al. [124] found that while 1000 mg supplemental calcium (i.e., total of 2549 mg from diet and supplement) reduced colonic crypt cell proliferation (indicated as the relative number of labeled cells) in patients with adenomatous polyps of the large bowel, 2000 mg of supplemental calcium was necessary to return proliferation rates to normal levels. Thus, a critical amount of calcium may be necessary to reduce risk of colon cancer in some individuals. Studies failing to show a calcium-induced reduction in colonic proliferation, such as the one reported by Gregoire et al. [133] that used 1200 mg calcium per day, may be explained by the low amount of calcium fed and the fact that the study subjects had portions of their colons surgically removed. Gregoire et al. [133], however, found that increased calcium intake by patients at risk of colon cancer resulted in a higher fecal pH and enhanced fecal bile acid concentration. Cats et al. [134] found that in individuals already consuming an adequate intake of dietary calcium,

TABLE 4.2
Effect of Calcium Supplements on Biomarker Response in Subjects at High Risk for Colon Cancer

Calcium Dose and Duration	Effect on Biomarker	P^b
1500 mg/day for 90 days ($n = 6$)	20% reduction in LI[a]	
2000 mg/day for 30 days ($n = 6$)	29% reduction in LI	0.08
2000 mg/day vs. placebo crossover for 4 to 30 days ($n = 20$)	Lower LI on calcium but not on placebo	0.004

[a] Labeling index (LI) from *in vitro* tritated thymidine uptake.
[b] Two-sided + test.
Source: Adapted from Wargovich, M. J. et al., *Gastroenterology*, 103, 92, 1992. With permission.

calcium supplementation has only a modest protective effect on cell proliferation. This was demonstrated in a randomized, double-blind placebo-controlled trial in individuals with a family history of colon cancer. Increasing calcium intake by 1500 mg/day in individuals who were already consuming 1250 mg calcium per day resulted in only a minor, insignificant reduction in epithelial cell proliferation [134].

Researchers in Arizona [135] found that increasing calcium intake by 1500 mg/day for 9 months significantly reduced fecal bile acids by 35% and deoxycholic fecal bile acid by 36% in patients with resected colon adenomas. In another investigation that involved 22 patients with a history of resected adenocarcinomas of the colon but who were currently free of cancer, increasing calcium intake by 2000 to 3000 mg/day for 16 weeks produced a healthier bile acid profile with respect to cancer [136]. Compared with baseline levels, calcium supplementation significantly decreased the proportion of water in the stool, doubled fecal excretion of calcium, increased excretion of organic phosphate, and decreased the proportion of the primary bile acid chenodeoxycholic acid in the bile and the ratio of lithocholate–deoxycholate in feces [136]. Buset et al. [118] found that a daily intake of 1500 mg calcium for 4 to 8 weeks reduced cellular hyperproliferation in six of nine patients with colon cancer or adenomas or with a family history of colon cancer. The three nonresponders may have had relatively quiescent epithelial cells similar to that in normal cells and which would not be further slowed by increased calcium [118]. Heterogeneity in response to calcium also may be explained by genetics [137–139]. Increased cellular calcium concentration may influence the expression of genetic mutations for predisposition for colon cancer [138]. Thus, early calcium intervention may delay the development of colon cancer in individuals who carry the gene for this disease.

Rozen et al. [140] reported a significant reduction in epithelial cell hyperproliferation (as indicated by the labeling index or LI) in the colonic mucosa when 1250 to 1500 mg calcium (as carbonate or a gluconate–lactate–carbonate preparation) was given for 3 months to 26 first-degree relatives of colorectal cancer patients and nine patients with sporadic adenomas. Calcium had no significant effect on epithelial proliferation in individuals with normal proliferation rates. The different sources of calcium used in this study did not influence the findings. After calcium treatment was discontinued for 6 to 8 weeks, colonic proliferation returned to high levels in individuals at risk of colon cancer [140]. Barsoum et al. [119] found that increased calcium intake (1250 mg/day) significantly reduced mucosal cell proliferation (measured by crypt cell production rate) in patients with adenomatous polyps (that is, patients at high risk of developing colorectal cancer).

Further evidence of calcium's role in regulation of mucosal cell proliferation is provided by measurement of ornithine decarboxylase. This enzyme is elevated in colon cancer. Dietary calcium (2500 mg/day) has been shown to suppress mucosal ornithine decarboxylase activity in elderly patients with adenomatous polyps [141], thus supporting findings in experimental animals [43,106].

Using another biomarker of cell differentiation, Yang et al. [142] demonstrated that soybean agglutinin (SBA) lectin binding of carbohydrate residues was greater in human colon biopsies of normal colonic epithelial cells than in colonic carcinomas. Quantitation of SBA lectin binding before and after supplementation of calcium (1500 mg/day, as calcium carbonate) was studied. In subjects with initial low SBA lectin binding, calcium supplementation for less than 3 months led to a nonsignificant increase in binding rates. When calcium supplementation continued for more than 3 months, there was a significant increase in SBA lectin binding towards levels observed in normal colonic epithelial cells [142]. Calcium supplementation had no effect on SBA lectin binding in subjects who had normal binding levels prior to calcium supplementation. This study not only demonstrates that calcium is beneficial for individuals at risk for colon cancer, but it also identifies a marker for people at increased risk of this disease. Further support for a protective effect of calcium on colon cancer comes from studies that have examined other risk markers for this disease [125,126,143,144]. Calcium has been demonstrated to normalize the distribution of proliferating cells within colorectal crypts [125]. In a randomized, double-blind, placebo-controlled trial, patients with sporadic colorectal adenomas received either a placebo or 1000 mg or 2000 mg calcium per day for 6 months. Increasing calcium intake normalized the distribution of proliferating cells within colorectal crypts without affecting the proliferation rate [125]. That is, calcium shifted the zone of proliferation from one that included the entire crypt to one that was confined to the lower 60%, or normal proliferative zone, of the crypt.

Calcium or dairy foods may also reduce the risk of colon cancer by decreasing the cytotoxicity of fecal water [20,126,143,144]. Substances such as bile acids and other surfactants in stool water have direct contact with the colonic mucosa where they can damage the epithelium and stimulate the proliferation of crypt cells. When 18 healthy adults received either a dairy product-rich or a dairy product-free diet for 1 week each in a crossover study, the cytotoxicity of fecal water increased when dairy products were excluded from the diet [144]. The subjects consuming the dairy-free diet consumed less calcium (i.e., from about 1500 to 400 mg/day), phosphate, vitamin D, and total and saturated fat than those who consumed the dairy product-rich diet. The researchers [144] suggest that the significant decrease in calcium and/or phosphate intake in the dairy-free diet likely contributed to the increase in cytotoxicity of fecal water. This explanation is supported by a study in The Netherlands that demonstrated that calcium in milk products precipitates cytotoxic surfactants in the colonic lumen, thereby inhibiting colonic cytotoxicity [20,126]. In this double-blind, crossover metabolic study, 13 healthy males consumed a typical Western-type diet containing either calcium-depleted milk products or calcium-rich milk products for 1 week each [20,126]. Subjects consumed 765 mg of calcium per day on the calcium-depleted diet and 1820 mg calcium per day on the diet with calcium-rich milk products. Milk calcium significantly increased fecal pH and the fecal excretion of phosphate, total fat, free fatty acids, and bile acids. These findings indicate that milk calcium precipitates luminal bile acids and free fatty acids inhibiting their absorption. Milk calcium also decreased fecal water concentration of long chain fatty acids, secondary bile acids, neutral sterols, and phospholipids by about half (Figure 4.7). The cytotoxicity of fecal water was reduced from 68 to 28% in subjects who consumed the diet high in dairy calcium.

Results from randomized clinical trials indicate that calcium may help prevent recurrent adenomas [127,128]. This finding is important considering that the majority of colorectal cancers are believed to originate from adenomatous polyps and that even after removal the recurrence rate for adenomas is approximately 50% [49]. The European Cancer Prevention Organization

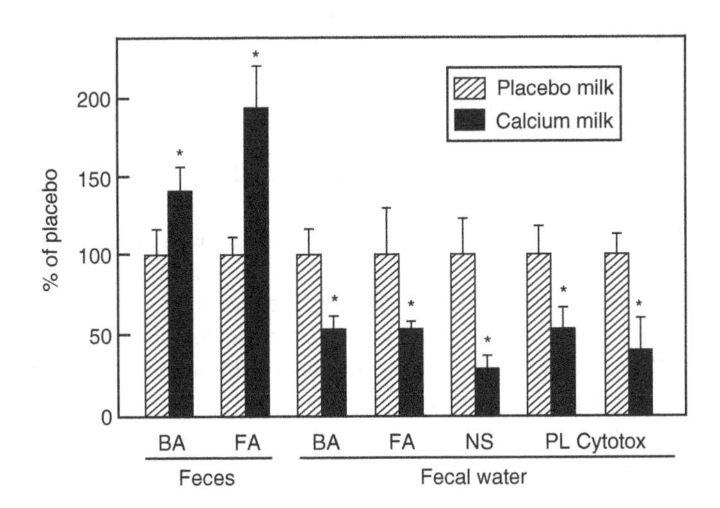

FIGURE 4.7 Effects of calcium milk vs. placebo milk in healthy subjects on fecal and fecal water bile acids (BA), and fatty acids (FA), on neutral sterols (NS), and phospholipids (PL) in fecal water and on cytotoxicity of fecal water (mean ± SE; $n = 13$; $^*P < 0.05$ vs. placebo). (Reprinted from Van der Meer, R. et al., *Cancer Lett.*, 114, 80, 1997. With permission from Elsevier Science.)

Intervention Study, a multicenter randomized trial to test the effect of increased calcium and fiber on adenoma recurrence in 655 patients with a history of this condition, found that in participants receiving calcium supplements (2000 mg/day) for 3 years, there was a modest, but not significant reduction in the risk of adenoma recurrence [128]. The 34% recurrence reduction in this trial did not reach statistical significance, possibly because of the lower compliance in the calcium group and fewer-than-expected number of participants [128]. In a larger blinded, placebo-controlled clinical study (the Calcium Polyp Prevention Study) of 930 patients who previously had a colorectal adenoma removed, increasing calcium intake for 4 years modestly but significantly reduced the risk of recurring colorectal adenomas [127]. The patients were randomized to receive either calcium carbonate (i.e., 1200 mg elemental calcium) or a placebo. In patients receiving the increased calcium, the risk of return of single tumors was reduced by 17% and the number of adenomas decreased by 25% [127]. A recent review and meta-analysis of randomized controlled trials examining the role of supplemental calcium in the recurrence of colorectal adenomas found a significant reduction of approximately 20% in the recurrence of colorectal adenomas in the calcium supplementation group compared to the control group [49]. In this meta-analysis, the researchers identified three trials including 1485 subjects with previously removed adenomas who were randomized to receive either increased calcium or a placebo. The study end point was recurrence of adenomas at the end of 3 to 4 years in 1270 subjects who completed the trials [49].

To learn more about the effect of calcium on the risk of different types of colorectal lesions (that is, hyperplastic polyps, tubular adenomas, adenomas with advanced histology or large size), or whether the protective effect of calcium extends beyond the early stages of carcinogenesis, and to determine if interactions occur between calcium supplementation and dietary fat and fiber intakes, Wallace and colleagues [131] conducted an analysis based on data from the above study of patients in the Calcium Polyp Prevention Study [127]. The results showed that, although increased calcium intake reduced the risk of all types of colorectal polyps, the protective effect was most pronounced for the advanced lesions that are considered to be most strongly associated with invasive colorectal cancer. The advanced colorectal polyps were reduced by approximately 35%, whereas the overall reduction was less than 20%. The finding that the protective effect of supplemental calcium was strongest in patients with high dietary calcium indicates that a total calcium intake greater than 1200 mg/day may be necessary to reduce the risk of colorectal cancer [131]. The researchers suggest that further investigation is needed to determine the optimal calcium intake to prevent colon cancer. Although a high fat intake partly inhibited the beneficial effect of calcium and a high intake of dietary fiber enhanced calcium's effectiveness, these interactions were not statistically significant [131]. In an accompanying editorial, the authors point out that this study did not have the statistical power to show differences between cancer stages or between calcium supplementation and dietary factors, but that studies are underway to provide the necessary statistical power to show a clear effect [145].

Grau et al. [130] found that calcium intake and vitamin D act synergistically to reduce recurrence of colorectal adenoma. This study examined the independent and joint effects of calcium supplementation (3 g calcium carbonate or 1200 mg of elemental calcium) and vitamin D status (serum vitamin D levels) on adenoma (colon polyp) recurrence in 803 adults who were enrolled in the Calcium Polyp Prevention Study, a multicenter, double-blind, placebo-controlled randomized clinical trial [130]. Among participants with blood levels of vitamin D (25-OHD) at or below the median, calcium supplementation was not associated with adenoma recurrence. However, for those with vitamin D levels above the median, calcium supplementation was associated with a statistically significant 29% reduced risk of recurrence. Blood levels of vitamin D were associated with a statistically significant 12% reduced risk only among participants receiving calcium supplements. These findings led the researchers to conclude that "calcium supplementation and vitamin D status appear to act largely together, not separately, to reduce the risk of colorectal adenoma recurrence" [130].

The findings of Grau et al. [130] indicating that calcium and vitamin D reduce the risk of colorectal cancer are consistent with studies by Holt et al. [129,146] who demonstrated that intake of low-fat dairy foods is associated with a significant reduction in the growth of abnormal cells that lead to colorectal polyps. In a randomized, single-blind controlled study, 70 adults at risk of colon cancer because of previous colonic adenomas were separated into two groups [146]. The control group consumed conventional diets, whereas the experimental group increased their intake of low-fat dairy foods to reach 1500 mg calcium per day. Participants were monitored for 1 year to evaluate changes in epithelial cells lining the colon and in other biomarkers of colon cancer. At both 6 and 12 months, significant positive changes were observed in the group receiving the increased intake of low-fat dairy foods. In this group, excess proliferative activity of colonic epithelial cells was reduced and markers of normal cellular differentiation improved [146]. The experimental group increased their calcium intake by a mean of 872 mg/day, bringing their total calcium intake to nearly 1500 mg/day. Although increased calcium intake was the major nutrient change, the researchers acknowledge that the beneficial effect of low-fat dairy foods on colon cancer risk may also be explained by other components in dairy foods such as vitamin D, butyrate, sphingomyelin, and CLA [146].

In a follow-up randomized, crossover, clinical trial, 40 men and women at high risk for colon cancer were randomly assigned to consume a diet supplemented with either calcium carbonate or low-fat dairy foods of their choice (that is, milk, yogurt, ice cream, cheeses) for 4 months [129]. After 4 months they switched to the opposite diet. During the dairy supplemented period, calcium intake increased from an average of 642 to 1309 mg/day. During supplementation, calcium intake increased from 644 to 1521 mg/day. Results showed a significant reduction in two markers of cell proliferation during both dairy food and calcium supplementation, when compared to baseline values. There was no significant difference between the treatments (that is, calcium supplements and dairy foods) or between the two markers of cell differentiation [129]. Based on the findings from this study [129], as well as their previous investigation [146], the researchers concluded that increasing calcium intake as supplements or low-fat dairy foods lowers epithelial cell proliferation indexes from a higher to a lower risk pattern [129].

Holt and coworkers [132] recently examined biological changes in adenomatous polyps and the rectal mucosa in 11 patients who received 1500 mg of calcium carbonate three times per day (i.e., 1800 mg elemental calcium) plus 400 IU of vitamin D3 per day, and in eight patients who received placebo tablets for 6 months. The researchers identified several changes in adenomatous tissue in patients receiving the calcium plus vitamin D supplements that may have contributed to reduced polyp formation [132].

The incidence of colorectal cancer was designated as a secondary outcome of the Women's Health Initiative trial of calcium and vitamin D supplementation to reduce the risk of bone fractures [147]. In this randomized, double-blind, placebo-controlled trial, more than 36,000 healthy post-menopausal U.S. women were randomly assigned to receive 500 mg of calcium carbonate plus 200 IU of vitamin D twice a day or a placebo for an average of 7 years [147]. The incidence of invasive colorectal cancer did not significantly differ between the women receiving the calcium plus vitamin D supplement and those receiving the placebo [147]. Several factors, including the initial higher than national average intakes of calcium (i.e., 1151 mg/day) and vitamin D (367 IU/day) in this population, as well as the long latency period of colorectal cancer, may have contributed to the failure to observe a protective effect of calcium and vitamin D against colorectal cancer in this study.

A review of large prospective studies and randomized controlled trials concludes that calcium has a modest protective effect of about 20% to 30% against colorectal cancer [77]. The beneficial effect of calcium against colorectal cancer may be greater for certain subgroups such as males, smokers, and people whose intake of vitamin D is low [77]. Although recent epidemiological and clinical studies support a modest protective effect of calcium, vitamin D and dairy foods against colorectal cancer endpoints, further investigation is needed to determine their beneficial effect on invasive colorectal cancer *per se* [145]. In particular, several questions need to be answered, including those related to confounding factors, calcium's role independent of vitamin D, the best form of calcium (that is, dietary vs. supplements), and the optimal amount of calcium to reduce colorectal cancer [145].

4.3 DAIRY FOODS AND BREAST CANCER

Breast cancer is the most common cancer diagnosed among American women and is second only to lung cancer as a cause of cancer deaths among women [1]. In 2005, an estimated 211,240 women will develop breast cancer and an estimated 40,410 are anticipated to die from this disease [1]. Although breast cancer primarily affects females, it can also occur in males.

Although an understanding of breast cancer is incomplete, a number of experimental animal and epidemiological studies have investigated a potential role for dairy foods and dairy food nutrients in protecting against or contributing to this disease [29,31,148–152]. Based on a comprehensive review of this evidence, including potential mechanisms, Moorman and Terry [31] concluded that, although animal data linking dairy food components with reduced risk of breast cancer is strong, human epidemiological evidence does not support a strong association between the consumption of milk or other dairy products and breast cancer risk.

Moorman and Terry [31] examined several postulated mechanisms whereby dairy products could either increase or decrease the risk of breast cancer. Hypotheses that dairy foods increase the risk of breast cancer focus on the total fat and saturated fat content of dairy foods, potential carcinogenic contaminants in milk (for example, pesticides), and the content of growth factors such as IGF-1. As mentioned above, and supported by studies examined by Moorman and Terry [31], investigations in experimental animals support the dietary fat hypothesis, but findings from epidemiological studies, especially prospective cohort studies, fail to support this hypothesis. Likewise, evidence is less than compelling that dairy products contribute to breast cancer because of the presence of contaminants or growth factors. Hypotheses that dairy food intake reduces the risk of breast cancer focus on the anticarcinogenic properties of dairy components such as vitamin D, calcium, and CLA [31,150]. Results of studies in breast cancer cells show that the active form of vitamin D (1,25(OH)D) reduces proliferation of cancer cells, down-regulates growth promoting factors, and causes cancer cells to shrink and die [31,148]. There is evidence that calcium alone or in conjunction with vitamin D has anticarcinogenic effects. In addition, animal studies indicate that CLA, a component of milk fat, offers protection against the development of mammary tumors [31,150].

Calcium and vitamin D, either independently or combined, may reduce the risk of breast cancer by their effect on mammographic breast density, a strong risk factor for breast cancer [151,153]. When relationships of dietary vitamin D and/or calcium intakes and breast densities were examined in 287 women with few breast densities and 256 women with extensive densities, increased intakes of vitamin D and calcium separately and in combination were associated with a reduction in breast densities [153]. The combination of higher intakes of vitamin D (100 IU/day or higher) and calcium (750 mg/day or higher) was significantly associated with fewer breast densities when compared to lower intakes of these nutrients [153]. Another study conducted by the same researchers found that higher intakes of vitamin D and calcium (from food and supplements) were associated with lower levels of breast density in premenopausal, but not postmenopausal, women [151].

Epidemiological studies show an inconsistent association between dairy food components and the risk of breast cancer [31,154]. In their review of three cohort studies and nine case-control studies of the relationship between intake of dairy products as a whole and breast cancer, Moorman and Terry [31] found a statistically significant inverse relationship between dairy product consumption and breast cancer in the cohort studies, although the effect was confined to premenopausal women in one of the studies [155], and an inconsistent effect in the case-control studies. In a recent case-control study of more than 800 postmenopausal women not included in the above review, increasing the intake of dairy products, particularly low-fat dairy products, was linked to a reduced risk of breast cancer [156].

When Moorman and Terry [31] examined epidemiological studies of specific types of dairy foods (for example, butter, milk, yogurt, cheese), including whole and reduced-fat milk, and breast cancer, none of the dairy products showed a consistent relationship to breast cancer risk. For example, inverse associations between milk intake and breast cancer were reported among premenopausal women in the U.S. Nurses' Health Study [155], in a Norwegian population [157], and among both premenopausal and postmenopausal women in a Finnish population [158], whereas other cohort and case-control studies found little or no association [31]. Reports that have combined data from a number of studies also support an inconsistent relationship between dairy food intake and breast cancer risk [149,154]. Boyd et al. [154], based on a meta-analysis of 45 observational, epidemiological studies, found that neither milk nor cheese consumption was significantly associated with breast cancer risk. A combined analysis of data from eight prospective cohort studies that included more than 35,000 women found no statistically significant association between consumption of any type of dairy food and breast cancer risk [149].

Based on their review, Moorman and Terry [31] acknowledge that dietary factors generally have relatively small effects on cancer risk, that assessing dietary factors is extremely difficult, and that different methods used to assess dietary intake may provide different results.

Following publication of the above review, McCullough et al. [152] reported that dietary calcium and consumption of two or more servings of dairy products per day were inversely associated with breast cancer in postmenopausal women. In this prospective study of more than 68,000 postmenopausal women from the American Cancer Society's Cancer Prevention Study II Nutrition Cohort, women who consumed more than 1250 mg of dietary calcium a day had a 20% lower risk of postmenopausal breast cancer than those who consumed less than 500 mg of dietary calcium per day [152]. Also, consumption of at least 2 servings of dairy foods daily was associated with a 19% lower risk for breast cancer compared to consumption of 1/2 a serving or less. When the type of breast tumor was considered, stronger inverse associations between dietary calcium or dairy products and breast cancer were found in women with estrogen receptor-positive tumors [152]. Parodi [150], in a comprehensive review of dairy product consumption and risk of breast cancer, suggests that, in addition to calcium, dairy products contain several components (for example, rumenic acid, CLA, butyric and branched chain fatty acids, whey protein, and vitamin D) with the potential to reduce the risk of breast cancer.

4.4 DAIRY FOODS AND PROSTATE CANCER

Prostate cancer is the most commonly diagnosed cancer in men and is the second (after lung cancer) leading cause of cancer deaths among men [1]. In 2005, an estimated 232,090 new cases are estimated to occur in the United States and as many as 30,350 men are anticipated to die from this disease [1]. Age, ethnicity, and a family history of the disease are the only established risk factors for prostate cancer [1]. During the past decade, a considerable amount of research has examined the association between dairy foods and dairy food nutrients such as calcium and vitamin D and risk of prostate cancer. In general, evidence to date provides little conclusive evidence that dairy foods or dairy food nutrients play a role in prostate cancer [41,159].

When researchers in The Netherlands reviewed prospective cohort studies of potential dietary risk factors for prostate cancer published between 1966 and September 2003, they found inconsistent effects between dairy products and dairy product nutrients (that is, calcium, vitamin D) and risk of prostate cancer [41]. Intake of milk and dairy products was either positively associated with or unrelated to risk of prostate cancer [41]. For calcium, although two cohort studies in which the highest quintiles of calcium intake were 1330 mg/day [160] and 1840 mg/day [161] showed no association, two other studies [37,162] showed an increased risk of prostate cancer at high calcium intakes (2000 mg/day) [41]. For example, in a prospective cohort of elderly men, high calcium intakes (2000 mg/day) were modestly associated with increased risk of prostate cancer, whereas no association was found for moderate levels of dietary calcium or dairy food (mainly milk) intake and prostate cancer risk [162]. In a 16-year follow-up of the Health Professionals Follow-up Study, a prospective cohort study of more than 47,000 male health professionals with no history of cancer at baseline, researchers found that a high calcium intake was not linked to total or nonadvanced prostate cancer [163]. However, the data indicated that calcium intakes exceeding 1500 mg/day may be associated with a higher risk of advanced and fatal prostate cancer [163].

Vitamin D intake has been shown to be inconsistently associated with prostate cancer risk [41]. In a prospective study that involved 3612 men who were followed in the National Health and Nutrition Examination Epidemiologic Follow-up Study from 1982 to 1992, higher intakes of calcium and low-fat milk, but not whole milk or any other dairy food, were associated with an increased risk of prostate cancer [164]. After adjusting for calcium intake, a higher intake of vitamin D was associated with a nonsignificant lower risk of prostate cancer. The researchers identified several limitations in their study, including the small number of prostate cancer cases (less than 4%) and failure to validate the diet questionnaire for estimating nutrient intake [164].

Epidemiological evidence related to calcium intake and prostate cancer remains equivocal. If calcium is positively associated with prostate cancer risk, it appears to occur at calcium intakes higher than current dietary calcium recommendations and may be stronger among older men as well as for those with advanced prostate cancer [38,41,165,166]. One proposed mechanism to explain the association between high dietary calcium intake and prostate cancer is that dietary calcium suppresses production of 1,25-dihydroxyvitamin D (calcitriol) from 25-dihydroxyvitamin D. Emerging findings from epidemiological, cell culture, and animal studies suggest that vitamin D, specifically calcitriol, the most active metabolite of vitamin D, may protect against prostate cancer, possibly by inducing cell apoptosis and differentiation and modulating the expression of growth factor receptors [167–170]. Vitamin D may suppress the spreading of prostate cancer by limiting the activity of selective protease enzymes that are involved in tumor invasion [171].

A new study on vitamin D and prostate cancer presented at the American Society of Clinical Oncology Multidisciplinary Prostate Cancer Symposium found that men with higher blood levels of vitamin D were less likely to develop aggressive forms of prostate cancer than those with lower amounts [172]. Moreover, among men with a specific polymorphism in the vitamin D receptor (VDR) gene called homozygous *Fokl*, high levels of both 25-hydroxyvitamin D and calcitriol were particularly effective in lowering the risk of prostate cancer, especially aggressive prostate cancer [172]. Based on findings that either low exposure to sun or vitamin D deficiency is associated with increased risk of prostate cancer at an earlier age as well as with a more aggressive progression, Chen and Holick [167] suggest that "adequate vitamin D nutrition should be a priority for men of all ages."

In the first randomized clinical trial to examine the effect of calcium supplementation on prostate cancer as the endpoint, the incidence of prostate cancer was not increased and was possibly lower among men whose calcium intake was increased [159]. In this study, 672 men were randomly assigned to receive either 1200 mg of calcium (calcium carbonate) or placebo daily for 4 years and were followed for up to 12 years for development of cancer. Participants' baseline dietary intake of calcium prior to supplementation was approximately 900 mg/day. After 4 years, blood was analyzed for 1,25-vitamin D, 25-vitamin D, and prostate specific antigen (PSA). During the first 6 years (4 years intervention plus 2 years posttreatment), there were significantly fewer cases of prostate cancer in the calcium group. The risk of converting to a PSA of less than 4 ng/mL (indicating high risk for prostate cancer) was 37% lower in the calcium group compared with the placebo group. Neither blood levels of vitamin D nor baseline calcium intakes were associated with risk of prostate cancer. Based on the findings, the researchers concluded that "our data do not support the hypothesis that calcium supplementation increases the overall risk of prostate cancer, and they raise the possibility that calcium may, in fact, lower risk for this cancer" [159].

The majority of studies examining the relationship between dairy foods and dairy food nutrients such as calcium and vitamin D and risk of prostate cancer are observational in character and do not establish causality. Inconsistent findings from different epidemiological studies examining dairy foods and dairy food nutrients and prostate cancer risk may be explained by several factors including differences in the size of studies, end points or outcome measures (for example, prostate cancer mortality vs. incidence), duration of follow-up, potential confounders (for example, energy intake), and methods used to assess dietary intake [41]. In some studies, dietary questionnaires are not validated and the relatively crude dietary exposure information collected by dietary questionnaires or interviews may lead to errors in dietary exposure. Further studies, particularly additional randomized controlled trials, are needed to determine the relationship between dairy foods, calcium, and vitamin D and prostate cancer risk [9]. Many questions remain to be answered, including whether low vitamin D rather than high calcium intake increases prostate cancer risk. In its review of risk factors for prostate cancer, the American Council on Science and Health concludes "drinking milk is not an established — or even reasonably suggestive — risk factor for prostate cancer. In fact, the evidence for a role of milk is merely speculative" [173].

4.5 DAIRY-FOOD CULTURES AND CANCER

A promising body of scientific evidence supports a protective role for fermented milks and probiotics against some cancers [31,35,48,174–176]. Probiotics are living microorganisms that, when consumed in sufficient amounts, provide health benefits beyond basic nutrition [176]. The majority of probiotics are lactic acid bacteria, especially strains of different species of *Lactobacillus*, *Bifidobacterium*, and *Streptococcus*. In the United States, food products containing these friendly probiotic bacteria are almost exclusively dairy products, particularly yogurt.

Recent analyses of epidemiological studies of dairy foods and colorectal cancer have found inconsistent associations between yogurt (or cheese) intake and colorectal cancer [35,48,176]. Based on an analysis of cohort studies, Cho et al. [35] observed that yogurt, cheese, or fermented dairy fluids as a whole were not strongly associated with colon cancer risk. However, the researchers suggest that the relatively low intake of these foods may have limited the ability to detect an association [35]. A prospective study of more than 61,000 women in Sweden found a moderate or weak association between the highest intake of fermented dairy foods and proximal colon cancer and between nonfermented dairy foods and distal colon cancer risk [70]. Saikali et al. [176] report that few cohort studies have identified beneficial effects of yogurt or fermented milks against colon cancer. However, some case-control studies show a protective effect of cultured milks. Inconsistencies in the type and concentration of probiotic strains, type of fermented milk product used, and bowel site examined, among other factors, contribute to inconsistencies in results from epidemiological studies [176]. Results from human intervention trials examining surrogate end points for colon cancer risk, as opposed to tumor occurrence, indicate that supplementation with fermented milk or probiotics for short periods can beneficially change markers (for example, fecal microflora modulation, mutagenicity decrease, and fecal pH decrease) of colon cancer risk [176]. However, continuous consumption of these products is necessary to maintain benefits.

In experimental animal studies, intake of probiotics reduces chemically induced colorectal tumor incidence and aberrant crypt formation [176]. For example, Perdigon et al. [177] report that feeding yogurt to mice treated with a chemical carcinogen inhibits the development of colorectal cancer and that this beneficial effect of yogurt is mediated in part by its ability to modulate the immune response and stimulate cellular apoptosis. A follow-up study found that yogurt inhibits tumor progression and promotion, as opposed to initiation [178]. Some studies suggest that probiotics may be most effective in reducing markers for colon cancer risk when administered together with high-fat diets [176].

In vitro studies are generally supportive of a protective effect of probiotics or fermented milks against colon cancer [176]. Furthermore, *in vitro* studies identify potential mechanisms whereby fermented milks and/or probiotic cultures exert anticancer effects. Some of the potential mechanisms may include alteration of the metabolic activities of intestinal microflora, binding and degrading of potential carcinogens, alterations in the intestinal microflora incriminated in producing carcinogens and promoters, production of antitumorigenic or antimutagenic compounds, and enhancement of the host's immune response [176,179].

A protective role for yogurt, other fermented milks, and probiotics against colon cancer risk is promising but as yet inconclusive [176]. Many questions remain such as which lactic acid bacteria are most effective and the amount of fermented milks containing probiotics to confer protection against colon cancer.

Few studies have examined the role of fermented dairy foods and probiotics in breast cancer risk and findings from these studies are inconsistent [31]. A Finnish prospective study found no association between fermented milk intake and breast cancer incidence [158]. However, a case-control study in The Netherlands observed a significantly lower intake of fermented milk products, mainly yogurt and buttermilk, among 113 subjects with breast cancer compared to 289 subjects without this disease [180]. In an *in vitro* study, milks fermented with one of five different lactic acid bacteria strains (that is, *Bifidobacterium infantis*, *Bifidobacterium bifidum*, *Bifidobacterium animalis*, *L. acidophilus*, *Lactobacillus paracasei*) inhibited the growth of human breast-cancer cells [181]. Although all of the fermented milks were effective, the greatest antiproliferative effect was found for milks fermented with *B. infantis* and *L. acidophilus* [181].

4.6 OTHER PROTECTIVE COMPONENTS IN DAIRY FOODS

4.6.1 Conjugated Linoleic Acid

Conjugated linoleic acid (CLA) is a collective term to describe one or more positional and geometric isomers of the essential fatty acid — linoleic acid [4–8,182]. While linoleic acid has been shown to have variable effects on tumor growth ranging from inhibition to promotion, *in vitro* and experimental animal studies indicate that CLA at very low concentrations inhibits the growth of tumors at a number of sites, particularly the mammary gland [4–8,150,182,183]. Animal products, specifically dairy products (milk, butter, yogurt, and cheese), are the principal dietary source of CLA (Table 4.3) [7,184,185]. Moreover, 90% of the CLA in milk fat is in the *cis*-9, *trans*-11, 18:2 isomeric form (called *rumenic acid*), that is, thought to be the biologically active CLA isomer [7,184]. Studies have demonstrated that the major source of rumenic acid in milk fat is vaccenic acid (*trans*-11, 18:1), the predominant *trans* monounsaturated fatty acid in milk fat [6,186–188].

Anticancer activity has been demonstrated for CLA mixed isomers and individual isomers such as rumenic acid in human tumor cell lines and in rodent models of carcinogenesis [7,188–193]. In cell culture studies, physiologic concentrations of CLA have been demonstrated to inhibit the proliferation of a wide range of human cancer cells, including those of the colon, breast, and prostate [7]. This CLA-induced growth inhibition is in contrast to the action of linoleic acid that promotes the growth of these cell lines [6,7].

In experimental animals, CLA, given as a chemically synthesized supplement or provided as a naturally enriched food (for example, butter) in the diet, has been shown to reduce the incidence of chemically induced aberrant crypt foci (a precancerous marker) in the colon, as well as the growth of human breast and prostate cancer cells [7,194]. The formation of some cancers in experimental animals fed a chemical carcinogen is reduced by as little as 0.5% CLA [7,195]. When laboratory rats were fed highly purified individual isomers of CLA, specifically rumenic acid and *trans*-10, *cis*-12 CLA at a level of 0.5%, both isomers equally prevented the development of chemically induced

TABLE 4.3
Conjugated Dienoic Isomers of Linoleic Acid in Dairy Products

Number Foodstuff Add Hair[a]	Total CLA of Samples[b]	c-9, t-11 (mg/g fat)[c]	%
Homogenized milk	3	5.5±0.30	92
Condensed milk	3	7.0±0.29	82
Cultured buttermilk	3	5.4±0.16	89
Butter	4	4.7±0.36	88
Butter fat	4	6.1±0.21	89
Sour cream	3	4.6±0.46	90
Ice cream	3	3.6±0.10	86
Nonfat frozen dairy dessert	2	0.6±0.02	n.d.[d]
Low-fat yogurt	4	4.4±0.21	86
Custard style yogurt	4	4.8±0.16	83
Plain yogurt	2	4.8±0.26	84
Nonfat yogurt	2	1.7±0.10	83
Frozen yogurt	2	2.8±0.20	85
Sharp Cheddar	3	3.6±0.18	93
Cream cheese	3	3.8±0.08	88
Colby	3	6.1±0.14	92
Cottage cheese	3	4.5±0.13	83
Cheez whiz™	4	5.0±0.07	92
Velveeta™	2	5.2±0.03	86

[a] Samples were from commercially available, uncooked edible portions.
[b] Values are means±SE for the number of samples indicated.
[c] Values are means for the number of samples indicated. All SE values are less than 3%. Data were expressed as % of total CLA isomers.
[d] n.d. = not detectable.
Source: From Chin, S. F. et al., *J. Food Compos. Anal.*, 5, 185, 1992. With permission.

premalignant lesions in the mammary gland and mammary tumor development [189]. Likewise in a study reported by Lavillonniere et al. [196], chemically induced mammary tumors were reduced in rats fed diets supplemented with 1% of either rumenic acid or a 1% mixture of CLA isomers compared to a control diet.

The mechanism(s) by which CLA influences carcinogenesis is under investigation in *in vitro* and experimental animal studies and may differ according to the site, age, duration of exposure, and stage of carcinogenesis [7,182]. CLA appears to reduce cancer risk by a mechanism different from that by which linoleic acid promotes cancer [195]. Possible mechanisms whereby CLA intake inhibits carcinogenesis include reduction of cell proliferation, induction of apoptosis (programmed cell death), regulation of gene expression, and modulation of the immune response [182,191–193].

In humans, feeding Cheddar cheese (112 g/day) for 4 weeks was shown to increase plasma CLA levels by 19% to 27% [197]. Aro et al. [198] reported lower dietary intakes of CLA and lower blood CLA concentrations in postmenopausal women with breast cancer than in those without this disease. However, other studies fail to support this inverse association [33,199]. A recent prospective study in Swedish women found that increased intake of CLA was associated with a reduced risk of colorectal cancer [85]. Human intervention studies using well defined isomers of CLA at different levels of intake are needed to clarify the effect of CLA on cancer risk [192].

4.6.2 Sphingolipids

Findings from experimental animal and cell culture studies indicate that sphingolipids, an important type of fat found in milk and other dairy foods, may protect against some cancers including those of the colon, breast, and prostate [6–8,200–207]. Sphingolipids are combinations of different compounds that include ceramides, sphingomyelin, cerebrosides, sulfatides, and gangliosides [200–203]. These compounds have a long-chain (sphingoid) base as the backbone. Sphingolipids regulate cell growth, differentiation, apoptosis, and transformation, and are important in cell-to-cell communication [7,201,202]. Because of the importance of these mechanisms in carcinogenesis, sphingolipids are referred to as *tumor suppressor lipids* [7]. Sphingolipids are found in small amounts in most foods and vary considerably from low amounts in fruits and some vegetables to higher amounts in dairy products [202,203]. Sphingomyelin, the most common sphingolipid, makes up about one-third of total milk phospholipids, although it can vary according to season and the cow's stage of lactation. Milk, butter, and cheese contain approximately 1 μmol of sphingolipids per gram [202,203]. Because sphingolipids are found mainly in cell membranes, rather than in fat droplets, nonfat, low-fat, and full-fat dairy products are all sources of sphingolipids [7,203].

Studies indicate that sphingolipids influence carcinogenesis by inhibiting cell growth and inducing cell death. According to *in vitro* investigations, sphingosine inhibits protein kinase C, which is thought to promote tumors [206]. Sphingosine also appears to reduce the metastatic potential and growth of several human cancer cell lines [201,204,205]. Studies demonstrate that sphingomyelin is broken down into biologically active compounds (that is, ceramide and sphingosine) throughout the gastrointestinal tract [207].

Studies in laboratory mice indicate a protective effect of dietary sphingomyelin on colon cancer [200,204,208,209]. In a study in which mice were fed a chemical carcinogen and sphingomyelin isolated from nonfat dried milk, the incidence of colon tumors (20%) was less than half that in the control animals fed the carcinogen only (47%) [200]. These findings were confirmed in another study that demonstrated that milk sphingolipids (1% of the diet) reduced the number of aberrant colonic crypt foci by 70% and aberrant crypts per focus by 30% (that is, early indicators of colon carcinogenesis) (Figure 4.8) [208]. Although the sphingomyelin-fed mice developed the same number of tumors as the mice that did not consume this compound, 31% of the tumors that formed in the sphingomyelin-fed mice were of the less dangerous form (that is, adenomas),

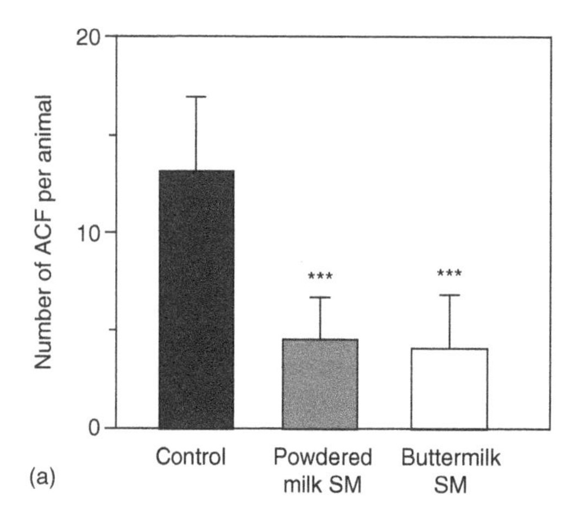

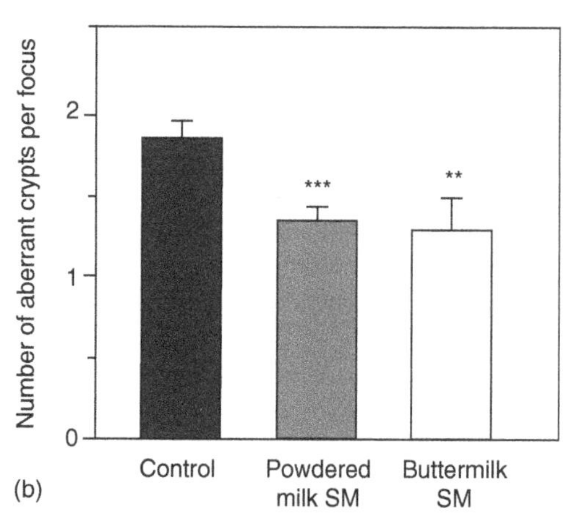

FIGURE 4.8 Effect of sphingomyelin on aberrant crypt foci (a) and number of aberrant crypts per focus (b). The significance of the differences from the control were $^{***}P<0.001$ and $^{**}P<0.01$. (From Schmelz, E. M. et al., *Cancer Res.*, 56, 4936, 1996. With permission.)

whereas all of the tumors that formed in the mice not fed sphingomyelin were the more dangerous type (that is, adenocarcinomas) [208]. The anticarcinogenic effect of sphingolipids is due to sphingomyelin and not to a contaminate [209]. Feeding sphingolipids in amounts that can be achieved in human diets reduced colon tumor formation in DMH-treated mice both when fed before and after tumor initiation [204]. Studies by Schmelz and colleagues [210] demonstrate an anticancer action of all the sphingolipid classes of milk in animal models of colon carcinogenesis.

The effect of sphingolipids on cancer prevention in humans is yet to be determined [7]. Findings that sphingolipids suppress tumor formation without apparent side effects in experimental animals make sphingolipids promising candidates for future studies in humans [7,203]. The presence of sphingolipids in dairy foods may help explain the anticarcinogenic effect of these foods [7].

4.6.3 Butyric Acid

Butyric acid, a four-carbon, short-chain fatty acid in milk fat, may protect against cancer, according to *in vitro* and experimental animal studies [6–8,150,211]. In a variety of human cancer cell lines, including those of the colon, breast, and prostate, physiological concentrations of butyric acid inhibit the proliferation and induce differentiation and programmed cell death (that is, apoptosis) [6–8,212–216]. At the molecular level, butyric acid is associated with down-regulation or inactivation of the expression of cancer genes [211]. Butyric acid also may inhibit tumor invasiveness and metastasis [7,211].

In addition to its presence in milk fat, butyric acid results from bacterial fermentation of unabsorbed carbohydrate (fiber) in the lower intestine [7,211]. Several studies indicate an anticarcinogenic effect of butyric acid against colon cancer [214–218]. In *in vitro* studies, the addition to butyric acid to colon cells from mice genetically at risk of colon cancer reduced cell proliferation by 28% and enhanced cell death by 350% compared to cell cultures not exposed to butyric acid [218]. When human cancer cell lines were treated with sodium butyrate, the proliferation of cancer cells was inhibited and morphological changes consistent with cell death occurred [214,215].

In laboratory animals fed a high-fiber diet and a carcinogen, the presence of high levels of butyric acid in the distal colon significantly reduced colon tumors [7,219]. Butyric acid has also been demonstrated to inhibit the development of chemically induced mammary tumors in rats [6,7]. The mechanism involved in the anticarcinogenic effect of butyric acid in milk fat is unknown. Milk short-chain fatty acids such as butyric acid are released in the upper gastrointestinal tract where they are immediately absorbed, processed, and released into circulation for transport to the liver where most of it is metabolized [211]. Because butyric acid from milk fat never reaches the lower intestine, it is unknown whether this source of butyric acid, unlike butyric acid derived from fiber, plays a protective role against cancer at this site. Butyric acid may inhibit mammary tumors by its ability to increase insulin-like growth factor binding protein-3 (IGFBP-3), the major circulating binding protein of insulin like growth factor-1 (IGF-1) [7]. Higher levels of IGF-1 and lower levels of IGFBP-3 have been associated with increased risk of cancer [7].

4.6.4 Milk Proteins

Findings from experimental animal and cell-culture studies indicate that milk proteins, such as casein and especially whey proteins, may protect against some cancers, including those of the colon, breast, and prostate [3,5,220,221]. Casein, which makes up nearly 80% of the protein in cow's milk, has been demonstrated to have anticarcinogenic properties [3,222,223]. Casein has been demonstrated to inhibit fecal beta-glucuronidase, an enzyme produced by intestinal bacteria that deconjugates procarcinogenic glucuronides to carcinogens [3]. Casein may also protect against colon cancer by its effect on the immune system, specifically by its ability to stimulate phagocytic activities and increase lymphocytes [3]. *In vitro* studies indicate that casein-derived peptides isolated from the microbial fermentation of milk inhibit colon cancer by altering cell kinetics

[222]. Other researchers suggest that the molecular structure of casein contributes to its anticarcinogenic properties [223].

Whey proteins (for example, lactoferrin, lactoperoxidase, alpha-lactalbumin) appear to have a potentially beneficial role in protecting against cancer [3,5,221]. Both experimental animal and *in vitro* studies demonstrate a protective effect of whey proteins against colon, breast, and prostate cancers [3,220–229]. In human prostate epithelial cells, whey protein, but not casein, was shown to increase glutathione (an important cancer-protective agent) synthesis and protect against oxidant-induced cell death [228]. In laboratory animals, whey-containing diets have been shown to reduce colon and mammary cancers [220,224]. Researchers in Australia reported decreased levels of aberrant crypt foci, precancer markers, in the proximal colon of rats fed whey protein concentrate and treated with a chemical carcinogen [225].

Among individual whey proteins, attention has focused on the cancer inhibitory effect of lactoferrin and lactoferricin [229,230]. In laboratory animals given chemical carcinogens, bovine lactoferrin inhibits colon and other cancers when administered orally in the post-initiation stage [229]. An *in vitro* study found that lactoferrin exerted significant cytotoxic activity against colon and other tumor cell lines by a direct antitumor mechanism [230].

The anticancer properties of bovine whey proteins may be attributed to their ability to increase cellular levels of glutathione, an antioxidant [3,5,228,231]. Whey proteins are rich in sulfur amino acids, cysteine, and methionine, which are precursors of glutathionine. Glutathionine is a substrate for two classes of enzymes, specifically selenium-dependent glutathione peroxidase and glutathione transferase, which appear to have anticancer activity [3]. Glutathione peroxidase may reduce substances such as hydrogen peroxide and free radicals that damage DNA [3]. Glutathione transferase may help eliminate mutagens and carcinogens from the body. Consumption of whey proteins (bovine lactoferrin) can increase plasma glutathione levels in humans [232]. Whey proteins may also reduce cancer risk by enhancing humoral and cell-mediated immune responses [3,221].

Few studies have investigated the role of milk proteins on cancer in humans. However, a prospective case-control study of colon cancer in women in New York found that protein primarily from dairy foods, followed by red meat, poultry, fish, and shellfish, was inversely associated with colon cancer [233]. The researchers speculate that the amino acid methionine may protect against colon cancer [233]. As mentioned above, whey protein is a rich source of cysteine and methionine, which are precursors of the anticarcinogenic tripeptide glutathionine. When dietary factors and the survival of women with breast cancer were examined, intake of protein from dairy foods was linked to an increased survival rate in women with this disease [234].

4.7 SUMMARY

Dietary recommendations to reduce cancer emphasize a reduction in total fat intake, especially from high-fat foods [51,235]. This recommendation should be interpreted cautiously to ensure that recommended intakes of animal foods such as dairy foods are not jeopardized. Although a high fat or calorie intake is associated with increased risk of some cancers, there is no scientific evidence that dairy foods *per se* contribute to cancer. On the contrary, components in dairy foods such as calcium, vitamin D, bacterial cultures (for example, *L. acidophilus*), CLA, sphingolipids, and others may protect against some cancers such as those of the colon, breast, and prostate.

Findings from epidemiological, experimental animal, *in vitro*, and clinical intervention studies support a modest protective effect of calcium and dairy foods against colorectal cancer [9,35,55,77,130,131]. Recent large prospective studies indicate an inverse association between calcium intake and risk of colorectal cancer [72,76–78]. However, this association appears to depend on variables such as the colon subsite, gender, source of calcium (dietary or supplemental), and vitamin D exposure. Experimental animal and *in vitro* studies suggest potential mechanisms underlying the protective effect of calcium and vitamin D against colorectal cancer [77]. Findings from clinical intervention trials indicate that increasing intake of low-fat dairy foods to reach more than 1200 mg calcium per day may reduce markers (for example, recurrence of colorectal cancer) for increased risk of colon cancer [49,127,129–131,146]. There is also evidence that intake of culture-containing dairy foods such as yogurt may protect against colon cancer, although more research is needed to confirm this finding, as well as to delineate the potential anticarcinogenic role of CLA, sphingolipids, and other components in dairy foods. Dairy foods are an important source of calcium, vitamin D, CLA, sphingolipids, and, if cultured, bacterial cultures, as well as proteins, each of which has been suggested to protect against colon as well as some other cancers [3–8,150].

Based on the evidence to date, meeting recommended intakes for calcium (1200 mg for adults over 50 years) [82] and vitamin D (10 to 15 μg/day for adults over 50 years) [82], especially from dairy foods that are major sources of these nutrients in our diets [236,237], appears to be a prudent measure to help reduce the risk of colon cancer. Unfortunately, calcium intake in the United States is generally lower than recommended [238]. According to NHANES (National Health and Nutrition Examination Survey) 2001 to 2002 nutrient intake data, among men ages 51 to 70 and 71+, half (50th percentile) consume less than 813 and 771 mg of calcium per day, respectively [238], compared to the 1200 mg calcium per day currently recommended [82]. Older women consume even less calcium than older men. Among women ages 51 to 70 and 71+, half (50th percentile) consume less than 661 and 613 mg of calcium per day, respectively [238], compared to the 1200 mg calcium per day currently recommended [82]. Americans' low dairy-food intake contributes to their low intake of calcium. On average, Americans consume only 1.7 servings of dairy foods per day [239] compared to the recommended 3 to 4 servings/day [240–242]. The National Medical Association, in a consensus report, recommends that the American public as a whole and African Americans in particular consume 3 to 4 servings/day of low-fat milk, cheese, and/or yogurt to help reduce the risk of certain chronic diseases, including colon cancer [242]. Based on a review of the science, researchers conservatively estimated that consuming 3 to 4 servings of dairy foods per day could reduce the risk of colorectal cancer by 5% annually after 3 years, resulting in health care cost savings of $0.75 billion over 5 years [243].

With respect to breast cancer, there is evidence from experimental animal studies that dairy food components reduce the risk of this cancer [31]. However, epidemiological evidence supporting an association between the consumption of milk or specific types of dairy products and risk of breast cancer is limited [31]. There is little evidence that dairy foods or dairy food components are associated with prostate cancer risk [41]. Some emerging findings indicate that calcium and vitamin D, especially calcitriol, the most active metabolite of vitamin D, may protect against prostate cancer [159,167,169].

There is no conclusive evidence that intake of dairy foods increases the risk of other cancers, for example, ovarian cancer [244–247]. Despite the suggestion that galactose (a simple sugar derived from lactose digestion and found naturally only in milk) may increase the risk of ovarian cancer, a recent meta-analysis of 20 case-control and two cohort studies found no association between milk/dairy products and ovarian cancer [244]. In this meta-analysis, the intake of milk had a borderline inverse association with ovarian cancer risk [244]. The researchers suggest that ovarian cancer risk may be reduced by some nutrients in milk such as vitamins A and D as well as calcium [244]. Another meta-analysis of 18 case-control and three prospective cohort studies reported inconsistent associations between milk, milk products, and lactose intake and ovarian cancer risk [245]. The researchers conclude that more research is needed, and in particular, that future studies consider individual subtypes of ovarian cancer. However, a pooled analysis of 12 prospective cohort studies of dairy and calcium intakes and three types of ovarian cancer found no statistically significant associations [246]. Likewise, a recent prospective study in The Netherlands found no association between dairy food intake and ovarian cancer risk [247].

Theoretically, consuming three servings of dairy foods/day may help reduce the risk of some cancers by their effect on body weight. Overweight or obesity is a risk factor for several cancers

[1,51,235,248]. Emerging research indicates that increasing intake of calcium or including three servings of dairy foods per day as part of a reduced-calorie diet helps adults lose more weight and body fat than calorie reduction alone [249]. See Chapter 7 for more information on dairy products and body-weight regulation.

REFERENCES

1. American Cancer Society, *Cancer Facts & Figures—2005*, American Cancer Society, Atlanta, GA, 2005.
2. Doll, R., Nature and nuture: possibilities for cancer control, *Carcinogenesis*, 17, 177, 1996.
3. Parodi, P. W., A role for milk proteins in cancer prevention, *Aust. J. Dairy Technol.*, 53, 37, 1998.
4. Parodi, P. W., Conjugated linoleic acid and other anticarcinogenic agents of bovine milk fat, *J. Dairy Sci.*, 82, 1339, 1999.
5. Parodi, P. W., Cow's milk components with anti-cancer potential, *Aust. J. Dairy Technol.*, 56, 65, 2001.
6. Parodi, P. W., Anti-cancer agents in milk fat, *Aust. J. Dairy Technol.*, 58, 114, 2003.
7. Parodi, P. W., Milk fat in human nutrition, *Aust. J. Dairy Technol.*, 59, 3, 2004.
8. German, J. B. and Dillard, C. J., Composition, structure and absorption of milk lipids: a source of energy, fat-soluble nutrients and bioactive molecules, *Crit. Rev. Food Sci. Nutr.*, 46, 57, 2006.
9. Holt, P. R., Calcium, vitamin D, and cancer, in *Calcium in Human Health*, Weaver, C. M. and Heaney, R. P., Eds., Humana Press, Totowa, NJ, 2006, chap. 25
10. Garland, C. F. et al., The role of vitamin D in cancer prevention, *Am. J. Public Health*, 96, 252, 2006.
11. Institute of Medicine of the National Academies, *Dietary Reference Intakes for Energy, Carbohydrate, Fiber, Fat, Fatty Acids, Cholesterol, Protein, and Amino Acids*, The National Academies Press, Washington, D.C., 2002.
12. Willett, W. C., Diet and cancer: one view at the start of the millennium, *Cancer Epidemiol. Biomarkers Prev.*, 10, 3, 2001.
13. Beresford, S. A. A., Low-fat dietary pattern and risk of colorectal cancer. The Women's Health Initiative Randomized Controlled Dietary Modification Trial, *JAMA*, 295, 643, 2006.
14. Prentice, R. L. et al., Low-fat dietary pattern and risk of invasive breast cancer: the Women's Health Initiative Randomized Controlled Dietary Modification Trial, *JAMA*, 295, 629, 2006.
15. Reddy, B. S., Dietary fat and colon cancer: animal model studies, *Lipids*, 27, 807, 1992.
16. Pence, B. C. et al., Protective effects of calcium from nonfat dried milk against colon carcinogenesis in rats, *Nutr. Res.*, 25, 35, 1996.
17. Rijnkels, J. M. et al., Interaction of dietary fat with a vegetables–fruit mixture on 1,2-dimethylhydrazine-induced colorectal cancer in rats, *Nutr. Cancer*, 27, 261, 1997.
18. Erickson, K. L. and Hubbard, N. E., Dietary fat and tumor metastasis, *Nutr. Rev.*, 48, 6, 1990.
19. Klurfeld, D. M. and Bull, A. W., Fatty acids and colon cancer in experimental models, *Am. J. Clin. Nutr.*, 66 (suppl.), 1530, 1997.
20. Van der Meer, R. et al. Mechanisms of the intestinal effects of dietary fats and milk products on colon carcinogenesis, *Cancer Lett.*, 114, 75, 1997.
21. Howe, G. R. et al., The relationship between dietary fat intake and risk of colorectal cancer: evidence from the combined analysis of 13 case-control studies, *Cancer Causes Control*, 8, 215, 1997.
22. Flood, A. et al., Meat, fat, and their subtypes as risk factors for colorectal cancer in a prospective cohort of women, *Am. J. Epidemiol.*, 158, 59, 2003.
23. Lieberman, D. A. et al., Risk factors for advanced colonic neoplasia and hyperplastic polyps in asymptomatic individuals, *JAMA*, 290, 2959, 2003.
24. Lin, J. et al. Dietary fat and fatty acids and risk of colorectal cancer in women, *Am. J. Epidemiol.*, 160, 1011, 2004.
25. Giovannucci, E. and Goldin, B., The role of fat, fatty acids, and total energy intake in the etiology of human colon cancer, *Am. J. Clin. Nutr.*, 66 (suppl.), 1564, 1997.
26. Slattery, M. L. et al., Eating patterns and risk of colon cancer, *Am. J. Epidemiol.*, 148, 4, 1998.
27. Shike, M., Body weight and colon cancer, *Am. J. Clin. Nutr.*, 63 (suppl.), 442, 1996.

28. Slattery, M. L. et al., Dietary energy sources and colon cancer risk, *Am. J. Epidemiol.*, 145, 199, 1997.
29. Newmark, H. L. and Suh, N., Mechanistic hypothesis for the interaction of dietary fat, calcium, and vitamin D in breast cancer, *Med. Hypotheses Res.*, 1, 67, 2004.
30. Welsch, C. W., Relationship between dietary fat and experimental mammary tumorigenesis: a review and critique, *Cancer Res.*, 52, 2040, 1992.
31. Moorman, P. G. and Terry, P. D., Consumption of dairy products and the risk of breast cancer: a review of the literature, *Am. J. Clin. Nutr.*, 80, 5, 2004.
32. Smith-Warner, S. A., Types of dietary fat and breast cancer: a pooled analysis of cohort studies, *Int. J. Cancer*, 92, 767, 2001.
33. Voorrips, L. E. et al., Intake of conjugated linoleic acid, fat, and other fatty acids in relation to postmenopausal breast cancer: The Netherlands Cohort Study on Diet and Cancer, *Am. J. Clin. Nutr.*, 76, 873, 2002.
34. Byrne, C., Rockett, H., and Holmes, M. D., Dietary fat, fat subtypes, and breast cancer risk: lack of an association among postmenopausal women with no history of benign breast disease, *Cancer Epidemiol. Biomarkers Prev.*, 11, 261, 2002.
35. Cho, E. et al., Premenopausal fat intake and risk of breast cancer, *J. Natl. Cancer Inst.*, 95, 1079, 2003.
36. Bingham, S. A. et al., Are imprecise methods obscuring a relation between fat and breast cancer? *Lancet*, 362, 212, 2003.
37. Giovannucci, E. et al., Calcium and fructose intake in relation to risk of prostate cancer, *Cancer Res.*, 58, 442, 1998.
38. Kristal, A. R. et al., Associations of energy, fat, calcium, and vitamin D with prostate cancer risk, *Cancer Epidemiol. Biomarkers Prev.*, 11, 719, 2002.
39. Ramon, J. M. et al., Dietary fat intake and prostate cancer risk: a case-control study in Spain, *Cancer Causes Control*, 11, 679, 2000.
40. Veierod, M. B., Laake, P., and Thelle, D. S., Dietary fat intake and risk of prostate cancer: a prospective study of 25,708 Norwegian men, *Int. J. Cancer*, 73, 634, 1997.
41. Dagnelie, P. C. et al., Diet, anthropometric measures and prostate cancer risk: a review of prospective cohort and intervention studies, *BJU Int.*, 93, 1139, 2004.
42. Lipkin, M., Application of intermediate biomarkers to studies of cancer prevention in the gastrointestinal tract: introduction and perspective, *Am. J. Clin. Nutr.*, 54 (suppl.), 188, 1991.
43. Newmark, H. L. and Lipkin, M., Calcium, vitamin D, and colon cancer, *Cancer Res.*, 52 (suppl.), 2067, 1992.
44. Wargovich, M. J., Lynch, P. M., and Liven, B., Modulating effects of calcium in animal models of colon carcinogenesis and short-term studies in subjects at increased risk for colon cancer, *Am. J. Clin. Nutr.*, 54 (suppl.), 202, 1991.
45. Van der Meer, R. et al., Milk products and intestinal health, *Int. Dairy J.*, 8, 163, 1998.
46. Holt, P. R., Dairy foods and prevention of colon cancer: human studies, *J. Am. Coll. Nutr.*, 18, 379s, 1999.
47. Parodi, P. W., An assessment of the evidence linking calcium and vitamin D to colon cancer prevention, *Aust. J. Dairy Technol.*, 56, 35, 2001.
48. Norat, T. and Riboli, E., Dairy products and colorectal cancer. A review of possible mechanisms and epidemiological evidence, *Eur. J. Clin. Nutr.*, 57, 1, 2003.
49. Shaukat, A., Scouras, N., and Schunemann, H. J., Role of supplemental calcium in the recurrence of colorectal adenomas: a metaanalysis of randomized controlled trials, *Am. J. Gastroenterol.*, 100, 390, 2005.
50. Garland, C. F. and Garland, F. C., Do sunlight and vitamin D reduce the risk of colon cancer? *Int. J. Epidemiol.*, 9, 227, 1980.
51. American Institute for Cancer Research, *Food, Nutrition and the Prevention of Cancer: A Global Perspective*, American Institute for Cancer Research, Washington, D.C., 1997.
52. Cho, E. et al., Dairy foods, calcium, and colorectal cancer: a pooled analysis of 10 cohort studies, *J. Natl. Cancer Inst.*, 96, 1015, 2004.
53. Slattery, M. L., Sorensen, A. W., and Ford, M. H., Dietary calcium intake as a mitigating factor in colon cancer, *Am. J. Epidemiol.*, 128, 504, 1988.

54. Sorensen, A. W., Slattery, M. L., and Ford, M. H., Calcium and colon cancer: a review, *Nutr. Cancer*, 11, 135, 1988.
55. Grant, W. B. and Garland, C. F., A critical review of studies on vitamin D in relation to colorectal cancer, *Nutr. Cancer*, 48, 115, 2004.
56. Garland, C. et al., Dietary vitamin D and calcium and risk of colorectal cancer: a 19-year prospective study in men, *Lancet*, 1, 307, 1985.
57. Peters, U. et al., Circulating vitamin D metabolites, polymorphism in vitamin D receptors, and colorectal adenoma risk, *Cancer Epidemiol. Biomarkers Prev.*, 13, 546, 2004.
58. Ghadirian, P. et al., Nutritional factors and colon carcinoma: a case-control study involving French Canadians in Montreal, Quebec, Canada, *Cancer*, 80, 858, 1997.
59. Peters, R. K. et al., Diet and colon cancer in Los Angeles County, California, *Cancer Causes Control*, 3, 457, 1992.
60. Arbman, G. et al., Cereal fiber, calcium, and colorectal cancer, *Cancer*, 69, 2042, 1992.
61. De Stefani, E. et al., Influence of dietary levels of fat, cholesterol, and calcium on colorectal cancer, *Nutr. Cancer*, 29, 83, 1997.
62. Kampman, E. et al., Calcium, vitamin D, sunshine exposure, dairy products and colon cancer risk (United States), *Cancer Causes Control*, 11, 459, 2000.
63. Ma, J. et al., Milk intake, circulating levels of insulin-like growth factor-1, and risk of colorectal cancer in men, *J. Natl. Cancer Inst.*, 93, 1330, 2001.
64. Peters, U. et al., Calcium intake and colorectal adenoma in a U.S. colorectal cancer early detection program, *Am. J. Clin. Nutr.*, 80, 1358, 2004.
65. Martinez, M. E. et al., Association of diet and colorectal adenomatous polyps: dietary fiber, calcium, and total fat, *Epidemiology*, 7, 264, 1996.
66. Martinez, M. E. et al., A case-control study of dietary intake and other lifestyle risk factors for hyperplastic polyps, *Gastroenterology*, 113, 423, 1997.
67. Bostick, R. M. et al., Relation of calcium, vitamin D, and dairy food intake to incidence of colon cancer among older women, *Am. J. Epidemiol.*, 137, 1302, 1993.
68. Hyman, J. et al., Dietary and supplemental calcium and the recurrence of colorectal adenomas, *Cancer Epidemiol. Biomarkers Prev.*, 7, 291, 1998.
69. Wu, K. et al., Calcium intake and risk of colon cancer in women and men, *J. Natl. Cancer Inst.*, 94, 437, 2002.
70. Terry, P. et al., Dietary calcium and vitamin D intake and risk of colorectal cancer: a prospective cohort study in women, *Nutr. Cancer*, 43, 39, 2002.
71. Martinez, M. E. et al., Calcium, vitamin D, and risk of adenoma recurrence (United States), *Cancer Causes Control*, 13, 213, 2002.
72. Hartman, T. J. et al., The association of calcium and vitamin D with risk of colorectal adenomas, *J. Nutr.*, 135, 252, 2005.
73. Martinez, M. E. et al., Calcium, vitamin D, and occurrence of colorectal cancer among women, *J. Natl. Cancer Inst.*, 88, 1375, 1996.
74. Kearney, J. et al., Calcium, vitamin D, and dairy foods and the occurrence of colon cancer in men, *Am. J. Epidemiol.*, 143, 907, 1996.
75. Bergsma-Kadijk, J. A. et al., Calcium does not protect against colorectal neoplasia, *Epidemiology*, 7, 590, 1996.
76. McCullough, M. L. et al., Calcium, vitamin D, dairy products, and risk of colorectal cancer in the Cancer Prevention Study II Nutrition Cohort (United States), *Cancer Causes Control*, 14, 1, 2003.
77. Chia, V. and Newcomb, P. A., Calcium and colorectal cancer: some questions remain, *Nutr. Rev.*, 62, 115, 2004.
78. Flood, A. et al., Calcium from diet and supplements is associated with reduced risk of colorectal cancer in a prospective cohort of women, *Cancer Epidemiol. Biomarkers Prev.*, 14, 126, 2005.
79. Lin, J. et al., Intake of calcium and vitamin D and risk of colorectal cancer in women, *Am. J. Epidemiol.*, 161, 755, 2005.
80. Larsson, S. C. et al., Calcium and dairy food intakes are inversely associated with colorectal cancer risk in the Cohort of Swedish Men, *Am. J. Clin. Nutr.*, 83, 667, 2006.

81. Kesse, E. et al., Dietary calcium, phosphorus, vitamin D, dairy products and the risk of colorectal adenoma and cancer among French women of the E3N-EPIC prospective study, *Int. J. Cancer*, 117, 137, 2005.
82. IOM (Institute of Medicine), *Dietary Reference Intakes for Calcium, Phosphorus, Magnesium, Vitamin D, and Fluoride,* Standing Committee on the Scientific Evaluation of Dietary Reference Intakes, Food and Nutrition Board, National Academies Press, Washington, D.C., 1997.
83. Garland, C. F. et al., Serum 25-hydroxyvitamin D and colon cancer: eight-year prospective study, *Lancet*, 2, 1176, 1989.
84. Phillips, R. L., Role of life-style and dietary habits in risk of colon cancer among Seventh-Day Adventists, *Cancer Res.*, 35, 3513, 1975.
85. Larsson, S. C., Bergkvist, L., and Wolk, A., High-fat dairy food and conjugated linoleic acid intakes in relation to colorectal cancer incidence in the Swedish Mammography Cohort, *Am. J. Clin. Nutr.*, 82, 894, 2005.
86. Oh, S.-Y. et al., Relationship of nutrients and food to colorectal cancer risk in Koreans, *Nutr. Res.*, 25, 805, 2005.
87. Mizoue, T. et al., Dietary patterns and colorectal adenomas in Japanese men. The Self-Defense Forces Health Study, *Am. J. Epidemiol.*, 161, 338, 2005.
88. Appleton, G. V. N., Bristol, J. B., and Williamson, R. C. N., Increased dietary calcium and small bowel resection have opposite effects on colonic cell turnover, *Br. J. Surg.*, 73, 1018, 1986.
89. Pence, B. C. and Buddingh, F., Inhibition of dietary fat-promoted colon carcinogenesis in rats by supplemental calcium or vitamin D3, *Carcinogenesis*, 9, 187, 1988.
90. Newmark, H. L., Lipkin, M., and Maheshwari, N., Colonic hyperplasia and hyperproliferation induced by a nutritional stress diet with four components of Western-style diet, *J. Natl. Cancer Inst.*, 82, 491, 1990.
91. Newmark, H. L., Lipkin, M., and Maheshwari, N., Colonic hyperproliferation induced in rats and mice by nutritional-stress diets containing four components of a human Western-style diet (series 2), *Am. J. Clin. Nutr.*, 54 (suppl.), 209, 1991.
92. Lapré, J. A. et al., An antiproliferative effect of dietary calcium on colonic epithelium is mediated by luminal surfactants and dependent on the type of dietary fat, *Cancer Res.*, 53, 784, 1993.
93. Lupton, J. R. et al., Rats fed high fat diets with increased calcium levels have fecal bile acid concentrations similar to those of rats fed a lowfat diet, *J. Nutr.*, 124, 188, 1994.
94. Risio, M. et al., Apoptosis, cell replication, and Western-style diet-induced tumorigenesis in mouse colon, *Cancer Res.*, 56, 4910, 1996.
95. Mokady, E. et al., A protective role of dietary vitamin D3 in rat colon carcinogenesis, *Nutr. Cancer*, 38, 65, 2001.
96. Newmark, H. L., Wargovich, M. H., and Bruce, W. R., Colon cancer and dietary fat, phosphate, and calcium: a hypothesis, *J. Natl. Cancer Inst.*, 72, 1323, 1984.
97. Appleton, G. N. V. et al., Effect of dietary calcium on the colonic luminal environment, *Gut*, 32, 1374, 1991.
98. Rafter, J. J. et al., Effects of calcium and pH on the mucosal damage produced by deoxycholic acid in the rat colon, *Gut*, 27, 1320, 1986.
99. Skrypec, D. J., Effect of dietary calcium on azoxymethane-induced intestinal carcinogenesis in male F344 rats fed high-fat diets, in *Calcium, Vitamin D, and Prevention of Colon Cancer*, Lipkin, M., Newmark, H. L., and Kelloff, G., Eds., CRC Press, Boca Raton, FL, pp. 241–247, 1991.
100. Lipkin, M., Biomarkers of increased susceptibility to gastrointestinal cancer: new application to studies of cancer prevention in human subjects, perspectives in cancer research, *Cancer Res.*, 48, 235, 1988.
101. Lipkin, M. D. and Newmark, H., Effect of added dietary calcium on colonic epithelial-cell proliferation in subjects at high risk for familial colonic cancer, *N. Engl. J. Med.*, 313, 1381, 1985.
102. Lipkin, M. et al., Colonic epithelial cell proliferation in responders and nonresponders to supplemental dietary calcium, *Cancer Res.*, 49, 248, 1989.
103. Wargovich, M. J., Eng, V. W. S., and Newmark, H. L., Calcium inhibits the damaging and compensatory proliferative effects of fatty acids on mouse colonic epithelium, *Cancer Lett.*, 23, 253, 1984.
104. Appleton, G. V. N. et al., Inhibition of intestinal carcinogenesis by dietary supplementation with calcium, *Br. J. Surg.*, 74, 523, 1987.

105. Beaty, M. M., Lee, E. Y., and Glauert, H. P., Influence of dietary calcium and vitamin D on colon epithelial cell proliferation and 1,2-dimethylhydrazine-induced colon carcinogenesis in rats fed high fat diets, *J. Nutr.*, 123, 144, 1993.
106. Behling, A. R. et al., Lipid absorption and intestinal tumour incidence in rats fed on varying levels of calcium and butterfat, *Br. J. Nutr.*, 64, 505, 1990.
107. Reshef, R. et al., Effect of a calcium-enriched diet on the colonic epithelial hyperproliferation induced by N-methyl-N-nitro-N-nitrosoquanidine in rats on a low calcium and fat diet, *Cancer Res.*, 50, 1764, 1990.
108. Wargovich, M. J. et al., Inhibition of the promotional phase of azoxymethane-induced colon carcinogenesis in the F334 rat by calcium lactate: effect of simulating two human nutrient density levels, *Cancer Lett.*, 53, 17, 1990.
109. Sitrin, M. D. et al., Dietary calcium and vitamin D modulate 1,2-dimethylhydrazine-induced colonic carcinogenesis in the rat, *Cancer Res.*, 51, 5608, 1991.
110. Karkare, M. R., Clark, T. D., and Glauert, H. P., Effect of dietary calcium on colon carcinogenesis induced by a single injection of 1,2-dimethylhydrazine in rats, *J. Nutr.*, 121, 568, 1991.
111. Comer, P. F., Clark, T. D., and Glauert, H. P., Effect of dietary vitamin D3 (cholecalciferol) on colon carcinogenesis induced by 1,2-dimethylhydrazine in male Fisher 344 rats, *Nutr. Cancer*, 19, 113, 1993.
112. Harris, D. M. and Go, V. L. W., Vitamin D and colon carcinogenesis, *J. Nutr.*, 134, 3463s, 2004.
113. Wargovich, M. J. and Lointier, P. H., Calcium and vitamin D modulate mouse colon epithelial proliferation and growth characteristics of a human colon tumor cell line, *Can. J. Physiol. Pharmacol.*, 65, 472, 1987.
114. Bird, R. P., Effect of dietary components on the pathobiology of colonic epithelium: possible relationship with colon tumorigenesis, *Lipids*, 21, 289, 1986.
115. Scalmati, A., Lipkin, M., and Newmark, H., Calcium, vitamin D, and colon cancer, *Clin. Appl. Nutr.*, 2, 67, 1992.
116. Govers, M. J. A. P., Termont, D. S. M. L., and Van der Meer, R., Mechanism of the antiproliferative effect of milk mineral and other calcium supplements on colonic epithelium, *Cancer Res.*, 54, 95, 1994.
117. Marchetti, M. C. et al., Possible mechanisms involved in apoptosis of colon tumor cell lines induced by deoxycholic acid, short-chain fatty acids, and their mixtures, *Nutr. Cancer*, 28, 74, 1997.
118. Buset, M. et al., Inhibition of human colonic epithelial cell proliferation *in vivo* and *in vitro* by calcium, *Cancer Res.*, 46, 5426, 1986.
119. Barsoum, G. H. et al., Reduction of mucosal crypt cell proliferation in patients with colorectal adenomatous polyps by dietary calcium supplementation, *Br. J. Surg.*, 79, 581, 1992.
120. Guo, Y.-S. et al., Differential effects of Ca2+ on proliferation of stomach, colonic, and pancreatic cancer lines *in vitro*, *Nutr. Cancer*, 14, 149, 1990.
121. Ichas, F. and Mazat, J. P., From calcium signaling to cell death: two conformations for the mitochondrial permeability transition pore. Switching from low-to high-conductance state, *Biochim. Biophys. Acta*, 1366, 33, 1998.
122. Brenner, B. M. et al., The effect of dietary vitamin D3 on the intracellular calcium gradient in mammalian colonic crypts, *Cancer Lett.*, 127, 43, 1998.
123. Wargovich, M. J. et al., Calcium supplementation decreases rectal epithelial cell proliferation in subjects with sporadic adenoma, *Gastroenterology*, 103, 92, 1992.
124. O'Sullivan, K. R. et al., Effect of oral calcium supplementation on colonic crypt cell proliferation in patients with adenomatous polyps of the large bowel, *Eur. J. Gastroenterol. Hepatol.*, 5, 85, 1993.
125. Bostick, R. M. et al., Calcium and colorectal epithelial cell proliferation in sporadic adema patients: a randomized, double-blinded, placebo-controlled clinical trial, *J. Natl. Cancer Inst.*, 87, 1307, 1995.
126. Govers, M. J. A. P. et al., Calcium in milk products precipitates intestinal fatty acids and secondary bile acids and thus inhibits colonic cytotoxicity in man, *Cancer Res.*, 56, 3270, 1996.
127. Baron, J. A. et al., for the Calcium Polyp Prevention Study Group, Calcium supplements for the prevention of colorectal adenomas, *N. Engl. J. Med.*, 340, 101, 1999.
128. Bonithon-Kopp, C. et al., Calcium and fibre supplementation in prevention of colorectal adenoma recurrence: a randomised intervention trial, *Lancet*, 356, 1300, 2000.

129. Holt, P. R. et al., Comparison of calcium supplementation or low-fat dairy foods on epithelial cell proliferation and differentiation, *Nutr. Cancer*, 41, 150, 2001.
130. Grau, M. V. et al., Vitamin D, calcium supplementation, and colorectal adenomas: results of a randomized trial, *J. Natl. Cancer Inst.*, 95, 1765, 2003.
131. Wallace, K. et al., Effect of calcium supplementation on the risk of large bowel polyps, *J. Natl. Cancer Inst.*, 96, 921, 2004.
132. Holt, P. R. et al., Calcium plus vitamin D alters preneoplastic features of colorectal adenomas and rectal mucosa, *Cancer*, 106, 287, 2006.
133. Gregoire, R. C. et al., Effect of calcium supplementation on mucosal proliferation in high risk patients for colon cancer, *Gut*, 30, 376, 1989.
134. Cats, A. et al., Randomized, double-blinded, placebo-controlled intervention study with supplemental calcium in families with hereditary nonpolyposis colorectal cancer, *J. Natl. Cancer Inst.*, 87, 598, 1995.
135. Alberts, D.-S. et al., Randomized, double-blinded, placebo-controlled study of effect of wheat bran fiber and calcium on fecal bile acids in patients with resected adenomatous colon polyps, *J. Natl. Cancer Inst.*, 88, 81, 1996.
136. Lupton, J. R. et al., Calcium supplementation modifies the relative amounts of bile acids in bile and affects key aspects of human colon physiology, *J. Nutr.*, 126, 1421, 1996.
137. Danes, B. S., Effect of increased calcium concentration on in vitro growth of human colonic mucosal lines, *Dis. Colon Rectum*, 34, 552, 1991.
138. Danes, B. S. et al., Heritable colon cancer: influence of increased calcium concentration on increased in vitro tetraploidy (IVT), *Med. Hypotheses*, 36, 69, 1991.
139. Llor, X. et al., K-ras mutations in 1,2-dimethylhydrazine-induced colonic tumors: effects of supplemental dietary calcium and vitamin D deficiency, *Cancer Res.*, 51, 4305, 1991.
140. Rozen, P. et al., Oral calcium suppresses increased rectal epithelial proliferation of persons at risk of colorectal cancer, *Gut*, 30, 650, 1989.
141. Lans, J. I. et al., Supplemental calcium suppresses colonic mucosal ornithine decarboxylase activity in elderly patients with adenomatous polyps, *Cancer Res.*, 51, 3416, 1991.
142. Yang, K., Cohen, L., and Lipkin, M., Lectin soybean agglutinin: measurements in colonic epithelial cells of human subjects following supplemental dietary calcium, *Cancer Lett.*, 56, 65, 1991.
143. Lupton, J. R., Dairy products and colon cancer: mechanisms of the protective effect, *Am. J. Clin. Nutr.*, 66, 1065, 1997.
144. Glinghammar, B. et al., Shift from a dairy product-rich to a dairy product-free diet: influence on cytotoxicity and genotoxicity of fecal water — potential risk factors for colon cancer, *Am. J. Clin. Nutr.*, 66, 1277, 1997.
145. Schatzkin, A. and Peters, U., Advancing the calcium-colorectal cancer hypothesis, *J. Natl. Cancer Inst.*, 96, 893, 2004.
146. Holt, P. R. et al., Modulation of abnormal colonic epithelial cell proliferation and differentiation by lowfat dairy foods, *JAMA*, 280, 1074, 1998.
147. Wactawski-Wende, J. et al., Calcium plus vitamin D supplementation and the risk of colorectal cancer, *N. Engl. J. Med.*, 354, 684, 2006.
148. Lipkin, M. and Newmark, H. L., Vitamin D, calcium and prevention of breast cancer: a review, *J. Am. Coll. Nutr.*, 18, 392s, 1999.
149. Missmer, S. A., Meat and dairy food consumption and breast cancer: a pooled analysis of cohort studies, *Int. J. Epidemiol.*, 31, 78, 2002.
150. Parodi, P. W., Dairy product consumption and the risk of breast cancer, *J. Am. Coll. Nutr.*, 24, 556s, 2005.
151. Berube, S. et al., Vitamin D and calcium intake from food or supplements and mammographic breast density, *Cancer Epidemiol. Biomarkers Prev.*, 14, 1653, 2005.
152. McCullough, M. L. et al., Dairy, calcium, and vitamin D intake and postmenopausal breast cancer risk in the Cancer Prevention Study II Nutrition Cohort, *Cancer Epidemiol. Biomarkers Prev.*, 14, 2898, 2005.
153. Berube, S. et al., Vitamin D, calcium, and mammographic breast densities, *Cancer Epidemiol. Biomarkers Prev.*, 13, 1466, 2004.

154. Boyd, N. F. et al., Dietary fat and breast cancer revisited: a meta-analysis of the published literature, *Br. J. Cancer*, 89, 1672, 2003.
155. Shin, M.-H. et al., Intake of dairy products, calcium, and vitamin D and risk of breast cancer, *J. Natl. Cancer Inst.*, 94, 1301, 2002.
156. Shannon, J., Cook, L. S., and Stanford, J. L., Dietary intake and risk of postmenopausal breast cancer (United States), *Cancer Causes Control*, 14, 19, 2003.
157. Hjartaker, A. et al., Childhood and adult milk consumption and risk of premenopausal breast cancer in a cohort of 48,844 women — the Norwegain women and cancer study, *Int. J. Cancer*, 93, 888, 2001.
158. Knekt, P. et al., Intake of dairy products and the risk of breast cancer, *Br. J. Cancer*, 73, 687, 1996.
159. Baron, J. A., Risk of prostate cancer in a randomized clinical trial of calcium supplementation, *Cancer Epidemiol. Biomarkers Prev.*, 14, 586, 2005.
160. Schuurman, A. G. et al., Animal products, calcium and protein and prostate cancer risk in The Netherlands Cohort Study, *Br. J. Cancer*, 80, 1107, 1999.
161. Chan, J. M. et al., Diet and prostate cancer risk in a cohort of smokers with a specific focus on calcium and phosphorus (Finland), *Cancer Causes Control*, 11, 859, 2000.
162. Rodriquez, C. et al., Calcium, dairy products, and risk of prostate cancer in a prospective cohort of U.S. men, *Cancer Epidemiol. Biomarkers Prev.*, 12, 597, 2003.
163. Giovannucci, E. et al., A prospective study of calcium intake and incident and fatal prostate cancer, *Cancer Epidemiol. Biomarkers Prev.*, 15, 203, 2006.
164. Tseng, M., Dairy, calcium, and vitamin D intakes and prostate cancer risk in the National Health and Nutrition Examination Epidemiologic Follow-up Study cohort, *Am. J. Clin. Nutr.*, 81, 1147, 2005.
165. Chan, J. M. and Giovannucci, E. L., Dairy products, calcium, and vitamin D and risk of prostate cancer, *Epidemiol. Rev.*, 23, 87, 2001.
166. Berndt, S. I. et al., Calcium intake and prostate cancer risk in a long-term aging study: the Baltimore Longitudinal Study of Aging, *Urology*, 60, 1118, 2002.
167. Chen, T. C. and Holick, M. F., Vitamin D and prostate cancer prevention and treatment, *Trends Endocrinol. Metab.*, 14, 423, 2003.
168. Peehl, D. M., Krishnan, A. V., and Feldman, D., Pathways mediating the growth-inhibiting actions of vitamin D in prostate cancer, *J. Nutr.*, 133, 2461s, 2003.
169. Trump, D. L. et al., Anti-tumor activity of calcitriol: pre-clinical and clinical studies, *J. Steroid Biochem. Mol. Biol.*, 89–90, 519, 2004.
170. Lou, Y.-R. et al., 25-hydroxyvitamin D3 is an active hormone in human primary prostatic stromal cells, *FASEB J.*, 18, 332, 2004.
171. Bao, B. Y., Yeh, S. D., and Lee, Y. F., 1 alpha, 25-dihydroxyvitamin D3 inhibits prostate cancer cell invasion via modulation of selective proteases, *Carcinogenesis*, 27, 32, 2006.
172. Li, H. et al., Prediagnostic Plasma Vitamin D Levels, Vitamin D Receptor Gene Polymorphisms, and Susceptibility to Prostate Cancer, Abstr. 2, Program and Abstracts of the 2005 Multidisciplinary Prostate Cancer Symposium, American Society of Clinical Oncology, February 17–20, Orlando, FL, 2005.
173. Meister, K., *Risk Factors for Prostate Cancer*, American Council on Science and Health, New York, 2002.
174. Parodi, P. W., The role of intestinal bacteria in the causation and prevention of cancer: modulation by diet and probiotics, *Aust. J. Dairy Technol.*, 54, 103, 1999.
175. Brady, L. J., Gallaher, D. D., and Busta, F. F., The role of probiotic cultures in the prevention of colon cancer, *J. Nutr.*, 130, 410s, 2000.
176. Saikali, J. et al., Fermented milks, probiotic cultures, and colon cancer, *Nutr. Cancer*, 49, 14, 2004.
177. Perdigon, G. et al., Role of yoghurt in the prevention of colon cancer, *Eur. J. Clin. Nutr.*, 56 (suppl. 3), 65s, 2002.
178. LeBlanc, A. and Perdigon, G., Yogurt feeding inhibits promotion and progression of experimental colorectal cancer, *Med. Sci. Monit.*, 10, BR96, 2004.
179. Rafter, J., Lactic acid bacteria and cancer: mechanistic perspective, *Br. J. Nutr.*, 88 (suppl. 1), 89s, 2002.
180. Van't Veer, P. et al., Consumption of fermented milk products and breast cancer: a case-control study in The Netherlands, *Cancer Res.*, 49, 4020, 1989.

181. Biffi, A. et al., Antiproliferative effect of fermented milk on the growth of a human breast cancer cell line, *Nutr. Cancer*, 28, 93, 1997.
182. Belury, M. A., Inhibition of carcinogenesis by conjugated linoleic acid: potential mechanisms of action, *J. Nutr.*, 132, 2995, 2002.
183. Maggiora, M. et al., An overview of the effect of linoleic acid and conjugated-linoleic acids on the growth of several human tumor cell lines, *Int. J. Cancer*, 112, 909, 2004.
184. Chin, S. F. et al., Dietary sources of conjugated dienoic isomers of linoleic acid, a newly recognized class of anticarcinogens, *J. Food Compos. Anal.*, 5, 185, 1992.
185. Lin, H. et al., Survey of the conjugated linoleic acid contents of dairy products, *J. Dairy Sci.*, 78, 2358, 1995.
186. Ip, C. et al., Conjugated linoleic acid-enriched butter fat alters mammary gland morphogenesis and reduces cancer risk in rats, *J. Nutr.*, 129, 2135, 1999.
187. Turpeinen, A. M., Bioconversion of vaccenic acid to conjugated linoleic acid in humans, *Am. J. Clin. Nutr.*, 76, 504, 2002.
188. Corl, B. A., *Cis*-9 *trans*-11 CLA derived endogenously from *trans*-11, 18:1 reduces cancer risk in rats, *J. Nutr.*, 133, 2893, 2003.
189. Ip, C. et al., Control of rat mammary epithelium proliferation by conjugated linoleic acid, *Nutr. Cancer*, 39, 233, 2001.
190. Banni, S. et al., Vaccenic acid feeding increases tissue levels of conjugated linoleic acid and suppresses development of premalignant lesions in rat mammary gland, *Nutr. Cancer*, 41, 91, 2001.
191. Field, C. J. and Schley, P. D., Evidence for potential mechanisms for the effect of conjugated linoleic acid on tumor metabolism and immune function: lessons from n-3 fatty acids, *Am. J. Clin. Nutr.*, 79, 1190s, 2004.
192. Wahle, K. W. J., Heys, S. D., and Rotondo, D., Conjugated linoleic acids: are they beneficial or detrimental to health? *Prog. Lipid Res.*, 43, 553, 2004.
193. Song, H.-J. et al., Conjugated linoleic acid inhibits proliferation and modulates protein kinase C isoforms in human prostate cancer cells, *Nutr. Cancer*, 49, 100, 2004.
194. Liew, C. et al., Protection of conjugated linoleic acid against 2-amino-3-methylimidazo[4,5-f]quinoline-induced colon carcinogenesis in the F344 rat: a study of inhibitory mechanisms, *Carcinogenesis*, 16, 3037, 1995.
195. Ip, C. and Scimeca, J. A., Conjugated linoleic acid and linoleic acid are distinctive modulators of mammary carcinogenesis, *Nutr. Cancer*, 27, 131, 1997.
196. Lavillonniere, F. et al., Dietary purified *cis*-9 *trans*-11 conjugated linoleic acid isomer has anticarcinogenic properties in chemically induced mammary tumours in rats, *Nutr. Cancer*, 45, 190, 2003.
197. Huang, Y.-C., Luedecke, L. O., and Shultz, T. D., Effect of cheddar cheese consumption on plasma conjugated linoleic acid concentrations in men, *Nutr. Res.*, 14, 373, 1994.
198. Aro, A., et al., Inverse association between dietary and serum conjugated linoleic acid and risk of breast cancer in postmenopausal women, *Nutr. Cancer*, 38, 151, 2000.
199. Chajes, V. et al., Conjugated linoleic acid content in breast adipose tissue is not associated with the relative risk of breast cancer in a population of French patients, *Cancer Epidemiol. Biomarkers Prev.*, 11, 672, 2002.
200. Dillehay, D. L. et al., Dietary sphingomyelin inhibits 1,2-dimethylhydrazine-induced colon cancer in CF1 mice, *J. Nutr.*, 124, 615, 1994.
201. Merrill, A. H. Jr. et al., Role of dietary sphingolipids and inhibitors of sphingolipid metabolism in cancer and other diseases, *J. Nutr.*, 125 (suppl.), 1677, 1995.
202. Merrill, A. H. Jr. et al., Importance of sphingolipids and inhibitors of sphingolipid metabolism as components of animal diets, *J. Nutr.*, 127 (suppl.), 830, 1997.
203. Vesper, H. et al., Sphingolipids in food and the emerging importance of sphingolipids to nutrition, *J. Nutr.*, 129, 1239, 1999.
204. Lemonnier, L. A. et al., Sphingomyelin in the suppression of colon tumors: prevention versus intervention, *Arch. Biochem. Biophys.*, 419, 129, 2003.
205. Schmelz, E. M. et al., Inhibition of colonic cell proliferation and aberrant crypt foci formation by dairy glycosphingolipids in 1,2 dimethylhydrazine-treated CF1 mice, *J. Nutr.*, 130, 22, 2000.

206. Hannun, Y. A. et al., Sphingosine inhibition of protein kinase C activity and of phorbol bibutyrate binding *in vitro* and in human platelets, *J. Biol. Chem.*, 261, 12604, 1986.
207. Schmelz, E. M., et al., Update and metabolism of sphingolipids in isolated intestinal loops of mice, *J. Nutr.*, 124, 702, 1994.
208. Schmelz, E. M. et al., Sphingomyelin consumption suppresses aberrant colonic crypt foci and increases the proportion of adenomas versus adenocarcinomas in CF1 mice treated with 1,2-dimethylhydrazine: implications for dietary sphingolipids and colon carcinogenesis, *Cancer Res.*, 56, 4936, 1996.
209. Schmelz, E. M. et al., Suppression of aberrant colonic crypt foci by synthetic sphingomyelins with saturated or unsaturated sphingoid base backbones, *Nutr. Cancer*, 28, 81, 1997.
210. Schmelz, E. M. et al., Modulation of intracellular B-catenin localization and intestinal tumorigenesis *in vivo* and *in vitro* by sphingolipids, *Cancer Res.*, 61, 6723, 2001.
211. Smith, J. G. and German, J. B., Molecular and genetic effects of dietary derived butyric acid, *Food Technol.*, 49, 87, 1995.
212. Chen, Z. and Breitman, T., Tributyrin: a prodrug of butyric acid for potential clinical application in differentiation therapy, *Cancer Res.*, 54, 3494, 1994.
213. Pouillart, P. et al., Enhancement by stable butyrate derivatives of antitumor and antiviral actions of interferon, *Int. J. Cancer*, 51, 596, 1992.
214. Hague, A. et al., Sodium butyrate induces apoptosis in human colonic cell lines in a p53-independent pathway. Implications for the possible role of dietary fibre in the prevention of large bowel cancer, *Int. J. Cancer*, 55, 498, 1993.
215. Hague, A. and Paraskeva, C., This short-chain fatty acid butyrate induces apoptosis in colorectal tumor cell lines, *Eur. J. Cancer Prev.*, 4, 359, 1995.
216. Lupton, J. R., Butyrate and colonic cytokinetics: differences between *in vitro* and *in vivo* studies, *Eur. J. Cancer Prev.*, 4, 373, 1995.
217. Boffa, L. C. et al., Modulation of colonic epithelial cell proliferation, histone acetylation, and luminal short chain fatty acids by variation of dietary fiber (wheat bran) in rats, *Cancer Res.*, 52, 5906, 1992.
218. Aukema, H. M. et al., Butyrate alters activity of specific cAMP-receptor proteins in a transgenic mouse colonic cell line, *J. Nutr.*, 127, 18, 1997.
219. McIntyre, A., Gibson, P. R., and Young, G. P., Butyrate production from dietary fibre and protection against large bowel cancer in a rat model, *Gut*, 34, 386, 1993.
220. McIntosh, G. H. and LeLeu, R. K., The influence of dietary proteins on colon cancer risk, *Nutr. Res.*, 21, 1053, 2001.
221. Walzem, R. L., Dillard, C. J., and German, J. B., Whey components: millennia of evolution create functionalities for mammalian nutrition: what we know and what we may be overlooking, *Crit. Rev. Food Sci. Nutr.*, 42, 353, 2002.
222. MacDonald, R. S., Thorton, W. H. Jr., and Marshall, R. T., A cell culture model to identify biologically active peptides generated by bacterial hydrolysis of casein, *J. Dairy Sci.*, 77, 1167, 1994.
223. Goeptar, A. R. et al., Impact of digestion on the antimutagenic activity of the milk protein casein, *Nutr. Res.*, 17, 1363, 1997.
224. Hakkak, R. et al., Dietary whey protein protects against azoxymethane-induced colon tumors in male rats, *Cancer Epidemiol. Biomarkers Prev.*, 10, 555, 2001.
225. Belobrajdic, D. P., McIntosh, G. H., and Owens, J. A., Whey proteins protect more than red meat against azoxymethane induced ACF in Wistar rats, *Cancer Lett.*, 198, 43, 2003.
226. Hakkak, R. et al., Diets containing whey proteins or soy protein isolate protect against 7,12-dimethylbenz(a) anthracene-induced mammary tumors in female rats, *Cancer Epidemiol. Biomarkers Prev.*, 9, 113, 2000.
227. Eason, R. R. et al., Dietary exposure to whey proteins alters rat mammary gland proliferation, apoptosis, and gene expression during postnatal development, *J. Nutr.*, 134, 3370, 2004.
228. Kent, K. D., Harper, W. J., and Bomser, J. A., Effect of whey protein isolate on intracellular glutathione and oxidant-induced cell death in human prostate epithelial cells, *Toxicol. In Vitro*, 17, 27, 2003.
229. Tsuda, H. et al., Cancer prevention by bovine lactoferrin and underlying mechanisms — a review of experimental and clinical studies, *Biochem. Cell Biol.*, 80, 131, 2002.

230. Eliassen, L. T. et al., Evidence for a direct antitumor mechanism of action of bovine lactoferricin, *Anticancer Res.*, 22, 2703, 2002.
231. Bounous, G., Whey protein concentrate (WPC) and glutathione modulation in cancer treatment, *Anticancer Res.*, 20, 4785, 2000.
232. Micke, P. et al., Oral supplementation with whey protein increases plasma glutathione levels of HIV-infected patients, *Eur. J. Clin. Invest.*, 31, 171, 2001.
233. Kato, I. et al., Prospective study of diet and female colorectal cancer: the New York University Women's Health Study, *Nutr. Cancer*, 28, 276, 1997.
234. Holmes, M. D. et al., Dietary factors and the survival of women with breast carcinoma, *Cancer*, 86, 826, 1999.
235. American Cancer Society, American Cancer Society guidelines on nutrition and physical activity for cancer prevention (2002), *CA Cancer J. Clin.*, 52, 92, 2002.
236. Cotton, P. A. et al., Dietary sources of nutrients among U.S. adults, 1994 to 1996, *J. Am. Diet. Assoc.*, 104, 921, 2004.
237. Weinberg, L. G., Berner, L. A., and Groves, J. E., Nutrient contributions of dairy foods in the United States, Continuing Survey of Food Intakes by Individuals, 1994–1996, 1998, *J. Am. Diet. Assoc.*, 104, 895, 2004.
238. Moshfegh, A., Goldman, J., and Cleveland, L., What We Eat in America, NHANES 2001–2002: Usual Nutrient Intakes from Food Compared to Dietary Reference Intakes. U.S. Department of Agriculture, Agriculture Research Service (www.ars.usda.gov/foodsurvey).
239. Cook, A. J. and Friday, J. E., Pyramid Servings Intakes in the United States 1999–2002, 1 Day, Agricultural Research Service, Community Nutrition Research Group, CNRG Table Set 3.0, 2004 (www.ba.ars.usda.gov/cnrg).
240. U.S. Department of Health and Human Services and U.S. Department of Agriculture, Dietary Guidelines for Americans, 2005, 6th ed., Government Printing Office, Washington, D.C. (www.healthierus.gov/dietaryguidelines).
241. Fulgoni, V. L. et al., Determination of the optimal number of dairy servings to ensure a low prevalence of inadequate calcium intake in Americans, *J. Am. Coll. Nutr.*, 23, 651, 2004.
242. Wooten, W. J. and Price, W., Consensus report of the National Medical Association, the role of dairy and dairy nutrients in the diet of African Americans, *J. Natl. Med. Assoc.*, 96 (suppl.), 1s, 2004.
243. McCarron, D. A. and Heaney, R. P., Estimated health care savings associated with adequate dairy food intake, *Am. J. Hypertens.*, 17, 88, 2004.
244. Qin, L.-Q. et al., Milk/dairy products consumption, galactose metabolism and ovarian cancer: meta-analysis of epidemiological studies, *Eur. J. Cancer Prev.*, 14, 13, 2005.
245. Larsson, S. C., Orsini, N., and Wolk, A., Milk, milk products and lactose intake and ovarian cancer risk: a meta-analysis of epidemiological studies, *Int. J. Cancer*, 118, 431, 2006.
246. Genkinger, J. M., Dairy products and ovarian cancer: a pooled analysis of 12 cohort studies, *Cancer Epidemiol. Biomarkers Prev.*, 15, 364, 2006.
247. Mommers, M. et al., Dairy consumption and ovarian cancer risk in the Netherlands Cohort Study on diet and cancer, *Br. J. Cancer*, 94, 165, 2006.
248. Calle, E. E. et al., Overweight, obesity, and mortality from cancer in a prospectively studied cohort of U.S. adults, *N. Engl. J. Med.*, 348, 1625, 2003.
249. Zemel, M. B., The role of dairy foods in weight management, *J. Am. Coll. Nutr.*, 24, 537s, 2005.

5 Dairy Foods and Bone Health

5.1 INTRODUCTION

Building and maintaining a healthy skeleton throughout life are essential to overall health and quality of life [1]. Osteoporosis, a skeletal disease characterized by reduced bone mass, structural deterioration, and excessive bone remodeling leading to increased bone fragility and susceptibility to fractures, is the most common bone disease [1,2]. Often called a silent disease, osteoporosis develops gradually over many years and before the occurrence of clinical symptoms such as loss of height, curvature of the spine, and fractures, especially of the spine, hip, and wrist [1–4]. For many individuals, a skeletal fracture is the first indication of osteoporosis.

Osteoporosis is a major public health problem in the United States, affecting 44 million adults over the age of 50 [1]. Although 80% of adults with osteoporosis are women, the disease also affects men and occurs in all races and ethnic groups [1,3]. An estimated 1.5 million adults will suffer an osteoporosis-related fracture each year and up to 20% of those with hip fractures will die from injury-related complications within a year [1]. Osteoporosis incurs direct health care costs of up to $18 billion a year [1]. By the year 2020, half of Americans over the age of 50 will have or be at high risk for osteoporosis if preventive measures are not taken [1]. The U.S. Surgeon General's first-ever report on *Bone Health and Osteoporosis* emphasizes that it is essential to develop effective strategies throughout life to prevent and manage this bone disease [1].

The cause(s) of osteoporosis, similar to other chronic diseases, is multifactorial, involving both genetic and environmental (nutrition, physical activity) factors [1–4]. Nutrition is an important modifiable factor in the development and maintenance of bones, as well as the prevention and treatment of osteoporosis [1]. Calcium and vitamin D have long been known to be beneficial for bone health [1–11]. This is understandable, considering that 99% of the body's calcium is stored in bones where it contributes to their strength and structure, and that vitamin D enhances calcium absorption [10]. In addition to calcium and vitamin D, other nutrients such as protein, phosphorus, magnesium, potassium, zinc, and vitamins A, C, and K support bone health [1,10,11]. Evidence indicates that consuming naturally nutrient-rich foods such as milk and other dairy products (cheese, yogurt) improves bone mineral status and helps to reduce the risk of osteoporosis [7].

Dairy foods such as milk, cheese, and yogurt are the major dietary source of calcium and vitamin D (if fortified) (Figure 5.1) [1,7,12–15]. Consuming at least the recommended number of servings of dairy foods each day not only increases calcium and other nutrients essential for building and maintaining healthy bones, but also improves the overall nutritional adequacy of the diet [15–19] (see Chapter 1). A diet without dairy products provides only about 250 to 300 mg calcium/day [1,15], an amount far less than the current recommendation [adequate intake (AI)] of 1000 to 1200 mg of calcium/day for adults (Table 5.1) [10]. The 2005 *Dietary Guidelines for Americans*, issued jointly by the U.S. Department of Health and Human Services and the U.S. Department of Agriculture (USDA), identifies seven nutrients low in the diets of children and adults [20]. Dairy foods, such as milk, cheese, and yogurt, supply four of these seven nutrients for adults (calcium, potassium, magnesium, and vitamin A) and three of these nutrients for children (calcium, magnesium, and potassium) [12,20].

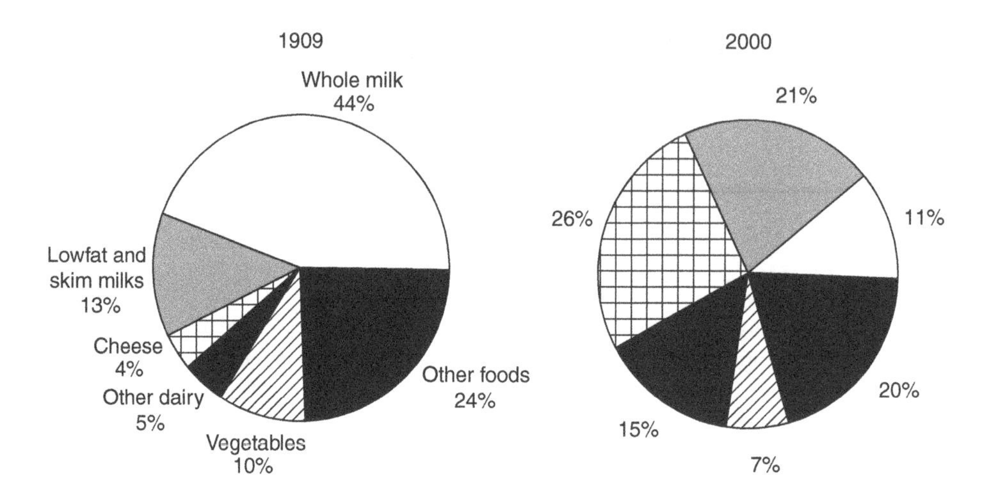

FIGURE 5.1 Sources of calcium in the U.S. food supply. (From Gerrior, S., Bente, L., and Hiza, L., *Nutrient Content of the U.S. Food Supply 1909–2000*, Home Economics Research Project No. 56, USDA, Center for Nutrition Policy and Promotion, 2004.)

An analysis of government food and nutrient consumption data determined that 3 to 4 servings of dairy foods a day is the optimal level to ensure AI of calcium for individuals older than 9 years of age [21]. Recognition of Americans' low intake of calcium and dairy foods, as well as the importance of dairy foods and dairy food nutrients in bone health, has led to the recommendation to consume at least 3 servings of dairy foods such as milk, cheese, or yogurt a day [1,20,22–24]. The 2005 *Dietary Guidelines for Americans* [20] and the USDA's *MyPyramid* [22] recommend 3 cups of low-fat or fat free milk or equivalent milk products (e.g., cheese, yogurt) a day for those 9 years of age and older, to improve nutrient intake and support bone health. Likewise, the 2004 Surgeon General's report on *Bone Health and Osteoporosis* [1] and the National Medical Association [23] recommend at least 3 daily servings of dairy foods a day. A report by the American Academy of Pediatrics [24] states, "most people can achieve the recommended dietary intake of calcium by eating 3 age-appropriate servings of dairy products per day (4 servings a day for adolescents) or the equivalent." Based on an analysis, researchers conservatively estimated that consuming 3 to 4 servings of dairy foods per day could reduce osteoporosis-related fractures by at least 20%, resulting in health care cost savings of more than $3.5 billion/year or $14 billion over 5 years [25].

This chapter reviews studies confirming and extending previous research findings which support the role of dairy foods or dairy food nutrients (i.e., calcium, vitamin D, etc.) in building and maintaining healthy bones throughout life. It should be appreciated that nutrition, particularly calcium and vitamin D, is among several factors influencing both optimal bone health and the risk of osteoporosis [1,9,17]. Also discussed is the importance of dairy foods as the preferred source of nutrients, particularly calcium, for healthy bones.

5.2 BONE BASICS

The skeleton is composed of two types of bone: cortical bone, the dense compact outer layer of bone which is the predominant bone in the shafts of long bones, and trabecular (cancellous) bone, which is the porous honeycomb-like structure in the interior of bones, especially in the vertebra and at the ends of all long bones [1]. About 75% of the adult skeleton is cortical (compact) bone, with the remaining 25% being trabecular bone [1]. However, the relative proportions of these two types of bone vary from one bone to another.

TABLE 5.1
Adequate Intakes (AI) or Recommended Dietary Allowances (RDA) and Tolerable Upper Intake Levels (UL) for Calcium, Vitamin D, Phosphorus, and Magnesium by Life-Stage Group for United States and Canada

Life-Stage Group	Calcium (mg/day)		Vitamin D (IU/day)		Phosphorus (mg/day)		Magnesium (mg/day)		
	AI	UL	AI	UL	RDA	UL	RDA		UL[a]
							Male	Female	
0–6 months	210	ND[b]	200	1000	100	ND[b]	30	30	ND[b]
7–12 months	270	ND[b]	200	1000	275	ND[b]	75	75	ND[b]
1–3 years	500	2500	200	2000	460	3000	80	80	*65*
4–8 years	800	2500	200	2000	500	3000	130	130	110
9–13 years	1300	2500	200	2000	1250	4000	240	240	350
14–18 years	1300	2500	200	2000	1250	4000	410	360	350
19–30 years	1000	2500	200	2000	700	4000	400	310	350
31–50 years	1000	2500	200	2000	700	4000	420	320	350
51–70 years	1200	2500	400	2000	700	4000	420	320	350
>70 years	1200	2500	600	2000	700	3000	420	320	350

[a] Upper Limit;
[b] Not Determined

Source: From Institute of Medicine, Dietary Reference Intakes of Calcium, Phosphorus, Magnesium, Vitamin D, and Fluoride, 1997.

Throughout life, bone is constantly remodeled, a process important for self-repair of skeletal tissue, as well as for maintaining calcium in extracellular fluid [1,26,27]. Bone remodeling is a complex, highly ordered sequence of cellular events, starting with activation of a quiescent bone surface, then a resorption phase whereby old bone is removed by osteoclasts, and finally, bone formation and mineralization. Bone mineralization is initiated by osteoblasts, but then it proceeds passively without further cellular activity. As a result of this remodeling process, most of the adult skeleton is replaced about every 10 to 12 years on average [1,27]. A number of interrelated hormonal, nutritional, mechanical, and genetic factors influence the bone remodeling rate and variance in bone mass [1]. For example, whenever dietary calcium is insufficient to meet adults' needs, the resorption component of bone remodeling exceeds the amount of new bone formed (i.e., bone is broken down and the released calcium helps to maintain a relatively constant concentration in the blood) [1]. Because actual mineralization of new bone is separated in time from the osteoblastic work that initiates the process, calcium entry into bone is not easily adjusted to meet the fluctuating demands of calcium homeostasis. For this reason, virtually all of the remodeling adjustment that is responsive to homeostatic need comes about minute-to-minute through regulation of the rate of bone resorption.

Bone mass increases during infancy, childhood, and adolescence [28]. However, it does not stop when longitudinal growth or adult height is achieved. It is generally accepted that following completion of longitudinal growth, consolidation of bone density continues until peak bone mass is reached, between 20 and 30 years of age or earlier [1,28]. Different bones reach peak bone mass at different ages [29]. For example, peak bone mass at the hip is reached before that of the spine [29]. In addition to attainment of peak bone mass, there is a slow increase in the periosteal diameter of most bones, which results in an increase in bone size. This mass slows during a woman's active reproductive life, but increases again after menopause. If bone mass remains the same, this increase in size results in a fall in bone density (as measured by bone mineral density, for example). But this decline in density does not mean a decrease in strength, as resistance to bending increases to the square of the radius. For the same reason, a decline in measured bone mineral density does not necessarily mean a decrease in bone mass. This is an important point, since it is bone mass, not bone density, which influences the susceptibility to osteoporotic fractures [30].

Achieving peak bone mass in the early years and preventing loss of bone due to extreme breakdown (resorption) in later adult years, reduces the risk of osteoporosis [1]. The amount of bone accumulated during growth depends in part on the amount of calcium consumed. Peak bone mass does not reach its genetic potential if calcium intake is deficient during skeletal formation. Variations in prevailing calcium intakes early in life may account for a 5% to 10% difference in peak bone mass and approximately a 25% to 50% difference in hip fracture rate later in life [28]. At menopause (i.e., between ages 45 and 55), bone loss, as measured by bone mineral density, accelerates (i.e., average of 3% a year) in women and remains elevated for about 4 to 8 years before slowing down to a rate similar to that in older men. Only a part of this is true loss, as periosteal expansion accelerates at menopause, resulting in a decline in density. The sharp decline in estrogen production at menopause is responsible for these changes after menopause [1,10]. In men, bone loss generally occurs after age 50, but is not as rapid or as great as womens [1]. Women's relatively lower peak bone mass and increased bone loss following menopause are a part of the reason why osteoporosis is two to three times more common in women than in men [1]. After age 65, women and men tend to lose bone at a similar rate. Decreases in levels of hormones (e.g., testosterone, estrogen) likely contribute to reduced bone mass and increased fracture risk in men [1].

Age-related bone loss in both sexes involves the gradual thinning of both cortex and trabeculae. The accelerated postmenopausal bone loss is mediated by osteoclasts. A gradual decrease in cortical thickness occurs with age and increases in women after menopause. The magnitude of peak bone mass and the rate and duration of postmenopausal and age-associated bone loss partially determine the likelihood of developing osteoporosis [1]. When bone mass is low, less trauma is necessary to cause a fracture. This is just as true in children as in adults. In addition to bone mass, bone geometry and microarchitecture, as well as bone remodeling, influence risk of bone fractures [26,27,31]. High bone remodeling activity is positively associated with osteoporotic bony fragility [31]. Research indicates that increasing calcium intake reduces homeostatic bone remodeling (i.e., remodeling to maintain blood calcium levels) and fracture risk prior to any perceptible change in bone mass [26,27]. That is, adequate calcium intake positively affects the quality, as well as the quantity of bone [26,27].

Although some age-related bone loss may be inevitable, osteoporotic fractures are not natural events. Throughout life, from early childhood through later adult years, measures can be taken to promote bone health [1]. For example, an AI of bone-related nutrients (e.g., calcium vitamin D, protein, etc.) benefits bones at all ages [1,7,8,32].

5.3 RISK FACTORS FOR OSTEOPOROSIS

A number of risk factors for osteoporosis have been identified (Table 5.2) [1,10]. Both genetics and environmental or lifestyle factors influence the likelihood of developing this disease [1]. Genetics (e.g., genetic polymorphisms related to vitamin D receptor) influences peak bone mass, skeletal structure, rate of bone loss, and the skeleton's response to environmental stimuli such as nutrients and physical activity [1,33,34]. Although genetics influences 50% to 90% of bone mass and other qualitative aspects of bone [35], it is important not to underestimate the key role of controllable lifestyle factors such as diet and physical activity, which are responsible for 10% to 50% of bone mass and structure [1].

Gender, ethnicity, age, hormonal status, and body frame/weight are other factors that influence bone mass and the development of osteoporosis [1,10]. Women, because of their generally smaller, lighter bones, their rapid loss of bone at menopause, and their lower calcium intake, are more likely to develop osteoporosis than are men [1]. Among U.S. adults age 50 and older, lifetime risk of fractures of the hip, spine, and wrist is about 40% in women and 13% in men [1]. Caucasians, particularly those of northern European ancestry, and Asians of Japanese and Chinese descent are at significantly higher risk of losing bone and developing osteoporosis than are Hispanic women or African American women, who generally have larger body frames [1,36]. Although African American women have a lower risk for osteoporosis than white or Hispanic women, African American

TABLE 5.2
Risk Factors for Osteoporosis

Family history	If a family member has had osteoporosis, other members may be at risk
Gender	Osteoporosis is more common in women than in men
Ethnicity	Caucasian (white) and Asian women are most susceptible; Hispanic and African American women are also at significant risk
Age	Osteoporosis is found mostly in older adults
Hormonal status	Estrogen deficiency at menopause or earlier (before age 45 years) in women, and hormonal reductions in men increase risk
Body frame/weight	A thin, small-boned frame increases risk of osteoporosis
Diet	A diet chronically low in calcium and vitamin D (if exposure to direct sunlight is limited) increases risk
Exercise	Lack of regular physical activity can reduce bone mass and in older adults also reduce muscle strength
Cigarette smoking	Smoking is linked to increased risk
Alcohol	Excess alcohol intake increases risk
Medications	Certain medications such as glucocorticoids used to treat asthma or arthritis can increase risk

women are still at significant risk for developing this disease [37]. The risk of osteoporosis also rises with advancing age because bones become more fragile, and the risk of falls increases with age in both men and women, and with the loss of estrogen at menopause (either natural or surgical) in women [1,10]. There is a linear decrease in calcium absorption efficiency from at least age 40, amounting to about 0.2% per year, with an additional 2.2% lost across menopause [38]. Between the ages of 40 and 60 years, the combination of increasing age and estrogen withdrawal reduces calcium absorption efficiency by 20% to 25% [39]. Age-related decreases in estrogen in women and testosterone and estrogen in men, contribute to increased risk of osteoporosis in later years [1].

Young women with amenorrhea resulting from anorexia nervosa or excessive exercise are at high risk for low bone mass and osteoporosis [40]. Low body weight may limit peak bone mass and in older women increase the risk of hip fractures [1]. Also, following weight loss diets may increase the risk of osteoporosis [41,42]. Investigations involving obese, postmenopausal women have found that increasing calcium intake by 1000 mg a day prevents the increase in bone turnover and bone loss associated with diet-induced weight loss [41,42]. In a study of overweight adults on a calorie-reduced diet, intake of a high dairy protein, higher calcium diet helped to minimize bone turnover during weight loss [43]. Increasing calcium or dairy food intake may not only protect bone health during weight loss, but also enhance weight loss efforts. Emerging scientific research indicates that overweight or obese adults can increase their body weight or fat loss by increasing calcium intake or consuming 3 servings of dairy products, such as milk, cheese, or yogurt, as part of a reduced calorie diet [44, see Chapter 7]. Diseases, surgery, and some medications (e.g., corticosteroids, anticonvulsants, aluminum-containing antacids) also increase risk of osteoporosis [1].

An individual's lifestyle choices may account for a substantial proportion of the variance in bone density and, in turn, fracture risk [1,10,45]. Lifestyle choices that increase the risk for osteoporosis include heavy cigarette smoking, excess alcohol intake, physical inactivity, high physical activity leading to sweat losses, and some dietary intakes, especially an inadequate intake of calcium and vitamin D. Although caffeine was once thought to adversely affect calcium status, research now indicates that moderate caffeine intake has a negligible effect on calcium metabolism, calcium status, or bone density when adequate levels of calcium are consumed [1,46]. Cigarette smoking may adversely affect the skeleton both directly and indirectly [1,47]. Nicotine and cadmium in cigarettes may have direct toxic effects on bone cells. Indirectly, smoking may harm bones by reducing intestinal calcium absorption, altering the body's handling of vitamin D and various hormones, or lowering body weight [1,48]. Studies associate smoking with increased bone loss and fracture risk [1,47,49]. A meta-analysis of data from 12 prospective studies worldwide found that current smoking, and to a lesser extent a history of smoking, was associated with a significantly increased risk of hip and other fractures in both men and women compared to nonsmokers [49].

Excess alcohol intake is another risk factor for osteoporosis [1,47,50]. High alcohol intake may damage bones directly and/or contribute to osteoporosis indirectly by its effect on consumption and losses of calcium and other nutrients, liver damage, and/or by increasing predisposition to falls. With respect to physical activity, a sedentary lifestyle is associated with bone loss, whereas weight-bearing activities and regular moderate activities such as walking are linked to increased bone mass and reduced fracture risk [1,10]. Physical activity improves bone mass at skeletal sites that receive the impact. This effect appears to be greater in individuals who are initially less active than in physically active individuals who increase their level of activity [1]. Also, bone is especially responsive to physical activity during the prepubertal period [1]. The benefit of physical activity on bone persists only if physical activity is maintained [1]. Further, physical activity is positively related to bone mineral content if calcium intake is sufficient to offset losses of calcium in sweat [51,52]. Studies in male athletes (e.g., triathletes, basketball players) have shown that sweat losses of calcium induced by intensive exercise, especially in warm climates, can be sufficient to decrease bone mass, potentially leading to bone loss [51,52]. However, increasing calcium intake can offset these harmful effects. Studies indicate a synergistic effect between physical activity and calcium intake on bone health in children and adults [1]. According to a meta-analysis of 17 trials in peri- and postmenopausal women, physical activity is more beneficial in increasing bone mineral density in individuals consuming adequate calcium intakes (i.e., > 1000 mg/day) than in those with lower calcium intakes [53].

As reviewed below, low calcium intake increases the risk of osteoporosis. In addition, some other nutrients or dietary components can influence risk of osteoporosis by their effect on the body's need for calcium. A high intake of sodium increases urinary calcium excretion [10,45]. In postmenopausal women, each 500 mg of sodium consumed increases urinary calcium excretion by about 10 mg [10,45]. According to a study by Matkovic et al. [54], sodium intake was the main determinant of urinary calcium loss in adolescent girls aged 8 to 13 years, a finding leading the researchers to suggest a potential adverse effect on bone mass. In postmenopausal women, high urinary sodium excretion, which is a measure of sodium intake, was associated with increased bone loss from the hip and ankle [55]. However, findings from an ancillary study of the Dietary Approaches to Stop Hypertension (DASH) — Sodium trial led the researchers to conclude that the effects of sodium intake on bone health are unclear [56]. The adverse effects of sodium on bone health can be offset by adequate calcium intake [1]. High potassium intake may also prevent the sodium-induced increase in urinary calcium excretion and help ameliorate the adverse effects of a high sodium intake on bone resorption [57,58]. Race also influences sodium-induced urinary calcium excretion [59]. Wigertz et al. [59] reported that African American adolescent girls excreted significantly less calcium in their urine in response to increased dietary sodium than did white girls.

Excess dietary protein (particularly purified proteins) may increase urinary calcium excretion [10,60]. However, the concept that protein-induced calciuria reflects an acceleration of bone resorption which could lead to net calcium loss, and eventually osteoporosis, is challenged [60,61]. The increased calciuria observed in response to increased intake of either animal or vegetable protein can be explained by stimulation of intestinal calcium absorption [60,62]. The actual amount of calcium absorbed depends on calcium intake. Therefore, it is useful to evaluate diets not on their protein intake per se, but on their calcium-to-protein ratios. A "good" calcium-to-protein ratio, or one that provides adequate protection for the skeleton, is 20:1 (mg:g) or higher [63]. The calcium to protein ratio of cow's milk is approximately 36. Accumulating evidence indicates that a high protein intake has a beneficial effect on bone and may help to speed the recovery and decrease mortality after a hip fracture [60,61].

Whether or not vegetarians — people who do not eat meat, fish, or fowl, or products containing these foods — are at unique risk for osteoporosis depends on a variety of factors, including the composition of their diets and lifestyle factors that influence bone health, such as physical activity and smoking [64]. There is no single definition of "vegetarian," a term often used to describe a whole range of diets. An individual who is a strict vegetarian or vegan eats no meat, fish, poultry, eggs, dairy, or anything derived from animals [65]. A lacto-ovo-vegetarian includes dairy and eggs, whereas a lacto-vegetarian includes dairy in the diet, but excludes eggs. Within these vegetarian patterns, there is considerable variation in the extent to which animal products are excluded. Because the components of a "vegetarian" diet vary, there are wide differences in the nutrient content of these diets. For example, vitamin D intake may be limited in some vegan diets, whereas a low intake of this vitamin is less likely among lacto- or lacto-ovo-vegetarians who consume vitamin D-fortified milk [66]. Also, some vegetarians, such as vegans, may be at risk for calcium deficiency because of their low calcium intake and/or high consumption of food components such as oxalates (e.g., in plant foods, such as spinach, rhubarb, red beans) or phytates (e.g., in wheat bran) which reduce the bioavailability of calcium [65–69].

A review of observational, clinical, and intervention studies of the impact of "vegetarian" diets on bone health found no differences in bone health indices between lacto-ovo-vegetarians and omnivores [64]. However, the analysis found that low protein vegan diets were detrimental to bone. The author acknowledges that this area of research is very complex and recommends more study on the effect of a vegetarian diet on bone health [64].

5.4 CALCIUM, DAIRY PRODUCTS, AND BONE HEALTH

5.4.1 Dietary Recommendations and Consumption

In 1997, the Food and Nutrition Board of the Institute of Medicine (IOM) issued Dietary Reference Intakes for calcium and several other related nutrients important to bone health [10]. The calcium recommendations, expressed as AI, are shown in Table 5.1. These recommendations are for healthy people, not those with osteoporosis who may need additional calcium [1]. For children and most adults, the calcium recommendations are based on intakes consistent with desirable calcium retention, randomized clinical trials, and a factorial approach [10]. For children (9 through 13) and adolescents (14 through 18), 1300 mg/day of calcium is recommended [10] to coincide with peak calcium accretion rates in bone, which occur at a mean age of 12.5 years for girls and 14 years for boys [70]. For adults aged 19 through 50 years, 1000 mg of calcium/day is recommended, whereas for both men and women over age 50, 1200 mg of calcium/day is recommended [10]. An age-related decline in calcium absorption, among other factors, supports the higher calcium recommendations for this older age group [10].

Unfortunately, calcium intake in the United States and many other countries throughout the world falls short of meeting calcium recommendations [71–73]. A review of dietary calcium intake recommendations and intakes around the world revealed that young men are the only group among adolescents and adults that are likely to have adequate calcium intakes [72]. In the United States, data from NHANES 2001–2002 reveal that females (especially adolescents and older women) and older adults consume less calcium than recommended (Figure 5.2) [71]. At all ages, males consume more calcium than females, presumably because of males' higher energy intake [71]. Low intake of dairy foods, which are the major source of calcium in the diet [15], contributes to low calcium intake [71,74,75].

In young children ages 1 to 8 years, the prevalence of an inadequate calcium intake is low — with 96% of children 1 to 3 years and 69% of children 4 to 8 years having a calcium intake greater than the AI level of 800 mg per day [71]. The same holds true for males aged 19 to 30 years — among whom 53% have calcium intakes that exceed their AI of 1000 mg/day. Among children 9 to 13 years, only 6% of girls and 28% of boys have a calcium intake greater than their AI of 1300 mg/day [71]. The median calcium intake (50th percentile) for boys 9 to 13 years is 1086 mg/day,

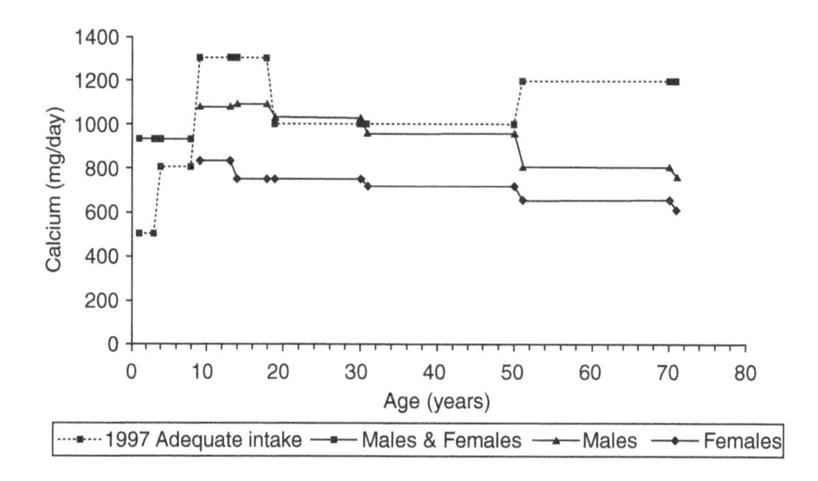

FIGURE 5.2 Median calcium intakes compared to recommended (adequate intake [AI]) levels. (From Moshfegh, A., Goldman, J., and Cleveland, L., *What We Eat in America, NHANES 2001–2002: Usual Nutrient Intakes Compared to Dietary Reference Intakes*, U.S. Department of Agriculture, Agricultural Research Service, 2005.)

whereas for similarly aged girls it is 837 mg/day [71]. Among boys and girls aged 14 to 18 years, 31% and 9%, respectively, have calcium intakes greater than the AI for this mineral [71]. Boys aged 14 to 18 years have a median calcium intake of 1094 mg/day, while girls of the same age have a median calcium intake of 735 mg/day [71]. It is estimated that nine out of ten girls aged 12 to 19 years and seven out of ten similar aged boys fail to consume recommended dietary intakes of calcium [73].

The AI of 1300 mg of calcium is equivalent to about 4 servings from the Milk Group (milk, cheese, or yogurt). On average, teenage boys are consuming only 2.4 servings a day from the Milk Group, while teenage girls are consuming 1.7 servings a day [75]. Low intake of dairy foods, which are the major dietary source of calcium, contributes to low calcium intake [15]. While possible, it is improbable that daily recommended dietary intakes of calcium will be met without including adequate amounts of dairy foods (i.e., at least 3 servings/day) in the diet [1,14,15].

Women are consuming more calcium than in past years, although their intake remains below recommended intake levels [71]. Median calcium intakes for women ages 19 to 30 and 31 to 50 are 755 and 722 mg/day, respectively — with 21% and 15%, respectively, consuming more than the AI for calcium [71]. The AI for calcium for adult women under age 50 is 1000 mg/day (an amount equivalent to 3 servings from the Milk Group) [10]. A survey conducted by the USDA found that, on average, women are consuming approximately 1.5 servings from the Milk Group each day [75].

Many older adults fail to meet their AI of 1200 mg/day of calcium — which is equivalent to about 4 servings from the Milk Group [71]. Calcium intakes continue to decline with advancing age. According to NHANES 2001 to 2002 nutrient intake data, among men ages 51 to 70 and 71+, half (50th percentile) consume less than 813 mg calcium/day and 771 mg of calcium/day, respectively. Only 16% and 12% of these age groups, respectively, consume more than the recommended amount of calcium [71]. Older women consume even less calcium than older men. Among women ages 51 to 70 and 71+, half (50th percentile) consume less than 661 and 613 mg of calcium per day, respectively. Only 5% and 4% of women at these ages, respectively, consume more than the recommended amount of calcium [71]. On average, both older men and women (ages 70 and over) consume little more than 1 serving from the Milk Group each day [75]. According to national consumption data, many older adults are not consuming the recommended amount of calcium needed to maintain bone health and minimize age-related bone loss.

The average American diet comes up short in servings from the Milk Group [75]. Overall, Americans (all individuals 2 years of age and over) are consuming an average of 1.7 servings each day from the Milk Group — about half of the 3 servings/day currently recommended [1,20,23,24,75]. African Americans consume 1.1 servings of dairy foods a day [76]. This is substantially lower than the National Medical Association's recommendation that African Americans consume 3 to 4 servings/day of low-fat milk, cheese, or yogurt [23].

Physiological and sociodemographic factors, as well as lifestyle choices, knowledge, and attitudes, influence intake of milk and milk products and as such, calcium intakes [16,77]. Among these factors are:

- *Taste*: Taste is an important factor influencing food choices and the decision to consume dairy products. People who enjoy the taste of dairy foods are likely to consume these foods more often and consequently have higher calcium intakes [78]. One study found that white girls were more likely to prefer the taste of milk than either Asian or Hispanic girls [79]. Also, white girls liked milk served cold, whereas Asian girls preferred milk warm and sweetened in combination with other beverages, such as milk [79]. Hispanic girls preferred milk in the form of shakes, puddings, and flan. A survey of 105 adolescent girls (mostly Asian Americans) found that liking the taste of milk and cheese was positively associated with calcium intakes [80]. Flavored milks are well-liked by children [18,81]. A study of elementary school children in Texas found that milk flavor (i.e., chocolate) was the most important factor influencing milk drinking [81]. Flavored milk has the potential to increase children's consumption of milk in school [18]. One study found that children who consumed flavored milk had higher calcium intakes but a similar percentage of energy from total and added sugars compared to children who did not drink flavored milk [18].

- *Availability of Soft Drinks and Other Beverages*: The availability of soft drinks and other beverages, such as fruit juices and/or fruit drinks, may be a barrier to AI of milk and calcium [24,82]. In 1945, Americans drank more than four times as much milk as carbonated soft drinks, whereas in 2001, they drank nearly 2.5 times more soft drinks than milk (Figure 5.3).
- *Fat and Weight Concerns*: Concern about body weight and the misperception that milk and other dairy foods are fattening may limit intake of dairy foods and dairy food nutrients such as calcium [24,83–85]. Frequent dieting has been associated with inadequate consumption of dairy products [84]. However, consumption of dairy foods improves the nutritional quality of the diet without significantly increasing total calories or fat intake, body weight, or percent body fat (see Chapter 1). Moreover, emerging scientific research indicates that consuming 3 servings of calcium-rich dairy foods (milk, cheese, yogurt) as part of a reduced calorie diet can increase weight and fat loss in overweight or obese adults (see Chapter 7) [44]. The *Dietary Guidelines for Americans* advises adults and children to not avoid milk and milk products because of concerns about weight gain [20]. The report of the Dietary Guidelines Advisory Committee on the 2005 *Dietary Guidelines for Americans* states that consuming 3 servings (equivalent to three cups) of milk and milk products each day "is not associated with increased body weight" [86]. The American Academy of Pediatrics [24] points out that "children, adolescents, and parents may not be aware that low-fat milk contains at least as much calcium as whole milk."
- *Lactose Maldigestion*: Some people who have lactose maldigestion or believe that they are lactose intolerant may restrict their dairy and calcium intake, thereby increasing their risk of osteoporosis and bone fractures [87–89]. A study in Finland involving more than 11,000 women linked self-reported lactose intolerance with both lower intakes of

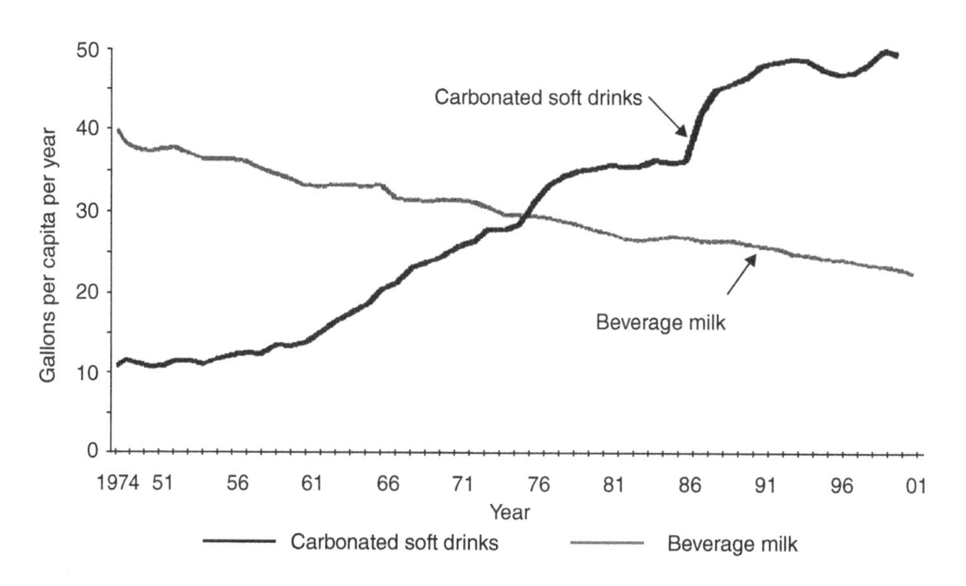

FIGURE 5.3 Trends in milk and carbonated soft drink consumption from 1945 to 2001. (From Weaver, C. M. and Heaney, R. P., In *Calcium in Human Health,* Humana Press, Totowa, NJ, p. 133, 2006.)

calcium from dairy foods (570 vs. 850 mg/day) and increased risk of fractures [89]. Low calcium intake from food sources was identified in a group of Canadian adults who said that they were lactose intolerant [88]. Research indicates that many individuals who are lactose maldigesters can consume dairy products, such as 1 or 2 cups of milk, especially in divided doses with meals, aged cheeses, and yogurt with active cultures, without developing symptoms (see Chapter 8) [90–92]. The 2005 *Dietary Guidelines for Americans* recommends dairy products, such as the above, as the primary strategy for individuals who are lactose intolerant [20]. A review of lactose intolerance in African Americans led to the conclusion that "African Americans, like other Americans, should not avoid consumption of dairy products due to concerns about lactose intolerance" [92].

- *Awareness and Knowledge*: Lack of awareness of the protective effect of calcium on bone health may contribute to low calcium intakes [93,94]. In a study involving 472 women aged 50 years and over, those who knew that calcium protects bone health consumed more calcium than women who were unaware of this association [93]. Similar findings were observed in an investigation involving 1117 adolescents in Rhode Island [94]. In this study, adolescents who were knowledgeable about their recommended intake of calcium, the beneficial effect of calcium on bone health, and the importance of adolescence as a time to build bone mass consumed more calcium than adolescents who were unaware of these facts [94]. Overall, only 10% of the adolescents knew the calcium content of various dairy foods and only 19% knew how many servings of dairy foods a day they should consume [94]. In a review of how family and social factors influence children's eating patterns, the authors report that adolescents whose parents were relatively more educated had higher intakes of calcium and were more likely to consume recommended daily servings of dairy foods [95].
- *Parental Influence*: Parents, through role modeling, expectations, and attitudes, can influence young children's intake of calcium and dairy products [96–98]. When intakes of milk, soft drinks, and calcium were examined in 180 pairs of mothers and their 5-year-old daughters over a 3 month period, researchers found that mothers who drank milk more frequently tended to have daughters who drank milk more often and who consumed fewer soft drinks [97]. These findings suggest that a mother's own beverage choices influence their young daughters' apparent trade-off between milk and soft drinks. For both mothers and daughters, consumption of soft drinks was linked to low intakes of milk and calcium [97]. In a study examining predictors of milk intake in children ages 5 to 17, the amount and type of milk consumed by mothers strongly predicted the amount and type of milk consumed by their school-aged children [96]. An investigation of 192 girls, followed from ages 5 to 9 years, and their mothers found that, at age 9, the girls who consumed recommended dietary intakes of calcium drank twice the amount of milk, had slightly higher bone mineral density, and had mothers who drank and served milk more frequently than girls with low calcium intakes [98]. The girls who consumed the recommended amounts of calcium also drank 18% less sweetened beverages than girls with low calcium intakes. In addition to mothers, others such as fathers, siblings, and peers, can influence children's milk and calcium intakes [80]. As stated by the American Academy of Pediatrics [24], "because of the influence of the family's diet on the diet of children and adolescents, adequate calcium intake by all members of the family is important."
- *Eating Away from Home*: Where food is consumed — at home, school, or at restaurants and fast food establishments — can influence intake of milk and milk products. Participating in school meal programs such as the National School Lunch Program and School Breakfast Program improves children's intake of dairy foods (milk, cheese) and dairy food nutrients such as calcium and vitamin D, both at these meals and over 24 hours [77,99]. A School Milk Pilot Test involving more than 100,000 students in 146 elementary and secondary schools found that a combination

of enhancements to school milk (i.e., upgrades in milk packaging to plastic containers, flavor variety, merchandising) increased students' milk intake and their participation in the National School Lunch Program [100]. Frequently eating at restaurants or fast food establishments may compromise intake of dairy foods and dairy food nutrients [77,101]. A study of more than 4700 adolescents in grades 7 through 12 found that eating at fast food restaurants was associated with a lower intake of milk, as well as other nutritious foods [101]. Adolescents participating in a focus group reported that they rarely order milk when eating out at fast food establishments because milk is unavailable, not promoted, or not as visible as other beverage options such as soft drinks [84].
- *Other*: Additional factors such as family meals [102,103] and eating breakfast [104,105] influence intake of calcium and dairy products. A survey of more than 16,000 children aged 9 to 14 found that children who frequently ate dinner with their family had substantially higher intakes of calcium and several other nutrients [102]. Greater frequency of family meals was associated with a higher intake of calcium-rich foods and lower consumption of soft drinks in a study of more than 4700 middle and high school students [103]. Studies also show that breakfast consumption improves children's calcium intake [104,105].

5.4.2 Prevention of Osteoporosis

There is general agreement that optimizing peak bone mass and reducing age-related bone loss later in life, especially after menopause, protects the skeleton and reduces fracture risk [1,2,5,6,10,45]. High calcium intake, especially from dairy foods, along with adequate vitamin D status, has been demonstrated to maximize genetically determined peak bone mass, which for most of the skeleton, is reached by age 30 or earlier; to maintain skeletal mass in adulthood; and to slow age-related bone loss and/or reduce fracture risk in later adult years [1,7–9]. In an analysis of 139 scientific papers published between 1975 and 2000, 50 out of 52 controlled calcium intervention studies showed a better bone balance, reduced bone loss, or decreased fracture risk at high calcium intakes [7]. In an updated analysis of 180 papers, a positive relationship between calcium intake and bone health was supported in 68 out of 70 intervention studies [8]. The majority (75% or more) of observational studies showed a positive association between calcium, dairy foods, and bone health [7,8], and all intervention studies that used dairy foods showed a beneficial effect on bone health [7].

Evidence supporting a protective role for calcium against osteoporosis led the U.S. Food and Drug Administration (FDA), in response to provisions of the Nutrition Labeling and Education Act of 1990, to authorize the use of health claims related to an association between calcium intake and osteoporosis on food labels [106]. The FDA concluded that a lifetime of "adequate calcium intake is important for maintenance of bone health and may help reduce the risk of osteoporosis particularly for individuals at greatest risk" [106]. To carry a health claim, a food must contain no more than 20% of the Daily Value (DV) of fat (13 g), saturated fat (4 g), cholesterol (60 mg), and sodium (480 mg). Therefore, nonfat, 1% low-fat, and 2% reduced fat milk and milk products (e.g., low-fat and nonfat yogurt) qualify for calcium-osteoporosis health claims [106].

Reviewed below are studies indicating that consuming an AI of dairy food nutrients and dairy foods, from periods of skeletal accumulation to maturity and beyond, protects against osteoporosis. Although the bulk of evidence supports calcium's or dairy food's beneficial effect on bone, some studies fail to support this finding. As reviewed by Heaney [45], reasons for such inconsistencies include the following:

- *The multifactorial nature of bone strength*: As mentioned previously, many factors (e.g., hormonal status, physical activity, smoking, medications) in addition to calcium intake influence bone health. Manipulating a single variable such as calcium may be ineffective if calcium is not the limiting factor [107]. For example, a high calcium intake alone cannot protect against bone loss caused by estrogen deficiency or physical inactivity [45].

- *The multifactorial nature of calcium deficiency*: In addition to calcium intake, calcium absorption and excretion also contribute to calcium status [107]. In general, fractional absorption of calcium is about 30%, although it varies with intake [107]. Some individuals may need to consume higher amounts of calcium because of their low absorption of it [45]. Dietary and nondietary factors influence calcium absorption and excretion and thus, the need for this nutrient [45,107]. The decline in calcium absorption associated with aging may be explained in part by low body stores of vitamin D, which help the body absorb calcium [10].
- *The menopausal effect*: In the early postmenopausal years, bone loss is specifically related to the cessation of estrogen production [1,10,39,45,107]. Calcium intake has a greater influence on bone mass after the first 5 years of the onset of menopause.
- *The threshold effect of calcium*: Several studies indicate threshold or saturation points above which there are no additional or limited benefits of calcium on bone (Figure 5.4) [8,27,107–110]. That is, individuals with an adequate calcium intake cannot be expected to derive further bone-preserving benefit from additional calcium intake. The nutritional response in terms of calcium balance or bone mass will occur at intakes below the threshold, but not above. For example, in a 2½ year randomized, controlled study in prepubertal children in New Zealand, the failure of increased calcium intake (i.e., calcium-enriched cocoa flavored dairy product) to increase bone mineral density or content was attributed to the children's high habitual dietary calcium [109]. Estimates of calcium threshold values for Caucasians are: 1350 to 1550 mg/day for adolescents; 800 to 1200 mg/day for mature adults; and 1400 to 1700 mg/day for older adults [8]. Because African Americans absorb calcium more efficiently than Caucasians during growth and retain it more efficiently at all ages, their calcium threshold for bone health may be about 400 to 600 mg/day lower [8].
- *Heterogeneity of the calcium response*: Skeletal sites differ in their degree of response to dietary calcium [107].
- *Duration of the study*: Because of the nature of bone remodeling, a period of at least 2 years and preferably longer is necessary to establish a positive effect of calcium on bone density [111–113].

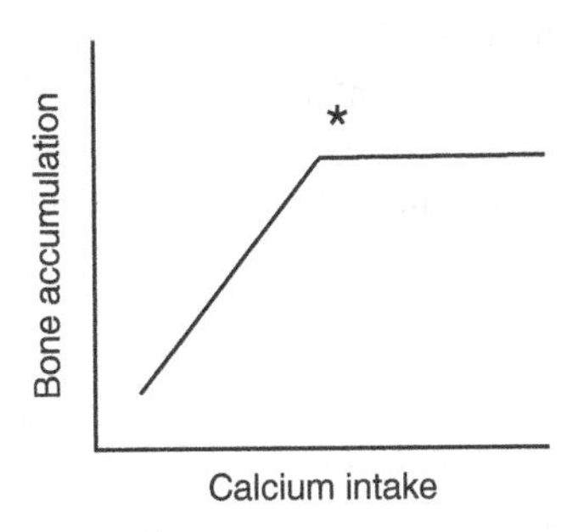

FIGURE 5.4 Threshold behavior of calcium intake. Theoretical relationship of bone accumulation to intake. Below a certain value (the threshold, indicated by an asterisk), bone accumulation is a linear function of intake (the ascending line); in other words, the amount of bone that can be accumulated is limited by the amount of calcium ingested. Above the threshold (the horizontal line), bone accumulation is limited by other factors and is no longer related to changes in calcium intake. (From Heaney, R. P., In *Calcium in Human Health,* Humana Press, Totowa, NJ, p. 9, 2006.)

- *Difficulties in accurately determining calcium intake and measuring bone mass*: The weakness of existing tools to accurately estimate calcium intake (e.g., food frequency questionnaires, 24-hour dietary recall) may contribute to a negative or inconsistent association between calcium intake and bone health. In many epidemiological studies, particularly observational studies, dietary calcium intake may be under- or overestimated [114,115]. Errors in food frequency questionnaires or dietary recalls, portion size estimations, and variability in the nutrient content of particular foods all contribute to inaccuracies in estimating actual calcium intake [115]. In addition, the bioavailability of calcium influences how much of a given nutrient is effectively used [115]. Calcium balance studies with or without isotopes are used to estimate calcium needs and to provide information on changes in calcium metabolism (e.g., urinary output, absorption). Direct measurements of bone mass indicate net retention of calcium over a long period. The advantage of the maximum calcium retention approach is that systematic errors of the balance method do not influence the ability to define the threshold value. A number of different noninvasive methods such as single and dual energy x-ray absorptiometry (DXA), peripheral dual energy absorptiometry, radiographic absorptiometry, quantitative computed tomography, and ultrasound are available to determine bone mass or density safely, conveniently, accurately, and at a relatively low cost [1,10]. Measurement of bone mineral density can detect osteoporosis before a fracture occurs, predict an individual's risk of fracture, and monitor the effectiveness of osteoporosis treatment.

5.4.2.1 Childhood and Adolescence

Childhood and adolescence are critical times to begin building optimal bone mass. Bone mass is important to future risk of osteoporosis. For this reason, a logical attempt to reduce the prevalence of this disease later in life is to optimize bone accretion during childhood and adolescence [1,7,10,24,28,116–118]. Consuming an adequate intake (AI) of calcium during childhood, and particularly during adolescence, is important for the development of peak bone mass, which may help reduce the risk of fractures in childhood and adolescence and the risk of osteoporosis in later years [1,3,5,6,10,24,119]. Although osteoporosis is typically a disease occurring in older adults, its prevention begins in childhood and adolescence by maximizing calcium retention and bone mass in the growing years [120].

Dietary calcium recommendations are 800 mg/day for children aged 4 to 8 years and 1300 mg/day for those aged 9 through 18 years [10]. For most children (under 8 years) and adolescents in the United States, calcium intakes are below these recommended levels [24,71]. The proportion of children achieving an AI of calcium is at its lowest point between the ages of 12 and 19 years, when accumulation of bone mineral is at its peak and the calcium requirement is highest [24].

Numerous studies indicate that increasing calcium or dairy food intake during childhood and adolescence benefits bone health at one or more skeletal sites [1,7,8,108,119,121–124]. According to a review of controlled trials of calcium's role in bone health during childhood, increases in bone mineral density associated with higher calcium intakes among children occurred primarily in cortical bone sites; spine bone mineral density increased more in pubertal than prepubertal children; and a bone health benefit was found mostly among populations with low calcium intakes [124].

Several studies demonstrate the benefits on young children's bone health from increased calcium intake. In a study at Indiana University involving 22 pairs of twins averaging 7 years of age, bone mass accumulation was 3% to 5% higher among children who consumed 1600 mg calcium a day than those who had an intake of 900 mg a day (Figure 5.5) [122]. In this 3-year, double-blind, placebo-controlled study of the effect of increased calcium intake, one twin served as the control for the other. The findings of this study led the researchers to suggest that increasing calcium intake of prepubertal children may reduce the risk of osteoporotic fractures later in life [122]. According to a placebo-controlled, double-blind study involving 149, 8-year old Caucasian females, increasing calcium intake from approximately 900 to 1750 mg per day for 1 year increased bone mineral density in the arm and hip, and, to a lesser degree, the spine [108]. This increase in bone mass in response to increased calcium intake was markedly dependent upon habitual calcium intake. There was a 3.5-fold (2.1% vs. 0.6% per year) greater benefit for below average calcium consumers (< 850 mg/day) than for above average calcium consumers [108]. This latter finding is explained by the fact that, at high calcium intakes, a larger fraction of the treated subjects will be replete, and therefore will not show any additional benefit from added calcium.

A 5 year prospective study of 192 non-Hispanic white girls, followed from ages 5 to 9, found that girls who met calcium intake recommendations had slightly higher bone mineral densities than girls who had inadequate calcium intakes [98]. Interestingly, girls who met calcium recommendations consumed almost twice the amount of milk daily and 18% less sweetened beverages than girls who did not meet calcium recommendations. Calcium intake showed moderate tracking from 5 to 9 years [98]. In a 6 year prospective study of 151 non-Hispanic white girls followed from ages 5 to 11, higher calcium intakes (provided mainly from dairy products) at ages 7 and 9 years were positively associated with total body bone mineral content at age 11 [125]. In a longitudinal study of young children aged 2 to 8 years, multiple nutrients (energy, calcium, phosphorus, protein, magnesium, and zinc) showed a positive and significant correlation with bone mineral content [126]. This finding led the researchers to suggest that children should consume a variety of nutrient-rich foods to protect their bone health [126].

Although bone mass may accumulate through the third decade of life, peak adult bone density may be reached as early as late adolescence in certain bones (proximal femur and vertebrae) [10,116]. Lu et al. [127] found that bone mineral density of the total body, lumbar spine, and femoral neck increased significantly until 17.5 years in males and 15.8 years in females. Meeting calcium needs is particularly important during adolescence [24]. Peak calcium accretion rate occurs at about age 12.5 years for girls and 14.0 years for boys [24,70]. During the few years of peak

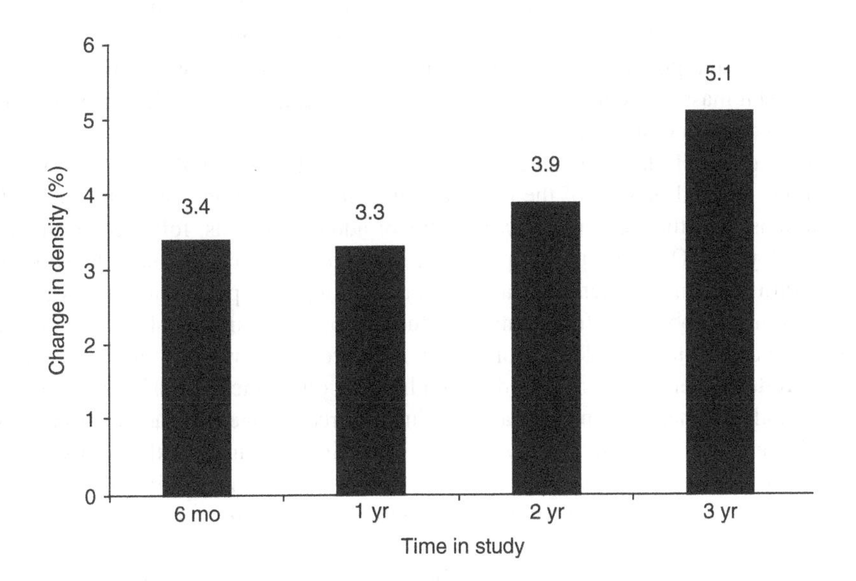

FIGURE 5.5 Mean differences within prepubertal twin pairs in the bone mineral density of the midshaft radius. (From Johnston, C. C., Jr. et al., *N. Engl. J. Med.*, 327, 82, 1992. With permission.)

skeletal growth, about 40% of adult bone mass is accrued [24,116]. The requirement for calcium is the highest during this pubertal growth spurt [10,116].

Increasing dietary calcium to at least 1300 mg/day, and even higher, has a positive effect on bone health in adolescents [98,121,128–134]. According to an 18-month, double-blind, placebo-controlled trial in Pennsylvania, involving 94 healthy Caucasian 12-year-old girls, increasing calcium intake from 935 mg/day to 1370 mg/day significantly increased total and spine bone mineral density [128]. Increasing calcium intake by the amount of calcium (i.e., 300 mg) in a one cup of milk or yogurt, or 1.5 ounces of hard cheese, increased skeletal mass between 1 and 3% [128]. Jackman et al. [129] found that adolescent females aged 12 to 15 years needed to consume at least 1300 mg calcium per day to maximize body calcium retention. This study of 35 girls found that a calcium intake of 1200 mg/day resulted in only 57% of maximum calcium retention [129]. An Australian study involving 42 pairs of 17-year-old twins, found that increasing calcium intake from about 800 mg a day to more than 1600 mg a day for 18 months increased spinal and hip bone mineral densities [130]. In the twins who consumed the additional calcium (i.e., 1000 mg/day), bone density increased by 1.3% at the hip and 1.5% at the spine [130]. In a more recent investigation of 51 pairs of premenarcheal female twins aged 8 to 13 years in Australia, increased calcium intake (1631 mg/day) resulted in a higher total body bone mineral content of 3.7% over 2 years, compared with that in the controls (718 mg calcium/day) [131]. A 1-year, double-blind, placebo-controlled calcium intervention study (1000 mg calcium carbonate/day) in 100 postmenarcheal girls with habitual low calcium intakes (<800 mg/day), found that calcium supplementation (1000 mg/day) enhanced bone mineral acquisition, especially in girls who were more than 2 years past the onset of menarche [134]. Calcium supplementation significantly reduced bone turnover and decreased serum parathyroid hormone levels [134].

In the only calcium supplement trial that spanned puberty — bone modeling (change in size and geometry) during the pubertal growth spurt and of bone consolidation during late adolescence — Matkovic et al. [133] found the benefits of calcium on bone were greater during the pubertal growth spurt than during bone consolidation. This 4-year, randomized, clinical trial evaluated the long-term effects of calcium accretion among 354 females from childhood to adolescence. The study was then extended for 3 years into late adolescence. The girls were randomly assigned to maintain their usual dietary intake of calcium (~830 mg/day over the 7 year period) or to receive a calcium supplement (670 mg/day) for a total calcium intake of about 1500 mg/day [133]. The results showed that calcium supplementation significantly increased total body and proximal radius bone density during the pubertal growth spurt (ages 8 to 13) – during which time ~37% of the entire adult skeletal mass is accumulated — but thereafter, a diminishing effect due to the catch-up phenomenon in bone mineral accretion [133].

Matkovic et al. [132] also evaluated the long-term effect of supplemental calcium and dairy products on bone mineral density of the hip and spine, and on the bone geometry and volumetric bone mineral density of the forearm, in two groups of adolescent girls, followed from an average age of 15 to 18 years. One group was part of a randomized, double-blind, placebo-controlled clinical trial with calcium supplements, and the other group was part of an observational study in which calcium was obtained from dairy products. Both calcium supplementation and dairy products increased bone mineral density of the hip and forearm. However, unlike calcium supplements, dairy products were also associated with a higher bone mineral density of the spine [132]. These findings indicate that calcium and dairy products increase bone mass acquisition, leading to a higher peak bone mass. Calcium influences bone accretion during growth mainly by affecting volumetric bone density, whereas dairy products may have an additional impact on bone growth and expansion, possibly due to their content of calcium, protein, and other bone-essential nutrients.

Increasing calcium intake for short periods has been shown to increase bone mineralization in children and adolescents. But whether or not there is a long-term benefit in attaining and maintaining maximum peak bone mass after the calcium intervention is stopped, has yet to be conclusively demonstrated [1,24,117]. Several follow-up investigations have indicated that the effects of calcium on gain in bone mineral density are maintained (i.e., from one to 7.5 years, depending on the study) after the calcium intervention is discontinued [108,135–139]. In other studies, no sustained effect has been observed [112,113,140,141]. Bonjour et al. [135] reported that the increase in bone mineralization in prepubertal girls (average age of eight) who received a milk-based calcium supplement for 1 year was maintained for 3.5 years after the supplement was discontinued. However, a follow-up study of the same cohort at a mean age of 16.4 years (7.5 years after discontinuation of the calcium supplement), found that the calcium supplement's lasting effect on bone mineral accrual was influenced by the timing of menarche [138]. A persistent, significant benefit of the calcium supplement on bone accrual was seen in the girls whose age at menarche was below, but not above, the median menarcheal age (13.0 years) [138]. It appears that several factors, such as the timing of pubertal maturation, source of calcium (food or supplement), and habitual calcium intake, may influence the lasting response to calcium supplementation. Because it is unknown whether a short-term increase in calcium results in a long-term benefit on bone health, it is important that dietary practices that promote adequate calcium intake throughout life be established in childhood [24].

Some studies demonstrate that increasing calcium intake enhances the positive effects of weight-bearing exercise on bone mineral status during growth [142–145]. A significant benefit to leg bone mineral content from combining calcium supplementation with physical activity was reported in 4-year old children [142]. Likewise, calcium supplementation increased the effect of physical exercise on bone mineral acquisition in healthy premenarcheal girls [143]. Both increased calcium intake (1000 mg/day) and regular exercise (3, 45-min classes/week) improved bone mineral status at several sites during late adolescence, according to a 15.5 month study in more than 130 older adolescents aged 16 to 18 [144]. A synergistic effect of habitual vigorous exercise and calcium intake on bone mass (but not total activity and calcium intake) was found in a study of 76 children aged 8 to 11 years in the United Kingdom [145]. A recent review of studies examining the effect of calcium and exercise on the growing skeleton led the authors to conclude that impact exercise can enhance skeletal growth and a calcium intake of at least 1300 mg/day during pubertal growth results in optimal calcium retention, but the combined effects of these interventions are unclear [146]. Based on their review, Welch and Weaver [146] conclude that "the best strategy for strong bones by the end of childhood may be either high-impact exercise with a moderate or adequate calcium intake, or a combination of moderate-impact exercise and adequate calcium during growth." The American Academy of Pediatrics [24] calls for additional research to determine the combined effects of calcium and exercise on bone mass during childhood and adolescence.

Several studies indicate that intake of milk and other dairy foods during childhood and adolescence is an important determinant of bone health [9,121,147–153]. In a classic study by Matkovic et al. [147], a comparison of two rural communities in Yugoslavia, which differed in their milk and dairy food consumption (and therefore calcium intake), identified a higher peak bone mass in residents of the community with a high milk intake than in those with a low milk intake [147]. Calcium intake of one area (950 mg/day) was more than twice that of the other area (450 mg/day). The greater bone mass and bone density reached by age 35 in residents of the high calcium district was maintained throughout life and was attributed to their larger bone mass formed in childhood (Figure 5.6). Of most importance, the incidence of hip fractures was lower among subjects in the high calcium district than in subjects in the low calcium district (Figure 5.7) [147].

Chan et al. [121] reported that, in a controlled study in Utah, involving 48 pubertal girls (9 to 13 years), increasing calcium intake from 728 to 1437 mg/day with dairy foods for a year, significantly increased total and spinal bone mineral density (Figure 5.8). The additional intake of dairy foods increased the girls' intake of calcium, phosphorus, vitamin D, and protein, but not their intake of total or saturated fat [121]. Body weight and fatness were similar between the dairy group and the controls [121]. Similar findings are reported by Cadogan et al. [148], who found bone mineral

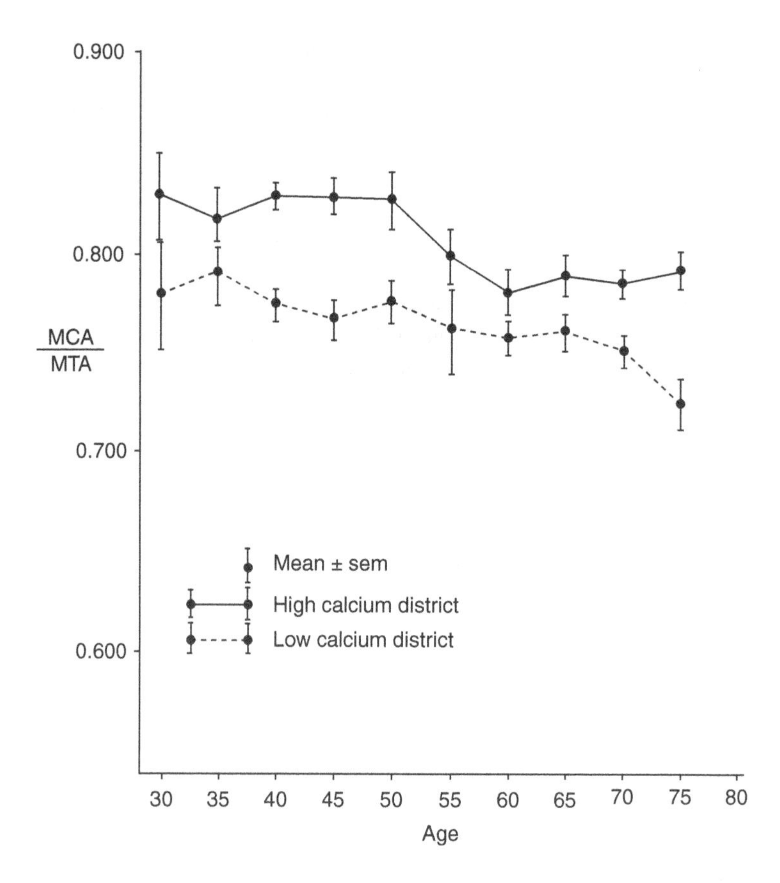

FIGURE 5.6 Bone density (MCA/MTA = metacarpal cortical/total area ratio of subjects accustomed to different calcium intakes over lifetime). (From Matkovic, V. et al., *Am. J. Clin. Nutr.*, 32, 540, 1979. With permission.)

content and bone mineral density were significantly increased in 80 girls aged 12 years, who consumed additional calcium in the form of whole or low-fat milk (i.e., 2 extra cups) for 18 months. Mean calcium in the milk group was 1125 mg per day compared with the baseline calcium intake of 746 mg per day [148]. Compared to the control group, the girls who increased milk intake gained an additional 37 g of bone mineral. No significant differences in height gain, weight gain, lean body mass, or fat mass were evident between the groups [148]. Girls in the milk group significantly increased their protein, phosphorus, magnesium, zinc, riboflavin, and thiamin intakes [148].

Volek et al. [149] found that increasing milk intake favorably affected bone mineral density responses to resistance training in adolescent boys. In this clinical trial, 28 boys between 13 and 17 years of age were randomly assigned to consume either 3 servings of 1% fluid milk/day or unfortified juice in addition to their usual diet while participating in a 12-week resistance training program. The main finding was that the increase in bone mineral density was twice as great in boys who drank 3 servings of milk/day than in those who drank juice [149]. Moreover, significant increases in whole body bone mineral density were seen as early as 6 weeks into the study. The researchers suggest that the enhanced positive impact on bone mineral density is due to the calcium and other nutrients in milk, together with the resistance training [149].

A 2-year, placebo-controlled intervention trial in Finland found that increasing calcium intake by consuming cheese appears to be more beneficial than consuming a similar amount of calcium from calcium supplements in bone mass accrual in girls aged 10 to 12 years [150]. A group of 195

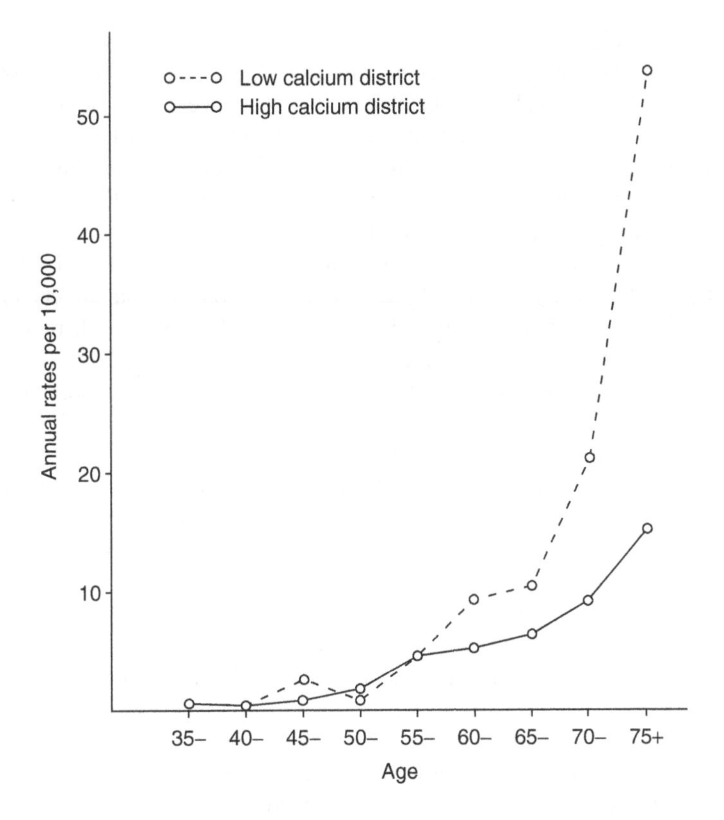

FIGURE 5.7 Annual hip fracture rates of subjects accustomed to different calcium intake over lifetime. (From Matkovic, V. et al., *Am. J. Clin. Nutr.*, 32, 540, 1979. With permission.)

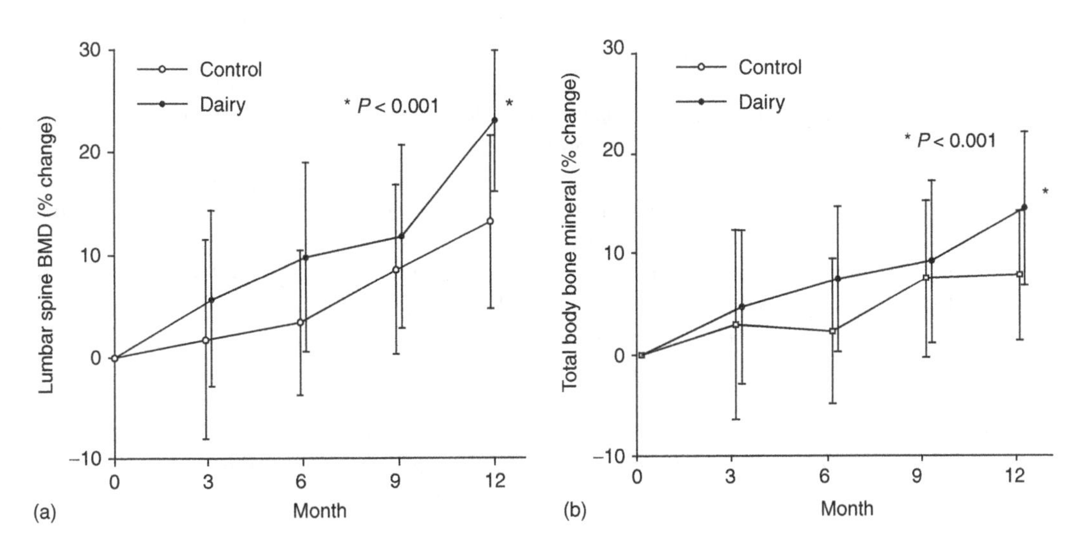

FIGURE 5.8 (a) Lumbar spine bone density change in the two groups. The dairy group had a higher percentage of change than the control groups. Means and standard deviations are presented. (b) Total body bone mineral change in the two groups. The dairy group had a higher percentage of change than the control group. Means and standard deviations are shown. (From Chan, G. M. et al., *J. Pediatr.*, 126, 551, 1995. With permission.)

healthy girls with habitual calcium intakes of <900 mg/day were randomly assigned to one of the following four groups: 1000 mg calcium tablets plus 200 IU of vitamin D a day; 1000 mg calcium tablets a day; cheese (1000 mg calcium); or placebo tablets. Cheese was the most beneficial treatment for bone growth, especially with regard to cortical thickness of the long bones (leg bone) and the secondary mineralization phase of bone growth. The researchers suggest that the possible bone benefits of cheese and habitual high calcium intake from foods may be the result of better absorption of calcium from dairy products, distribution of calcium intake throughout the day, and higher intakes of protein, magnesium, and other nutrients supplied by dairy products [150]. After adjusting for differences in growth velocity among subjects, there were no beneficial effects on bone with any of the treatments. The researchers speculate that the large effect of growth may have masked a smaller effect of diet in this modestly sized cohort [150].

Several studies in Asian children support a beneficial effect of milk on bone health [151–154]. A cross-sectional study of 649 girls aged 12 to 14 years in the area of Beijing, found that milk consumption was associated with a significantly greater bone mineral density in three out of four forearm sites measured [151]. After accounting for factors affecting bone mineral density, milk was the only food group with a significant positive effect on bone mineral density. The researchers attribute the positive effects of milk consumption on bone health to the integration of several nutrients, particularly calcium, vitamin D, and protein [151]. In a 2-year, school milk intervention trial involving 757 Chinese girls aged 10 to 12 years in Beijing, increased intake of milk, with or without added vitamin D, significantly increased total body bone mineral content (1.2%) and bone mineral density (3.2%) [152]. Significantly greater increases in change in total body bone mineral content (2.4% vs. 1.2%) and bone mineral density (5.5% vs. 3.2%) were found in the girls consuming milk with added vitamin D than milk without added vitamin D. A subsequent study of this population demonstrated that the milk supplementation positively affected periosteal apposition and cortical bone accretion, which, if maintained, could increase bone strength [154]. Lau et al. [153] reported that milk powder supplements increased bone accretion in a study of 344 children aged nine to 10 years in Hong Kong. The children were randomly chosen to receive a milk powder equivalent to 1300 mg of calcium, 650 mg of calcium, or to a control group. After 18 months, children who received the milk powder equivalent to 1300 mg of calcium had a significantly greater increase in bone mineral density at both the total hip and spine than did the control group [153]. Children receiving the lower amount of milk and calcium (half the amount of the high group) experienced significantly greater increases in bone mineral density of the total body than did the control group, with smaller increases in bone mineral density at the hip and spine [153].

Children who avoid milk products for a prolonged period of time are at potential risk of low bone mineral content and density and increased risk of fractures [155–161]. Risk of inadequate bone mass accrual has been shown to increase in children who avoid milk because of specific conditions such as cow's milk allergy or short-bowel syndrome [155,157].

In a study in New Zealand, Goulding et al. [162] found that bone density was 3% to 5% lower at different skeletal sites in girls aged three to 15 years who had a recent forearm fracture, compared to those who had never broken a bone. A similar finding was observed in a cohort of boys aged 3 to 19 years [158]. When the researchers evaluated dietary calcium intakes and bone health in 50 milk avoiders aged 3 to 10 years and 200 milk-drinking control children from the same community, they found the children who avoided milk had poor bone health, short stature, and high adiposity compared to the controls [156]. The milk avoiders had smaller bones, a significantly lower total body bone area and bone mineral content, and lower bone mineral density scores at the hip, spine, and arm when compared to the children in the control group [156]. In a subsequent study, Goulding et al. [159] compared the frequency of bone fractures in 50 milk avoiding children with a birth cohort of more than 1000 children from the same city in New Zealand. More of the children who avoided milk reported fractures (16 observed vs. 6 expected) and experienced more total fractures (22 observed vs. 8 expected) when compared with the birth cohort (Table 5.3) [159]. All of the fractures occurred before 7 years of age and the majority (82%) of them were the result of minor

TABLE 5.3
Number of Fractures Observed in Children Who Avoid Cow's Milk Compared with Total Fractures Expected from Community Data

Age (y)	Time Exposed (y)	Observed Fractures (*n*)	Expected Fractures (*n*)	Fracture Rate per 1000 Person Years in Community
0–2.9	150	9	1.97	13.1
3–4.9	96.1	5	2.08	21.7
5–6.9	83.4	4	1.99	23.8
7–8.9	44	4	1.15	26.0
9–10.9	16.2	0	0.80	49.3
11–13	6.3	0	0.45	72.4
0–13	396.0	22	8.44	

Source: From Goulding, A. et al, *J. Am. Diet. Assoc.*, 104, 250, 2004. Goodness of fit $X^2 = 33.57$, $P < 0.001$, degrees of freedom = 5.

trips and falls. The researchers state that "this study is the first to demonstrate that young children who avoid milk sustain more fractures than community controls of similar age and sex" [159].

An investigation of 90 New Zealand children and adolescents aged 5 to 19 years with repeated forearm fractures, demonstrated that this group had lower bone mineral content and weighed more — two factors that increase fracture risk — than fracture-free children of the same age and gender [160]. Children and adolescents with multiple forearm fractures were also more likely than those who were fracture-free to have a fracture at an earlier age, to have a history of symptoms related to milk intake, and to have a low dietary calcium intake [160]. A longitudinal study of young children, with an average age of 8 years and a history of avoiding cow's milk, demonstrated persisting height reduction, overweight, and low bone mineral content at the ultradistal radius (forearm) and lumbar spine over 2 years of follow-up, despite modest increases in milk consumption and calcium intake from all sources [161].

Several retrospective studies link increased milk intake during early years with greater bone density in adulthood [119,163–169]. A retrospective study among middle-aged and elderly women found that bone mineral density in the hip and spine was significantly higher in women who reported drinking one or more servings of milk a day up to age 25 [164]. Soroko et al. [165] reported that milk intake during adolescence was positively associated with increased bone mineral density at the spine and midradius in postmenopausal women. The findings of a beneficial effect of milk intake in early life on bone health in later years in these two studies were independent of other factors such as age, body mass, smoking, and physical activity [164,165]. New et al. [166] reported higher spine and hip bone mineral densities in premenopausal women who consumed more than 2.5 cups of milk per day during their childhood and early teenage years than in those who reported low milk intakes (1 cup or less per day). An earlier study found that a calcium intake of 1600 mg/day during adolescence was associated with increased hip bone density in women aged 30 to 39 years [163].

According to data from more than 3200 white women aged 20 years and older surveyed in NHANES III, reported frequency of milk intake during both childhood and adolescence was significantly associated with increased bone mineral content and bone mineral density of the hip in those aged less than 50 years [168]. Among women 50 years and older, those with low milk intakes during childhood had a twofold greater risk of osteoporotic fractures than women with high milk intake during childhood [168]. Wang et al. [169], using data from 161 African American and 180 white females aged 21 to 24 years, found that an intake of at least 1000 mg of calcium a day during midpuberty (age 12) was associated with higher bone mass during young adulthood. Moreover, calcium intake during midpuberty was more strongly associated with bone mass during young adulthood than was calcium intake during early puberty or late puberty [169]. Teegarden et al. [167], based on a study of 224 young women aged 18 to 31 years, reported that drinking more milk during adolescence was associated with not only increased total body and radius bone mineral density, but also increased likelihood of a high milk intake in young adulthood. Childhood and adolescent milk intakes were positively correlated, and childhood and adolescent milk intakes were correlated with current calcium intakes [167]. The findings of this study led the researchers to suggest that early establishment of milk drinking behaviour may contribute to a similar habit of milk drinking in later years.

Health professional organizations and government agencies, such as the American Academy of Pediatrics [24], the American Dietetic Association (ADA) [170], and the U.S. Surgeon General [1], recognize the importance of calcium and calcium-rich foods such as milk, cheese, and yogurt for children's and adolescents' bone health. The 2005 *Dietary Guidelines for Americans* [20] states that "the consumption of milk products is especially important for children and adolescents who are building their peak bone mass and developing lifelong habits." In a position statement on dietary guidance for healthy children, the ADA recognizes that children's "failure to meet calcium requirements in combination with a sedentary lifestyle in childhood can impede the achievement of maximal skeletal growth and bone mineralization, thereby increasing the diet-related risk of developing osteoporosis later in life" [170]. The position statement identifies the decline in milk consumption and the increase in carbonated soft drinks among children as a health concern, especially because milk drinking habits in childhood can affect lifetime milk consumption. The American Academy of Pediatrics, in a position statement on soft drinks in schools, urges pediatricians and others to work to eliminate soft drinks from schools and to recommend healthful alternatives such as low-fat white or flavored milk [171]. The statement recognizes that a high intake of sweetened beverages may displace milk from the diet, resulting in calcium deficiency and increased risk of osteoporosis and fractures. In its report on optimizing bone health and calcium intakes of infants, children, and adolescents, the American Academy of Pediatrics [24] states that "drinking three 8-ounce glasses of milk per day (or the equivalent ...) will achieve the recommended AI of calcium in children 4 to 8 years of age, and four 8- to 10-ounces of milk (or the equivalent) will provide the adequate calcium intake for adolescents. Yogurt and cheese are also good sources of calcium. Flavored milks, cheeses and yogurts containing reduced fat or no fat and modest amounts of sweeteners (both caloric and noncaloric) are generally recommended" [24].

5.4.2.2 Adulthood

5.4.2.2.1 Young Adulthood

In the early adult years (19 through 30), there is continued accumulation of bone mass. This retention of bone mass occurs for approximately 10 years after longitudinal growth has stopped, but generally at a lower rate than during adolescence [10,172]. Although data are limited, 1000 mg calcium per day is recommended for men and women aged 19 through 30 years to maximize calcium retention [10]. Several studies in young adults report positive correlations between dietary calcium and bone measurements [172–176]. A review of both prospective and cross-sectional studies of the effects of calcium intake on bone mineral content in females between the ages of 20 and 40 years indicates a positive effect of calcium intakes at or greater than 1000 mg/day on bone health [176].

A high daily dietary calcium (i.e., 1000 mg) intake and physical activity (i.e., >90 min of moderate activity a week) increased radial bone mineral content and density in 24 to 28 year old Caucasian women participating in a cross-sectional study [173]. In a longitudinal prospective study (up to 5 years) involving 156 healthy women in their twenties (18 to 26 years), increasing dietary calcium intake to 1400 mg or higher and increasing physical activity each had a positive effect on bone density [172].

In a cross-sectional analysis of 215 women aged 18 to 31 years, calcium, protein, phosphorus, and the calcium-protein or calcium-phosphorus ratios together, had a significant effect on spine and total body bone mineral densities and bone mineral contents [177]. Another cross-sectional study in this population group found that current calcium intakes were positively associated with spine bone mineral density [167]. When the effect of nutrition and mild hyperparathyroidism on bone mineral density was examined in 108 female Japanese nursing students aged 19 to 25 years, a low calcium intake and mildly elevated levels of parathyroid hormone (partly explained by low vitamin D nutrition and low calcium and protein intakes) were identified as important independent predictors of low bone mineral density [178]. In this study, nutrient intakes were analyzed directly from food consumed, which is more accurate than assessing intake using food records or dietary recall. Calcium intake was the primary factor predicting bone mineral density of the hip [178].

Intake of dairy foods is beneficial to bones in young adults [175,179,180]. When factors related to peak bone mass were examined in 421 women ages 25 to 34 living in Hawaii, milk intake was positively associated with forearm bone mass index [179]. In a study of 705 healthy, Caucasian college women (18 to 22 years), radial bone mineral content and density were positively associated with intake of calcium from milk and cheese [175]. Distal radial bone mineral content and density were 1.8% and 2.7% higher, respectively, in women with high long-term calcium intakes (i.e., calcium intakes close to 1200 mg/day, both during high school and college) than in women who consumed less than 1 serving of milk or cheese a day since age 14 [175]. Findings of this study also indicate a significant positive association between long-term physical activity patterns (greater then 4 hours a week for 8 or more months of the year) and distal bone mineral content and bone mineral density. Moderate long-term dairy calcium intake combined with moderate long-term physical activity was especially beneficial to bone mass. Conversely, a low calcium intake was most detrimental to bone mass when physical activity also was low (less than 1 hour a week). "Both regular physical activity and adequate calcium intake may be positive modulators of the distal radius from the perimenarcheal period through mid-adulthood," concluded Tylavsky et al. [175].

A cross-sectional study of 963 healthy Norwegian women aged 19 to 35 years, found that after controlling for age and weight, women who did not consume milk daily had twice the odds of low forearm bone mineral density [180]. On the other hand, milk consumption, which was a significant source of calcium, was associated with higher bone mineral density of the wrist and forearm [180].

A recent randomized controlled intervention in physically active, healthy, young women aged 18 to 30 years, with a low dietary intake of calcium (<800 mg/day), found that increasing intake of dairy products to achieve recommended intake levels of calcium improved hip bone mineral density and content and helped to protect oral contraceptive users from total hip and spine bone mineral density loss [181]. Use of oral contraceptives without adequate calcium intake may prevent young women from reaching peak bone mass and increase their risk of osteoporosis in later years. In this 1-year study, the women (oral contraceptive users and nonusers) were randomized to one of three diet intervention groups: control (<800 mg calcium/day), medium dairy (1000 to 1100 mg calcium/day) or high dairy (1200 to 1300 mg calcium/day). Throughout the year, bone mineral density measurements and 3-day food records were periodically collected. At the end of the year, oral contraceptive users consuming the medium or high dairy diets had significantly higher bone mineral density in their hips and spines compared to the low dairy group (Figure 5.9) [181]. Oral contraceptive users consuming low calcium intakes lost bone at both spine and hip sites compared to nonusers, but this loss was prevented with the medium or high dairy intakes. Findings of this study indicate that women taking oral contraceptives should consume dairy products at levels necessary to achieve recommended intakes of calcium to optimize their bone health.

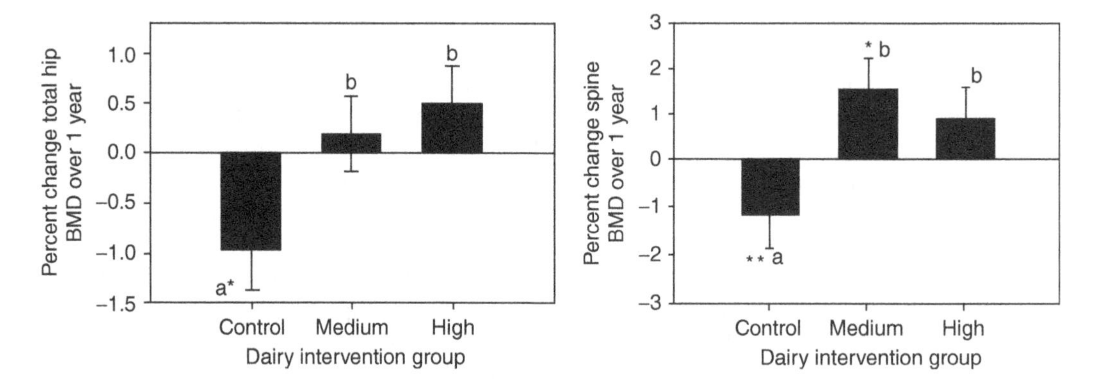

FIGURE 5.9 Increased intake of dairy products protects women consuming oral contraceptives from spine and hip bone loss. For the spine and total hip bone mineral density, the significance of diet intervention by use of oral contraceptives interaction was $P = 0.03$ and $P = 0.36$, respectively. Asterisk (*) and double asterisk (**) indicates difference ($P < 0.05$) from zero (paired t) or a trend ($0.1 > P > 0.05$), respectively. (From Teegarden, D. et al. *J. Clin. Endocrinol. Metab.*, 90, 5127, 2005.)

5.4.2.2.2 Between Peak Bone Mass and Menopause

Adequate calcium intake continues to be important to offset calcium losses and maintain bone health in the years after peak bone mass has been reached and before menopause [45,182]. For premenopausal women ages 31 through 50 years, 1000 mg calcium per day is recommended to maximize calcium retention [10]. According to a meta-analysis of 27 well-designed cross-sectional studies involving women between 18 and 50 years of age, a calcium intake of approximately 1000 mg/day or higher is positively associated with bone mass [183].

Increasing calcium intake from dairy products has been shown to benefit bone health in premenopausal women [184]. In a 3-year prospective trial involving premenopausal women 30 to 42 years of age, 20 women were randomly assigned to consume more dairy products (an increase of 610 mg calcium for a total of 1572 mg, plus or minus 920 mg), while 17 women continued their usual diet (810 mg, ±367 mg calcium) [184]. Vertebral bone mineral density was significantly greater in the women consuming the higher than lower dairy calcium diets [184]. Based on these findings, the authors suggested that the increase in the bone mass of women entering menopause might reduce their risk of osteoporosis as they age [184]. As mentioned above, a randomized, controlled intervention demonstrated that increasing dairy food intake to meet dietary calcium recommendations positively impacted bone health in premenopausal women taking oral contraceptives [181].

5.4.2.2.3 Postmenopausal Years

Calcium intake has a variable effect on bone health in women during the early postmenopausal years, a period of rapid bone loss [10,185]. Due to the loss of estrogen at menopause, women lose spinal bone mineral at a rate of an average of about 3% a year for about 5 years after menopause and then more slowly (1% a year) thereafter [186]. During this time, the prevalence of bone loss at one or more sites is relatively high in women not taking estrogen or increasing their calcium intake [187]. During the first 5 years of menopause, calcium is less effective in protecting the skeleton than in later menopausal years [10,45,185,188]. In an 8-year study of 154 healthy women with a mean age of 53 years, rate of cortical bone loss was unaffected by habitual calcium intake (75% derived from dairy products), ranging from less than 800 mg to more than 1350 mg in early postmenopausal years [188]. In contrast, dietary calcium influenced bone mass in women more than 5 years postmenopausal (Figure 5.10). Dawson-Hughes et al. [185] also showed that increasing calcium intake had little or no benefit on bone health in women during the first 5 years of menopause, but provided substantial protection thereafter. The profound and rapid loss of estrogen in the early postmenopausal years is responsible for the bone loss at this time. As a result of the initial rapid decline in estrogen at menopause, women lose about 15% of the bone they had before menopause [45]. Estrogen replacement therapy has been used to help prevent postmenopausal bone loss, but its use is controversial because of the potential risk for other health problems [1].

Although increased calcium intake has only a modest effect on the rapid bone loss that occurs immediately after menopause, studies indicate that even early postmenopausal women benefit from calcium intakes at or greater than recommended intakes [1,185,189,190]. Support for a beneficial effect of increased calcium intake on bone health in early postmenopausal years is provided by Aloia et al. [189]. In their study, 118 healthy Caucasian women between 3 and 6 years past menopause were randomly assigned to one of three treatment groups for 3 years: (1) 1700 mg calcium a day from diet and calcium carbonate supplement; (2) estrogen-progesterone replacement therapy plus 1700 mg calcium a day; and (3) placebo. All subjects received 400 IU of vitamin D a day. The placebo group lost bone density in the arm, spine, and three areas of the hip [189]. However, increased calcium intake slowed age-related bone loss in the skeletal sites

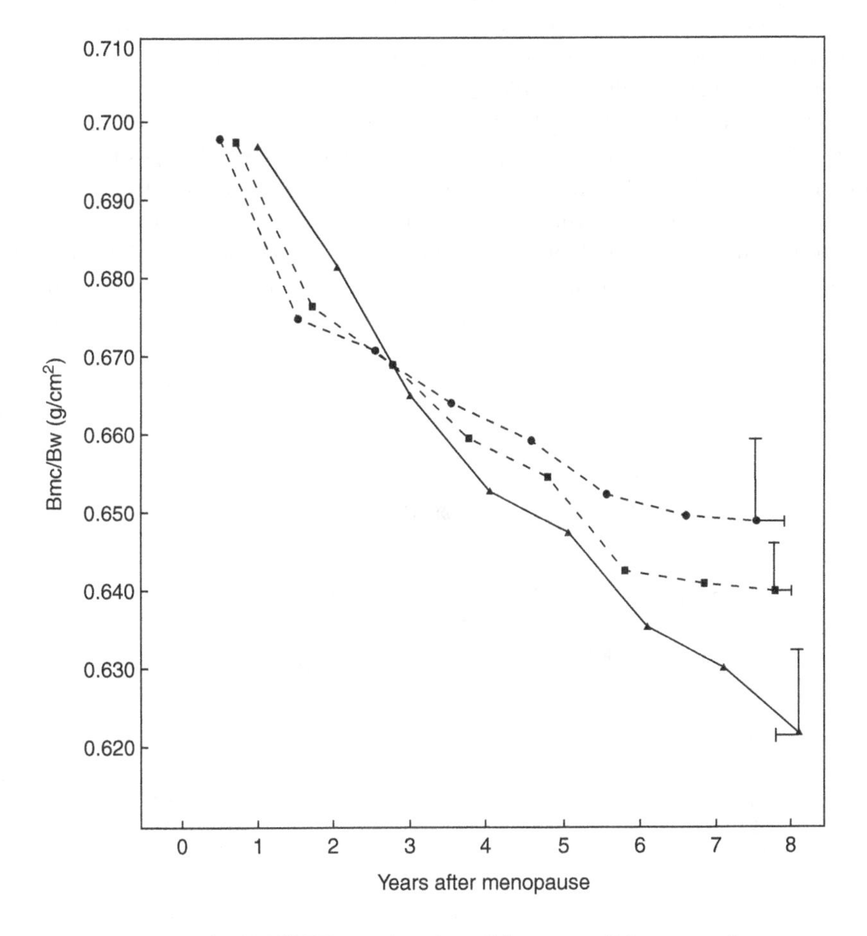

FIGURE 5.10 Mean changes in BMC/BW as a function of the mean of the years after menopause in 154 perimenopausal women subdivided according to habitual dietary calcium intake. Bars are 1 SEM. (BMC/BW first measured in 1980.) (●) Ca intake <800 mg/day ($n = 28$); (■ Ca intake 800–1350 mg/day ($n = 95$); (▲) Ca intake > 1350 mg/day ($n = 31$). (From Van Beresteijn, E. C. H. et al., *Calcif. Tissue Int.*, 47, 338, 1990. With permission.)

measured. The estrogen-progesterone-calcium treatment was more effective in reducing bone loss and improving calcium balance than calcium alone. The findings nevertheless support a significant beneficial effect of calcium in reducing bone loss, especially in the neck of the femur, around the time of menopause (Figure 5.11) [189]. Although calcium is less effective than estrogen in slowing the rapid bone loss that occurs immediately after menopause, studies show that increasing calcium or dairy food intake augments the bone protective effect of estrogen replacement therapy [189,191–195].

Beginning about 5 years after the onset of menopause, calcium once again resumes relatively more importance in bone health than in early postmenopausal years [10,185]. The difference in calcium's role in bone health between early and late menopause can best be explained by the effect of estrogen on the bone mass "set point." When estrogen declines at menopause, bone initially adjusts its mass downward, releasing calcium. The result is that during the first few years after menopause, there is a modest dependence on external (dietary) calcium sources [45]. After a period of adjustment, however, dependence on dietary calcium increases [45].

For postmenopausal women ages 51 through 70 years, 1200 mg of calcium per day is recommended [10]. This calcium recommendation is 200 mg/day higher than the recommendation for 31 through 50 year adults because of the decrease in calcium absorption with advancing age [10]. Evidence is insufficient to support different calcium recommendations for women depending on their menopausal status or use of hormone replacement therapy [10].

Findings from calcium balance studies and calcium intervention trials support a calcium recommendation of at least 1200 mg/day for postmenopausal women [10,196–200]. Michaelsson et al. [200] found that bone mineral density significantly improved in Swedish postmenopausal women who consumed more than 1400 mg calcium per day. This 4-year prospective study divided 115 women into the following three groups based on their estimated mean dietary intakes of calcium: low (465 mg), medium (1006 mg), and high (1645 mg) [200]. The group with the highest calcium intake had significantly greater hip, lumbar spine, and total body bone mineral densities than women in either the low or the intermediate calcium groups [200]. Another 4-year follow-up study involving 84 women aged 54 to 74 years who were more than 10 years past menopause, found that a calcium intake of almost 2 g/day was necessary to slow or stop bone loss and reduce fracture risk [198]. Women consuming 1988 mg calcium/day for 4 years did not lose bone at the

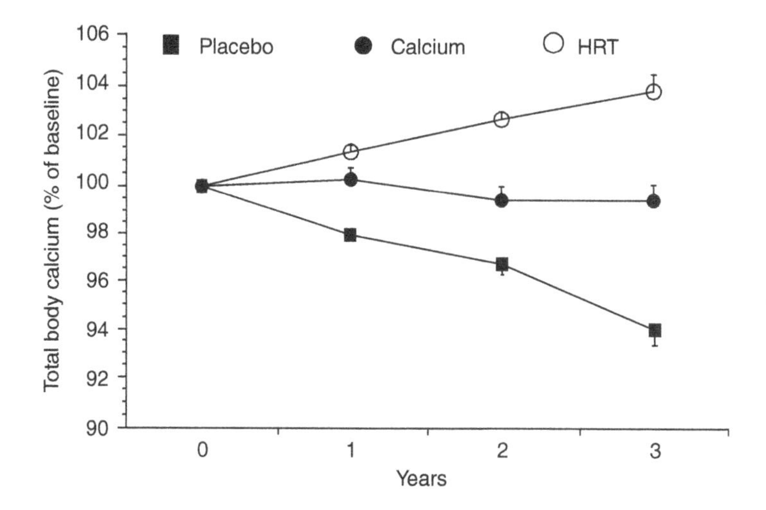

FIGURE 5.11 The change in total body calcium with time. Calcium augmentation remained intermediate in effect between placebo and estrogen-progesterone-calcium throughout the 3 years of the study. HRT = hormone replacement therapy. (From Aloia, J. F., *Ann. Intern. Med.*, 120, 97, 1994. With permission.)

hip or ankle, whereas significant bone loss occurred from these sites in the control group which consumed 952 mg calcium/day (Figure 5.12) [198]. Compared to the calcium supplemented group, significantly more bone was lost at all sites of the ankle in 49 women who were treated with increased calcium for 2 years, but then stopped [198]. This indicates that continuation of increased calcium intake is important to maintain a positive effect on bone density. The researchers suggest that the findings are consistent with a growing body of evidence indicating that more than 1500 mg of calcium/day is associated with bone health and reduced risk of fractures [198]. An earlier 2-year, placebo-controlled study in women 10 years past menopause by these same investigators demonstrated that calcium supplementation (1800 mg/day) as milk powder or as tablets completely prevented bone loss at some areas of the hip [199].

In contrast to the above studies, findings from the Nurses' Health Study failed to provide evidence that increasing calcium intake reduces the risk of bone fractures in postmenopausal women [201,202]. An 18-year prospective analysis of more than 72,000 postmenopausal women who participated in this study found that an AI of vitamin D was associated with a lower risk of osteoporotic hip fractures, but the effect of calcium or milk intake was not significant [202]. Higher total calcium intake from food and supplements was associated with a significantly lower risk of hip fracture when adjusted for age. However, this relationship was no longer significant after adjusting for other factors (e.g., body mass index, hormone use, physical activity, smoking, multivitamin use, intakes of vitamin K, alcohol, caffeine, protein, retinol, and vitamin D). After adjusting for calcium, vitamin D, and retinol supplement use, women consuming 1.5 or more cups of milk per day had a

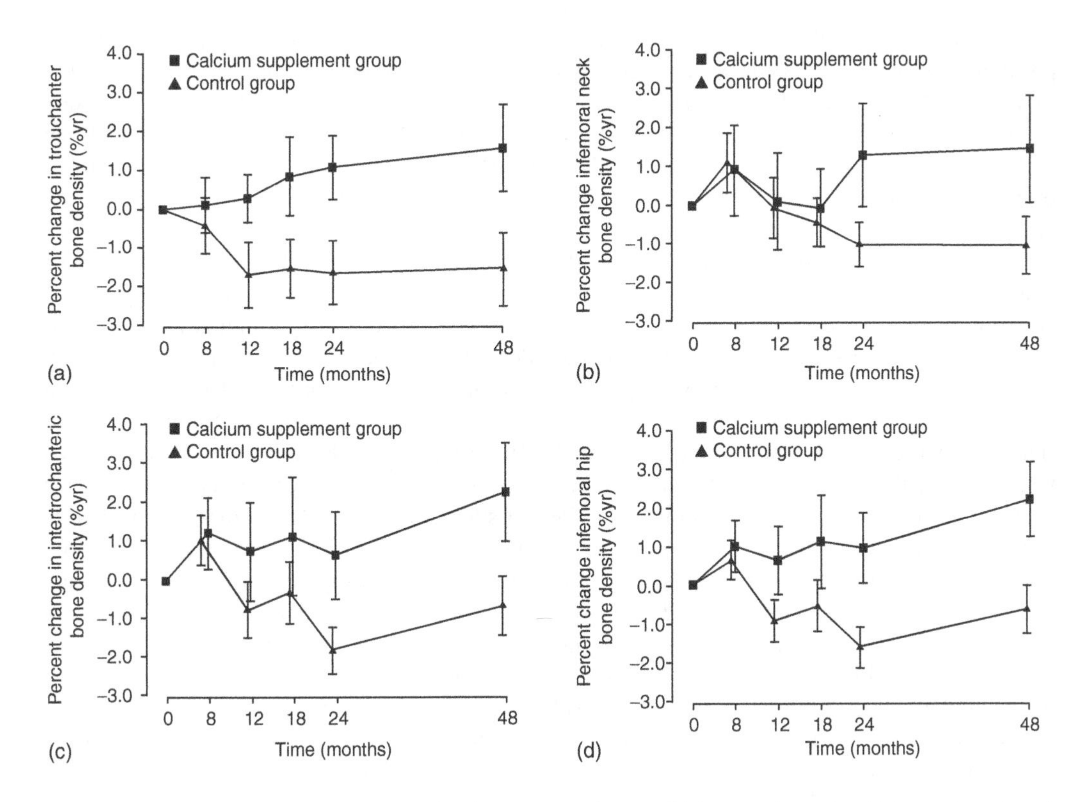

FIGURE 5.12 Percentage change in bone density at (a) trochanter, (b) intertrochanteric, (c) femoral neck and (d) total hip sites. Results are the mean plus or minus SEM. The 4-year change in bone density determined from the slope of the least squares regression analysis was significantly different between the control group (*triangles*; $n = 21$) and calcium supplemented group (*squares*; $n = 14$). (From Devine, A. et al., *Osteoporosis Int.*, 7, 23, 1997, European Foundation for Osteoporosis and the National Osteoporosis Foundation.)

nonsignificant 17% lower risk of hip fracture than those consuming less than 1 cup per week [202]. It is important to note that this is an observational study and the failure to show a significant benefit for calcium or dairy foods may be due to the weak method for estimating long-term calcium intake (i.e., a semiquantitative food frequency questionnaire).

In a cross-sectional study in which a food frequency questionnaire was employed, McCabe et al. [203] found no relationship between calcium, or dairy food intake, and bone mineral density in postmenopausal women, but a positive relationship was observed in men. Yet, a 4-year calcium intervention study found it was effective in preventing a decline in bone mineral density in both the men and women [203]. According to the researchers, this discrepancy may suggest that women are more likely to under-report calcium consumption than are men [203].

According to a randomized clinical trial of 122 healthy postmenopausal New Zealand women, increasing calcium intake from 750 to 1750 mg/day (i.e., 1000 mg calcium from calcium lactate-gluconate and calcium carbonate) for 2 years reduced age-related bone loss by one-third to one-half in several bones as compared with the placebo group [196]. Increasing calcium intake reduced the rate of loss of total body mineral density by 43% [196]. At most skeleton sites, the placebo group lost bone at a rate of approximately 1% a year. When 86 postmenopausal women participated in a 2-year extension to this study, a sustained beneficial effect on bones over the 4 years occurred with calcium supplementation [197]. However, the effect of increased calcium differed according to the specific bone site [197]. In the lumbar spine and femoral neck, bone loss was reduced in the calcium group in the first year with only a small positive effect of increased calcium over the remaining years. In contrast, the rate of bone loss of total body bone mineral density in the calcium group was maintained over the 4 years [197].

A carefully conducted meta-analysis of 15 randomized, controlled trials, representing 1806 postmenopausal women with an average calcium intake of about 700 mg/day, found calcium supplementation alone reduced bone loss at all skeletal sites (i.e., hip, lumbar spine, total body, and distal radius) by a small (~ 2%) but significant amount after two or more years of treatment compared to the placebo [204]. The results also demonstrated a trend toward reduction in vertebral fractures, although calcium's effect on reducing the incidence of nonvertebral fractures was unclear [204].

The Women's Health Initiative Study in the United States found that intake of calcium plus vitamin D supplements helped to preserve bone mass and prevent hip fractures in certain groups of postmenopausal women, although the effects were less than expected [205]. In this 7-year double-blind, placebo-controlled trial of more than 36,000 healthy postmenopausal women aged 50 to 79 years (average age of 62), women were randomly assigned to receive either 1000 mg of calcium carbonate with 400 IU of vitamin D a day, or a placebo. Calcium with vitamin D supplementation significantly increased hip bone mineral density by 1% [205]. The 12% reduction in hip fractures in women taking the calcium plus vitamin D supplements was not statistically significant. However, in a subgroup of women who consistently took the full supplement dose and in those older than 60 years, there was a significant reduction in hip fractures. Intake of calcium and vitamin D supplements had no significant effect on spine or total fractures. Moreover, supplement use was associated with increased risk of kidney stones [205]. Several factors attributed to the finding that the reduction in hip fracture rate in response to calcium and vitamin D therapy was half of what had been predicted [206]. Most of the women in the study already had AIs of calcium before the intervention. As mentioned above, there is a threshold level for calcium above which additional calcium is unlikely to confer further benefit for bones. The calcium with vitamin D supplement may be more effective for bone health in women with initially low intakes of these nutrients [206]. Also, the bone health benefit of the supplement may be greater for women with osteoporosis than in this study population, which was not selected on the basis of low bone mineral density or risk factors for osteoporosis. In addition, the dose of vitamin D (400 IU a day) may have been too low, and half of the women in the study were receiving hormone replacement therapy (i.e., a fairly potent antiresorptive regimen) [206]. This study examined the impact of supplements, not food.

Food sources of calcium and vitamin D, such as dairy foods, have been demonstrated to benefit bone health [7]. Also, in contrast to calcium supplements, which have been associated with increased risk of kidney stones [205], calcium-rich dairy foods have been shown to be associated with reduced risk of kidney stones [207–209].

Calcium combined with physical activity has also been shown to benefit bone health in postmenopausal women. A 2-year, placebo-controlled study involving 168 postmenopausal women in Australia found that increasing calcium intake from 800 to 1800 mg/day by consuming either milk powder or calcium supplements, reduced bone loss in the hip and leg [199]. Adding an extra 4 hours a week of weight-bearing exercise to increased calcium intake was more effective in reducing hip bone loss than calcium alone [199]. The findings led the authors to conclude that "… a lifestyle regimen of increased dietary intake of calcium to ~1.8 g of calcium/day plus an exercise regimen of a 10% increase in the average exercise undertaken will significantly reduce bone loss at the clinically important hip site" [199]. Researchers in England also demonstrated that both calcium intake and physical activity benefit bone health in women 5 to 12 years into menopause [210]. A study of 126 postmenopausal women (average age of 60) found that calcium supplementation (600 mg/day) and strength training three times a week, using progressively heavier weights, significantly increased total hip bone mineral density [211].

A number of studies have investigated dairy food intake and bone health in postmenopausal women [7]. More than 20 years ago, Recker and Heaney [212] reported that increased milk intake (24 ounces/day) improved calcium balance in 13 healthy postmenopausal women compared to that in nine control subjects who did not receive the milk supplement. Milk consumption also resulted in less bone remodeling than that found with calcium supplements [212]. More recently, intake of yogurt was demonstrated to benefit bone health in postmenopausal American women with low calcium intakes (average of 466 mg/day) [213]. In this controlled clinical trial, 29 postmenopausal women (61 years) were randomly assigned to consume fruit-flavored yogurt or a jellied fruit-flavored snack, three times a day for a period of 7 to 10 days. After a 2-week washout period, the participants were switched to the opposite snack. Intake of the yogurt snack consumed three times a day significantly increased the women's intake of calcium and other nutrients and decreased the rate of bone resorption as indicated by urinary excretion of N-telopeptide [213].

Several studies in Asian postmenopausal women indicate that consuming milk has a positive effect on bone health [214–216]. Hu et al. [214] examined associations between dietary calcium, from both dairy and nondairy sources, and bone status in 843 Chinese women aged 35 to 75 years and living in five different counties where dietary calcium varied widely. Peak bone mass at skeletal maturity was the same for the women before menopause. However, women in pastoral and semipastoral areas who consumed higher dairy calcium had a slower decline in bone mass after menopause than women residing in nonpastoral areas without dairy calcium [214]. Women in dairy calcium areas lost 8.6% bone per decade, whereas bone loss in women in nondairy areas was 9.2%. In a separate analysis involving women living in pastoral areas, bone mineral content and density at the distal and midradius were positively associated with intake of milk, hard cheese, and other dairy foods [214]. These findings indicate that dietary calcium, especially from dairy sources, increases bone mass in postmenopausal women and helps to reduce the risk of osteoporosis.

In a 2-year randomized controlled trial, 173 healthy postmenopausal Chinese women aged 55 to 65 years, living in Malaysia, were randomly chosen to supplement their diets with high-calcium, skimmed milk powder (which when reconstituted provided 1200 mg of calcium taken as two glasses of milk a day) or to continue eating their regular low calcium diet (473 mg/day) [215]. Results showed that the high calcium milk supplement taken for 2 years reduced bone loss at the total body, lumbar spine, and regions of the hip (femoral neck and total hip) (Figure 5.13). Chee and colleagues [215] reported that "at all sites, the control groups experienced significant bone loss over time compared to the baseline while bone density was maintained in the milk-supplemented group." Compared to the control group which continued to consume their usual diet, the milk treatment group had significantly higher intakes of dietary calcium, improved vitamin D status, and lower bone loss rates, despite not gaining weight [215].

The findings of Chee et al. [215] support those of an earlier investigation of postmenopausal women aged 55 to 59 years in Hong Kong [216]. In this 2-year randomized controlled trial, 200 women were randomly assigned to an intervention group receiving a milk powder containing 800 mg calcium per day, or to a control group. Compared to the control group, the milk supplemented group lost significantly less height and bone mineral density at all sites measured, including the lumbar spine, two areas of the hip, across the hip, and total body after 24 months [216].

In a position statement on nutrition and women's health, the ADA and Dietitians of Canada point out that calcium and vitamin D are the nutrients most important for bone health [217]. Low-fat dairy products are identified as the "most desirable way to meet calcium goals" [217]. Further, these organizations state, "it is difficult to achieve an AI [of calcium] when dairy products are eliminated from the diet" [218]. A report from the North American Menopause Society (NAMS) emphasizes the important role of calcium, both before and after menopause, in preventing diseases such as osteoporosis [218]. The NAMS states that dairy products are among the best sources of calcium due to their high calcium content, high calcium bioavailability, and low cost relative to their total nutritional value [218].

5.4.2.2.4 Men

Although osteoporosis is more prevalent in women than men, it is now recognized as an increasingly important public health problem in men [1,3]. An estimated two million American men have osteoporosis [3]. After age 50, 6% of all American men will experience a hip fracture and 5% will have an osteoporosis-related vertebral fracture [3]. Women lose bone mass rapidly during the first few years of menopause (3% per year), however by age 65 or 70, women and men lose bone mass at

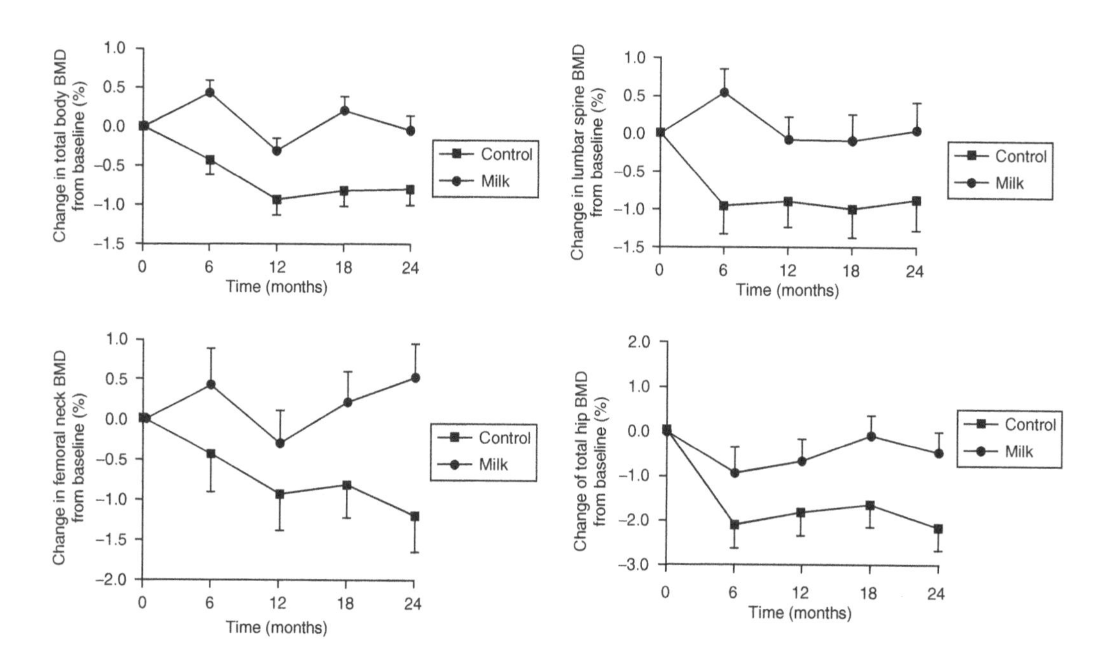

FIGURE 5.13 Effect of milk supplementation on bone mineral density (mean +/− SE percentage change) in postmenopausal women in Malaysia. (From Chee, W. S. S. et al., *Osteoporos. Int.*, 14, 828, 2003.)

the same slower rate of about 1% per year and calcium absorption decreases in both sexes [3,219]. About 30% of hip fractures occur in men [220]. However, the mortality rate in men from hip fractures is reported to be about twice that of women, perhaps because such fractures tend to occur at older ages in men than in women, and fewer men than women are treated for osteoporosis [3,221]. The lower risk of osteoporosis in men than in women is explained by men's larger bones and higher bone mineral content, their shorter lifespan (i.e., less time to lose bone), and hormonal changes [222]. Similar to women, men with low peak bone mass are vulnerable to osteoporosis. Also, peak bone mass and subsequent bone loss in men, like in women, is influenced by genetics and lifestyle factors including physical activity, alcohol consumption, smoking, disease, and use of some medications (e.g., bone-resorbing medications such as glucocorticoids) [3,223].

Because negative calcium balance can accompany aging in men as a result of low calcium intake, reduced efficiency of intestinal calcium absorption, and low synthesis of 1,25-dihydroxy-vitamin vitamin D_3 (i.e., the metabolically active form of vitamin D), it is important that men consume recommended intakes of calcium and vitamin D [224]. As there are few data suggesting that calcium and vitamin D needs of men are different from those of women, recommendations for these nutrients are the same for similar aged men and women [10]. The calcium recommendation is 1300 mg/day for men 9 through 18 years, 1000 mg/day for 19 through 50 year olds, and 1200 mg/day for men 51 years and older [10].

Relatively few studies have examined the relationship between calcium (and vitamin D) intake and bone health in men. However, low dietary calcium or dairy intake is identified as a risk factor for osteoporosis in men [225–228]. A prospective analysis that included 739 Australian men over the age of 60 identified low dietary calcium intake as an independent predictor of arm fracture [225]. An analysis of some risk factors for accelerated bone loss in Spanish men aged 50 years and older found low milk consumption to be an independent risk factor for loss of bone mass [227]. The researchers suggest that ensuring an AI of milk may prevent the loss of bone mass in men.

Kroger and Laitinen [229] reported that hip bone mineral density, but not spinal bone density, was higher in Finnish men who consumed calcium intakes greater than 1200 mg/day than in those whose calcium intake was less than 800 mg/day. A cross-sectional analysis to determine factors associated with bone mineral density of the lumbar spine and proximal femur in nearly 6000 men aged 65 years and older who were enrolled in the Osteoporosis Fractures in Men Study ("Mr.OS"), found that dietary calcium was positively related to bone mineral density [228]. Dawson-Hughes et al. [224] reported that calcium and vitamin D supplementation reduced total body bone loss in both elderly men and women in a 3-year randomized trial, but the effect on femoral neck was significant only in men.

An analysis of the Health Professionals Follow-up Study, that followed more than 43,000 men aged 40 to 75 years for 8 years, linked higher reported intakes of calcium from dairy foods in general (but not from milk) with decreased risk of forearm and hip fractures [230]. Researchers at the University of Pittsburgh reported that bone mineral density was higher in men who drank milk from ages 18 to 50, and/or after age 50, than for men who drank milk less frequently [231]. High intakes of milk, and particularly cheese, were linked to decreased risk of hip fractures in a study of more than 1800 men in Southern Europe [223].

In a cross-sectional study which included 116 white and 75 black men (average age of 72 years), intake of calcium from dairy products was positively correlated with bone mineral density at the total hip and femoral neck after adjusting for age, race, and weight [203]. In a nested, longitudinal study of white men, increasing calcium intake by 750 mg/day reduced bone loss from the total hip and femoral neck in those who consumed less than 1.5 servings of dairy products per day and were younger than 72 year of age [203]. A 2-year randomized, controlled trial in 149 Australian men over age 50 who were assigned to an intervention of reduced fat milk containing 1000 mg of calcium plus 800 IU of vitamin D_3 a day or no additional milk (control), found that age-related bone loss was reduced at several sites (e.g., femoral neck, total hip, ultradistal radius) in men who received the milk supplement compared to the controls [232].

Whiting et al. [233] report that several dairy food nutrients are beneficial for men's bone. In a cross-sectional study of 57 Canadian men ages 39 to 42 years, a dietary pattern of adequate calcium intake (1200 mg/day), moderate protein (100 g/day or 1.17 g/kg body weight), generous potassium (~3800 mg/day), and phosphorus (~1700 mg/day), contributed to higher bone mineral densities than a pattern in which calcium is adequate but protein and potassium are low [233]. The researchers suggest that incorporating dairy foods, fruits, and vegetables into the diet can help men achieve the benefits provided by the bone-boosting nutrients [233].

5.4.2.2.5 Elderly

Osteoporosis and related fractures are a major cause of morbidity and mortality in the elderly [1,10]. Twenty percent of older adults who suffer a hip fracture die within 1 year [1]. Due primarily to the aging of the population and previous limited attention to bone health, the number of hip fractures in the United States is estimated to double, or even triple, by the year 2020 [1]. The important role of calcium and vitamin D in decreasing bone loss and osteoporotic fractures in elderly men and women is widely recognized [234,235]. Many older adults have low bone mass and continue to lose bone (i.e., 0.5% to 1.0% per year) with further aging [45]. Moreover, calcium deficiency and low vitamin D status are frequently identified in this population [10,71,73].

For adults over 70 years of age, a calcium intake of 1200 mg/day is recommended [10]. Studies indicate that a calcium intake of at least this amount, either alone or in combination with vitamin D, is necessary to protect older adults' bone health [7,114,198,224,235–238]. According to a review by Heaney [235], a calcium intake of 1300 to 1700 mg/day appears to be needed to arrest age-related bone loss and reduce fracture risk in the elderly, because of the decline in their ability to adapt to a low calcium intake. Even higher intakes (i.e., 2400 mg/day) of calcium may be necessary to restore bone remodeling levels to those found in young adults [235]. High levels of parathyroid hormone are associated with elevated levels of bone remodeling, which is a recognized fragility factor (apart from bone mass) [234,235]. High intakes of calcium have been demonstrated to reduce these high levels of parathyroid hormone [27].

In a landmark double-blind, placebo-controlled investigation in France, involving 1765 ambulatory elderly women 69 to 106 years of age (mean age of 84), women who increased their calcium intake from 500 to 1700 mg/day and consumed an additional 800 IU of vitamin D_3 (cholecalciferol) for 18 months, increased their hip bone density and reduced their rate of hip fractures by 41%, and other nonvertebral fractures by 30% (Figure 5.14) [236]. Hip bone density increased almost 3% (2.7%) in the women who increased their intake of calcium and vitamin D, whereas the control group lost almost 5% (4.6%) of their bone density [236]. When this study was extended for an additional 18 months, risk of hip fractures was reduced by 29% and risk of all nonvertebral fractures was reduced by 24% [239]. These studies clearly indicate the peril that low calcium intake presents for older adults and the importance of consuming AIs of calcium and vitamin D to prevent bone loss and subsequent fractures, even in the very old.

Recker et al. [238], in a 4-year randomized, controlled trial in vitamin D replete elderly women (mean age 73.5 years), found that increasing calcium intake by 1200 mg/day (total of about 1600 mg/day) reduced both femoral bone loss and the incidence of vertebral fractures. Women who experienced a previous fracture and were not treated with calcium were 2.8 times more likely to experience a fracture than other women [238]. Similar findings are reported by Chevalley et al. [237]. In this study involving vitamin D replete elderly women, some of whom had suffered a hip fracture, increasing calcium intake by 800 mg/day (total of 1500 mg/day) for 18 months reduced femoral bone loss and the rate of vertebral fractures.

An investigation by Dawson-Hughes et al. [224] demonstrated that increasing calcium intake by 500 mg/day (total of about 1400 mg/day) and vitamin D by about 700 IU/day for 3 years, reduced

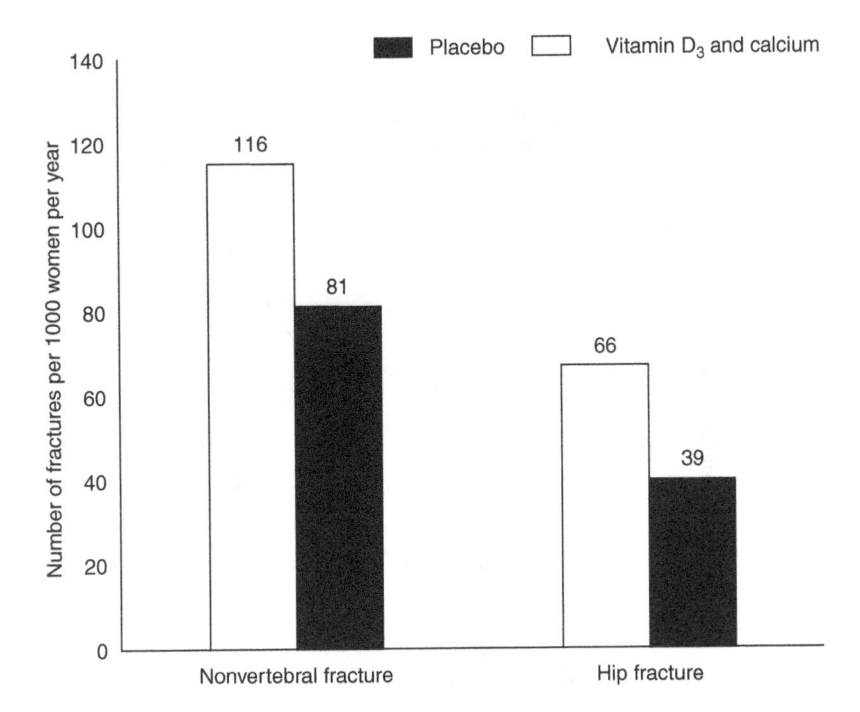

FIGURE 5.14 Incidence of fractures among elderly women treated with either vitamin D_3 and calcium or a placebo after 12 to 18 months of follow-up. (Adapted from Chapuy, M. C. et al., *N. Engl. J. Med.*, 327, 1637, 1992. With permission.)

bone loss in the hip, spine, and total body. Nonvertebral fractures were reduced by 50% in adults 65 years and older (Figure 5.15) [224]. According to a meta-analysis of seven calcium intervention studies and 30 epidemiological trials in elderly women, increasing calcium intake by 1000 mg/day decreased hip fracture risk by 24% [114]. The researchers state that this translates into "... an 8% reduction in hip fracture risk for every glass of milk [consumed] per day" [114]. As mentioned above, findings from the Women's Health Initiative clinical trial, involving more than 36,000 postmenopausal women aged 50 to 79 years, revealed that intake of calcium (1000 mg/day) and vitamin D (400 IU/day) supplements helped to preserve bone mass and prevent hip fractures in certain groups of older women, but the supplements did not prevent other types of fractures [205].

The importance of adequate calcium intake in later years is supported by studies of age-related changes in the calcium economy [239,240]. Elevated blood levels of parathyroid hormone, which increases bone resorption, are thought to be typical of advancing age. However, increasing older adults' calcium intake has been shown to decrease parathyroid hormone levels and biochemical markers of bone breakdown [27,239–242]. In elderly women who had abnormally high blood levels of parathyroid hormone, increasing calcium intake by 1200 mg/day normalized blood parathyroid hormone levels [239]. McKane et al. [240], in a double-blind calcium supplementation study in healthy older adults treated with either 800 or 2400 mg calcium a day for 3 years, found that a calcium intake of 2400 mg/day was necessary to normalize parathyroid hormone levels and reduce bone remodeling to levels found in healthy young adult women [240]. According to an 8-week double-blind, controlled trial in Germany, involving 148 women (mean age 74 years), increasing intake of calcium by 1200 mg/day and vitamin D by 800 IU/day was effective in normalizing blood parathyroid hormone levels and reducing body sway, both of which may help prevent falls and hip fracture in older women [243]. In another randomized controlled trial, researchers in Switzerland reported that supplementation with calcium (1200 mg/day) and vitamin D (800 IU/day) over 3

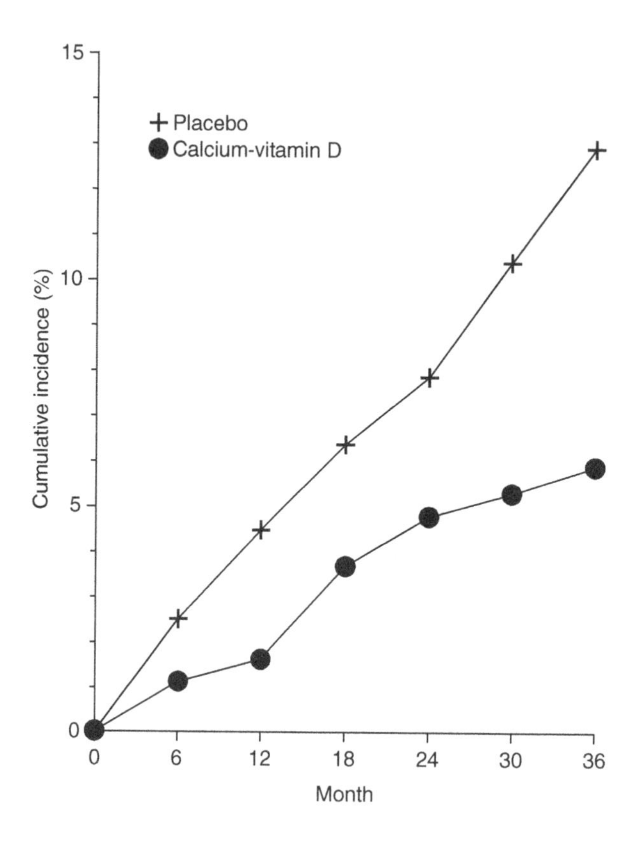

FIGURE 5.15 Cumulative percentage of all 389 subjects with a first nonvertebral fracture, according to study group. By 36 months, 26 of 202 subjects in the placebo group and 11 of 187 subjects in the calcium-vitamin D group had had a fracture ($P = 0.02$). (From Dawson-Hughes, B. et al., *N. Engl. J. Med.*, 337, 670, 1997. With permission.)

months, reduced parathyroid hormone and biochemical markers of bone resorption, improved musculoskeletal function, and significantly reduced falls by 49%, compared to calcium alone in 122 frail elderly women with vitamin D deficiency [242]. Increased calcium intake combined with physical activity has a beneficial effect on older adults' bones [244]. A population-based study of 1363 older women (mean age of 75 years) in Australia demonstrated that the combination of high calcium intake and high physical activity increased total hip bone mineral density by 5.1% compared to that in individuals who consumed a low calcium diet and had a low level of physical activity [244].

Food sources of calcium, such as milk and other dairy products, have been demonstrated to favorably affect bone health in older adults. Hu et al. [214] found that increasing dietary calcium, especially from dairy sources, increased bone mass in elderly women. Heaney et al. [241] reported that older adults could significantly improve their skeletal health by consuming 3 servings/day of fat free or low-fat milk [241]. In this 12-week multicenter, randomized, controlled trial involving 204 healthy adults, aged 55 to 85 years, who habitually consumed less than 1.5 servings of dairy foods per day, participants were randomly assigned to an intervention group in which they received three 8-ounce servings of fluid milk/day in addition to their usual diet or to a control group in which they consumed their usual diet. The high calcium intake from dairy foods resulted in changes in indexes of bone remodeling and the calcium economy indicative of positive bone balance [241]. In the milk group, parathyroid hormone and bone resorption (as reflected by N-telopeptide excretion) levels significantly decreased by 9% and 13%, respectively, and serum insulin-like growth factor-1 rose by 10% (Table 5.4). There was little change in the level of bone-specific alkaline phosphatase, a marker of bone formation. The decline in the resorption marker in the milk group, and no difference between groups in the formation marker, indicate a shift in bone remodeling in the direction of a more positive bone balance [241]. The findings of this study led the researchers to conclude that increasing milk intake is an effective, cost-efficient way to improve calcium nutrition [241]. Adding 3 servings of fluid milk (skim or 1%) a day to older adults' diets has been demonstrated to substantially improve their nutrient intakes, particularly calcium and vitamin D, with no adverse effect on blood pressure, glucose level, lipid metabolism, or body weight [17].

5.4.3 Treatment of Osteoporosis

Increasing calcium and vitamin D intakes in adults will slow or stop age-related bone loss and reduce fracture risk. However, intake of these nutrients rarely leads to appreciable bone gain [8]. By contrast, medications such as bisphosphonates (e.g., alendronate), raloxifene (a selective estrogen receptor modulator or SERM), and estrogen, although primarily antiresorptive drugs, increase bone gain at the spine at a rate of about 0.5% to 1.0% per year after the remodeling transient phase is over [8]. But this effect occurs only when adequate calcium is available. The full therapeutic potential of many medications used to treat osteoporosis cannot be realized without increasing calcium intake by 500 to 1000 mg/day or more above average dietary calcium intakes [8,234,245].

The importance of ensuring an adequate calcium intake has been demonstrated most clearly for estrogen [8,189,191–194]. According to a meta-analysis of 31 estrogen studies and seven calcitonin (an antiresorptive drug) trials, an adequate calcium intake potentiates the beneficial effect of estrogen and possibly calcitonin on bone mass [192]. In postmenopausal women who took estrogen combined with calcium (1183 mg/day) to treat osteoporosis, bone mass increased by 3.3% per year in the lumbar spine, by 2.4% per year in the femoral neck, and by 2.1% per year in the forearm (Figure 5.16) [192]. Thus, bone mass increased two to five times more when the women taking estrogen also consumed nearly 1200 mg calcium/day. The findings indicate that the effectiveness of osteoporosis treatments such as estrogen may not be fully realized unless adequate calcium is consumed. The results also underscore the conclusion that women taking estrogen after menopause need just as much calcium (i.e., 1200 mg/day) as women not taking estrogen [246]. All patients with osteoporosis are encouraged to consume intakes of calcium and vitamin D meeting at least the amounts recommended [247].

5.5 VITAMIN D AND BONE HEALTH

Adequate vitamin D status is important for bone health throughout the life cycle [1,10,248,249]. Vitamin D affects bone health by increasing calcium absorption and by reducing the risk for bone loss [10,20]. In a vitamin D sufficient state, 30% of dietary calcium is typically absorbed, whereas in a vitamin D deficient state, intestinal calcium absorption drops to about 10% to 15% [249]. In children, vitamin D deficiency results in inadequate mineralization of the skeleton causing rickets, a bone-softening disease leading to bone deformity [10,248,249]. A deficiency of vitamin D may also prevent children from reaching their genetically programmed height and peak bone mass [10,248,249]. In adults, vitamin D deficiency leads to a mineralization defect of the collagen matrix causing osteomalacia. In addition, increased parathyroid activity associated with vitamin D deficiency mobilizes calcium from bone to maintain blood calcium concentrations in the normal range, thus reducing bone mineral density and ultimately precipitating or exacerbating osteoporosis [248].

Vitamin D is obtained from cutaneous synthesis upon exposure of the skin to sunlight and from the diet [10,248,249]. Vitamin D_3 (cholecalciferol) is synthesized from 7-dehydrocholesterol in the epidermis when the skin is exposed to ultraviolet light. Cholecalciferol then is successively hydroxylated in the liver and kidney to 1,25-dihydroxyvitamin D_3, the metabolically active form

TABLE 5.4
Milk-Related Changes in Indexes of Bone and the Calcium Economy in Older Adults

Measure	Milk Group		Control Group		P^b
	No. of Subjects	Mean ± SE[a]	No. of subjects	Mean ± SE	
N-telopeptide (nmol/mmol creatinine)	97	−4.6 ± 1.0[c]	102	+1.1 ± 1.0	<0.0001
Bone-specific alkaline phosphatase (U/L)	97	−1.6 ± 0.4[c]	101	−1.1 ± 0.4[c]	NS
Parathyroid hormone (ng/L)	98	−3.9 ± 1.1[c]	102	+0.7 ± 1.1	<0.005
1,25-dihydroxycholecalciferol (pg/mL)	98	−2.6 ± 0.[c]	102	−0.5 ± 0.8	0.06
Urine calcium (mg/d)	94	+21 ± 7.6[c]	96	−15 ± 9.8	<0.01
Insulin-like growth factor-1 (ng/mL)	98	+12 ± 2.4[c]	102	−2.0 ± 2.1	<0.001
Insulin-like growth factor binding protein-4 (ng/mL)	98	−8 ± 15[c]	102	+36 ± 16	<0.05

[a] SE, Standard error.

[b] Difference between groups. NS, not significant.

[c] Significantly different from baseline.

Source: From Heaney, R. P. et al., *J. Am. Diet. Assoc.*, 99, 1228, 1999.

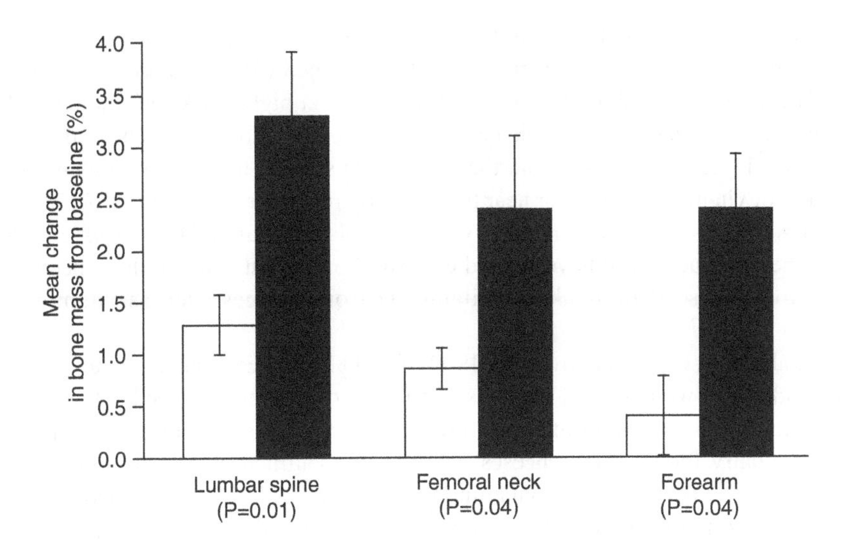

FIGURE 5.16 Mean ($\pm$SEM) annual percentage change in bone mass at the lumbar spine, femoral neck, and forearm in postmenopausal women treated with estrogen alone (□ total average calcium intake: 563 mg/d) compared with women treated with estrogen and calcium ■ total average calcium intake: 1183 mg/day). (From Nieves, J. W. et al., *Am. J. Clin. Nutr.*, 67, 18, 1998. With permission.)

of vitamin D which stimulates intestinal absorption of calcium [248,249]. Skin biosynthesis of vitamin D is influenced by a number of factors, including latitude, sun (UV) exposure, age, dress, season of the year, and skin melanin pigment [10,248–250]. Few foods naturally contain vitamin D, including fatty fish (salmon, mackerel, sardines) and some fish liver oils. Almost all of dietary intake of vitamin D comes from fortified milk products (milk, some cheeses, and yogurts) and a few other fortified foods such as some breads, cereals, and juices [249]. In the United States, virtually all milk, regardless of its fat content, is voluntarily fortified with vitamin D at the level of 400 IU (10 μg) per quart [10]. Two cups of vitamin D fortified milk provides 200 IU of vitamin D, the amount recommended for children and adults to age 50.

Current dietary recommendations for vitamin D, as established in 1997 by the Food and Nutrition Board of the IOM are 200 IU (i.e., 5 μg/day) for children, adolescents, and adults up to 50 years of age [10] (Table 5.1). Vitamin D recommendations are twice as high for adults 51 through 70 years (i.e., 400 IU/day or 10 μg/day) and three times higher for adults over 70 years (i.e., 600 IU/day or 15 μg/day) than in earlier adulthood and childhood years [10]. An upper level of vitamin D intake is set at 2000 IU/day (50 μg/day). However, intakes twice as high (4000 IU/day) have been shown to have no adverse health effects and may in fact be more desirable [251,252]. In recent years, accumulating evidence has indicated that the current dietary vitamin D recommendations are inadequate to protect bone health when exposure to sunlight is limited [253–256]. An individual's vitamin D status is determined by measuring serum concentrations of 25-hydroxyvitamin D (25(OH)D), the major circulating form of vitamin D. Optimal blood levels of 25(OH)D may be as high as 80 nmol/L (32 ng/mL) [248,251,253,254]. Some individuals may require higher levels of dietary vitamin D (i.e., $>$ 2200 IU or 55 μg/day) to achieve serum 25(OH)D levels necessary for optimal calcium absorption and bone health [252–254].

The introduction of vitamin D-fortified milk in the 1930s virtually eliminated vitamin D deficiency rickets in the United States. However, there has been a recent resurgence of rickets, especially among African American children, and of increased vitamin D insufficiency among several population groups, including adolescent girls, women, older adults, and some ethnic groups (i.e., dark pigmented persons and Asians due to a reduced ability to produce vitamin D in the skin) [257–262]. Gordon et al. [260], based on a study of a group of 307 multiethnic, healthy adolescents attending a medical clinic in Boston, reported that the prevalence of vitamin D deficiency for the group was 24.1%, with the highest prevalence (35.9%) among African American teenagers. The adolescents who selected soft drinks were at higher risk for vitamin D deficiency, whereas the consumption of milk or cold cereal was protective [260]. A 3-year study of adolescent girls aged 9 to 11 years in Maine found that vitamin D status was low even though the reported dietary intakes of vitamin D were at or near the currently recommended level [257]. The finding led the researchers to suggest that current dietary intake goals for vitamin D are insufficient for people living in northern latitudes who have limited exposure to sunlight and that these people should be encouraged to increase their intake of vitamin D from sources such as vitamin D-fortified milk [257].

Moore et al. [262], using data from the 1999 to 2000 NHANES, found that among adults, only 4% of men and 1% of women aged 51 years of age and older met or exceeded the current dietary recommendation for vitamin D from food sources (Figure 5.17). Low intake of vitamin D fortified milk and other dairy foods (some cheeses, yogurts) is identified as a factor contributing to the increase in vitamin D deficiency and vitamin D-related rickets [263]. The American Academy of Pediatrics, recognizing the continued occurrence of vitamin D-deficiency rickets in children, recommends a dietary intake of 200 IU of vitamin D per day [264]. For children and adolescents who are not regularly exposed to sunlight, do not consume at least 2 cups/day of vitamin D fortified milk, or do not take a daily multivitamin supplement containing at least 200 IU of vitamin D, a supplement of 200 IU of vitamin D/day is recommended [264].

Studies of the effect of vitamin D status or vitamin D supplementation on bone mass in adolescents have yielded inconsistent findings due to differences in study design, means to assess bone, and stage of puberty [265]. Although serum levels of 25(OH)D are used to indicate a person's total vitamin D exposure, there is no consensus regarding the optimum level that would

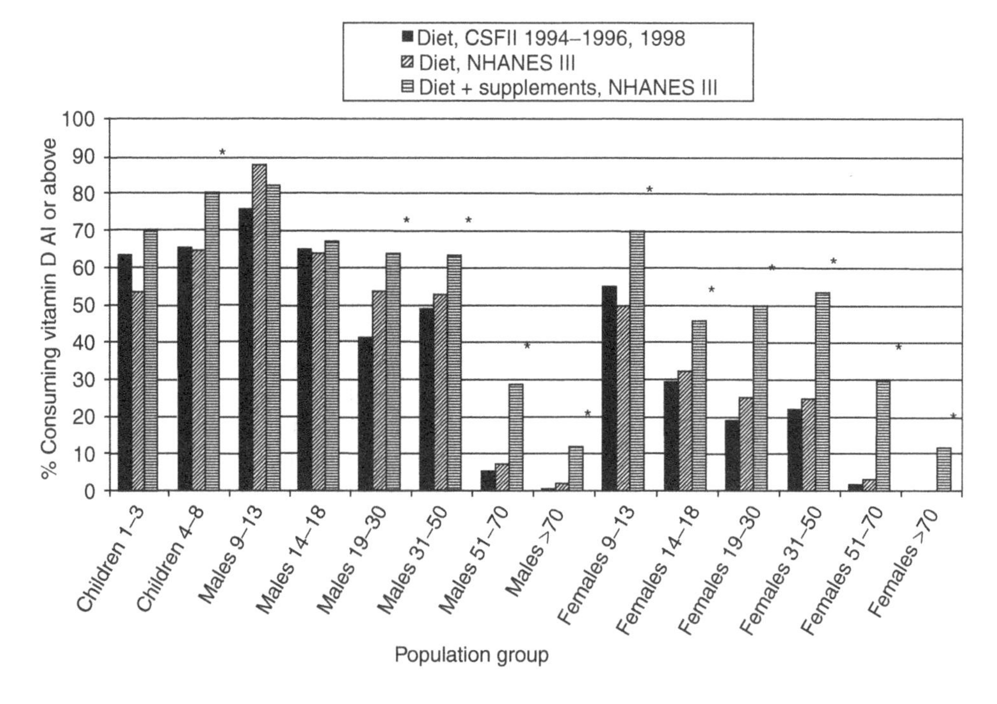

FIGURE 5.17 Percentage of U.S. populations with usual intake of vitamin D from diet alone or diet plus supplements at or above the vitamin D Adequate Intake (AI). (From Moore, C. et al., *J. Am. Diet. Assoc.*, 104, 980, 2004.)

most benefit bone health or that is required to achieve optimum peak bone mass [265,266]. Outila et al. [267], in a cross-sectional study of 178 female adolescents in Finland, found that the girls with serum 25(OH)D levels above 40 nmol/L had greater bone mineral densities at the radial and ulnar sites than did girls with lower levels of 25(OH)D. Cheng and colleagues [268], using the same cut-points for 25(OH)D, showed a progressive increase in cortical bone mineral density with increasing serum levels of 25(OH)D at both the distal radius and tibia shaft. However, this relationship was not observed at other sites when a different method was used to assess bone mineral density. Other researchers have demonstrated that the relationship between 25(OH)D status and bone mineral density in adolescent girls is primarily evident during the premenarcheal, not postmenarcheal, years [269,270]. A cross-sectional investigation of the determinants of peak bone mass in young Finnish men aged 18 to 21 years identified low vitamin D levels in the winter and an association between these low levels and bone mineral content at several sites [271].

Studies indicate that many older adults are at risk of vitamin D deficiency [10,252,272–275]. The aging population, especially those who are housebound, residents of nursing homes, or live in northern climates, may be at risk for vitamin D deficiency because of inadequate dietary intake and/or limited exposure to sunlight without a compensatory increase in dietary vitamin D [249,252,272–277]. Also, several age-related physiological changes in vitamin D metabolism potentially compromise vitamin D status and/or increase the requirement for this vitamin [252]. With advancing age, the capacity of the skin to make cholecalciferol dramatically declines [252]. Also behavioral factors can limit older adults' vitamin D status [252]. Low intake of vitamin D due to decreased consumption of vitamin D enriched-dairy products can contribute to suboptimal vitamin D status in older adults.

Research indicates that vitamin D deficiency in older adults may be more widespread than previously suspected [249,262]. Thomas et al. [278] reported that more than half of 290 hospitalized patients were deficient in vitamin D, even including some patients with high intakes of vitamin D. These findings indicate that even higher vitamin D intakes (i.e., 800 to 1000 IU/day) than currently recommended [10] may be beneficial for some individuals.

Several studies indicate that increasing vitamin D intake of older adults enhances calcium absorption and reduces age-related bone loss or osteoporotic-related bone fractures [202,236,253,279–281]. A meta-analysis of 25 randomized trials of the effect of vitamin D, with or without calcium supplementation, on bone density and fractures in postmenopausal women found that vitamin D reduced the risk of spine fractures by 37% and showed a trend toward reduced incidence of nonvertebral fractures [279]. Ooms et al. [281] reported that increasing vitamin D by 400 IU/day for 2 years slightly decreased parathyroid hormone secretion and increased bone mineral density at the femoral hip. In a study in Finland, where vitamin D deficiency among the aging population is common during the winter months, intramuscular vitamin D injections of single, yearly doses equivalent to 400 to 800 IU/day maintained blood levels of 25-hydroxyvitamin D and reduced the incidence of fractures of the upper limb, but not the lower limb [280].

In a 4-year, placebo-controlled, double-blind trial in older adults, increasing 25(OH) vitamin D_3 by 15 μg/day was more effective than the placebo in reducing bone loss at the hip, but less effective than increasing calcium intake by 750 mg/day [282]. The finding that the effects of vitamin D supplementation were observed only at low calcium intakes suggests that the mechanism for vitamin D's beneficial effect on bone is to reverse calcium insufficiency [282].

A number of the studies examining the effect of vitamin D on bone health have investigated the effect of a combination of vitamin D and calcium intake. Harwood and colleagues [283] found that a combination of vitamin D and calcium was more effective than vitamin D alone in terms of suppressing parathyroid hormone, increasing bone mineral density, and reducing falls in elderly women who had suffered a hip fracture. A double-blind, randomized controlled trial in 120 peri- and postmenopausal Italian women aged 45 to 55 years, demonstrated a beneficial effect of vitamin D and calcium combined on bone mineral density [284].

As discussed above, nonvertebral and hip fractures were reduced by 30% and 41%, respectively, within 2 years in healthy ambulatory elderly women (mean age 84 years) in nursing homes in France, who were supplemented with 800 IU (20 μg) vitamin D and 1200 mg calcium, compared to women receiving a placebo (Figure 5.14) [236]. In a 3-year study of men and women aged 65 years and older, living in New England, increasing calcium intake by 500 mg/day and vitamin D intake by 700 IU/day moderately reduced bone loss at several sites (i.e., hip, spine, total body) and the incidence of nonspine fractures [224].

A meta-analysis that pooled results from five randomized, controlled trials for hip fracture and seven randomized, controlled trials for nonvertebral fracture risk, found that trials using 700 to 800 IU/day of oral vitamin D, with or without calcium supplementation, significantly reduced the risk of hip fractures by 26% and nonvertebral fractures by 23% compared to calcium or a placebo [255]. A vitamin D supplement of 400 IU/day was insufficient to prevent fractures [255]. Because vitamin D intakes in the range of 700 to 800 IU/day are higher than the current vitamin D recommendations of 400 to 600 IU/day for older adults, the researchers suggest that their results support increasing dietary vitamin D intake recommendations. The role of additional calcium together with 700 to 800 IU/day of vitamin D was not clearly defined, but dietary calcium intakes greater than 700 mg/day appeared to be necessary to prevent nonvertebral fractures [255]. Two randomized trials of calcium (1000 mg) plus vitamin D (800 IU) supplements failed to reduce the risk of nonvertebral fractures among older adults with one or more risk factors for fractures or with a previous fracture [285,286]. However, both these trials had very low compliance rates and one study [285] failed to achieve therapeutic blood levels of 25(OH)D. The less than expected benefit of calcium (1000 mg) and vitamin D (400 IU) supplements on hip bone density and hip fractures in certain groups of postmenopausal and older women participating in the Women's Health Initiative clinical trial may be attributed in part to in AI of vitamin D, although a more likely explanation is that there was no calcium control group [205,206].

The decline in fracture risk with vitamin D may be explained in part by vitamin D's ability to reduce the risk of falls [287]. A meta-analysis based on five randomized, controlled trials involving 1237 older adults (average age of 60 years) found that vitamin D supplementation reduced the risk of falls by a statistically significant 22% when compared with patients receiving calcium supplements or a placebo [287]. Adding another five randomized, controlled trials to the analysis reduced the risk reduction to 13%, but the result remained statistically significant.

Clearly, more research is needed to determine the optimal intake of vitamin D, with and without calcium, needed to support bone health in both younger and older people. However, based on available evidence, ensuring an AI of both calcium and vitamin D throughout life is recommended to support bone health [1,10]. Vitamin D-fortified milk and other dairy products (some cheeses and yogurts) are major dietary sources of both these nutrients.

5.6 PROTEIN AND BONE HEALTH

In addition to calcium and vitamin D, dietary protein is an essential nutrient for bone health and osteoporosis prevention [60,61]. About 50% of the volume of bone is protein, and because of extensive, posttranslational modification of the amino acids in protein (e.g., cross-linking), many amino acids released in bone resorption cannot be recycled into new protein synthesis. For this reason, bone repair requires a continuous supply of dietary protein. The dietary protein recommendation is 0.80 g/kg/day for males (56 g/day) and females (46 g/day) aged 19 years and older [288]. Accumulating scientific evidence indicates that increasing protein intake increases bone mineral mass and reduces the incidence of osteoporotic fractures [60,289–294]. When dietary protein (mostly animal protein) and bone mineral density were examined in a 4-year follow-up study of 615 older adults in the Framingham Osteoporosis Study, high protein intake (i.e., within the range commonly consumed) was found to be protective against loss of bone mineral density at the hip and spine compared to low protein intakes [290]. Higher intakes of total and animal protein were significantly associated with increased bone mineral density of the hip and total body in older women participating in a 4-year prospective study in California (291]. According to an epidemiological study of 1077 elderly Australian women (aged 75 years), those who consumed the lowest tertile of protein (<66 g/day) had significantly lower qualitative ultrasound of the heel (1.3%) and hip bone mineral density (2.6%) than did women in the higher tertiles of protein intake (>87 g/day) [294]. These findings led the researchers to suggest that older women may need higher protein intakes than currently recommended to optimize their bone mass [294].

In a 3-year prospective study of more than 30,000 postmenopausal women who participated in the Iowa Women's Health Study, higher protein intake, particularly animal protein, was associated with a 70% reduction in hip fractures, even after controlling for major confounding factors [289]. In an observational case-control study in Utah, higher intakes of protein were shown to reduce the risk of hip fractures in adults aged 50 to 69 years, but not in older adults [292]. Increased protein intake may also help in the healing of fractures and the prevention of bone loss following a fracture [293]. In a 6-month randomized, controlled trial, older adults with a hip fracture and habitually low protein intakes, all received calcium and vitamin D and either a protein supplement (20 g/day) or a placebo [293]. Compared to the placebo group, patients given the protein supplement had less bone loss, improved muscle strength, and a shorter hospital stay [293]. A prospective study in 229 healthy children and adolescents, aged 6 to 18 years, demonstrated that dietary protein was significantly associated with beneficial changes in bone modeling, remodeling, and strength during growth [295].

Some evidence suggests that protein's favorable effect on bone depends on an AI of calcium and vitamin D [296–299]. A study in 342 healthy adults aged 65 years and over, who had completed a 3-year randomized, double-blind, placebo-controlled trial of calcium (500 mg/day) and vitamin D (700 IU/day) supplementation, found that a higher protein intake (20% of energy) resulted in a greater gain in hip and total body bone mineral density if dietary calcium and vitamin D recommendations were also met [296]. Changes in bone mineral density by tertile of protein intake for the calcium and vitamin D supplemented groups (upper panels) and placebo groups (lower panels) are shown in Figure 5.18. The researchers suggest that a higher calcium intake may reduce the negative effect of protein on calcium retention [296]. In a cohort of women enrolled in a 3-year osteoporosis intervention trial, higher (71 g/day) vs. lower (54 g/day) baseline protein intakes were associated with higher bone mineral densities of the spine, arm, and total body in those who consumed more than 408 mg calcium/day [299]. However, findings from other studies fail to support these findings [291,300]. Additional research is therefore needed to clarify the interaction between protein and calcium intake on bone health [60,301].

Although the mechanism(s) is unknown, protein's favorable effect on bone may be explained by its ability to provide amino acid substrates for bone formation and remodeling [301]. Another mechanism may relate to dietary protein's ability to increase the production of insulin-like growth factor-1 (IGF-1), a hormone that stimulates bone formation [293,302]. Dawson-Hughes et al. [302], in a study of the effect of protein on calcium excretion in healthy older adults, found that increased protein intake increased the circulating level of IGF-1 and significantly reduced the urinary excretion of N-telopeptide, a marker of bone resorption.

Milk is a unique source of protein because its calcium content is high in relation to its protein content (i.e., 36:1). A dietary calcium to protein ratio equal to or greater than 20:1 (mg/g) is thought to provide adequate protection for the skeleton [63]. Because protein exists in close association with other nutrients in the diet (e.g., calcium, phosphorus, magnesium, vitamin D, and potassium), the overall dietary pattern impacts protein's effect on bone health [11,233,295,303].

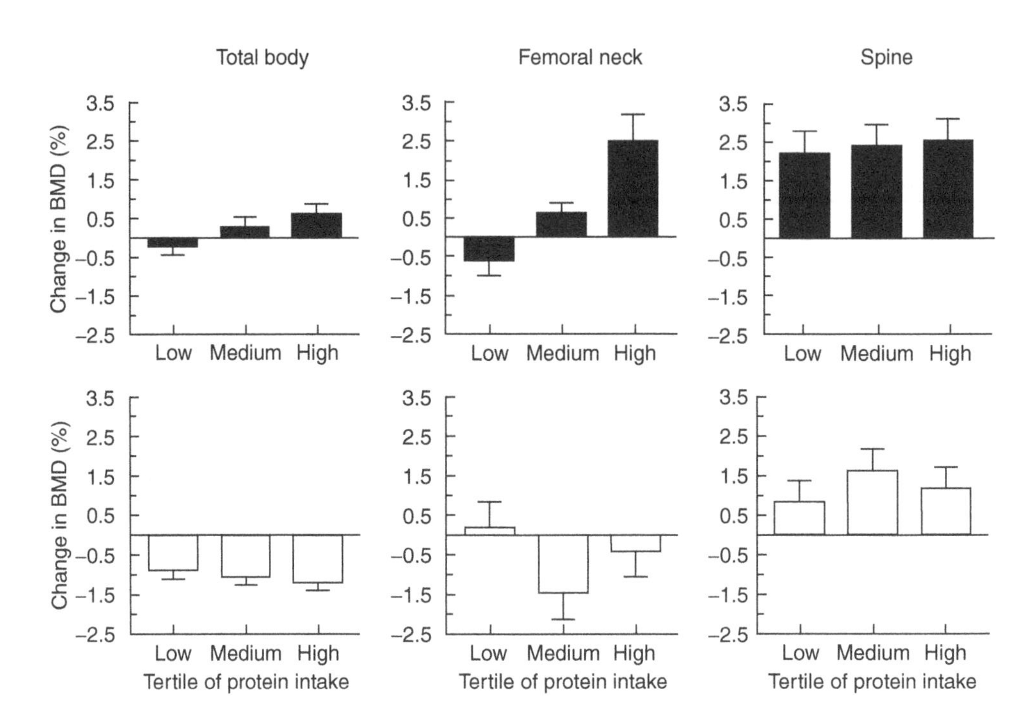

FIGURE 5.18 The association of protein intake with rates of bone loss in older adults treated for 3 years with 500 mg of calcium as calcium citrate malate and 700 IU of vitamin D (as solid bars) and with placebo (open bars). For the total body there was a significant interaction of treatment group x protein tertile ($P = 0.044$). (From Dawson-Hughes, B. and Harris, S. S., *Am. J. Clin. Nutr.*, 75, 773, 2002.)

5.7 ADDITIONAL NUTRIENTS AND BONE HEALTH

In addition to calcium, vitamin D, and protein, milk and other dairy foods are an important source of several other bone-supporting nutrients, such as phosphorus, magnesium, potassium, vitamin B_{12}, and trace elements such as zinc [1,10,11,304]. For information on dairy's contribution to intake of these nutrients, refer to Chapter 1. As mentioned above, interactions among calcium, vitamin D, and protein impact their individual effect on bone health. The same holds true for other nutrients discussed below, although these have been investigated to a lesser extent [233,305]. Prevention of osteoporosis through diet is complex and involves many nutrients and other food components [306].

Bone mineral consists of calcium phosphate, and phosphorus is as important as calcium for both mineralization and maintenance of the skeleton [1,10]. Phosphorus intake does not appear to influence skeletal homeostasis within normal ranges of intake [304]. Whiting et al. [233] reported that in adult men consuming adequate dietary calcium (1200+/− 515 mg/day), a diet plentiful in phosphorus (1741+/− 535 mg/day) was beneficial for maintaining bone mineral density. However, excess phosphorus intake (particularly when combined with a low calcium intake) or a low phosphorus intake may be deleterious to the skeleton [307,308]. Epidemiological studies have demonstrated lower bone mineral density in population groups (i.e., postmenopausal women, peri-menopausal women, men) consuming high phosphorus, low calcium diets. Although most attention has focused on the effect of excess phosphorus intake on bone health, a low phosphorus intake is also a concern [307,308]. Researchers at Creighton University in Omaha, Nebraska, found that an increase in calcium primarily from supplements that did not contain phosphorus reduced dietary phosphorus absorption, thereby increasing the risk of phosphorus insufficiency [308].

Because many older adults have diets low in phosphorus and older patients with osteoporosis often consume calcium supplements without phosphorus, which can decrease dietary phosphorus absorption, the researchers recommend a combination of calcium and phosphorus (e.g., calcium phosphate supplements instead of calcium carbonate or citrate) [308]. The ratio of phosphorus to calcium is thought to be more important for bone health than the intake of phosphorus alone [308,309]. Milk and many other dairy products are not only a rich source of calcium, but also a major source of phosphorus in the diet [14].

Magnesium appears to play a role in calcium and bone metabolism [1,10,11,304,305]. Animal studies demonstrate that magnesium deficiency adversely affects bone development, and some epidemiological studies have found that magnesium intake is positively associated with bone health [11,304,310,311]. Tucker et al. [310] found that magnesium intake was positively associated with hip bone mineral density in a cohort of elderly men and women participating in the Framingham Heart Study. In a cross-sectional study of more than 2000 adults aged 70 to 79 years, higher magnesium intakes (from food and supplements) were associated with a greater bone mineral density among Caucasian, but not African American, adults [311]. More research, particularly well-controlled clinical trials, is needed to better determine magnesium's effect on bone health in humans [10,11].

Potassium also has a role in bone health [1,312]. Americans' dietary intake of potassium is considerably lower than the recommended intake of 4.7 g/day (120 mmol/day) [312]. A number of epidemiological studies and a few intervention investigations indicate that increased potassium intake is associated with increased bone mineral density [1,312]. In longitudinal studies, potassium intake has been shown to be positively associated with bone mineral density at various sites [310,313]. A Western diet (i.e., high in protein and low in calcium) generates a large amount of acid, which, without sufficient alkaline-forming foods in the diet (i.e., potassium-containing foods such as dairy foods, fruits, vegetables), may adversely affect bone health. Because measurement of acid-base balance is not practical in large population studies, algorithms based on the ratio of protein to potassium have been used to estimate net endogenous acid production (NEAP). NEAP may be related to potassium intake and bone density. In the United Kingdom, MacDonald et al. [313] investigated the relationship between dietary potassium and protein, NEAP, and potential renal acid load, and markers of bone health in more than 3000 perimenopausal and early postmenopausal women. Low dietary potassium and high dietary estimates of NEAP were associated with low bone mineral density in premenopausal women and increased markers of bone resorption in postmenopausal women. The researchers conclude that dietary potassium may modestly influence markers of bone health, which over time may contribute to decreased risk of osteoporosis [314].

Dietary potassium (i.e., potassium citrate) has been shown to ameliorate the hypercalciuria and concomitant higher bone resorption seen with high salt diets [58,312,315]. Much remains to be learned about potassium's potential bone protective effect. Increasing potassium intake decreases urinary calcium excretion [1,304]. However, a study in a cohort of about 650 women, with a mean age of 50.2 years, found that dietary potassium also reduced intestinal calcium absorption [316]. Thus, potassium may not exert any beneficial effect on calcium balance because the reduced calciuria is offset by the reduction in calcium absorption. Potassium's benefit for bones may be related to its alkaline producing characteristic (i.e., its ability to buffer the acid load from Western type diets).

Vitamin B_{12} is another nutrient found in dairy products which may have a beneficial role in bone health [317,318]. Tufts University researchers measured vitamin B_{12} levels and bone mineral density in more than 2500 adults participating in the Framingham Offspring Osteoporosis study [317]. Both men and women with low vitamin B_{12} levels had lower bone mineral densities than those with higher vitamin B_{12} levels. A study of frail elderly adults in The Netherlands found that osteoporosis occurred more often in women (but not men) with marginal or deficient vitamin B_{12} status than in those with normal vitamin B_{12} status [318]. Considering that vitamin B_{12} deficiency is common in older adults, it is important that additional studies be conducted to learn more about the role of this vitamin in bone health.

Trace elements and other components in dairy foods may also contribute to bone health [304]. The role of zinc in bone formation is well documented in animal models, and low zinc intakes and reduced blood zinc concentrations have been reported to be associated with osteoporosis in humans [11,304,319]. Certain fatty acid components in milk fat may contribute to bone health. In the first study to evaluate the relationship between dietary conjugated linoleic acid (CLA) and bone health in humans, dietary CLA, particularly the c9t11-CLA isomer (rumenic acid), which is abundant in dairy products that contain fat, was positively associated with bone mineral density in postmenopausal women [320]. In this cross-sectional analysis of 136 Caucasian, healthy, postmenopausal women, average age of 69 years, usual intake of dietary CLA — i.e., 63 mg/day or the amount found in two cups of 1% milk plus 1 ounce of Cheddar cheese — was associated with higher hip and forearm bone mineral densities [320].

Because many nutrients in addition to calcium and vitamin D are related to bone health, it is important to consume a well-balanced diet containing a variety of foods, rather than focusing on single nutrients, to achieve and maintain a healthy skeleton [1,126]. Intake of a dietary pattern such as the DASH diet — a low-fat, calcium-rich diet that emphasizes fruits, vegetables, and 3 servings of dairy products a day — has been shown to significantly decrease bone turnover in adults aged 23 to 76 years, which immediately reduces fragility and, if sustained, may improve bone mineral status [56]. The researchers speculate that the skeletal benefit of the DASH diet is due to the presence of multiple bone-active nutrients (e.g., calcium, protein, potassium, magnesium) together in foods [56].

5.8 THE DAIRY ADVANTAGE

As indicated above, many nutrients are essential for bone health. For this reason, it is important to consume a well-balanced diet containing a variety of foods, including dairy products and other calcium-rich foods, fruits and vegetables, grains, and meat or beans each day [1,20]. Among the nutritional factors involved in bone health, calcium — a nutrient in short supply in many Americans' diets [71] — is identified as the nutrient most important for preventing and treating osteoporosis [1,2,10]. Calcium can be obtained from foods naturally rich in this nutrient, calcium-fortified foods and beverages, and/or supplements [1,82]. Foods naturally containing nutrients such as calcium are considered to be the best source of calcium for health. Calcium-fortified foods and calcium supplements are a supplement to, not a substitute for, foods naturally containing calcium such as dairy foods.

5.8.1 Foods Naturally Containing Calcium

Government and health professional organizations, as well as leading nutrition and medical experts, recommend foods, particularly dairy foods, as the preferred source of calcium, primarily because bone health is not a mononutrient issue.

A 1994 National Institutes for Health (NIH) Consensus Panel on Optimal Calcium Intake [5] stated that "... the preferred approach to attaining optimal calcium intake is through dietary sources." The panel specifically identified dairy products as the ideal source of calcium in the diet. The NIH's National Institute of Child Health and Human Development encourages consumption of at least three cups of low-fat or fat-free milk and milk products every day for strong bones and lifelong health [321]. This government agency has undertaken an educational effort called "Milk Matters" to increase calcium awareness among pediatricians and other health care professionals, as well as children, adolescents, and their parents [321]. The IOM, in its dietary recommendations for calcium and related nutrients, recognizes the importance of "unfortified foodstuffs" as the major source of calcium [10]. The IOM explains that meeting calcium needs through foods offers such advantages as providing intake of other beneficial nutrients and unidentified food components and possibly enhancing the body's use of nutrients through nutrient interactions [10].

The U.S. Department of Health and Human Services' report, *Healthy People 2010,* also recognizes dietary sources of calcium [322]. This report states that "with current food selection practices, use of dairy products may constitute the difference between getting enough calcium in one's diet or not" [322]. The 2005 *Dietary Guidelines for Americans*, issued jointly by the U.S. Department of Health and Human Services and the U.S. Department of Agriculture, recommends that Americans 9 years of age and older consume 3 cups a day of fat-free or low-fat milk, or equivalent milk products [i.e., cheese, yogurt], as part of a healthful diet [20]. For children 2 through 8 years, 2 cups a day of fat-free or low-fat milk, or equivalent milk products, is recommended [20]. The 2005 *Dietary Guidelines for Americans* recognizes that consumption of milk products is associated with "overall diet quality and adequacy of intake of many nutrients" and is "especially important to bone health during childhood and adolescence" [20]. The 2004 U.S. Surgeon General's report on *Bone Health and Osteoporosis* recommends 3 daily servings of low-fat milk to help build better bodies and stronger bones [1].

Several health professional organizations recommend food, and in particular milk and other dairy products, as the preferred source of calcium. The American Medical Association states that "... inclusion of low-fat dairy products in the diet is the most desirable way to meet calcium goals" [6]. The ADA recognizes that the best strategy to meet nutrient needs is to choose wisely from a wide variety of foods [323]. In a position statement on nutrition and women's health, ADA and Dietitians of Canada state that "Inclusion of low-fat dairy products in the diet is the most desirable way to meet calcium goals. With the recent increases in requirements, it is difficult to achieve an AI when dairy products are eliminated from the diet" [217]. The National Medical Association, the nation's oldest and largest organization representing African American physicians, recommends that the American public in general, and African Americans in particular, consume 3 to 4 servings of low-fat milk, cheese, or yogurt a day to help reduce the risk of nutrient-related chronic diseases, including osteoporosis, and to improve health [23]. The NAMS recommends dietary sources of calcium as the preferred way to meet adequate calcium needs because of the presence of other essential nutrients found in high-calcium foods [218]. The Society states that dairy products are among the best sources of calcium due to their high calcium content and bioavailability, and their relatively low cost [218]. The American Academy of Pediatrics, in its report on optimizing bone health and calcium intakes of infants, children, and adolescents, recommends three 8-ounce glasses of milk a day or the equivalent (cheese, yogurt) for children 4 to 8 years of age, and four 8- to 10-ounce glasses of milk (or the equivalent) for adolescents [24]. Flavored milks, cheeses, and yogurts containing reduced fat or no fat and modest amounts of added sweeteners (caloric and noncaloric) are recommended [24]. The American Academy of Pediatrics recognizes dairy foods as the preferred source of calcium for children and adolescents [24]. For children and adolescents who do not drink milk, the American Academy of Pediatrics recommends alternative sources, such as nondairy calcium rich foods and supplements, but cautions that "these products do not offer the benefits of other associated nutrients, and compliance may be a problem" [24].

Numerous nutrition and medical experts recommend foods as the best source of calcium for health [7,9,16,82,241]. According to Robert Heaney, M.D., a noted calcium researcher, "While it is possible to arrange an adequate diet using available Western foods, it is usually difficult to do so without including dairy produces. Few individuals succeed and, in general, a diet low in dairy foods means a diet that is poor in several respects beyond insufficiency of calcium" [7]. Also, dairy foods, particularly milk and yogurt, are considered to be an economical way to get calcium and other nutrients in a single package [7,9].

Dairy foods such as milk, cheese, and yogurt are the major dietary source of calcium (Table 5.5) [1,12]. These foods provide 72% of the calcium available in the U.S. food supply [13]. A diet without dairy foods provides only about 250 to 300 mg calcium a day [1,15]. Not only are milk and

TABLE 5.5
Selected Food Sources of Calcium

Food	Calcium (mg)	%DV[a]
Sardines, canned in oil, with bones, 3 oz	324	32%
Cheddar cheese, 1½ oz shredded	306	31%
Milk, nonfat, 8 fl oz	302	30%
Yogurt, plain, low-fat, 8 oz	300	30%
Milk, reduced fat (2% milk fat), no solids, 8 fl oz	297	30%
Milk, whole (3.25% milk fat), 8 fl oz	291	29%
Milk, buttermilk, 8 fl oz	285	29%
Milk lactose reduced 8 fl oz (content varies according to fat content; average = 300 mg)	285–302	29–30%
Cottage cheese, 1% milk fat, 2 cups unpacked	276	28%
Mozzarella, part skim 1½ oz	275	28%
Tofu, firm, w/calcium, ½ cup[b]	204	20%
Orange juice, calcium fortified, 6 fl oz	200–260	20–26%
Salmon, pink, canned, solids with bone, 3 oz	181	18%
Pudding, chocolate, instant, made with w/2% milk, ½ cup	153	15%
Tofu, soft, w/calcium, ½ cup[b]	138	14%
Breakfast drink, orange flavor, powder prepared with water, 8 fl oz	133	13%
Frozen yogurt, vanilla, soft serve, ½ cup	103	10%
Ready to eat cereal, calcium fortified, 1 cup	100–1000	10 to 100%
Turnip greens, boiled, ½ cup	99	10%
Kale, raw, 1 cup	90	9%
Kale, cooked, 1 cup	94	9%
Ice cream, vanilla, ½ cup	85	8.5%
Soy beverage, calcium fortified, 8 fl oz	80–500	8–50%
Chinese cabbage, raw, 1 cup	74	7%
Tortilla, corn, ready to bake/fry, 1 medium	42	4%
Tortilla, flour, ready to bake/fry, one 6" diameter	37	4%
Sour cream, reduced fat, cultured, 2 tbsp	32	3%
Bread, white, 1 oz	31	3%
Broccoli, raw, ½ cup	21	2%
Bread, whole wheat, 1 slice	20	2%
Cheese, cream, regular, 1 tbsp	12	1%

Daily Values (DV) were developed to help consumers determine if a typical serving of a food contains a lot or a little of a specific nutrient. The DV for calcium is based on 1000 mg. The percent DV (% DV) listed on the nutrition facts panel of food labels tells you what percentages of the DV are provided in one serving. For instance, if you consumed a food that contained 300 mg of calcium, the DV would be 30% for calcium on the food label. A food providing 5% of the DV or less is a low source while a food that provides 10% to 19% of the DV is a good source and a food that provides 20% of the DV or more is an excellent source for a nutrient. For foods not listed in this table, see the U.S. Department of Agriculture's Nutrient Database Web site: www.nal.usda.gov/fnic/cgi-bin/nut_search.pl.

[a] DV, Daily Value.

[b] Calcium values are only for tofu processed with a calcium salt. Tofu processed with a noncalcium salt will not contain significant amounts of calcium.

Source: From Department of Health and Human Services; Office of the Surgeon General, Bone Health and Osteoporosis. A Report of the Surgeon General, Rockville, MD, 2004, p. 161.

other dairy products calcium-dense foods, providing about 300 mg calcium per serving, but these foods also contain other nutrients important for bone health such as vitamin D (if fortified), protein, phosphorus, magnesium, potassium, vitamin B_{12}, and trace elements such as zinc [12]. Consuming at least the recommended number of servings of dairy foods each day improves the overall nutritional adequacy of the diet [15–19,213] (see Chapter 1). Additionally, dairy foods can improve the nutritional quality of the diet without significantly increasing total calorie or fat intake, body weight, or percent body fat [16–18] (see Chapter 1).

Although consuming recommended servings of dairy foods is the easiest way to meet calcium needs, a number of nondairy foods such as salmon with bones, some green leafy vegetables such as broccoli, beans (pinto, red, white), bok choy, sweet potatoes, rhubarb, and corn tortillas naturally contain calcium (Table 5.5) [12,69]. However, these foods generally contain less calcium per serving than do milk and other dairy products [12,69]. Therefore, larger servings of many nondairy foods containing calcium may be needed to equal the calcium intake from a typical serving of milk or other dairy food. Also, the bioavailability of calcium from foods varies widely, from a low of approximately 5% in spinach to more than 50% in some vegetables such as bok choy and broccoli (Table 5.6) [69,82]. However, the high absorbability of calcium from a particular food cannot overcome its low calcium content [10]. The bioavailability of calcium from some nondairy foods is lower than that from dairy foods because of the presence of food components such as phytates and oxalates [69,82]. Phytates in unleavened bread, seeds, nuts, and most cereals, and oxalates in spinach, rhubarb, and sweet potatoes can form insoluble complexes with calcium, reducing its bioavailability [1,69,82]. Researchers at Purdue University found that an individual would need to consume 16 servings (8 cups) of spinach, nearly 10 servings (5 cups) of red beans, or 4.5 servings (2¼ cups) of broccoli to obtain the same amount of calcium *absorbed* from 1 cup of milk (Table 5.6) [69,82]. A food's contribution to meeting calcium needs depends on its calcium content, calcium bioavailability, and frequency of consumption.

5.8.2 Calcium-Fortified Foods

For individuals who have difficulty meeting their calcium needs from foods naturally containing calcium (e.g., dairy products) and want to supplement their intake, a number of calcium-fortified foods and beverages are available [1,2]. Orange juice, juice drinks, cereals, waffles, snack foods, spreads/margarines, candy, water, and dairy products are among the foods fortified with calcium. Calcium-fortified foods and beverages can be a reasonable option to help some people increase their low calcium intake [323]. However, concerns have been raised regarding the widespread availability and types of calcium-fortified foods and beverages [82,324–326]. These concerns center on the inability of calcium-fortified foods to correct a poor dietary pattern, the risk of calcium excess, unknown calcium bioavailability, and potential negative effects of excessive high calcium diets on other nutrients such as trace elements.

Low calcium diets are generally low in several other nutrients and are the result of poor food choices, not the unavailability of calcium-rich foods in the food supply. Fortification of a food or beverage with a single nutrient such as calcium will not correct a poor dietary pattern [16]. The American Academy of Pediatrics, in a statement on the use and misuse of fruit juice for healthy infants and young children, cautions that calcium-fortified juices provide a bioavailable source of calcium, but lack other nutrients found in cow's milk [327]. Individuals using calcium-fortified foods, particularly low nutrient foods such as candy, snack foods, or water, may be misled into believing that these calcium-fortified foods are an adequate substitute for milk and other dairy foods and that they ensure a healthy diet. The FDA discourages fortification of low nutrient dense foods because of the risk that people consuming such fortified products will ignore the rest of their diet, resulting in nutrient deficiencies [328].

TABLE 5.6
Comparison of Sources for Bioavailable Calcium

Source	Serving Size[a] (g)	Calcium Content[b] (mg/serving)	Estimated Absorption Efficiency[c](%)	Absorbable C a/Serving[d] (mg)	Servings Needed to = 1 Cup Milk
Foods					
Milk	240	290	32.1		1.0
Beans, pinto	86	44.7	26.7	11.9	8.1
Beans, red	172	40.5	24.4	9.9	9.7
Beans, white	110	113	21.8	24.7	3.9
Bok choy	85	79	53.8	42.5	2.3
Broccoli	71	35	61.3	21.5	4.5
Cheddar cheese	42	303	32.1	97.2	1.0
Cheese food	42	241	32.1	77.4	1.2
Chinese cabbage flower leaves	85	239	39.6	94.7	1.0
Chinese mustard green	85	212	40.2	85.3	1.1
Chinese spinach	85	347	8.36	29	3.3
Kale	85	61	49.3	30.1	3.2
Spinach	85	115	5.1	5.9	16.3
Sugar cookies	15	3	91.9	2.76	34.9
Sweet potatoes	164	44	22.2	9.8	9.8
Rhubarb	120	174	8.54	10.1	9.5
Whole wheat bread	28	20	82.0	16.6	5.8
Wheat bran cereal	28	20	38.0	7.54	12.8
Yogurt	240	300	32.1	96.3	1.0
Fortified foods					
Tofu, calcium set	126	258	31.0	80.0	1.2
Orange juice with Ca citrate malate	240	300	36.3	109	0.88
Soy milk with tricalcium phosphate	240	300	24	72	1.3
Bread with calcium sulfate	16.8	300	43.0	129	0.74

[a] Based on a one-half cup serving size (~85 g for green leafy vegetables) except for milk and fruit punch (1 cup or 240 mL) and cheese (1.5oz).

[b] Taken from refs. 10 and 11 (averaged for beans and broccoli processed in different ways) except for the Chinese vegetables, which were analyzed in out laboratory.

[c] Adjusted for load using the equation for milk (fractional absorption = 0.889 − 0.0964 In load [23]) then adjusting for the ratio of calcium absorption of the test food relative to milk tested at the same load, the absorptive index.

[d] Calculated as calcium content × fractional absorption.

Source: From Weaver, C. M. and Heaney, R. P., In: *Calcium in Human Health*, Weaver, C. M. and Heaney, R. P., Eds., Humana Press, Totawa, NJ, 2006, p. 137.

The widespread availability of many calcium-fortified foods and beverages, many of which are fortified at high levels and/or are not normally a source of this mineral, may lead to calcium excess [82,324–326,329]. The window between dietary recommendations for calcium (i.e., 1000 to 1300 mg/day) and the "Tolerable Upper Intake Level," or UL of 2500 mg calcium/day, is relatively small [10]. In particular, excess calcium intake could readily result if calcium-fortified foods are added to a diet already containing generous amounts of calcium-rich foods such as milk and cheese [324,325,329]. Risk of calcium excess from calcium-fortified foods, for certain subgroups of the population already meeting or close to meeting their calcium recommendations (e.g., adolescent and young adult men), is increased [325]. The National Academy of Sciences, IOM, recognizing the increase in the availability of calcium-fortified foods, states that "... it is important to maintain surveillance of the calcium-fortified products in the marketplace and monitor their impact on calcium intake" [10]. To be safe and effective, calcium-fortified foods should reach individuals in need, without contributing to excess calcium intakes in others.

Another consideration is the bioavailability of calcium from calcium-fortified foods. Few calcium-fortified foods have been tested for bioavailability, and even fewer have been tested for their effectiveness on bone [82]. In general, calcium absorption is most efficient when consumed in doses of 500 mg or less [1]. Some cereals are fortified with calcium levels as high as 600 and 1000 mg/cup. A serving of these cereals with ½ cup of milk provides either 750 or 1150 mg calcium. Calcium absorption from this high intake consumed at a single time is likely to be lower than multiple calcium intakes of 500 mg or less.

A variety of calcium salts are used to fortify foods and beverages. Although the bioavailability of calcium form various salts is similar to that from milk [330], calcium bioavailability from calcium-fortified foods may differ from that expected. For example, calcium-fortified soy beverages may not be comparable to cow's milk as a source of calcium [331], although it depends on the fortificant used [332]. Because soy beverages naturally contain very little calcium (i.e., about 10 mg per serving), they are often fortified with calcium, with levels varying from 80 to 500 mg per serving [333]. In a study of healthy men, Heaney et al. [331] found that calcium absorption from a tricalcium phosphate-fortified soy beverage was 25% lower than that of cow's milk. In contrast, in a study in healthy young adult women, calcium bioavailability from calcium carbonate fortified soy beverage was similar to that of cow's milk [332]. Heaney et al. [333] compared the calcium content and solubility of 14 calcium-fortified beverages (i.e., soy and rice beverages, orange juice) and unfortified, fat-free milk. Milk was rated as the most reliable calcium source. In contrast, much of the calcium in fortified soy and rice beverages settled to the bottom of the containers and could not be resolubilized even after shaking [333]. Based on their findings, the researchers concluded that the quality of calcium fortification is "uneven at best, with the result that consumers are likely to be misled with respect to ... any calcium benefit" [333]. Initial analysis of the physical state of fortificants in some beverages showed that the total calcium content would fall short of the labeled content. The researchers recommended that the beverage industry develop standards to ensure a uniform, high quality of calcium fortification [333].

Although there is some concern that fortifying foods with large quantities of calcium may adversely affect the utilization of other essential nutrients such as iron, zinc, and magnesium, the evidence is inconclusive [10]. More research is needed to determine whether or not a high intake of calcium results in calcium-mineral interactions that adversely affect the mineral status of vulnerable populations.

5.8.3 Supplements

Nutrients such as calcium should be obtained from food first whenever possible [1,9,20,24,82,323,326]. However, calcium supplements may help some individuals meet their recommended intakes of calcium if they do not consume an AI of dairy products or other calcium-rich foods [1,10,323].

Individuals who are considering taking calcium supplements should determine whether or not supplements are necessary and, if so, which calcium supplement is best [16]. Other considerations include the elemental calcium content, absorption, dose and timing, potential side effects, and compliance [16,326]. There are many different forms (caplets, tablets, chewables, liquids) and formulations of calcium supplements. Calcium carbonate is the most common preparation; others include tricalcium phosphate, dicalcium phosphate, calcium citrate-malate, calcium lactate, and calcium gluconate [334]. Calcium preparations differ widely in their percentage of calcium. Calcium carbonate contains 40% calcium, whereas only 9% of calcium gluconate is calcium [16,334]. Some calcium supplements may contain vitamin D, which helps the body absorb calcium, as well as other nutrients such as magnesium. Several factors such as solubility, timing of intake, and meal conditions can influence the bioavailability of calcium from calcium supplements [16,334]. In general, all major forms of calcium (e.g., carbonate, citrate) are absorbed well when taken with meals [1]. Calcium from supplements (or fortified foods) is best absorbed when taken in several small doses (e.g., 500 mg at a time) throughout the day [1,16].

Cost is another factor that can influence the choice of a calcium supplement [1,16]. The cost of calcium supplements of comparable quality can vary by fivefold [1]. Calcium carbonate supplements tend to be the least expensive. Use of calcium supplements may contribute to potential side effects including constipation and bloating, especially at intakes over two g/day, as well as nutrient imbalances [324,334]. Also, intake of calcium supplements may increase the risk of kidney stones, whereas consumption of dairy products may be protective [207–209]. High intakes of calcium from supplements (and fortified foods) which do not contain phosphorus (as do dairy products) could potentially reduce phosphorus absorption and the effectiveness of bone-enhancing agents currently used to prevent and treat osteoporosis [308]. Because some calcium supplements can diminish the effectiveness of some medications, individuals should talk to their physician or pharmacist regarding drug-nutrient interactions [16,323].

When choosing a calcium supplement, check the label for U.S.P. (U.S. Pharmacopia) designation, which signifies that the calcium supplement meets voluntary standards for quality (i.e., purity, composition) [16,323]. Also, increasing reliance on calcium supplements to meet calcium needs presupposes a relatively high level of compliance. In addition, if calcium supplements are substituted for calcium-rich foods such as dairy products to meet calcium needs, attention should be given to other nutrients provided by foods [16]. As pointed out by Lichtenstein and Russell [326], an advantage of food sources of nutrients, as opposed to supplements, is that foods may contain beneficial nutrients or biologically active factors that have yet to be identified.

Educating the public about how to best meet calcium needs is of high importance. The public needs to understand how to evaluate the nutritional adequacy of their diets using food labels, how to improve their intake of foods naturally containing calcium, and, if necessary, how to use calcium-fortified foods and/or calcium supplements to help close the calcium gap without risk of calcium toxicity or other adverse health effects.

5.9 SUMMARY

Building and maintaining a healthy skeleton throughout life reduces the risk of osteoporosis, the most common bone disease [1]. Osteoporosis is characterized by reduced bone mass, structural deterioration, and excessive bone remodeling leading to increased bone fragility and susceptibility to fractures. This disease affects 44 million U.S. adults over the age of 50 and incurs direct health care costs of up to $18 billion a year [1]. Given the aging population, these health care costs will continue to escalate if preventive measures are not taken to decrease osteoporosis. According to the U.S. Surgeon General's first-ever report on *Bone Health and Osteoporosis*, it is never too early or too late to take measures to improve your bone health [1]. The report calls for effective strategies, particularly improved nutrition and physical activity, throughout life to prevent and manage osteoporosis.

Calcium and vitamin D are the major contributors to bone health for individuals of all ages [1]. Unfortunately, intake of these nutrients falls below the levels recommended for many population groups [71]. Consumption of dairy foods such as milk, cheese, and yogurt, which are the major dietary source of calcium and vitamin D (if fortified), enhance intakes of calcium and vitamin D [14,15,75]. In addition to these nutrients, milk and other dairy foods are an important source of several other nutrients which have a beneficial role in bone health [1].

As reviewed in this chapter, studies at all stages of the lifecycle — from childhood to later adult years — support the role of dairy foods and dairy food nutrients, especially calcium and vitamin D, in building and maintaining healthy bones. A high intake of calcium, especially from dairy foods, has been demonstrated to maximize genetically determined peak bone mass, which for most of the skeleton is reached by age 30 or earlier; to maintain skeletal mass in adulthood; and to slow age-related bone loss and/or reduce fracture risk in later adult years. AI of vitamin D-fortified milk and other dairy foods (i.e., some cheeses, yogurts) may help prevent rickets in young children and vitamin D insufficiency in some population groups, and reduce the risk of osteoporosis in adults. Studies also indicate a beneficial role for other nutrients in dairy foods such as protein, phosphorus, magnesium, potassium, vitamin B_{12}, and zinc in skeletal health.

Because multiple nutrients, and perhaps unidentified components in foods, are involved in skeletal health, government and health professional organizations and leading nutrition and medical experts recommend foods (e.g., dairy foods) as the preferred source of nutrients for bone health. In recent years, there has been a growing body of scientific evidence in support of consuming at least 3 servings of dairy foods a day for healthy bones. The 2005 *Dietary Guidelines for Americans* acknowledges the important role of dairy foods in the diet and recommends that Americans 9 years of age and older consume 3 cups/day of fat-free or low-fat milk, or equivalent milk products (i.e., cheese, yogurt), as part of a healthful diet [20]. This recommendation is consistent with that in other reports. The U.S. Surgeon General's report on *Bone Health and Osteoporosis* [1] recommends 3 daily servings of low-fat milk to help build better bodies and stronger bones. In a consensus report, the National Medical Association, the nation's oldest and largest organization representing African American physicians, recommends that the American public in general, and African Americans in particular, consume 3 to 4 servings of low-fat milk, cheese, or yogurt a day to help reduce the risk of nutrient-related chronic diseases, including osteoporosis [23]. The American Academy of Pediatrics, in a report on optimizing bone health and calcium intakes of infants, children, and adolescents, recommends three 8-ounce glasses of milk a day or the equivalent (i.e., cheese, yogurt) for children 4 to 8 years of age, and four 8-to-10 ounce glasses of milk (or the equivalent) for adolescents [24].

Although significant strides have been made in recent years in our understanding of how nutrition impacts bone health, too few people consume healthful diets and follow lifestyles supportive of a healthy skeleton. Therefore, the dairy industry, with leading health professional organizations, launched a multiyear campaign called 3-A-Day of Dairy for Stronger Bones (www.3aday.org) as a call to action to establish positive eating behaviors including 3 daily servings of calcium-rich milk, cheese, or yogurt. This health and wellness campaign is supported by the following health professional organizations: the American Academy of Family Physicians, the American Academy of Pediatrics, the ADA, and the National Medical Association. To optimize bone health, a total healthful diet, including 3 servings a day of dairy foods, as well as recommended servings of a variety of foods from the other major food groups, and a healthful lifestyle which includes physical activity, are recommended [1].

REFERENCES

1. U.S. Department of Health and Human Services, *Bone Health and Osteoporosis: A Report of the Surgeon General*, U.S. Department of Health and Human Services, Office of the Surgeon General, Rockville, MD, 2004.
2. National Institutes of Health (NIH), Consensus Development Panel on Osteoporosis Prevention, Diagnosis, and Therapy, Osteoporosis prevention, diagnosis, and therapy, *JAMA*, 285, 785, 2001.
3. National Institutes of Health, *Osteoporosis and Related Bone Diseases,* National Resource Center (www.osteo.org).
4. National Osteoporosis Foundation, *Physicians' Guide to Prevention and Treatment of Osteoporosis*, National Osteoporosis Foundation, Washington, D.C., 2003.

5. U.S. Department of Health and Human Services, Public Health Service, National Institutes of Health, Consensus Development Conference Statement, Optimal Calcium Intake, June 6–8, 12 (4), 1994.
6. American Medical Association, Council on Scientific Affairs, Intake of dietary calcium to reduce the incidence of osteoporosis, *Arch. Fam. Med.*, 6, 495, 1997.
7. Heaney, R. P., Calcium, dairy products and osteoporosis, *J. Am. Coll. Nutr.*, 19, 83s, 2000.
8. Heaney, R. P., The importance of calcium intake for lifelong skeletal health, *Calcif. Tissue Int.*, 70, 70, 2002.
9. Heaney, R. P. and Weaver, C. M., Calcium and vitamin D, *Endocrinol. Metab. Clin. N. Am.*, 32, 181, 2003.
10. IOM (Institute of Medicine), Dietary Reference Intakes for Calcium, Phosphorus, Magnesium, Vitamin D, and Fluoride, Standing Committee on the Scientific Evaluation of Dietary Reference Intakes, Food and Nutrition Board, Institute of Medicine National Academy Press, Washington, D.C., 1997.
11. Ilich, J. Z. and Kerstetter, J. E., Nutrition in bone health revisited: a story beyond calcium, *J. Am. Coll. Nutr.*, 19, 715, 2000.
12. U.S. Department of Agriculture, Agricultural Research Service, *U.S.D.A. National Nutrient Database for Standard Reference, Release 18*, Nutrient Data Laboratory, 2005, Home Page, www.ars.usda.gov/ba/bhnrc/ndl.
13. Gerrior, S., Bente, L., and Hiza, H., *Nutrient Content of the U.S. Food Supply, 1999–2000*, Home Economics Research Report No. 56, U.S. Department of Agriculture, Center for Nutrition Policy and Promotion, Washington, D.C., 2004.
14. Cotton, P. A. et al., Dietary sources of nutrients among U.S. adults, 1994 to 1996, *J. Am. Diet. Assoc.*, 104, 921, 2004.
15. Weinberg, L. G., Berner, L. A., and Groves, J. E., Nutrient contributions of dairy foods in the United States, Continuing Survey of Food Intakes by Individuals, 1994–1996, 1998, *J. Am. Diet. Assoc.*, 104, 895, 2004.
16. Miller, G. D., Jarvis, J. K., and McBean, L. D., The importance of meeting calcium needs with foods, *J. Am. Coll. Nutr.*, 20, 168s, 2001.
17. Barr, S. I. et al., Effects of increased consumption of fluid milk on energy and nutrient intake, body weight, and cardiovascular risk factors in healthy older adults, *J. Am. Diet. Assoc.*, 100, 810, 2000.
18. Johnson, R. K., Frary, C., and Wang, M. Q., The nutritional consequences of flavored milk consumption by school-aged children and adolescents in the United States, *J. Am. Diet. Assoc.*, 102, 853, 2002.
19. Rajeshwari, R. et al., The nutritional impact of dairy product consumption on dietary intakes of young adults (1995–1996): The Bogalusa Heart Study, *J. Am. Diet. Assoc.*, 105, 1391, 2005.
20. U.S. Department of Health and Human Services and U.S. Department of Agriculture, *Dietary Guidelines for Americans, 2005*, 6th ed., U.S. Government Printing Office, Washington, D.C., January 2005, www.healthierus.gov/dietaryguidelines.
21. Fulgoni, V. L. III et al., Determination of the optimal number of dairy servings to ensure a low prevalence of inadequate calcium intake in Americans, *J. Am. Coll. Nutr.*, 23, 651, 2004.
22. U.S. Department of Agriculture, Center for Nutrition Policy and Promotion, *MyPyramid Steps to a Healthier You, 2005*, MyPyramid.gov.
23. Wooten, W. J. and Price, W., Consensus report of the National Medical Association, The role of dairy and dairy nutrients in the diet of African Americans, *J. Natl. Med. Assoc.*, 96, 1s, 2004.
24. Greer, F. R., Krebs, N. F., and The Committee on Nutrition, American Academy of Pediatrics, Optimizing bone health and calcium intakes of infants, children, and adolescents, *Pediatrics*, 117, 578, 2006.
25. McCarron, D. A. and Heaney, R. P., Estimated healthcare savings associated with adequate dairy food intake, *Am. J. Hypertens.*, 17, 88, 2004.
26. Heaney, R. P. and Weaver, C. M., Newer perspectives on calcium nutrition and bone quality, *J. Am. Coll. Nutr.*, 24, 574s, 2005.
27. Heaney, R. P., Bone as the caclium nutrient reserve, in *Calcium in Human Health*, Weaver, C. M. and Heaney, R. P., Eds., Humana Press, Inc., Totowa, NJ, 2006.
28. Heaney, R. P. et al., Peak bone mass, *Osteoporos. Int.*, 11, 985, 2000.

29. Lin, Y. C. et al., Peak spine and femoral neck bone mass in young women, *Bone*, 32, 546, 2003.
30. Heaney, R. P., BMD: the problem, *Osteoporos. Int.*, 16, 1013, 2005.
31. Heaney, R. P., Is the paradigm shifting? *Bone*, 33, 457, 2003.
32. Miller, G. D., Groziak, S. M., and DiRienzo, D., Age considerations in nutrient needs for bone health, *J. Am. Coll. Nutr.*, 15, 553, 1996.
33. Hunter, D. et al., Genetic contribution to bone metabolism, calcium excretion, and vitamin D and parathyroid hormone regulation, *J. Bone Miner. Res.*, 16, 371, 2001.
34. Abrams, S. A. et al., Vitamin D receptor Fok1 polymorphisms affect calcium absorption, kinetics, and bone mineralization rates during puberty, *J. Bone Miner. Res.*, 20, 945, 2005.
35. Recker, R. R. and Deng, H. W., Role of genetics in osteoporosis, *Endocrine*, 17, 55, 2002.
36. Barrett-Connor, E. et al., Osteoporosis and fracture risk in women of different ethnic groups, *J. Bone Miner. Res.*, 20, 185, 2005.
37. Siris, E. S. et al., Identification and fracture outcomes of undiagnosed low bone mineral density in postmenopausal women: results from the National Osteoporosis Risk Assessment, *JAMA*, 286, 2815, 2001.
38. Heaney, R. P. et al., Calcium absorption in women: relationships to calcium intake, estrogen status, and age, *J. Bone Miner. Res.*, 4, 469, 1989.
39. Weaver, C. M., Age-related calcium requirements due to changes in absorption and utilization, *J. Nutr.*, 124, 1418s, 1994.
40. International Olympic Committee Medical Commission Working Group, Women in Sport, Position standard on the female athlete triad, 2004, http://multimedia.olympic.org/pdf/en_report_917.pdf.
41. Ricci, T. A. et al., Calcium supplementation suppresses bone turnover during weight reduction in postmenopausal women, *J. Bone Miner. Res.*, 13, 1045, 1998.
42. Jensen, L. B. et al., Bone mineral changes in obese women during a moderate weight loss with and without calcium supplementation, *J. Bone Miner. Res.*, 16, 141, 2001.
43. Bowen, J., Noakes, M., and Clifton, P. M., A high dairy protein, high-calcium diet minimizes bone turnover in overweight adults during weight loss, *J. Nutr.*, 134, 568, 2004.
44. Zemel, M. B., The role of dairy foods in weight management, *J. Am. Coll. Nutr.*, 24, 537s, 2005.
45. Heaney, R. P., Bone mass, nutrition, and other lifestyle factors, *Nutr. Rev.*, 54 (4), 3, 1996.
46. Massey, L. K., Is caffeine a risk factor for bone loss in the elderly? *Am. J. Clin. Nutr.*, 74, 569, 2001.
47. Alekel, D. L. and Matvienko, O., Influence of lifestyle choices on calcium homeostasis, in *Calcium in Human Health*, Weaver, C. M. and Heaney, R. P., Eds., Humana Press, Inc., Totowa, NJ, 2006, chap. 13.
48. U.S. Department of Health and Human Services, The health consequences of smoking: A report of the Surgeon General, U.S. Department of Health and Human Services, Centers for Disease Control and Prevention, National Center for Chronic Disease Prevention and Health Promotion, Office on Smoking and Health, Atlanta, GA, 2004.
49. Kanis, J. A. et al., Smoking and fracture risk: a meta-analysis, *Osteoporos. Int.*, 16, 155, 2005.
50. Kanis, J. A. et al., Alcohol intake as a risk factor for fracture, *Osteoporos. Int.*, 16, 737, 2005.
51. Klesges, R. C. et al., Changes in bone mineral content in male athletes. Mechanisms of action and intervention effects, *JAMA*, 276, 226, 1996.
52. Guillemant, J. et al., Acute effects of an oral calcium load on markers of bone metabolism during endurance cycling exercise in male athletes, *Calcif. Tissue Int.*, 74, 407, 2004.
53. Specker, B. L., Evidence for an interaction between calcium intake and physical activity on changes in bone mineral density, *J. Bone Miner. Res.*, 11 (10), 1539, 1996.
54. Matkovic, V. et al., Urinary calcium, sodium and bone mass of young females, *Am. J. Clin. Nutr.*, 62, 417, 1995.
55. Devine, A. et al., A longitudinal study of the effect of sodium and calcium intakes on regional bone density in postmenopausal women, *Am. J. Clin. Nutr.*, 62, 740, 1995.
56. Lin, P.-H. et al., The DASH diet and sodium reduction improve markers of bone turnover and calcium metabolism in adults, *J. Nutr.*, 133, 3130, 2003.
57. Sellmeyer, D. E., Schloetter, M., and Sebastian, A., Potassium citrate prevents increased urine calcium excretion and bone resorption induced by a high sodium chloride diet, *J. Clin. Endocrinol. Metab.*, 87, 2008, 2002.

58. Harrington, M. and Cashman, K. D., High salt intake appears to increase bone resorption in postmenopausal women, but high calcium intake ameliorates this adverse effect, *Nutr. Rev.*, 61, 179, 2003.
59. Wigertz, K. et al., Racial differences in calcium retention in response to dietary salt in adolescent girls, *Am. J. Clin. Nutr.*, 81, 845, 2005.
60. Bonjour, J.-P., Dietary protein: an essential nutrient for bone health, *J. Am. Coll. Nutr.*, 24, 526s, 2005.
61. Spence, L. A. and Weaver, C. M., New perspectives on dietary protein and bone health: preface, *J. Nutr.*, 133, 850s, 2003.
62. Kerstter, J. E., The impact of dietary protein on calcium absorption and kinetic measures of bone turnover in women, *J. Clin. Endocrinol. Metab.*, 90, 26, 2005.
63. Heaney, R. P., Dietary protein may not adversely affect bone, *J. Nutr.*, 128, 1054, 1998.
64. New, S. A., Do vegetarians have a normal bone mass? *Osteoporos. Int.*, 15, 679, 2004.
65. The American Dietetic Association and Dietitians of Canada, position of the American Dietetic Association and Dietitians of Canada: vegetarian diets, *J. Am. Diet. Assoc.*, 103, 748, 2003.
66. Barr, S. I. and Broughton, T. M., Relative weight, weight loss efforts and nutrient intakes among health-conscious vegetarian, past vegetarian and nonvegetarian women ages 18 to 50, *J. Am. Coll. Nutr.*, 19, 781, 2000.
67. Barr, S. I. et al., Spinal bone mineral density in premenopausal vegetarian and nonvegetarian women: cross-sectional and prospective comparisons, *J. Am. Diet. Assoc.*, 98, 760, 1998.
68. Larsson, C. L. and Johansson, G. K., Dietary intake and nutritional status of young vegans and omnivores in Sweden, *Am. J. Clin. Nutr.*, 76, 100, 2002.
69. Weaver, C. M., Proulx, W. R., and Heaney, R., Choices for achieving a vegetarian diet, *Am. J. Clin. Nutr.*, 70, 543s, 1999.
70. Bailey, D. A., et al., Calcium accretion in girls and boys during puberty: a longitudinal analysis, *J. Bone Miner. Res.*, 15, 2245, 2000.
71. Moshfegh, A., Goldman, J., and Cleveland, L., *What We Eat in America, NHANES 2001–2002: Usual Nutrient Intakes from Food Compared to Dietary Reference Intakes*, U.S. Department of Agriculture, Agricultural Research Service, 2005, www.ars.usda.gov/foodsurvey.
72. Looker, A. C., Dietary calcium recommendations and intakes around the world, in *Calcium in Human Health*, Weaver, C. M. and Heaney, R. P., Eds., Humana Press, Inc., Totowa, NJ, 2006, chap. 8.
73. U.S. Department of Agriculture, Agricultural Research Service, *Data Tables: Results from U.S.D.A.'s 1994–96 Continuing Survey of Food Intakes by Individuals* (recalculated to reflect % of 1997 AI for calcium), ARS Food Surveys Research Group, December 1997.
74. Basiotis, P.P. et al., *The Healthy Eating Index: 1999–2000*, U.S. Department of Agriculture, Center for Nutrition Policy and Promotion, CNPP-12, December 2002, www.cnpp.usda.gov.
75. Cook, A.J. and Friday, J.E., *Pyramid Servings Intakes in the United States 1999–2002, 1 Day*, CNRG Table Set 3.0., USDA Agricultural Research Service, Community Nutrition Research Group, Beltsville, MD, March 2005, www.barc.usda.gov/bhnrc/cnrg.
76. U.S. Department of Agriculture, Agricultural Research Service, Data Tables: Food and Nutrient Intakes by Race, 1994–1996, Table Set 11, 1998, www.barc.usda.gov/bhnrc/foodsurvey/home.htm.
77. Nicklas, T. A., Calcium intake trends and health consequences from childhood through adulthood, *J. Am. Coll. Nutr.*, 22, 340, 2003.
78. Novotny, R., Han, J.-S., and Biernacke, I., Motivators and barriers to consuming calcium-rich foods among Asian adolescents in Hawaii, *J. Nutr. Educ.*, 31, 99, 1999.
79. Auld, G. et al., Perspectives on intake of calcium-rich foods among Asian, Hispanic, and white preadolescent and adolescent females, *J. Nutr. Educ. Behav.*, 34, 242, 2002.
80. Lee, S. and Reicks, M., Environmental and behavioral factors are associated with the calcium intake of low-income adolescent girls, *J. Am. Diet. Assoc.*, 103, 1526, 2003.
81. Conners, P., Bednar, C., and Klammer, S., Cafeteria factors that influence milk-drinking behaviors of elementary school children: grounded theory approach, *J. Nutr. Educ.*, 33, 31, 2001.
82. Weaver, C. M. and Heaney, R. P., Food sources, supplements and bioavailability, in *Calcium in Human Health*, Weaver, C. M. and Heaney, R. P., Eds., Humana Press, Inc., Totowa, NJ, 2006, chap. 9.

83. Barr, S. I., Associations of social and demographic variables with calcium intakes of high school students, *J. Am. Diet. Assoc.*, 94, 260–269, 1994.
84. Newmark-Sztainer, D. et al., Factors influencing food choices of adolescents: findings from focus-group discussions with adolescents, *J. Am. Diet. Assoc.*, 99, 929, 1999.
85. Barr, S. I. et al., Eating attitudes and habitual calcium intake in peripubertal girls are associated with initial bone mineral content and its change over 2 years, *J. Bone Miner. Res.*, 16, 940, 2001.
86. Dietary Guidelines Advisory Committee, *Report of the Dietary Guidelines Advisory Committee on the Dietary Guidelines for Americans*, 2005, U.S. Department of Agriculture, Agricultural Research Service, August 2004, p. 182.
87. Savaiano, D., Lactose intolerance: a self-fulling prophecy leading to osteoporosis? *Nutr. Rev.*, 61, 221, 2003.
88. Lovelace, H. Y. and Barr, S. I., Diagnosis, symptoms, and calcium intakes of individuals with self-reported lactose intolerance, *J. Am. Coll. Nutr.*, 24, 51, 2005.
89. Honkanen, R. et al., Lactose intolerance associated with fractures of weight-bearing bones in Finnish women aged 38–57 years, *Bone*, 21, 473, 1997.
90. McBean, L. D. and Miller, G. D., Allaying fears and fallacies about lactose intolerance, *J. Am. Diet. Assoc.*, 98, 671, 1998.
91. Jarvis, J. K. and Miller, G. D., Overcoming the barrier of lactose intolerance to reduce health disparities, *J. Natl Med. Assoc.*, 94, 55, 2002.
92. Byers, K. G. and Savaiano, D. A., The myth of increased lactose intolerance in African Americans, *J. Am. Coll. Nutr.*, 24, 569s, 2005.
93. Tepper, B. J. and Nayga, R. M. Jr, Awareness of the link between bone disease and calcium intake is associated with higher dietary calcium intake in women aged 50 years and older: results of the 1991 CSFII-DHKS, *J. Am. Diet. Assoc.*, 98, 196, 1998.
94. Harel, Z. et al., Adolescents and calcium: what they do and do not know and how much they consume, *J. Adol. Health*, 22, 225, 1998.
95. Patrick, H. and Nicklas, T. A., A review of family and social determinants of children's eating patterns and diet quality, *J. Am. Coll. Nutr.*, 24, 83, 2005.
96. Johnson, R. K., Panely, C. V., and Wang, M. Q., Associations between the milk mothers drink and the milk consumed by their school-aged children, *Fam. Econ. Nutr. Rev.*, 13, 27, 2001.
97. Fisher, J. O. et al., Maternal milk consumption predicts the tradeoff between milk and soft drinks in young girls' diets, *J. Nutr.*, 131, 246, 2001.
98. Fisher, J. O. et al., Meeting calcium recommendations during middle childhood reflects mother-daughter beverage choices and predicts bone mineral status, *Am. J. Clin. Nutr.*, 79, 698, 2004.
99. Gleason, P., Suitor, C. *Children's Diets in the Mid-1990s. Dietary Intake and Its Relationship with School Meal Participation*, Nutrition Assistance Program Report Series, Report No. CN-01-CD1, January 2001.
100. National Dairy Council and American School Food Service Association, *The School Milk Pilot Test*, Beverage Marketing Corporation for National Dairy Council and American School Food Service Association, 2002, www.nationdairycouncil.org.
101. French, S. A. et al., Fast food restaurant use among adolescents; associations with nutrient intakes, food choices and behavioral and psychosocial variables, *Int. J. Obes.*, 25, 1823, 2001.
102. Gillman, M. W. et al., Family dinner and diet quality among older children and adolescents, *Arch. Fam. Med.*, 9, 235, 2000.
103. Neumark-Sztainer, D. et al., Family meal patterns: associations with sociodemographic characteristics and improved dietary intake among adolescents, *J. Am. Diet. Assoc.*, 103, 317, 2003.
104. Nicklas, T. A., O'Neil, C., and Myers, L., The importance of breakfast consumption to nutrition of children, adolescents, and young adults, *Nutr. Today*, 39, 30, 2004.
105. Affenito, S. G., Breakfast consumption by African Americans and White adolescent girls correlates positively with calcium and fiber intake and negatively with body mass index, *J. Am. Diet. Assoc.*, 105, 938, 2005.
106. U.S. Department of Health and Human Services, Food and Drug Administration, Food labeling: health claims; calcium and osteoporosis, *Fed. Register*, 58 (3), 2665, 1993, January, 6.

107. Heaney, R. P., Nutritional factors in bone health in elderly subjects: methodological and contextual problems, *Am. J. Clin. Nutr.*, 50, 1182, 1989.
108. Bonjour, J.-P. et al. Calcium-enriched foods and bone mass growth in prepubertal girls: a randomized, double-blind, placebo-controlled trial, *J. Clin. Invest.*, 99, 1287, 1997.
109. Gibbons, M. J. et al. The effects of a high calcium dairy food on bone health in pre-pubertal children in New Zealand, *Asia Pac. J. Clin. Nutr.*, 13, 341, 2004.
110. Barger-Lux, M. J., Davies, K. M., and Heaney, R. P., Calcium supplementation does not augment bone gain in young women consuming diets moderately low in calcium, *J. Nutr.*, 135, 2362, 2005.
111. Heaney, R. P., The bone remodeling transient: implications for the interpretation of clinical studies of bone mass change, *J. Bone Miner. Res.*, 9, 1515, 1994.
112. Lee, W. T. K. et al. A follow-up study on the effects of calcium-supplement withdrawal and puberty on bone acquisition of children, *Am. J. Clin. Nutr.*, 64, 71, 1996.
113. Lee, W. T. K. et al. Bone mineral acquisition in low calcium intake children following the withdrawal of calcium supplement, *Acta Paediatr.*, 86, 570, 1997.
114. Cumming, R. G. and Nevitt, M. C., Calcium for prevention of osteoporotic fractures in postmenopausal women, *J. Bone Miner. Res.*, 12, 1321, 1997.
115. Heaney, R. P., Nutrient effects: discrepancy between data from controlled trials and observational studies, *Bone*, 21, 469, 1997.
116. Matkovic, V. et al. Timing of peak bone mass in Caucasian females and its implication for the prevention of osteoporosis, *J. Clin. Invest.*, 93, 799, 1994.
117. Abrams, S. A., Calcium supplementation during childhood: long-term effects on bone mineralization, *Nutr. Rev.*, 63, 251, 2005.
118. Whiting, S. J. et al. Factors that affect bone mineral accrual in the adolescent growth spurt, *J. Nutr.*, 134, 696s, 2004.
119. Weaver, C. M., Prepuberty and adolescence, in *Calcium in Human Health*, Weaver, C. M. and Heaney, R. P., Eds., Humana Press, Inc., Totowa, NJ, 2006, chap. 17.
120. Fassler, A.-L. and Bonjour, J.-P., Osteoporosis as a pediatric problem, *Pediatr. Clin. N. Am.*, 42, 811, 1995.
121. Chan, G. M., Hoffman, K., and McMurray, M., Effects of dairy products on bone and body composition in pubertal girls, *J. Pediatr.*, 126, 551, 1995.
122. Johnston, C. C. Jr. et al. Calcium supplementation and increases in bone mineral density in children, *N. Engl. J. Med.*, 327, 82, 1992.
123. Lee, W. T. K. et al. Double-blind controlled calcium supplementation and bone mineral accretion in children accustomed to low calcium diet, *Am. J. Clin. Nutr.*, 60, 744, 1994.
124. Wosje, K. S. and Specker, B. L., Role of calcium in bone health during childhood, *Nutr., Rev.*, 58, 253, 2000.
125. Fiorito, L. M. et al. Girls' calcium intake is associated with bone mineral content during middle childhood, *J. Nutr.*, 136, 1281, 2006.
126. Bounds, W. et al. The relationship of dietary and lifestyle factors to bone mineral indexes in children, *J. Am. Diet. Assoc.*, 105, 735, 2005.
127. Lu, P. W. et al. Bone mineral density of total body, spine, and femoral neck in children and young adults: a cross-sectional and longitudinal study, *J. Bone Miner. Res.*, 9, 1451, 1994.
128. Lloyd, T. et al. Calcium supplementation and bone mineral density in adolescent girls, *JAMA*, 270, 841, 1993.
129. Jackman, L. A. et al. Calcium retention in relation to calcium intake and postmenarcheal age in adolescent females, *Am. J. Clin. Nutr.*, 66, 327, 1997.
130. Nowson, C. A. et al. A co-twin study of the effect of calcium supplementation on bone density during adolescence, *Osteoporosis Int.*, 7, 219, 1997.
131. Cameron, M. A. et al. The effect of calcium supplementation on bone density in premenstrual females: a co-twin approach, *J. Clin. Endocrinol. Metab.*, 89, 4916, 2004.
132. Matkovic, V. et al. Nutrition influences skeletal development from childhood to adulthood: a study of hip, spine, and forearm in adolescent females, *J. Nutr.*, 134, 701s, 2004.
133. Matkovic, V. et al. Calcium supplementation and bone mineral density in females from childhood to young adulthood: a randomized controlled trial, *Am. J. Clin. Nutr.*, 81, 175, 2005.

134. Rozen, G. et al. Calcium supplementation provides an extended window of opportunity for bone mass accretion after menarche, *Am. J. Clin. Nutr.*, 78, 993, 2003.
135. Bonjour, J. P. et al. Gain in bone mineral mass in prepubertal girls 3.5 years after discontinuation of calcium supplementation: a follow-up study, *Lancet*, 358, 1208, 2001.
136. Dibba, B. et al. Bone mineral contents and plasma osteocalcin concentrations of Gambian children 12 and 24 mo after the withdrawal of a calcium supplement, *Am. J. Clin. Nutr.*, 76, 681, 2002.
137. Dodiuk-Gad, R. P. et al. Sustained effect of short-term calcium supplementation on bone mass in adolescent girls with low calcium intake, *Am. J. Clin. Nutr.*, 81, 168, 2005.
138. Chevalley, T. et al. Interaction between calcium intake and menarcheal age on bone mass gain: an eight-year follow-up study from prepuberty to postmenarche, *J. Clin. Endocrinol. Metab.*, 90, 44, 2005.
139. Chevalley, T. et al. Skeletal site selectivity in the effects of calcium supplementation on areal bone mineral density gain: a randomized, double-blind, placebo-controlled trial in prepubertal boys, *J. Clin. Endocrinol. Metab.*, 90, 3342, 2005.
140. Slemenda, C. W. et al. Reduced rates of skeletal remodeling are associated with increased bone density during the development of peak skeletal mass, *J. Bone Miner. Res.*, 12, 676, 1997.
141. Zhu, K. et al. Growth, bone mass, and vitamin D status of Chinese adolescent girls 3 y after withdrawal of milk supplementation, *Am. J. Clin. Nutr.*, 83, 714, 2006.
142. Specker, B. and Binkley, T., Randomized trial of physical activity and calcium supplementation on bone mineral content in 3- to 5-year old children, *J. Bone Miner. Res.*, 18, 885, 2003.
143. Courteix, D. et al. Cumulative effects of calcium supplementation and physical activity on bone accretion in premenarcheal children: a double-blind randomized placebo-controlled trial, *Int. J. Sports Med.*, 26, 332, 2005.
144. Stear, S. J. et al. Effect of a calcium and exercise intervention on the bone mineral status of 16–18-year-old adolescent girls, *Am. J. Clin. Nutr.*, 77, 985, 2003.
145. Rowlands, A. V. et al. Interactive effects of habitual physical activity and calcium intake in boys and girls, *J. Appl. Physiol.*, 97, 1203, 2004.
146. Welch, J. M. and Weaver, C. M., Calcium and exercise affect the growing skeleton, *Nutr. Rev.*, 63, 361, 2005.
147. Matkovic, V. et al. Bone status and fracture rates in two regions of Yugoslavia, *Am. J. Clin. Nutr.*, 32, 540, 1979.
148. Cadogan, J. et al. Milk intake and bone mineral acquisition in adolescent girls: randomized, controlled intervention trial, *Br. Med. J.*, 315, 1255, 1997.
149. Volek, J. S., Increasing fluid milk favorably affects bone mineral density responses to resistance training in adolescent boys, *J. Am. Diet. Assoc.*, 103, 1353, 2003.
150. Cheng, S. et al. Effects of calcium, dairy product, and vitamin D supplementation on bone mass accrual and body composition in 10–12-y-old girls: a 2-y randomized trial, *Am. J. Clin. Nutr.*, 82, 1115, 2005.
151. Du, X. Q. et al. Milk consumption and bone mineral content in Chinese adolescent girls, *Bone*, 30, 521, 2002.
152. Du, X. et al. School-milk intervention trial enhances growth and bone mineral accretion in Chinese girls aged 10–12 years in Beijing, *Br. J. Nutr.*, 92, 159, 2004.
153. Lau, E. M. C. et al. Benefits of milk powder supplementation on bone accretion in Chinese children, *Osteoporos. Int.*, 15, 654, 2004.
154. Zhu, K. et al. Effects of school milk intervention on cortical bone accretion and indicators relevant to bone metabolism in Chinese girls aged 10–12 years in Beijing, *Am. J. Clin. Nutr.*, 81, 1168, 2005.
155. Infante, D. and Tormo, R., Risk of inadequate bone mineralization in diseases involving long-term suppression of dairy products, *J. Pediatr. Gastroenterol. Nutr.*, 30, 310, 2000.
156. Black, R. E. et al. Children who avoid drinking cow milk have low dietary calcium intakes and poor bone health, *Am. J. Clin. Nutr.*, 76, 675, 2002.
157. Hidvegi, E. et al. Slight decrease in bone mineralization in cow milk-sensitive children, *J. Pediatr. Gastroenterol. Nutr.*, 36, 44, 2003.
158. Goulding, A. et al. Bone mineral density and body composition in boys with distal forearm fractures. A dual energy X-ray absorptiometry study, *J. Pediatr.*, 139, 509, 2001.

159. Goulding, A. et al. Children who avoid drinking cow's milk are at increased risk of prepubertal bone fractures, *J. Am. Diet. Assoc.*, 104, 250, 2004.
160. Goulding, A., Grant, A. M., and Williams, S. M., Bone and body composition of children and adolescents with repeated forearm fractures, *J. Bone Miner. Res.*, 20, 2090, 2005.
161. Rockell, J. E. et al. Two-year changes in bone and body composition in young children with a history of prolonged milk avoidance, *Osteoporos. Int.*, 16, 1016, 2005.
162. Goulding, A. et al. Bone mineral density in girls with forearm fractures, *J. Bone Miner. Res.*, 13, 143, 1998.
163. Nieves, J. W. et al. Teenage and current calcium intakes are related to bone mineral density of the hip and forearm in women aged 30–39, *Am. J. Epidemiol.*, 141, 342, 1995.
164. Murphy, S. et al. Milk consumption and bone mineral density in middle aged and elderly women, *Br. Med. J.*, 308, 939, 1994.
165. Soroko, S. et al. Lifetime milk consumption and bone mineral density in older women, *Am. J. Public Health*, 84, 1319, 1994.
166. New, S. A. et al. Nutritional influences on bone mineral density: a cross-sectional study in premenopausal women, *Am. J. Clin. Nutr.*, 65, 1831, 1997.
167. Teegarden, D. et al. Previous milk consumption is associated with greater bone density in young women, *Am. J. Clin. Nutr.*, 69, 1014, 1999.
168. Kalkwarf, H. J., Khoury, J. C., and Lanphear, B. P., Milk intake during childhood and adolescence, adult bone density, and osteoporotic fractures in U.S. women, *Am. J. Clin. Nutr.*, 77, 257, 2003.
169. Wang, M.-C. et al. Diet in midpuberty and sedentary activity in prepuberty predict peak bone mass, *Am. J. Clin. Nutr.*, 77, 495, 2003.
170. The American Dietetic Association, Position of the American Dietetic Association: dietary guidance for healthy children ages 2 to 11 years, *J. Am. Diet. Assoc.*, 104, 660, 2004.
171. American Academy of Pediatrics, Committee on School Health, Soft drinks in schools, *Pediatrics*, 113, 152, 2004.
172. Recker, R. R. et al. Bone gain in young adult women, *JAMA*, 268, 2403, 1992.
173. Metz, J. A., Anderson, J. J. B., and Gallagher, P. N. Jr, Intakes of calcium, phosphorus, and protein, and physical activity level are related to radial bone mass in young adult women, *Am. J. Clin. Nutr.*, 58, 537, 1993.
174. Hirota, T. et al. Effect of diet and lifestyle on bone mass in Asian young women, *Am. J. Clin. Nutr.*, 55, 1168, 1992.
175. Tylavsky, F. A. et al. Are calcium intakes and physical activity patterns during adolescence related to radial bone mass of white college-age females? *Osteoporosis Int.*, 2, 232, 1992.
176. Anderson, J. J. B. and Rondano, P. A., Peak bone mass development of females: can young adult women improve their peak bone mass? *J. Am. Coll. Nutr.*, 15, 570, 1996.
177. Teegarden, D. et al. Dietary calcium, protein, and phosphorus are related to bone mineral density and content in young women, *Am. J. Clin. Nutr.*, 68, 749, 1998.
178. Nakamura, K. et al. Nutrition, mild hyperparathyroidism and bone mineral density in young Japanese women, *Am. J. Clin. Nutr.*, 82, 1127, 2005.
179. Davis, J. W. et al. Anthropometric, lifestyle and menstrual factors influencing size-adjusted bone mineral content in a multiethnic population of premenopausal women, *J. Nutr.*, 126, 2968, 1996.
180. Hawker, G. A. et al. Correlates of forearm bone mineral density in young Norwegian women. The Nord-Trondelag health study, *Am. J. Epidemiol.*, 156, 418, 2002.
181. Teegarden, D. et al. Dietary calcium intake protects women consuming oral contraceptive from spine and hip bone loss, *J. Clin. Endocrinol. Metab.*, 90, 5127, 2005.
182. Anderson, J. J. B., Calcium, phosphorus, and human bone development, *J. Nutr.*, 126, 1153, 1996.
183. Welten, D. C. et al. A meta-analysis of the effect of calcium intake on bone mass in young and middle aged females and males, *J. Nutr.*, 125, 2802, 1995.
184. Baran, D. et al. Dietary modification with dairy products for preventing vertebral bone loss in premenopausal women: a three-year prospective study, *J. Clin. Endocrinol. Metab.*, 70, 264, 1990.
185. Dawson-Hughes, B. et al. A controlled trial of the effect of calcium supplementation on bone density in postmenopausal women, *N. Engl. J. Med.*, 323, 878, 1990.
186. Dawson-Hughes, B., Calcium and vitamin D nutritional needs of elderly women, *J. Nutr.*, 126, 1165s, 1996.

187. Masse, P. G. et al. Bone mineral density and metabolism at an early stage of menopause when estrogen and calcium supplements are not used and without the interference of major confounding variables, *J. Am. Coll. Nutr.*, 24, 354, 2005.
188. Van Beresteijn, E. C. H. et al. Habitual dietary calcium intake and cortical bone loss in perimenopausal women: a longitudinal study, *Calcif. Tissue Int.*, 47, 338, 1990.
189. Aloia, J. F. et al. Calcium supplementation with and without hormone replacement therapy to prevent postmenopausal bone loss, *Ann. Intern. Med.*, 120, 97, 1994.
190. Suzuki, Y. et al. Total calcium intake is associated with cortical bone mineral density in a cohort of postmenopausal women not taking estrogen, *J. Nutr. Health & Aging*, 7, 296, 2003.
191. Davis, J. W. et al. Estrogen and calcium use among Japanese–American women: effects upon bone loss when used singly and in combination, *Bone*, 17 (4), 369, 1995.
192. Nieves, J. W. et al. Calcium potentiates the effect of estrogen and calcitonin on bone mass: review and analysis, *Am. J. Clin. Nutr.*, 67, 18, 1998.
193. Haines, C. J. et al. Calcium supplementation and bone mineral density in postmenopausal women using estrogen replacement therapy, *Bone*, 16, 529, 1995.
194. Recker, R. R. et al. The effect of low-dose continuous estrogen and progesterone therapy with calcium and vitamin D on bone health in elderly women, *Ann. Intern. Med.*, 130, 897, 1999.
195. Sirola, J. et al. Interaction of nutritional calcium and HRT in prevention of postmenopausal bone loss: a prospective study, *Calcif. Tissue Int.*, 72, 659, 2003.
196. Reid, I. R. et al. Effect of calcium supplementation on bone loss in postmenopausal women, *N. Engl. J. Med.*, 328, 460, 1993.
197. Reid, I. R. et al. Long-term effects of calcium supplementation on bone loss and fractures in postmenopausal women: a randomized controlled trial, *Am. J. Med.*, 98, 331, 1995.
198. Devine, A. et al. A 4-year follow-up study of the effects of calcium supplementation on bone density in elderly postmenopausal women, *Osteoporosis Int.*, 7, 23, 1997.
199. Prince, R. et al. The effects of calcium supplementation (milk powder or tablets) and exercise on bone density in postmenopausal women, *J. Bone Miner. Res.*, 10, 1068, 1995.
200. Michaelsson, K. et al. A high dietary calcium intake is needed for a positive effect on bone density in Swedish postmenopausal women, *Osteoporosis Int.*, 7, 155, 1997.
201. Feskanich, D. et al. Milk, dietary calcium, and bone fractures in women: a 12-year prospective study, *Am. J. Public Health*, 87, 992, 1997.
202. Feskanich, D., Willett, W. C., and Colditz, G. A., Calcium, vitamin D, milk consumption, and hip fractures: a prospective study among postmenopausal women, *Am. J. Clin. Nutr.*, 77, 504, 2003.
203. McCabe, L. D. et al. Dairy intakes affect bone density in the elderly, *Am. J. Clin. Nutr.*, 80, 1066, 2004.
204. Shea, B. et al. Meta-analysis of calcium supplementation for the prevention of postmenopausal osteoporosis, *Endocrine Rev.*, 23, 552, 2002.
205. Jackson, R. D. et al. For the Women's Health Initiative Investigators, Calcium plus vitamin D supplementation and the risk of fractures, *N. Engl. J. Med.*, 354, 669, 2006.
206. Finkelstein, J. S., Calcium plus vitamin D for postmenopausal women — bone appetite? *N. Engl. J. Med.*, 354, 750, 2006.
207. Curhan, G. C. et al. A prospective study of dietary calcium and other nutrients and the risk of symptomatic kidney stones, *N. Engl. J. Med.*, 328, 833, 1993.
208. Curhan, G. C. et al. Comparison of dietary calcium with supplemental calcium and other nutrients as factors affecting the risk for kidney stones in women, *Ann. Intern. Med.*, 126, 497, 1997.
209. Curhan, G. C. et al. Dietary factors and the risk of incident kidney stones in younger women, Nurses' Health Study II, *Arch. Intern. Med.*, 164, 885, 2004.
210. Suleiman, S. et al. Effect of calcium intake and physical activity level on bone mass and turnover in healthy, white, postmenopausal women, *Am. J. Clin. Nutr.*, 66, 937, 1997.
211. Kerr, D. et al. Resistance training over 2 years increases bone mass in calcium-replete postmenopausal women, *J. Bone Miner. Res.*, 16, 175, 2001.
212. Recker, R. R. and Heaney, R. P., The effect of milk supplements on calcium metabolism, bone metabolism and calcium balance, *Am. J. Clin. Nutr.*, 41, 254, 1985.
213. Heaney, R. P., Rafferty, K., and Dowell, M. S., Effect of yogurt on a urinary marker of bone resorption in postmenopausal women, *J. Am. Diet. Assoc.*, 102, 1672, 2002.

214. Hu, J.-F. et al. Dietary calcium and bone density among middle-aged and elderly women in China, *Am. J. Clin. Nutr.*, 58, 219, 1993.
215. Chee, W. S. S. et al. The effect of milk supplementation on bone mineral density in postmenopausal Chinese women in Malaysia, *Osteoporos. Int.*, 14, 828, 2003.
216. Lau, E. M. C. et al. Milk supplementation of the diet of postmenopausal Chinese women on a low calcium intake retards bone loss, *J. Bone Miner. Res.*, 16, 1704, 2001.
217. The American Dietetic Association and Dietitians of Canada, Position of the American Dietetic Association and Dietitians of Canada: nutrition and women's health, *J. Am. Diet. Assoc.*, 104, 984, 2004.
218. North American Menopause Society, The role of calcium in peri- and postmenopausal women: consensus opinion of the North American Menopause Society, *Menopause*, 8, 84, 2001.
219. Hannan, M. T., Felson, D. T., and Anderson, J. J., Bone mineral density in elderly men and women: results from the Framingham Osteoporosis Study, *J. Bone & Miner. Res.*, 7, 547, 1992.
220. Campion, J. M. and Maricic, M. J., Osteoporosis in men, *Am. Fam. Physician*, 67, 1521, 2003.
221. Kiebzak, G. M. et al. Undertreatment of osteoporosis in men with hip fractures, *Arch. Intern. Med.*, 162, 2217, 2002.
222. Anderson, D. C., Osteoporosis in men, *Br. Med. J.*, 305, 489, 1992.
223. Kanis, J. et al. Risk factors for hip fracture in men from Southern Europe: the MEDOS Study, *Osteoporos. Int.*, 9, 45, 1999.
224. Dawson-Hughes, B. et al. Effect of calcium and vitamin D supplementation on bone density in men and women 65 years of age or older, *N. Engl. J. Med.*, 337, 670, 1997.
225. Nguyen, T. V. et al. Risk factors for proximal humerus, forearm, and wrist fractures in elderly men and women, *Am. J. Epidemiol.*, 153, 587, 2001.
226. Olszynski, W. P. et al. Osteoporosis in men: epidemiology, diagnosis, prevention, and treatment, *Clin. Ther.*, 26, 15, 2004.
227. Naves, M. et al. Prevalence of osteoporosis in men and determinants of changes in bone mass in a non-selected Spanish population, *Osteoporos. Int.*, 16, 603, 2005.
228. Cauley, J. A., for the Mr. Os Research Group, et al., Factors associated with the lumbar spine and proximal femur bone mineral density in older men, *Osteoporos. Int.*, 16, 1525, 2005.
229. Kroger, H. and Laitinen, K., Bone mineral density measured by dual-energy X-ray absorptiometry in normal men, *Europ. J. Clin. Invest.*, 22, 454, 1992.
230. Owusu, W. et al. Calcium intake and the incidence of forearm and hip fractures among men, *J. Nutr.*, 127, 1782, 1997.
231. Glynn, N. W. et al. Determinants of bone mineral density in older men, *J. Bone Miner. Res.*, 10, 1769, 1995.
232. Daly, R. M. et al. Calcium and vitamin D_3-fortified milk reduces bone loss at clinically relevant skeletal sites in older men: a 2-year randomized controlled trial, *J. Bone Miner. Res.*, 21, 397, 2006.
233. Whiting, S. J. et al. Dietary protein, phosphorus, and potassium are beneficial to bone mineral density in adult men consuming adequate dietary calcium, *J. Am. Coll. Nutr.*, 21, 402, 2002.
234. Dawson-Hughes, B., Calcium throughout the life cycle. The later years, in *Calcium in Human Health*, Weaver, C. M. and Heaney, R. P., Eds., Humana Press, Inc., Totowa, NJ, 2006, chap. 24.
235. Heaney, R. P., Calcium needs of the elderly to reduce fracture risk, *J. Am. Coll. Nutr.*, 20, 192s, 2001.
236. Chapuy, M. C. et al. Vitamin D_3 and calcium to prevent hip fractures in elderly women, *N. Engl. J. Med.*, 327, 1637, 1992.
237. Chevalley, T. et al. Effects of calcium supplements on femoral bone mineral density and vertebral fracture rate in vitamin D-replete elderly patients, *Osteoporosis Int.*, 4, 245, 1994.
238. Recker, R. R. et al. Correcting calcium nutritional deficiency prevents spine fractures in elderly women, *J. Bone Miner. Res.*, 11, 1996, 1961.
239. Chapuy, M. C. et al. Effect of calcium and cholecalciferol treatment for three years on hip fractures in elderly women, *Br. Med. J.*, 308, 1081, 1994.
240. McKane, W. R. et al. Role of calcium intake in modulating age-related increases in parathyroid function and bone resorption, *J. Clin. Endocrinol. Metab.*, 81, 1699, 1996.
241. Heaney, R. P. et al. Dietary changes favorably affect bone remodeling in older adults, *J. Am. Diet. Assoc.*, 99, 1228, 1999.

242. Bischoff, H. A. et al. Effects of vitamin D and calcium supplementation on falls: a randomized controlled trial, *J. Bone Miner. Res.*, 18, 343, 2003.
243. Pfeifer, M. et al. Effects of short-term vitamin D and calcium supplementation on body sway and secondary hyperparathyroidism in elderly women, *J. Bone Miner. Res.*, 15, 1113, 2000.
244. Devine, A. et al. Physical activity and calcium consumption are important determinants of lower limb bone mass in older women, *J. Bone Miner. Res.*, 19, 1634, 2004.
245. McClung, M., for the Alendronate Osteoporosis Prevention Study Group, et al., Alendronate prevents postmenopausal bone loss in women without osteoporosis, *Ann. Intern. Med.*, 128, 253, 1998.
246. Dawson-Hughes, B., Osteoporosis treatment and the calcium requirement, *Am. J. Clin. Nutr.*, 67, 5, 1998.
247. Packard, P. T. and Heaney, R. P., Medical nutrition therapy for patients with osteoporosis, *J. Am. Diet. Assoc.*, 97, 414, 1997.
248. Holick, M. F., The vitamin D epidemic and its health consequences, *J. Nutr.*, 135, 2739s, 2005.
249. Holick, M. F., Sunlight and vitamin D for bone health and prevention of autoimmune diseases, cancers, and cardiovascular disease, *Am. J. Clin. Nutr.*, 80, 1678s, 2004.
250. Dawson-Hughes, B., Harris, S. S., and Dallal, G. E., Plasma calcidiol, season, and serum parathyroid hormone concentrations in healthy elderly men and women, *Am. J. Clin. Nutr.*, 65, 67, 1997.
251. Vieth, R., Critique of the considerations for establishing the tolerable upper intake level for vitamin D: critical need for revision upwards, *J. Nutr.*, 136, 1117, 2006.
252. Heaney, R. P., Barriers to optimizing vitamin D_3 intake for the elderly, *J. Nutr.*, 136, 1123, 2006.
253. Heaney, R. P., The vitamin D requirement in health and disease, *J. Steroid Biochem. Mol. Biol.*, 97, 13, 2005.
254. Dawson-Hughes, B. et al. Estimates of optimal vitamin D status, *Osteoporosis. Int.*, 16, 713, 2005.
255. Bischoff-Ferrari, H. A. et al. Fracture prevention with vitamin D supplementation: a meta-analysis of randomized controlled trials, *JAMA*, 293, 2257, 2005.
256. Whiting, S. J. and Calvo, M. S., Dietary recommendations for vitamin D: a critical need for functional end points to establish an estimated average requirement, *J. Nutr.*, 135, 304, 2005.
257. Sullivan, S. S. et al. Adolescent girls in Maine are at risk for vitamin D insufficiency, *J. Am. Diet. Assoc.*, 105, 971, 2005.
258. Calvo, M. S. and Whiting, S. J., Prevalence of vitamin D insufficiency in Canada and the United States: importance to health status and efficacy of current food fortification and dietary supplement use, *Nutr. Rev.*, 61, 107, 2003.
259. Weisberg, P. et al. Nutritional rickets among children in the United States: a review of cases reported between 1986 and 2003, *Am. J. Clin. Nutr.*, 80, 1697s, 2004.
260. Gordon, C. M. et al. Prevalence of vitamin D deficiency among healthy adolescents, *Arch. Pediatr., Adolesc. Med.*, 158, 531, 2004.
261. Nesby-O'Dell, S. et al. Hypovitaminosis D prevalence and determinants among African American and White women of reproductive age: third National Health and Nutrition Examination Survey, 1968–1994, *Am. J. Clin. Nutr.*, 76, 187, 2002.
262. Moore, C. E., Murphy, M. M., and Holick, M. F., Vitamin D intakes by children and adults in the United States differ among ethnic groups, *J. Nutr.*, 135, 2478, 2005.
263. Raiten, D. J. and Picciano, M. F., Vitamin D and health in the 21st century: bone & beyond: executive summary, *Am. J. Clin. Nutr.*, 80, 1673s, 2004.
264. Gartner, L. M., Greer, F. R., and The Section on Breastfeeding and Committee on Nutrition, American Academy of Pediatrics, Prevention of rickets and vitamin D deficiency: new guidelines for vitamin D intake, *Pediatrics*, 111, 908, 2003.
265. Tylavsky, F. A. et al. Vitamin D, parathyroid hormone, and bone mass in adolescents, *J. Nutr.*, 135, 2735s, 2005.
266. Willett, A. M., Vitamin D status and its relationship with parathyroid hormone and bone mineral status in older adolescents, *Proc. Nutr. Soc.*, 64, 193, 2005.
267. Outila, T. A., Karkkainen, U. M., and Lamberg-Allardt, C. J. E., Vitamin D status affects serum parathyroid hormone concentrations during winter in female adolescents: associations with forearm bone mineral density, *Am. J. Clin. Nutr.*, 74, 206, 2001.

268. Cheng, S. et al. Association of low 25-hydroxyvitamin D concentrations with elevated parathyroid hormone concentrations and low cortical bone density in early pubertal and prepubertal Finnish girls, *Am. J. Clin. Nutr.*, 78, 485, 2003.
269. Lehtonen-Veromaa, M. K. M. et al. Vitamin D and attainment of peak bone mass among peripubertal Finnish girls: a 3-y prospective study, *Am. J. Clin. Nutr.*, 76, 1446, 2002.
270. El-Hajj Fuleihan, G. et al. Effect of vitamin D replacement on musculoskeletal parameters in school children: a randomized controlled trial, *J. Clin. Endocrinol. Metab.*, 91, 405, 2005.
271. Valimaki, V. V. et al. Vitamin D status as a determinant of peak bone mass in young Finnish men, *J. Clin. Endocrinol. Metab.*, 89, 76, 2004.
272. Gloth, F. M. et al. Vitamin D deficiency in homebound elderly persons, *JAMA*, 274, 1683, 1995.
273. Chapuy, M. C. et al. Healthy elderly French women living at home have secondary hyperparathyroidism and high bone turnover in winter, *J. Clin. Endocrinol. Metab.*, 81, 1129, 1996.
274. Chapuy, M.-C. et al. Prevalence of vitamin D insufficiency in an adult normal population, *Osteoporosis. Int.*, 7, 439, 1997.
275. Jacques, P. F. et al. Plasma 25-hydroxyvitamin D and its determinants in an elderly population sample, *Am. J. Clin. Nutr.*, 66, 929, 1997.
276. Kinyamu, H. K. et al. Dietary calcium and vitamin D intake in elderly women: effect on serum parathyroid hormone and vitamin D metabolites, *Am. J. Clin. Nutr.*, 67, 342, 1998.
277. Kinyamu, H. K. et al. Serum vitamin D metabolites and calcium absorption in normal young and elderly free-living women and in women living in nursing homes, *Am. J. Clin. Nutr.*, 65, 790, 1997.
278. Thomas, M. K. et al. Hypervitaminosis D in medical inpatients, *JAMA*, 338, 777, 1998.
279. Papadimitropoulos, E., Meta-analyses of therapies for postmenopausal osteoporosis. VIII: Meta-analysis of the efficacy of vitamin D treatment in preventing osteoporosis in postmenopausal women, *Endocr. Rev.*, 23, 560, 2002.
280. Heikinheimo, R. J. et al. Annual injection of vitamin D and fractures of aged bones, *Calcif. Tissue Int.*, 51 (2), 105, 1992.
281. Ooms, M. E. et al. Prevention of bone loss by vitamin D supplementation in elderly women: a randomized double blind trial, *J. Clin. Endocrinol. Metab.*, 80, 1052, 1995.
282. Peacock, M. et al. Effect of calcium or 25OH vitamin D_3 dietary supplementation on bone loss at the hip in men and women over the age of 60, *J. Clin. Endocrinol. Metab.*, 85, 3011, 2000.
283. Harwood, R. H. et al. A randomized, controlled comparison of different calcium and vitamin D supplementation regimens in elderly women after hip fracture: The Nottingham Neck of Femur (NoNOF) Study, *Age & Ageing*, 33, 45, 2004.
284. DiDaniele, N. et al. Effect of supplementation of calcium and vitamin D on bone mineral density and bone mineral content in peri- and postmenopausal women; a double-blind, randomized, controlled trial, *Pharmacol. Res.*, 50, 637, 2004.
285. Grant, A. M. et al. Oral vitamin D3 and calcium for secondary prevention of low-trauma fractures in elderly people (Randomised Evaluation of Calcium or Vitamin D, RECORD): a randomized placebo-controlled trial, *Lancet*, 365, 1621, 2005.
286. Porthouse, J. et al. Randomised controlled trial of calcium and supplementation with cholecalciferol (vitamin D3) for prevention of fractures in primary care, *Br. Med. J.*, 330, 1003, 2005.
287. Bischoff-Ferrari, H. A. et al. Effect of vitamin D on falls, *JAMA*, 291, 2004, 1999.
288. Institute of Medicine of the National Academies, *Dietary Reference Intakes for Energy, Carbohydrate, Fiber, Fat, Fatty Acids, Cholesterol, Protein and Amino Acids*, The National Academies Press, Washington, D.C., 2002.
289. Munger, R. G., Cerhan, J. R., and Chiu, B. C., Prospective study of dietary protein intake and risk of hip fracture in postmenopausal women, *Am. J. Clin. Nutr.*, 69, 147, 1999.
290. Hannan, M. T. et al. Effect of dietary protein on bone loss in elderly men and women: the Framingham Osteoporosis Study, *J. Bone Miner. Res.*, 15, 2504, 2000.
291. Promislow, J. H. et al. Protein consumption and bone mineral density in the elderly: the Rancho Bernardo Study, *Am. J. Epidemiol.*, 155, 636, 2002.
292. Wengreen, H. J. et al. Dietary protein intake and risk of osteoporotic hip fracture in elderly residents in Utah, *J. Bone Miner. Res.*, 19, 537, 2004.

293. Schurch, M. A., Protein supplements increase serum insulin-like growth factor-1 levels and attenuate proximal femur bone loss in patients with recent hip fracture. A randomized, double-blind, placebo-controlled trial, *Ann. Intern. Med.*, 128, 801, 1998.
294. Devine, A. et al. Protein consumption is an important predictor of lower limb bone mass in elderly women, *Am. J. Clin. Nutr.*, 81, 1423, 2005.
295. Alexy, U. et al. Long-term protein intake and dietary potential renal acid load are associated with bone modeling and remodeling at the proximal radius in healthy children, *Am. J. Clin. Nutr.*, 82, 1107, 2005.
296. Dawson-Hughes, B. and Harris, S. S., Calcium intake influences the association of protein intake with rates of bone loss in elderly men and women, *Am. J. Clin. Nutr.*, 75, 773, 2002.
297. Dawson-Hughes, B., Interaction of dietary calcium and protein in bone health in humans, *J. Nutr.*, 133, 852s, 2003.
298. Heaney, R. P., Protein and calcium: antagonists or synergists? *Am. J. Clin. Nutr.*, 75, 609, 2002.
299. Rapuri, P. B., Gallagher, J. C., and Haynatzka, V., Protein intake: effects on bone mineral density and the rate of bone loss in elderly women, *Am. J. Clin. Nutr.*, 77, 1517, 2003.
300. Roughead, Z. K., The effects of interaction on dietary protein and calcium on calcium retention: a controlled feeding study, *J. Bone Miner. Res.*, 19, 302s, 2004.
301. Roughead, Z. K., Is the interaction between dietary protein and calcium destructive or constructive for bone? Summary, *J. Nutr.*, 133, 866s, 2003.
302. Dawson-Hughes, B. et al. Effect of dietary protein supplements on calcium excretion in healthy older men and women, *J. Clin. Endocrinol. Metab.*, 89, 1169, 2004.
303. Massey, L. K., Dietary animal and plant protein and human bone health: A whole foods approach, *J. Nutr.*, 133, 862s, 2003.
304. Nieves, J. W., Osteoporosis: the role of micronutrients, *Am. J. Clin. Nutr.*, 81, 1232s, 2005.
305. Ilich, J. Z., Brownbill, R. A., and Tamborini, L., Bone and nutrition in elderly women: protein, energy, and calcium as main determinants of bone mineral density, *Europ. J. Clin. Nutr.*, 57, 554, 2003.
306. Tucker, K. L., Dietary intake and bone status with aging, *Current Pharmaceut. Design*, 9, 2687, 2003.
307. Heaney, R. P., Phosphorus nutrition and the treatment of osteoporosis, *Mayo Clin. Proc.*, 79, 91, 2004.
308. Heaney, R. P. and Nordin, B. E., Calcium effects on phosphorus absorption: implications for the prevention and co-therapy of osteoporosis, *J. Am. Coll. Nutr.*, 21, 239, 2002.
309. Shapiro, R. and Heaney, R. P., Co-dependence of calcium and phosphorus for growth and bone development under conditions of varying deficiency, *Bone*, 32, 532, 2003.
310. Tucker, K. L. et al. Potassium, magnesium, and fruit and vegetable intakes are associated with greater bone mineral density in elderly men and women, *Am. J. Clin. Nutr.*, 69, 727, 1999.
311. Ryder, K. M., Magnesium intake from food and supplements is associated with bone mineral density in healthy older white subjects, *J. Am. Geriatr. Soc.*, 53, 1875, 2005.
312. Institute of Medicine of the National Academies, *Dietary Reference Intakes for Water, Potassium, Sodium, Chloride, and Sulfate*, The National Academies Press, Washington, D.C., 2004.
313. Macdonald, H. M. et al. Nutritional associations with bone loss during the menopausal transition: evidence of a beneficial effect of calcium, alcohol, and fruit and vegetable nutrients and of a detrimental effect of fatty acids, *Am, J. Clin. Nutr.*, 79, 155, 2004.
314. Macdonald, H. M. et al. Low dietary potassium intakes and high dietary estimates of net endogenous acid production are associated with low bone mineral density in premenopausal women and increased markers of bone resorption in postmenopausal women, *Am. J. Clin. Nutr.*, 81, 923, 2005.
315. Sellmeyer, D. E., Schlotter, M., and Sebastian, A., Potassium citrate prevents increased urine calcium excretion and bone resorption induced by high sodium chloride diet, *J. Clin. Endocrinol. Metab.*, 87, 2008, 2002.
316. Rafferty, K., Davies, K. M., and Heaney, R. P., Potassium intake and the calcium economy, *J. Am. Coll. Nutr.*, 24, 99, 2005.
317. Tucker, K. L. et al. Low plasma vitamin B_{12} is associated with lower BMD: the Framingham Osteoporosis Study, *J. Bone Miner. Res.*, 20, 152, 2005.

318. Dhonukshe-Rutten, R. A. et al. Vitamin B_{12} status is associated with bone mineral content and bone mineral density in frail elderly women but not in men, *J. Nutr.*, 133, 801, 2003.
319. Hyun, T. H., Barrett-Connor, E., and Milne, D. B., Zinc intakes and plasma concentrations in men with osteoporosis: the Rancho Bernardo Study, *Am. J. Clin. Nutr.*, 80, 715, 2004.
320. Brownbill, R. A., Petrosian, M., and Ilich, J. Z., Association between dietary conjugated linoleic acid and bone mineral density in postmenopausal women, *J. Am. Coll. Nutr.*, 24, 177, 2005.
321. U.S. Department of Health and Human Services, National Institutes of Health, National Institute of Child Health and Human Development, *Milk Matters*, NIH Publ., No., 05-4521, September 2005, www.nichd.nih.gov/milk.
322. U.S. Department of Health and Human Services, *Healthy People 2010*, Washington, D.C., January 2000, www.health.gov/healthypeople.
323. The American Dietetic Association, Position of The American Dietetic Association: fortification and nutritional supplements, *J. Am. Diet. Assoc.*, 105, 1300, 2005.
324. Whiting, S. J. and Wood, R. J., Adverse effects of high-calcium diets in humans, *Nutr. Rev.*, 55, 1, 1997.
325. Johnson-Down, L. et al. Appropriate calcium fortification of the food supply presents a challenge, *J. Nutr.*, 133, 2232, 2003.
326. Lichtenstein, A. H. and Russell, R. M., Essential nutrients: food or supplements? Where should the emphasis be? *JAMA*, 20 (294), 351, 2005.
327. American Academy of Pediatrics, Committee on Nutrition, The use and misuse of fruit juice in pediatrics, *Pediatrics*, 107, 1210, 2001.
328. Food and Drug Administration, Health and Human Services, Fortification Policy, 21 *Code of Federal Regulations*, Ch.1, 104.20, p. 184, 2004.
329. Suojanen, A., Raulio, S., and Ovaskainen, M.-L., Liberal fortification of foods: the risks. A study relating to Finland, *J. Epidemiol. Community Health*, 56, 259, 2002.
330. Gueguen, L. and Pointillart, A., The bioavailability of dietary calcium, *J. Am. Coll. Nutr.*, 19, 119s, 2000.
331. Heaney, R. P. et al. Bioavailability of the calcium in fortified soy imitation milk, with some observations on method, *Am. J. Clin. Nutr.*, 71, 1166, 2000.
332. Zhao, Y. et al. Calcium bioavailability of calcium carbonate fortified soymilk is equivalent to cow's milk in young women, *J. Nutr.*, 135, 2379, 2005.
333. Heaney, R. P. et al. Not all calcium-fortified beverages are equal, *Nutr. Today*, 40, 39, 2005.
334. Marcason, W., How much calcium is really in that supplement? *J. Am. Diet. Assoc.*, 102, 1647, 2002.

6 Dairy Foods and Oral Health

6.1 INTRODUCTION

Dental caries (tooth decay) and periodontal (gum) diseases are the two most prevalent, but preventable, infectious oral health diseases in industrialized nations [1–6]. Although the prevalence and severity of dental caries in children and periodontal diseases in adults has been declining in developed countries over the last three decades [2], these diseases nevertheless remain major public health concerns and pose a substantial economic burden on Americans [1–6]. Among children, dental caries is the single most common chronic childhood disease [1,2]. As shown in Figure 6.1, dental caries among children still exceeds the U.S. Department of Health and Human Services' *Healthy People 2010* objectives [4,6]. Nearly 20% of young children, almost 80% of young adults, and approximately 95% of older adults have experienced tooth decay [2]. Older adults are at high risk of developing root caries and periodontal disease, both of which can lead to tooth loss [5]. The prevalence of periodontal disease increases with age, from 6% among persons aged 25 to 34 years to 41% among those aged 65 years and older [5]. About one-third of older adults (>65 years) have lost all of their natural teeth compared to 46% 20 years ago [1,5]. The nation's total bill for dental services was estimated at $74 billion in 2003 [7].

In recognition of the substantial social and economic consequences of poor oral health, the first U.S. Surgeon General's report on oral health calls for a national effort to improve oral health among all Americans [1]. More recently, the Office of the U.S. Surgeon General released a national call to action to promote oral health [8].

The causes of dental caries and periodontal disease are multifactorial, involving genetic and environmental (e.g., diet, microbial) factors. Diet and nutrition have long been recognized as contributing factors to these infectious oral health diseases [1,9–13].

Nutrition or nutritional status systemically influences the pre-eruptive development of teeth and oral tissues (e.g., the composition, size, and morphology of teeth, and the quantity and composition of saliva) [9–16]. Nutritional deficiencies during the pre-eruptive development of teeth could directly and indirectly influence caries susceptibility by affecting the formation of enamel, composition and function of saliva, and immunological responses [17]. Epidemiological studies have demonstrated that a single episode of mild to moderate malnutrition during the first year of life is associated with increased risk of developing carious lesions in both deciduous and permanent teeth [16]. It is therefore important that children consume sufficient amounts of tooth-forming nutrients such as calcium, phosphorus, magnesium, fluoride, trace minerals, and others such as vitamin D. Once teeth have erupted, it is the local effects of food and composition of saliva and plaque that are critical to the development of oral diseases such as dental caries [11].

This chapter reviews scientific findings regarding the role of dairy foods in dental caries, including tooth enamel erosion, and periodontal disease. Research indicates that several varieties of cheese (e.g., aged Cheddar, Monterey Jack, Swiss) have caries protective properties and that milk is a healthy food for teeth.

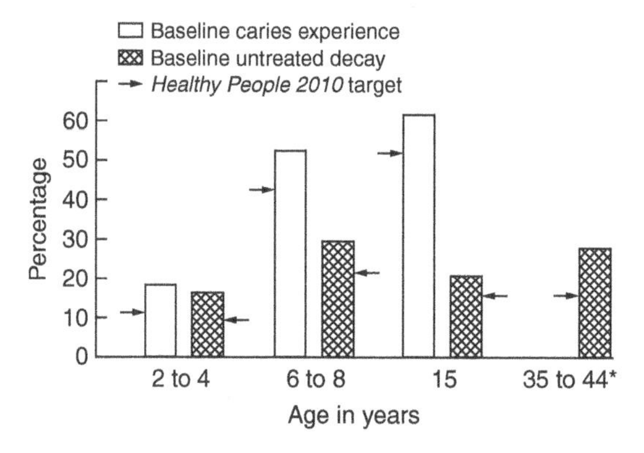

	Ages 2 to 4 %	Ages 6 to 8 %	Age 15 %	Ages 35 to 44 %
Baseline caries experience	18	52	61	
Healthy People 2010 Target: baseline caries	11	42	51	*
Baseline untreated decay	16	29	20	27
Healthy People 2010 Target: baseline untreated decay	9	21	15	15

*There is no *Healthy People 2010* objective for adult caries; 94% of adults who have one or more natural teeth have experienced tooth decay.

Source: U.S. Department of Health and Human Services, *Healthy People 2010, 2nd* Ed. Vol. II, U.S. Government Printing Office, Washington, D.C., pp. 21–11; 21–15, 2000.

FIGURE 6.1 Prevalence of dental caries compared to *Healthy People 2010* targets. (From National Center for Chronic Disease Prevention and Health Promotion, *Fact Sheet, Preventing Dental Caries*, 2002.)

6.2 DENTAL CARIES AND TOOTH ENAMEL EROSION

Foods *per se* do not cause dental caries. Dental caries is the result of complex interactions involving the host (e.g., nutrition, genetics, behavior, race, age), plaque bacteria (e.g., *Streptococcus mutans*, *S. sorbrinus*), saliva flow and composition, and environment (Figure 6.2) [15]. Diet is only one environmental factor in this process, albeit an important one. Dental caries is a diet-bacterial disease. Plaque, which forms on tooth surfaces, results from the interaction of bacteria on tooth surfaces with dietary constituents, usually sucrose and starches. Plaque is composed of viable bacteria embedded in a matrix of polysaccharides. Following exposure to sugars, plaque may form acid rapidly.

The caries process is considered to be a dynamic equilibrium involving alternating periods of demineralization of enamel or dentine (i.e., release of calcium and phosphate from teeth) and remineralization (i.e., replacement of calcium and phosphate) (Figure 6.3). Caries occurs when demineralization exceeds remineralization. Following intake of food containing fermentable carbohydrates (e.g., sugars and cooked starches), bacteria in dental plaque on either smooth surfaces, or within pits and fissures, metabolize the carbohydrate producing organic acids. When organic acids cause plaque pH to fall from its usual level of around neutrality (i.e., pH 7.0) to a so-called "critical

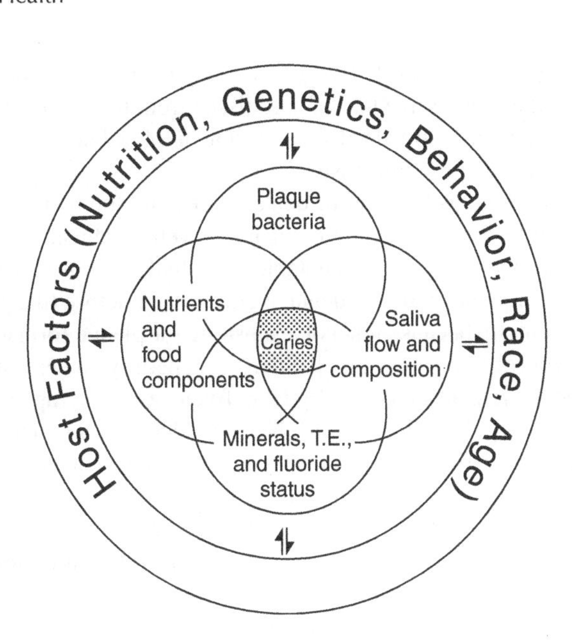

FIGURE 6.2 Multifactorial interactions in the etiology of dental caries. (From Navia, J. M., *Am. J. Clin. Nutr.*, 61 (suppl.), 407, 1995. With permission.)

pH" in the range of 5.2 to 5.7 (i.e., an acidic environment), demineralization of tooth enamel occurs as calcium and phosphate are lost from the tooth surface. Over time (i.e., 6 months to 2 years), acid penetrates tooth enamel and acid and bacteria invade enamel and dentin resulting in carious lesions. Fortunately, caries is usually not a continuous process of mineral loss from the tooth. The protective effects of saliva, fluoride, and remineralization help to offset the many episodes of acid attack. For example, saliva is super-saturated with calcium and phosphate at pH 7, which favors the deposition of calcium and remineralization of enamel. However, remineralization may be hampered by the presence of dental plaque.

Multiple factors influence both demineralization and remineralization [11]. Dental caries results when the following conditions are present simultaneously: a susceptible tooth, cariogenic (caries promoting) microorganisms in plaque that adheres to the tooth, and a fermentable carbohydrate substrate, especially if consumed frequently throughout the day or before bedtime without cleansing. Prevention of caries involves increasing tooth resistance (e.g., by fluoride), reducing or interfering with oral microorganisms (e.g., by fluoride, oral hygiene), and changing the oral

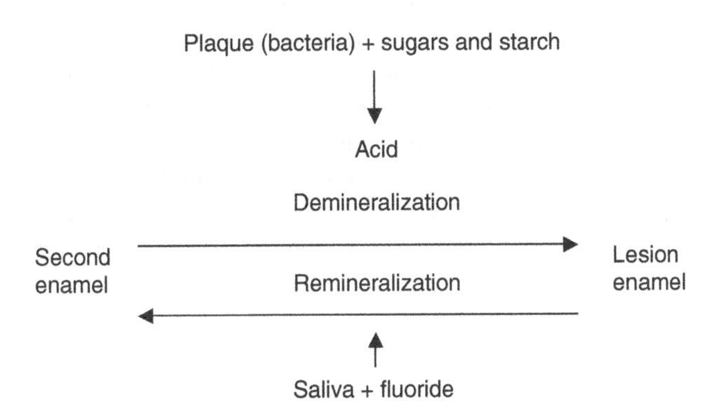

FIGURE 6.3 The caries process: an equilibrium of demineralization and remineralization.

environment (e.g., dietary intervention) [11,14,18]. Unlike dental caries, tooth enamel erosion (or dental erosion), which is the progressive loss of hard tissue from the enamel of the tooth surface by acids (e.g., in fruits, fruit juices, soft drinks), may not involve bacteria or sugars. Frequently, erosion and dental caries occur simultaneously.

Food intake can affect the development of dental caries and tooth erosion [11,14]. The cariogenicity (ability to promote caries) of simple sugars is well established [11,14,19]. Sucrose is identified as the most cariogenic of all fermentable carbohydrates, in part because oral bacteria quickly convert this sugar into the matrix of dental plaque [19]. Lactose (the primary sugar in milk) has relatively low cariogenicity because it is not a substrate for plaque formation and is not rapidly fermented by oral microorganisms [9–11,17]. Sucrose generally lowers plaque pH below 5.0, whereas lactose may reduce it to around 6.0 [20]. High fructose corn syrup used in the manufacture of carbonated beverages is highly cariogenic [9]. Not only does the amount of fermentable carbohydrate in a food influence its cariogenicity, but also the food's physical consistency, how often it is consumed, the intervals between exposures, how long it remains in the mouth, and other foods with which it is consumed [10,11,14,19]. Sucrose in a retentive or sticky form (e.g., dried fruits) and eaten between meals is potentially more cariogenic than sugars that are rapidly cleared from the mouth (e.g., in liquids such as chocolate milk) [14]. The longer fermentable carbohydrates remain in the mouth or on tooth surfaces where they are exposed to microorganisms, the greater the risk of dental caries. Ingestion of fermentable carbohydrates before bedtime without cleansing may be hazardous for oral health.

Diet, particularly intake of carbonated soft drinks, citrus fruit juices, and acidic sports drinks, contribute to dental erosion and to the development of dental caries [9,11,17,21–23]. Of recent concern is the high intake of soft drinks among children and adolescents because of the potential of these beverages to increase erosion of dental enamel and caries [22–24]. Both regular and diet soft drinks are acidic (pH 2.5 to 3.5), which can result in enamel erosion or demineralization [22]. The high amounts of sucrose and fructose corn syrup in regular (nondiet) soft drinks contribute to dental caries. The increased consumption of soft drinks has paralleled a decline in the consumption of cow's milk, a beverage that has been shown repeatedly to be noncariogenic (i.e., neither promotes nor reduces dental caries) [22]. The American Academy of Pediatrics, concerned about potential health problems such as dental erosion and caries resulting from children's high intake of soft drinks in schools, recommends that pediatricians work to eliminate soft drinks in schools and encourage healthful alternatives such as low-fat white or flavored milk [24]. Because excessive intake of fruit juice can contribute to caries and dental erosion, the American Academy of Pediatrics recommends that children aged 1 to 6 years consume no more than 4 to 6 ounces of fruit juice/day and children aged 7 to 18 years consume no more than 8 to 12 ounces of fruit juice/day [25].

Some foods or food components have the potential to prevent or reduce dental caries in the presence of a cariogenic challenge as well as tooth erosion. A review of sugars and dental caries led the researchers to conclude, "the caries risk of foods may be modified by combining cariogenic foods with dairy products that may reduce the acidogenic effect and promote remineralization" [19]. As discussed below, findings from laboratory animal and human studies (e.g., plaque pH, enamel demineralization/remineralization, epidemiological, clinical) indicate that dairy foods such as milk and cheese do not promote dental caries or tooth erosion. Moreover, dairy foods, particularly certain cheeses, may even protect against dental caries [20,26–28]. Because dairy foods such as milk have low acidogenic potential, they do not contribute to tooth erosion [9,22].

6.2.1 Animal Studies

While findings from experimental animal studies cannot be causally extrapolated to humans, foods that are cariogenic for animals are generally thought to be cariogenic for humans [29]. Animal experiments also provide evidence of the relative cariogenicity of different foods [29].

Studies in laboratory animals indicate that several varieties of cheese inhibit the formation of caries even when the animals consume diets high in sugars or cooked starches [20,28]. Few smooth surface carious lesions developed in laboratory rats when selected exposures to a high sucrose diet were followed by cheese intake [30]. The incidence of smooth surface caries has been demonstrated to be reduced in rats fed Cheddar cheese, a cheese spread, Mozzarella cheese, and cream cheese [30,31]. Cheese intake also has been demonstrated to reduce the incidence of root caries, a common form of dental caries in older adults. When experimental desalivated animals (i.e., animals at high risk of caries development because of their lack of saliva) were fed Cheddar- or Swiss-type cheeses as between meal snacks, along with a cariogenic diet, the animals developed fewer and less severe carious lesions on crowns and root surfaces than when fed cariogenic snacks alone or not fed additional snacks, thereby demonstrating the ability of cheese to actually prevent the development of lesions [32]. These findings may be of relevance for older adults who are at high risk for root-surface caries and for whom loss of saliva gland function may occur due to certain medications [14].

Experimental animal studies not only indicate that cheese prevents dental caries, but also that cow's milk is noncariogenic (i.e., not caries promoting) [20,27,28,33–40]. In 1961, Dreizen et al. [33] reported that nonfat dry cow's milk fed to laboratory rats was noncariogenic. In 1966, Stephan [34] identified whole milk as a noncariogenic food. Similar findings were reported in 1981 by Reynolds and Johnson [36] who suggested that a cariogenic diet with milk (4% to 5%) substantially reduced the incidence of caries in rats. When three casein-free milk mineral concentrates with various levels of whey protein, calcium, and phosphate were included in a caries-producing diet containing 20% sucrose, significant reductions in caries occurred on the smooth surfaces of rat molars [37].

Studies in desalivated rats have shown that milk is essentially noncariogenic [38,41,42]. When desalivated rats were given cow's milk, one of three popular infant formulas marketed in Brazil, or water with added sucrose, cow's milk had the lowest cavity-producing potential [41]. In another investigation in which desalivated rats were given 2% milk (4% lactose) or lactose-reduced milk, the animals remained essentially caries free [38]. In contrast, animals which drank sucrose (10%) solutions developed many and severe lesions and those that drank lactose (4%) solutions developed a few small carious lesions. This study demonstrates that milk with lactose, in contrast to sucrose, is either noncariogenic or minimally caries-promoting. The authors of the study suggest that because milk has many of the physical properties of saliva and is negligibly cariogenic, this food may be a good saliva substitute for older people who have decreased salivary flow (i.e., hyposalivation) and, as such, experience difficulty in chewing, tasting, and swallowing food. Hyposalivation can result from use of medications, or degenerative physiological changes, or treatment of head and neck cancer by radiation [18]. Milk may buffer oral acidity, reduce enamel solubility, and contribute to enamel remineralization [43].

Using desalivated rats, Bowen and Lawrence [42] compared the cariogenicity of various fluids (i.e., sucrose, cola drink, honey, human milk, cow milk, and water) frequently fed to infants and toddlers. The rats were fed the above beverages through a feeding method simulating the way infants ingest fluid through a bottle or nipple. The highest incidence of dental caries was found in the animals receiving a cola beverage, water with 10% sugar, or water with 10% honey [42]. Considerable tooth erosion developed in the animals receiving the cola or honey beverages. Rats receiving human milk developed slightly more decay (but not more than found with infant formulas in other studies) than those given cow's milk [42]. The researchers suggest that human milk may be more cariogenic than cow milk because of the higher amount of lactose and lower mineral (calcium, phosphorus) content of human milk. Based on their findings, the researchers discourage the use of honey, cola, and sucrose water in nursing bottles [42]. They also discourage prolonged exposure to human milk or formula through allowing infants to sleep on the nipple. After tooth eruption, oral hygiene is encouraged [42].

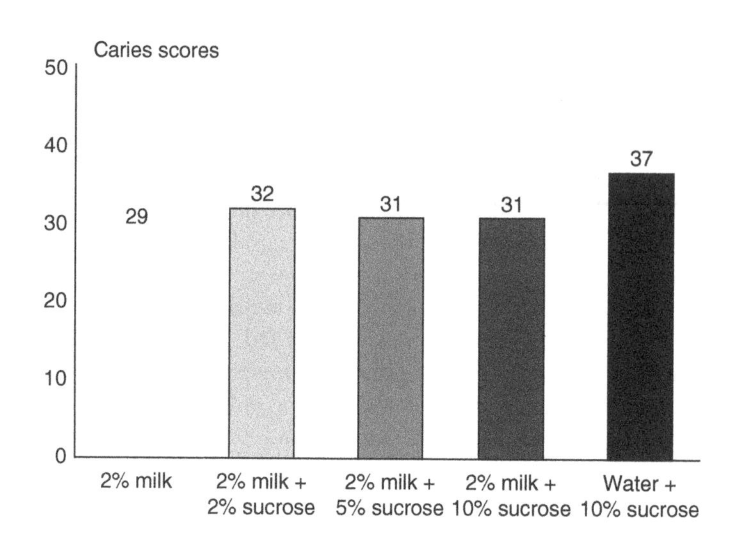

FIGURE 6.4 Sucrose-milk solutions are significantly less cariogenic in rats than a sucrose–water solution. Note that milk protects against the cariogenic challenge of sucrose. (Adapted from Bowen, W. H. and Pearson, S. K., *Caries Res.*, 27, 461, 1993. With permission.)

Several studies demonstrate that milk exerts some protection against the cariogenic challenge of sucrose [39,40]. When the cariostatic properties of milk were examined in laboratory rats, the relative noncariogenicity of milk was maintained despite the addition of sucrose in concentrations of 2%, 5%, and 10% [39]. Animals given milk containing as much as 10% sucrose developed 70% less smooth surface caries than animals given a 10% aqueous solution of sucrose (Figure 6.4) [39]. However, milk containing sucrose was more cariogenic than milk alone [39]. When desalivated rats received a sucrose solution (5%) or one of several commonly used infant formulas or 2% milk, cow's milk was found to be the least cariogenic of all the products tested [40]. In contrast, sucrose was by far the most cariogenic [40]. In fact, sucrose was 2.5 times more cariogenic than the most cariogenic infant formulas and at least 20 times more cariogenic than milk [40]. Experimental animal studies have identified yogurt as a food with low cariogenic potential [44], thus supporting earlier findings [45].

6.2.2 Human Studies

6.2.2.1 Plaque pH

Plaque acidity studies, which indicate pH changes following food intake, are another important measure of relative food cariogenicity [46]. Human dental plaque pH studies have shown that a number of cheeses including aged Cheddar, Swiss, blue, Monterey Jack, Mozzarella, Brie, and Gouda do not cause plaque pH to fall to a level conducive to the development of caries (Table 6.1) [28,47–50]. When a variety of foods were fed to humans and interproximal plaque pH was measured by telemetry, all foods except aged cheddar cheese and skim milk caused plaque pH to fall close to 4.0 (i.e., a pH conducive to caries) [48]. Some cheeses, including aged Cheddar, Monterey Jack, and Swiss have been demonstrated to eliminate sucrose-induced decreases in plaque pH when consumed just prior to [48] or after [50] sucrose intake. A study of plaque pH changes demonstrated a beneficial effect of American processed cheese [51]. When processed cheese was eaten alone or before sucrose (10%), plaque pH stayed above 5.7 (Figure 6.5) [51]. In this study, processed cheese alone was not acidogenic and prevented the low pH produced with the sucrose rinse [51]. Linke and Riba [52] reported that when subjects consumed Cheddar cheese immediately after a sugar-containing food, the amount of acid produced in the oral cavity was

TABLE 6.1
Foods Which Do Not Cause the Interproximal Plaque pH to Fall to 5.5 within 30 minutes after Ingestion

Eggs	Chewing Gums
Cheeses	Mannitol
Blue	Sorbitol
Brie	Xylitol
Cheddar, aged	Meats
Gouda	Ham
Monterey Jack	Nuts
Mozzarella	Peanuts
Swiss	Walnuts
	Swiss Products[a]

[a] Approximately 90 sweet confectionary products formulated to be nonacidogenic in humans.

Source: From Schachtele, C. F. and Harlander, S. K., *J. Can. Dent. Assn.*, 3, 213, 1984. With permission.

significantly reduced compared to the amount of acid obtained from the sugar-containing food alone.

Early studies evaluating changes in plaque pH in humans following intake of specific foods suggested that fat-free milk is relatively noncariogenic [49]. When Dodds and Edgar [53] ranked seven foods (apple drink, caramel, chocolate, cookie, skimmed milk powder, snack cracker, and wheat flake) according to their plaque pH response in 12 volunteers, skimmed milk powder was ranked as the food with the lowest potential cariogenicity.

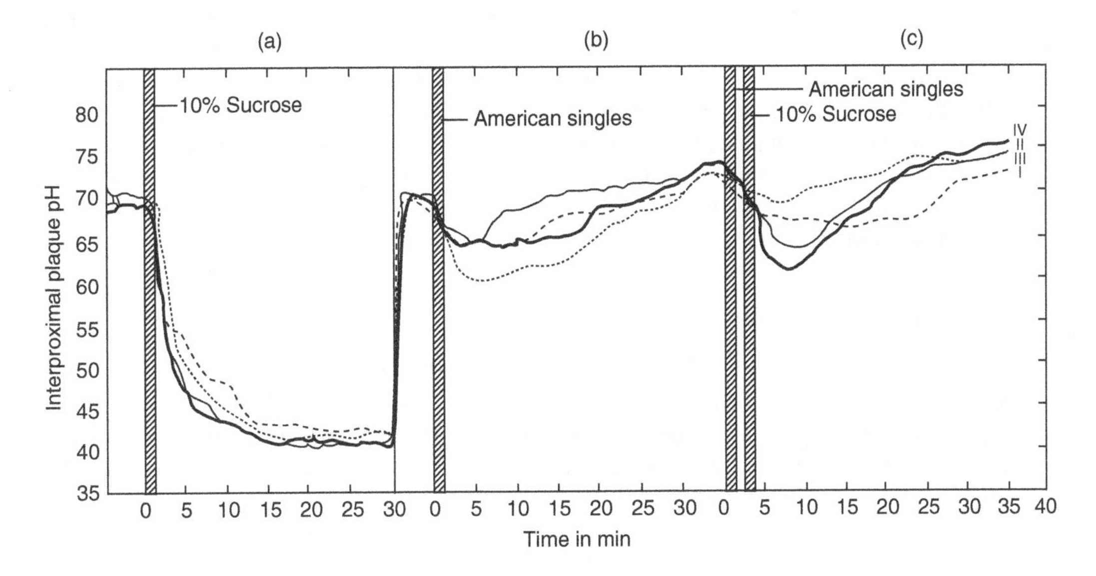

FIGURE 6.5 Effects of processed cheese on human plaque pH. (a) Demonstrates the acidogenicity with sucrose (pH 4.26). (b) Shows that when cheese is eaten alone, the plaque pH stays above a "safe for teeth" (pH 5.7) level. (c) Shows that cheese intake prevents the acid challenge when followed by sucrose. (From Jensen, M. E. and Wefel, J. S., *Am. J. Dent.*, 3 (5), 217, 1990. With permission.)

6.2.2.2 Demineralization/Remineralization Studies

Several studies indicate that dairy foods such as cheese and milk prevent demineralization of enamel and that cheese favors remineralization of carious lesions [28]. Silva et al. [54], using intraoral caries models (i.e., models that use sections of human or bovine enamel often placed at interproximal sites in fixed appliances), found that consumption of 5 g of aged Cheddar cheese immediately following sucrose intake (i.e., a 10% sucrose challenge) reduced, by an average of 71%, sucrose-induced demineralization of experimental enamel slabs. Similarly, cheese [55] and a dairy product (derived from the whey of cow's milk) containing 26% calcium and 39% phosphorus [56] were identified as foods of low cariogenic potential in *in vivo* intraoral tests carried out in New Zealand. The enamel-softening effect of toasted breadcrumbs was substantially reduced when cheese (aged Cheddar) was added [55]. Similarly, the addition of whey mineral to fruit juice reduced the enamel softening effect of fruit juice [56]. Processed cheese also has been shown to prevent demineralization and enhance remineralization of enamel and root lesions in a human in situ caries model [51]. In this model, processed cheese reduced the cariogenic potential on root surfaces by 52%. When researchers evaluated the cariogenic potential of four different processed cheeses by enamel demineralization and plaque pH tests, all were shown to be noncariogenic or safe for teeth [57].

A study in Israel involving ten subjects demonstrated that chewing hard cheese significantly increased in situ remineralization of previously softened (by a cola-type drink) tooth enamel surfaces [58]. The researchers speculated that the calcium and phosphate in cheese may be partly responsible for the remineralization. Likewise, using an in situ caries model developed by Featherstone and Zero [59], enamel demineralization occurred in the absence of Cheddar cheese. In contrast, in the presence of cheese, a significant trend toward remineralization of enamel was evident [59].

Early *in vitro* studies demonstrated that the presence of milk solids reduced the ability of a fermentable food to demineralize enamel [45]. Moreover, whole milk solids offered more protection against demineralization than skim milk solids [45], possibly because of the inclusion of fat, which has been demonstrated to have protective effects. Other investigations indicate that phosphoproteins in milk are adsorbed into enamel *in vitro* and inhibit acid dissolution of enamel [60,61]. Milk also has been shown to remineralize enamel *in vitro* [62]. Gedalia and coworkers [63] reported that milk (and saliva) enhanced remineralization of previously softened tooth enamel surfaces.

When the relative potential of different foods to contribute to caries was assessed by a combination of tests (i.e., two plaque pH models, an experimental animal study, and an *in vitro* enamel demineralization model), skimmed milk was found to be the least cariogenic and apple juice the most cariogenic of the seven foods tested (i.e., apple juice, chocolate, caramel, wheat flake, cookie, cracker, skimmed milk) [46].

6.2.2.3 Epidemiological and Clinical Studies

Epidemiological studies associate intake of cheese and milk with a reduced incidence of caries [23,64–68]. The only significant difference in the diets of 23 caries-prone and 19 caries-free English schoolchildren over a 2-year period was average intake of cheese, according to an early epidemiological study [65]. The caries-free group consumed twice as much cheese (8 g daily) as did the caries-prone group (4 g daily) [65].

Milk intake has been associated with a low incidence of caries in 14-year-old Danish schoolchildren [66]. In a survey of preschool children of different ethnic origins in Fort Worth, Texas, average decayed, extracted, or filled teeth (DEF) decreased with increased daily milk intake (as determined by a 24-hour dietary recall), especially for black and Hispanic children [67]. When the effect of milk intake on dental caries was studied in Italian schoolchildren aged 6- to 11-years, milk was shown to protect against caries in children who did not use fluoride, whose oral hygiene was poor, and who frequently had a high daily sucrose intake [68]. A study of 642 young children enrolled in the Iowa Fluoride Study and followed from age 1 to age 5 found that a change in beverage patterns, specifically decreased consumption of milk and increased intake of soft drinks and 100% juices was associated with increased risk of dental caries [23]. In this study, milk intake had a neutral association with caries, whereas consumption of soft drinks and, to a lesser extent 100% juice, was associated with increased caries risk [23].

Epidemiological investigations support a protective effect of cheese against root surface caries [64,69]. Root surface caries affects about two-thirds of the U.S. elderly [64]. Given that the size of this population is increasing, combined with the use of prescription drugs, many of which suppress saliva gland function, root caries can be expected to become an even greater problem. When food intake was assessed in 275 adults aged 44 to 64 years who were grouped according to their root caries status, those without root caries consumed more cheese, dairy products, fruits and fruit juices, and less sugars and starches than did subjects with root caries [69]. In another investigation of the relationship between diet and root caries in 141 adults aged 47 to 83 years, individuals in the lowest quartile for root caries consumed approximately twice as much cheese as those in the highest quartile (Table 6.2) [64]. Individuals who were free from root caries consumed 50% more cheese and 25% more of other dairy products than did subjects who experienced the most root caries [64]. Additionally, root caries-free subjects had higher daily intakes of fiber, protein, calcium, phosphorus, and magnesium and lower sugar intakes than subjects with root caries (Table 6.3) [64].

A protective effect of cheese has also been demonstrated in a clinical trial involving 179 Israeli children aged 7 to 9 years [70]. In this 2-year clinical trial, the incidence of dental caries was significantly reduced (by 26%) in children who consumed 5 g of Edam cheese a day following breakfast compared to children who did not consume this extra cheese (Table 6.4).

6.2.3 Caries Protective Components in Dairy Foods

Available evidence indicates that cheese is cariostatic and that milk is noncariogenic [27]. Researchers have identified several possible components in dairy foods to explain these beneficial effects, as indicated in Table 6.5 [20,26–28,30,37,38,71,72]. Cheese, for example, may stimulate the flow of alkaline saliva and reduce the number of plaque bacteria [26,28]. Enamel demineralization can be prevented by stimulating the production of saliva, which increases plaque pH (i.e., increases its alkalinity) and the clearance of fermentable carbohydrate from the oral cavity

TABLE 6.2
Frequency of Consumption of Specific Food Items (Based on the Food Diaries), with Groups Separated by Caries Experience

Food Item[a]	Lower Quartile Root DFS/100 Teeth	Upper Quartile Root DFS 100 Teeth
Liquid sugars	4.23 ± 5.74	8.50 ± 7.26
Sticky sugars	2.81 ± 1.81	8.41 ± 1.81[b]
Cheese	4.77 ± 3.00	2.20 ± 2.00[c]

$x \pm SD$; $n = 13$, lower quartile; $n = 16$, upper quartile. DFS, decayed and filled surfaces.

[a] There were no differences in the total number of food items eaten by the two groups.
[b] Significantly different from lower quartile, $P < 0.02$.
[c] Significantly different from lower quartile, $P < 0.03$.

Source: From Papas, A. S. et. al., *Am. J. Clin. Nutr.*, 61 (suppl.), 423, 1995. With permission.

TABLE 6.3
Comparison of Daily Intakes in Subjects with Root Caries Compared with Those Who Were Root-Caries Free

	Subjects with Caries	Subjects without Caries
Crude fiber (g)	4	5
Protein (g)	76	87
Calcium (mg)	727	828
Phosphorus (mg)	1136	1331[a]
Magnesium (mg)	241	297
Sucrose (g)	11	72
Refined sugar (g)	22	15

$N = 66$, with caries; $n = 42$, without caries.

[a] Significantly different from caries-laden subjects, $P = 0.02$.

Source: From Papas, A. S. et. al., *Am. J. Clin. Nutr.*, 61 (suppl.), 423, 1995. With permission.

(Figure 6.6) [47,54]. However, the finding that cheese may inhibit dental caries in the absence of saliva indicates that there may be other mechanisms involved in addition to its effect on saliva [32].

Components in cheese or milk such as protein (casein and whey), lipids, calcium, phosphorus, and other constituents may be partly responsible for the beneficial effects of these dairy foods on oral health [20,26–28,37,38,71–75]. Casein and whey proteins in dairy foods may help reduce enamel demineralization and enhance remineralization [26,28]. Using an intraoral caries model, Reynolds [61] found that casein prevented enamel demineralization and that this effect was related to casein's incorporation into plaque. Minor milk proteins or milk-derived bioactive peptides such as casein phosphopeptide (CPP) and glycomacropeptide (GMP) may contribute to the cariostatic properties of cheese by inhibiting the growth of cariogenic bacteria, concentrating calcium and phosphate in plaque, reducing enamel demineralization, and favoring remineralization [26,75].

TABLE 6.4
Mean and Number of DMF Surfaces for Groups 1 and 2 at the Start of the Study and after 2 Years

Group	No. of Children	Baseline DMFS (SE)	At 2 Years DMFS (SE)	Caries Increment	% Reduction
Control (no cheese)	136	0.55[a]	2.90	2.35[b]	
		(0.16)	(0.31)	(0.35)	
Cheese (5 g/day)	84	0.62[a]	1.24	0.62[b]	26.4
		(0.25)	(0.15)	(0.19)	

(SE) ± not standard error.

[a] Not significant.

[b] Significant, $P < 0.001$.

Source: From Gedalia, I. et. al., *Am. J. Dent.*, 7, 331, 1994. With permission.

TABLE 6.5
Proposed Mechanisms by Which Cheese Reduces Cariogenicity

Effect	Consequence	Mechanism
Stimulation of salivary flow	Buffering effect	Neutralizes plaque acids
	Enhances food clearance	Removes source of fermentable carbohydrate
Inhibition of plaque bacteria	May reduce bacterial load	Reduces acid production
Delivery of high amounts of calcium and inorganic phosphate	Reduces demineralization	By adsorbed proteins, by casein phosphopeptides, i.e., bound Ca and Pj
	Enhances remineralizalion	By casein phosphopeptides, i.e., bound Ca and Pi

Source: From Kashket, S. and DePaola, D. P., *Nutr. Rev.*, 60, 102, 2002.

Reynolds and colleagues [74] have suggested that casein phosphopeptides stabilize calcium phosphate through the formation of casein phosphopeptide–calcium phosphate complexes (CPP–CP) and facilitate the uptake of calcium and phosphate by plaque. Studies in rats investigated the cariostatic effect of CPP–CP on caries. Animals were fed a cariogenic diet free of dairy products and solutions of CPP–CP (0.1, 0.2, 0.5, and 1.0% w/v) were applied to molar teeth twice daily. Control groups received solutions of 500 parts per million (ppm) fluoride or nonphosphorylated peptides of a casein digest (0.5% w/v). CPP-CP reduced caries in a dose response manner and the anticariogenic effects of fluoride and CPP–CP were additive [74]. The researchers suggest that the anticariogenicity of CPP–CP complexes may be explained by the increase in calcium phosphate in plaque, reducing enamel demineralization and increasing remineralization [74]. A double-blind, randomized clinical trial in ten subjects found that the addition of casein phosphopeptide amorphous calcium phosphate nanocomplexes (CPP–ACP) to milk substantially increased milk's ability to remineralize enamel subsurface lesions and that the effect was dose-dependent [76]. Water-soluble proteose-peptones in the whey fraction of milk protein may provide protection against tooth demineralization, according to an *in vitro* study [77]. Also, other constituents in milk

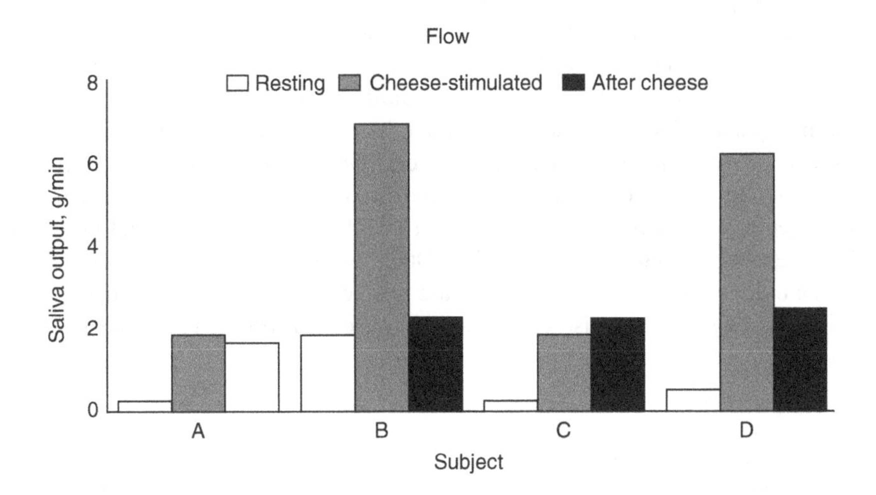

FIGURE 6.6 Salivary flow rate (g/min) for four subjects during pre-experimental resting period (3 minutes), during cheese stimulation (1 minute) and during post cheese period (2 minutes). (From Silva, M. F., de A., Jenkins, G. N., Burgess, R. C., and Sandham, H. J., *Caries Res.*, 20, 263, 1986. With permission.)

and milk products such as glycoproteins and proteoglycans may play a role in inhibiting dental caries [77].

Milk proteins such as lactoferrin and enzymes isolated from milk (e.g., lysozyme and lactoperoxidase) may protect against caries by inhibiting the ability of cavity-causing bacteria to adhere to tooth surfaces [20,27,75]. Milk proteins, particularly kappa casein, have been demonstrated to reduce the adherence of *Streptococcus mutans* to the saliva-coated hydroxyapatite surfaces of teeth [20,27,78,79]. Milk and the milk protein, kappa casein, also may protect against caries by decreasing the activity of the plaque-promoting enzyme, glucosyltransferase produced by *S. mutans*, and the ability of this enzyme to adhere to tooth surfaces or saliva-coated hydroxyapatite [79]. Guggenheim and coworkers [80] reported that the specific form or macromolecular configuration of casein in milk contributes to its caries-protective effect. In a series of three studies in laboratory rats, micellar casein from skim milk powder reduced fissure and smooth surface caries, as well as the ability of *S. sobrinus* to form colonies [80]. Soluble casein did not exhibit the caries-protective effect of micellar casein. The researchers state that this is the first finding demonstrating that a dietary component, specifically micellar casein, selectively modifies the microbial composition of dental plaque consistent with reducing its cariogenic potential [80].

Lipids in cheese, by forming a protective coating on enamel surfaces, may retard the dissolution of enamel surfaces. An antibacterial effect of fatty acids in cheese also may explain cheese's protective effect against dental caries [26,32]. Also, fats may increase the oral clearance of food particles [9].

The high calcium and phosphorus content of cheese and milk may contribute in part to the anticariogenic effect of these foods [20,26–28,37,63,71,72,77,81,82]. Cheese may increase calcium and phosphorus concentrations in dental plaque thus increasing its buffering capacity and favoring remineralization of preformed lesions [26,57,71,72,81,82]. A significant increase in plaque calcium, but not plaque phosphate, was reported in subjects who ate 5 g of several different varieties of cheese (mild Cheddar, Cheshire, Danish blue, double Glouster, Edam, Gouda, Stilton, Wensleydale) (Figure 6.7) [72]. The findings led the authors to suggest that eating cheese at the end of a meal might be an effective way to reduce dental caries [72]. A study of 16 British adults found that consuming cheese alone, or as part of a cooked mixed meal (e.g., pasta in cheese sauce), significantly increased the calcium concentration in dental plaque when compared to a meal not containing cheese [82]. Subjects with the lowest baseline calcium intake exhibited the largest increases in plaque calcium [82]. Based on these findings, the researchers suggest that cheese-containing meals may protect against dental caries.

In studies reported by Gedalia et al. [58,63], the remineralizing effects of hard cheese and cow's milk on enamel surfaces previously softened by an acidic beverage were attributed to the uptake of calcium and phosphate salts by the surface enamel. These findings support earlier observations from *in vitro* and *in vivo* experiments that cheese's calcium and phosphorus content contributes to this food's ability to inhibit demineralization and favor remineralization, thus, reducing the potential cariogenicity of sucrose [71]. However, it is unlikely that calcium and phosphate alone account for cheese's cariostatic properties [27]. Other components in cheese such as tyramine, which could be used by microorganisms to increase plaque pH, and fatty acids, many of which are potent antimicrobial agents, may also contribute to cheese's cariostatic properties [27].

6.2.4 Chocolate Milk

There is some evidence that foods containing cocoa, milk fat, and other components such as calcium and phosphorus found in chocolate milk may be less likely to contribute to dental caries than either sucrose alone or snack foods such as potato chips, cookies, and raisins [83]. Cocoa powder has been shown to be noncariogenic [84,85]. Water-soluble components of cocoa have been found to inhibit plaque accumulation and caries by reducing the biosynthesis of extracellular

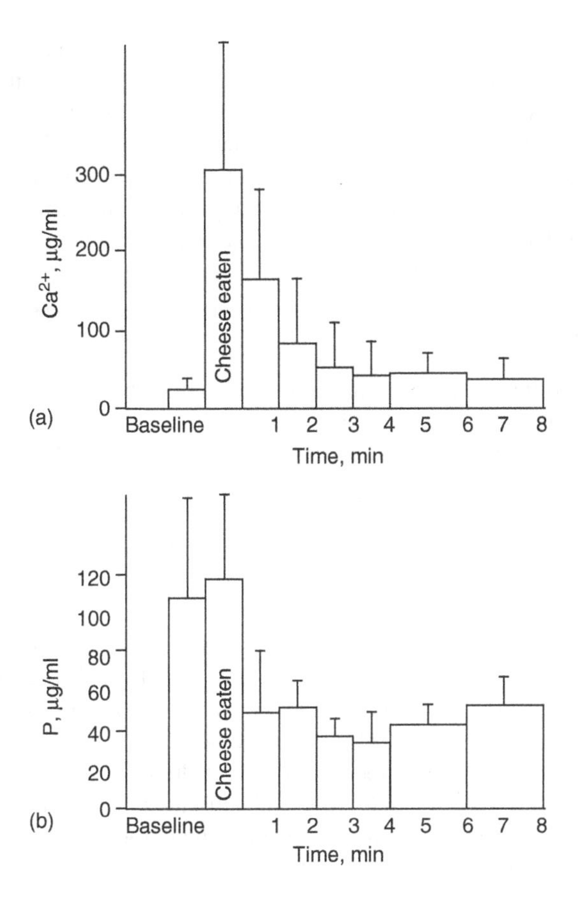

FIGURE 6.7 Mean Ca^{2+} (a) and soluble phosphate (b) concentrations in saliva before, during, and after eating 5 g of edam cheese. (From Jenkins, G. N. and Hargreaves, J. A., *Caries Res.*, 23, 159, 1989. With permission.)

polysaccharide by selected human plaque-forming microorganisms (e.g., *Streptococcus mutans*) [85].

The moderate amount of sucrose in chocolate milk is unlikely to cause dental caries [67]. As discussed above, the inclusion of sugar in milk is less likely to contribute to dental caries than sugar in water [39,40]. The cariogenicity of chocolate milk has yet to be established in humans. However, liquids such as chocolate milk tend to clear the mouth faster than carbohydrate-containing solids, and therefore may be less likely to cause tooth decay. Levine [86], based on a review of flavored milk products and caries, concludes that the cariogenicity of flavored milk products is "negligible to low and consumed in moderation they are a preferable alternative to similarly sweetened soft drinks." The American Academy of Pediatric Dentistry states that "chocolate milk is OK for children's teeth," is highly nutritious, and because children like it, they drink more of it [87].

6.2.5 Early Childhood Caries

Early childhood caries is the presence of one or more decayed, missing, or filled tooth surfaces in any primary tooth in a preschool child between birth and 71 months of age [88]. Baby bottle tooth decay, one of the more severe manifestations of this syndrome, is rampant dental caries in infants and toddlers caused by prolonged contact with almost any liquid other than water [13,88]. For example, allowing infants and young children to use a nursing bottle containing a fermentable carbohydrate (e.g., fruit juice, soda, other sweetened drinks, honey) while sleeping can lead to early childhood caries [14,42,88]. Milk given in a bottle has been claimed to contribute to nursing bottle caries or early childhood caries. However, Bowen [27,89] argues that there is no evidence to support this suggestion. All of the available scientific evidence indicates that cow's milk is noncariogenic [27,42]. A small study in Puerto Rico found that when cow's milk was the only substrate in young children's nursing bottles, none of the children developed evidence of dental caries [90]. Other factors in addition to the contents of the nursing bottle, such as the physical effect of the nipple, which obstructs the flow of saliva, and the intake of solid food (e.g., sweetened cereals), may contribute to nursing bottle caries [27,89].

6.2.6 Fluoridation

Nearly 100 national and international organizations recognize the public health benefit of community water fluoridation to prevent tooth decay [91]. When consumed in optimal amounts in water (0.7 to 1.2 ppm) and food and used topically (e.g., toothpastes, mouth rinses), fluoride increases tooth mineralization, helps reduce dental enamel demineralization and promote enamel remineralization, and helps reduce dentin hypersensitivity [91]. Fluoridation of water supplies reduces enamel caries in children by 20% or more and helps prevent root surface caries and tooth loss in adults [91]. Widespread use of fluoride in water and dentifrices is the major factor responsible for the recent decline in dental caries in developed countries [11].

However, excessive intake of fluoride during enamel formation, for example, from prolonged use of powdered infant formulas reconstituted with fluoridated water, may lead to dental fluorosis [91,92]. Fluorosis is a defect in tooth enamel that generally is not harmful but may lead to chalky white spots to brown discoloration [87,91]. Although cow's milk is not recommended before 1 year of age, intake after infancy could help reduce the risk of fluorosis in permanent teeth, suggest the authors of a recent study [92]. In this study, food and nutrient intakes of 677 children were analyzed periodically at 6 weeks through 16 months of age and primary tooth fluorosis was assessed at 4.5 to 6.9 years of age. The increased percentage of children consuming cow's milk and the quantities of cow's milk consumed were associated with reduced risk of fluorosis [92].

Many countries do not have adequate exposure to fluoride, placing populations at risk of dental caries [93]. The World Health Organization recommends that adequate exposure to fluoride provided by appropriate vehicles including milk should be promoted in these countries [93]. A caries-protective effect of fluoridated milk has been shown in experimental animals [94,95], *in vitro* studies of human dental enamel and plaque [96–99], and human studies [100,101]. When laboratory rats were given frequent feedings of fluoridated milk, plain milk, fluoridated water, and plain distilled water via an automatic feeding machine, the lowest caries scores occurred in animals given the fluoridated milk, followed by the plain milk [94]. *In vitro* studies demonstrate that fluoridated milk inhibits demineralization of tooth enamel [96,97], helps protect against root surface caries [98], and increases fluoride concentrations in saliva and dental plaque [99]. Community-based milk fluoridation studies in Chinese and Bulgarian children describe a caries-reducing effect of fluoridated milk [100,101]. These studies suggest that fluoridation of milk may be a potential source of fluoride for populations at risk of caries who do not receive adequate fluoride from public water supplies and/or other sources.

6.3 PERIODONTAL DISEASE

Periodontal disease is an oral infectious disorder characterized by inflammation and progressive loss of soft tissues supporting the teeth, as well as resorption of hard (alveolar bone) tissues [13,102,103]. Actually, periodontal disease is a collection of several diseases of soft and hard tissues surrounding the teeth: gingivitis (inflammatory gum changes without loss of bone) and periodontitis (inflammatory and destructive changes in the soft tissues and in alveolar bone supporting the teeth) [13,14]. Most Americans will develop gingivitis in which there is mild periodontal disease. Severe periodontitis with risk of tooth loss is less prevalent [14,102]. Because of the potential for severe consequences in terms of tooth loss and treatment costs, as well as ensuing nutritional problems, prevention of periodontal disease is emphasized [14,102,103].

Periodontal disease is initiated by a bacterial infection, but can be modified by host response factors including those that affect bone remodeling [14,102,103]. Certain individuals are at high risk of periodontal disease because of a genetic predisposition, diseases such as autoimmune diseases, diabetes mellitus, alcoholism, and endocrine disorders; use of certain drugs (e.g., anti-epileptic, cancer therapy, corticosteroids); and lifestyle choices such as cigarette smoking, chewing tobacco, and consumption of a nutritionally inadequate diet (e.g., low intake of calcium, vitamin C) [13,14,102,103].

Unlike dental caries, for which a strong role for diet is suggested, the role of diet, specific foods, or single nutrients in the development of periodontal disease is less clear [13,103,104]. Theoretically, diet may modulate the progression of periodontal disease in several ways. The composition of the diet can affect accumulation of plaque. Specific nutrients may influence periodontal disease by their effect on wound healing processes [104]. Diet may also affect host defense mechanisms important in oral health. Periodontal disease is an infectious disorder and it is well known that dietary imbalances alter inflammatory and immunologic responses and thus resistance to infection [13,105].

The role of specific foods such as dairy foods in immune processes and periodontal disease is unknown. In one study, cheese intake was associated with reduced bone loss (root-surface exposure) in experimental animals receiving a cariogenic diet, leading the authors to suggest that cheese may be important in the prevention of periodontal disease [32].

Diet may influence the pathogenesis of periodontal disease by its effect on the metabolism of collagen and alveolar bone. Dietary calcium, the nutrient most important for preventing and treating osteoporosis, may influence periodontal disease [102–104]. Some experimental animal and human epidemiological studies of calcium intake, bone mineral density, and tooth loss suggest that low dietary intake of calcium increases the risk for periodontal disease [102]. Studies have shown that increasing intake of calcium and vitamin D is associated with a lower risk of tooth loss in post-menopausal women and older men [106,107]. However, periodontal disease was not evaluated in these studies.

Nishida et al. [108], using data from (National Health and Nutrition Examination Survey) NHANES III, examined the association between dietary calcium intake and severity of periodontal disease in more than 12,000 adults 20 years and older. The odds ratio (OR) for periodontal disease was determined for each of three levels of calcium intake (low, medium, and high) after adjusting for age, tobacco use, and gingival bleeding. Low calcium intake (i.e., 2 to 499 mg/day) almost doubled the risk of periodontal disease in young males (OR 1.84), young females (OR 1.99), and in older males (OR 1.90). Compared to females with a calcium intake of 800 mg/day, females with the lowest intake of calcium (i.e., 2 to 499 mg/day) had a 54% greater risk of periodontal disease, while those with a moderate calcium intake of 500 to 799 mg/day had a 27% higher risk of periodontal disease (Figure 6.8). The researchers suggest that low calcium intake indirectly leads to loss of alveolar bone by disturbing the calcium/phosphorus balance and increasing the production of parathyroid hormone [108]. Vitamin D may have a beneficial role in periodontal health through its effects on bone health and/or modulation of the immune response [102]. Using data from NHANES III, researchers found an association between low blood levels of 25-hydroxyvitamin D3 and increased periodontal disease, independent of bone mineral density [109].

Increased intake of dairy foods, a major source of calcium and vitamin D (if fortified), has been shown to be associated with a low prevalence of periodontal disease [110]. Dairy food consumption (categorized into quintiles) and the prevalence of periodontal disease were examined in 12,764 adults aged 18 years and older who participated in NHANES III [110]. Individuals who were in the highest quintile of dairy products (4.7 servings/day) were 20% less likely to have periodontal

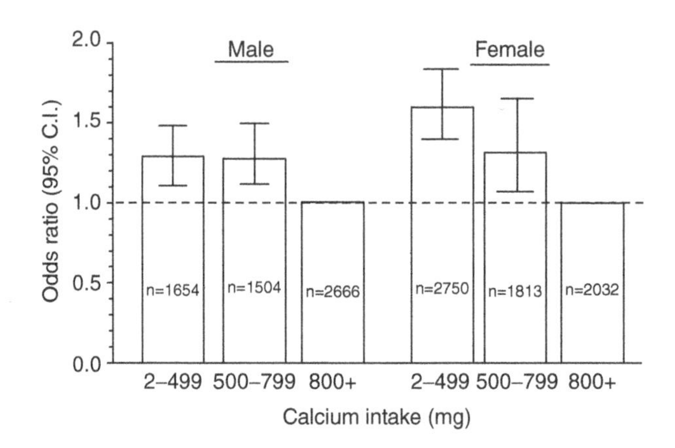

FIGURE 6.8 Odds ratio for periodontal disease by level of dietary calcium intake in males and females after adjusting for age decade, tobacco use status, and gingival bleeding in NHANES III. (From Nishida, M., Grossi, S. G., Dunford, R. G., Ho, A. W., Trevisan, M., and Genco, R. J., *J. Periodontal.*, 71, 1057, 2000.)

disease than those in the lowest quintile of dairy products (0.2 servings/day) after adjusting for major risk factors for this oral health disease.

Bone loss is a "common denominator" for both periodontal disease and osteoporosis [13]. Findings from some studies indicate an association between low systemic bone density and loss of teeth, alveolar bone loss, and periodontal disease [14,102–104]. In a cross-sectional study of more than 300 healthy postmenopausal women, significant correlations were found between the number of teeth retained and bone mineral density of the forearm, spine, and hip [111]. In a prospective observational study, rates of systemic bone loss were more rapid in postmenopausal women who lost teeth than in those who retained teeth [106]. A study in Japanese postmenopausal women showed that the risk of low spinal bone density was almost four times greater in subjects with tooth erosion, leading the researchers to suggest that dental x-rays may be able to detect osteoporosis [112]. However, not all studies support an association between oral bone loss and osteoporosis [102–104]. Although the two conditions share several of the same risk factors (e.g., advancing age, cigarette smoking) and common mechanisms for bone loss may be involved, a causal relationship remains to be established [13,102–104].

Prevention of the progression of periodontal diseases involves removal of soft and hard deposits and keeping teeth free of bacterial plaque [6]. To help reduce the risk of and/or severity of periodontal disease, consumption of a nutritionally balanced diet containing recommended dietary intakes of calcium and vitamin D is encouraged [13,103]. However, more studies, particularly randomized, controlled clinical trials, are necessary to determine the role of dairy foods and dairy food nutrients (e.g., calcium, vitamin D) in the prevention of periodontal disease [102,110].

6.4 SUMMARY

Given the number of genetic and environmental (diet) factors that contribute to oral health, it is difficult to establish how a particular food (e.g., single dairy food), consumed as part of a complex diet, influences dental caries and periodontal diseases. There is substantial scientific evidence (i.e., from animal testing, human plaque pH measurements, *in vitro* caries models) supporting the protective effect of a variety of cheeses against dental caries. Consuming cheese alone or in combination with foods may reduce the risk of dental caries.

Evidence indicates that milk (whole, low-fat, chocolate), consumed as usual or as part of a diet, does not contribute to dental caries. Further, research findings indicate that milk may be a good saliva substitute for individuals with hyposalivation such as may occur in older adults receiving certain medications.

Considering the growing population of older adults in the United States many of whom are at risk of periodontal diseases, more research on the role of specific nutrients such as calcium and vitamin D and foods such as dairy foods in this condition seems warranted. Also, the relationship, if any, between oral bone density, periodontal disease, and osteoporosis needs to be clarified.

The American Academy of Pediatric Dentistry encourages parents to serve nutritious snacks such as cheese, chocolate milk, yogurt, and vegetables to protect children's dental health. Likewise, the American Academy of Pediatrics, concerned about potential health problems such as dental caries and enamel erosion resulting from children's high intake of soft drinks in schools, recommends that pediatricians work to eliminate sweetened drinks in schools and recommend healthful alternatives such as low-fat white or flavored milk. The beneficial effect of milk and milk products on oral health is yet another reason to encourage intake of 3 or more servings of dairy foods such as milk, cheese, or yogurt a day. Research supporting the caries-protective effects of dairy products should be incorporated into dietary recommendations to help reduce the risk of dental caries.

REFERENCES

1. U.S. Department of Health and Human Services, U.S. Public Health Service, *Oral Health in America: A Report of the Surgeon General*, National Institute of Dental and Craniofacial Research, National Institutes of Health, Rockville, MD, 2000, www.nidcr.nih.gov/sgr/execsumm.htm.
2. National Institutes of Health, *Diagnosis and Management of Dental Caries Throughout Life*, NIH Consensus Statement, March 26–28, 18 (1), 1, 2001.
3. Dental, Oral and Craniofacial Data Resource Center, Oral Health U.S., Bethesda, MD, 2003.
4. National Center for Chronic Disease Prevention and Health Promotion, Fact Sheet, *Preventing Dental Caries with Community Programs*, 2005, www.cdc.gov/oralhealth/factsheets/dental_caries.htm.
5. Vargas, C. M., Kramarow, E. A., and Yellowitz, J. A., The Oral Health of Older Americans, *Aging Trends* 3, National Center for Health Statistics, Hyattsville, MD, 2001, www.cdc.gov/nchs/data/agingtrends/03oral.pdf.
6. U.S. Department of Health and Human Services, *Healthy People 2010*, Vol. II, U.S. Government Printing Office, Washington, D.C., 21, 2000.
7. National Center for Chronic Disease Prevention and Health Promotion, *Oral Health: Preventing Cavities, Gum Disease, and Oral Cancers*, At a Glance, 2004, www.cdc.gov/nccdphp/aag/aag_oh.htm.
8. U.S. Department of Health and Human Services, *National Call to Action to Promote Oral Health*, NIH Publication No. 03-5303, Public Health Service, National Institutes of Health, National Institute of Dental and Craniofacial Research, Rockville, MD, 2003.
9. Palmer, C. A., Important relationships between diet, nutrition, and oral health, *Nutr. Clin. Care*, 4, 4, 2001.
10. Mobley, C. C., Nutrition and dental caries, *Dent. Clin. North Am.*, 47 (2), 319, 2003.
11. Moynihan, P. and Petersen, P. E., Diet, nutrition and the prevention of dental diseases, *Pub. Health Nutr.*, 7, 201, 2004.
12. Mobley, C. and Dodds, M. W., Diet, nutrition and teeth, in *Diet and Nutrition in Oral Health,* Palmer, C. A., Prentice Hall, NJ, 182, 2003.
13. The American Dietetic Association, Position of the American Dietetic Association: oral health and nutrition, *J. Am. Diet. Assoc.*, 103, 615, 2003.
14. DePaola, D. P. et al. Nutrition and dental medicine, in *Modern Nutrition in Health and Disease*, 10th ed., Shils, M.E. et al., Ed., Lippincott Williams, Wilkins, Philadelphia, 2006, chap. 2.
15. Navia, J. M., A new perspective for nutrition: the health connection, *Am. J. Clin. Nutr.*, 61 (suppl.), 407s, 1995.
16. Alvarez, J. O., Nutrition, tooth development, and dental caries, Am, *J. Clin. Nutr.*, 61, 410s, 1995.
17. Nunn, J., Nutrition and dietary challenges in oral health, *Nutrition*, 17, 426, 2001.

18. Bowen, W. H., Tabak, L. A., Eds., *Cariology for the Nineties*, University of Rochester Press, Rochester, NY, 1993.
19. Touger-Decker, R. and van Loveren, C., Sugars and dental caries, *Am. J. Clin. Nutr.*, 78, 881s, 2003.
20. Johansson, I., Milk and dairy products: possible effects on dental health, *Scand. J. Nutr.*, 46, 119, 2002.
21. Parry, J. et al., Investigation of mineral waters and soft drinks in relation to dental erosion, *J. Oral Rehabil.*, 28, 766, 2001.
22. Shenkin, J. D. et al., Soft drink consumption and caries risk in children and adolescents, *General Dentistry*, 51, 30, 2003.
23. Marshall, T. A. et al., Dental caries and beverage consumption in young children, *Pediatrics*, 112, e184, 2003.
24. American Academy of Pediatrics, Committee on School Health, Soft drinks in schools, *Pediatrics*, 113, 152, 2004.
25. American Academy of Pediatrics, Committee on Nutrition, The use and misuse of fruit juice in pediatrics, *Pediatrics*, 107, 1210, 2001.
26. Herod, E. L., The effect of cheese on dental caries: a review of the literature, *Aust. Dent. J.*, 36 (2), 120, 1991.
27. Bowen, W. H., Effects of dairy products on oral health, *Scand. J. Nutr.*, 46, 178, 2002.
28. Kashket, S. and DePaola, D. P., Cheese consumption and the development and progression of dental caries, *Nutr. Rev.*, 60, 97, 2002.
29. Tanzer, J. M., Testing food cariogenicity with experimental animals, *J. Dent. Res.*, 65, 1491, 1986.
30. Edgar, W. M. et al., Effects of different eating patterns on dental caries in the rat, *Caries Res.*, 16, 384, 1982.
31. Harper, D. S. et al., Cariostatic evaluation of cheeses with diverse physical and compositional characteristics, *Caries Res.*, 20, 123, 1986.
32. Krobicka, A. et al., The effects of cheese snacks on caries in desalivated rats, *J. Dent. Res.*, 66 (6), 1116, 1987.
33. Dreizen, S., Dreizen, J. G., and Stone, R. E., The effect of cow's milk on dental caries in the rat, *J. Dent. Res.*, 1025, 1961.
34. Stephan, R. M., Effects of different types of human foods on dental health in experimental animals, *J. Dent. Res.*, 45 (5), 1551, 1966.
35. Navia, M. and Lopez, H., Rat caries assay of reference foods and sugar-containing snacks, *J. Dent. Res.*, 62 (8), 893, 1983.
36. Reynolds, E. C. and Johnson, I. H., Effect of milk on caries incidence and bacterial composition of dental plaque in the rat, *Archs. Oral Biol.*, 26, 445, 1981.
37. Harper, D. S. et al., Modification of food cariogenicity in rats by mineral-rich concentrates from milk, *J. Dent. Res.*, 66 (1), 42, 1987.
38. Bowen, W. H. et al., Influence of milk, lactose-reduced milk, and lactose on caries in desalivated rats, *Caries Res.*, 25 (4), 283, 1991.
39. Bowen, W. H. and Pearson, S. K., Effect of milk on cariogenesis, *Caries Res.*, 27, 461, 1993.
40. Bowen, W. H. et al., Assessing the cariogenic potential of some infant formulas, milk and sugar solutions, *J. Am. Dent. Assoc.*, 128, 865, 1997.
41. Peres, R. C. R. et al., Cariogenicity of different types of milk: an experimental study using animal model, *Braz. Dent. J.*, 13, 27, 2002.
42. Bowen, W. H. and Lawrence, R. A., Comparison of the cariogenicity of cola, honey, cow milk, human milk, and sucrose, *Pediatrics*, 116, 921, 2005.
43. Herod, E. L., The use of milk as a saliva substitute, *J. Publ. Health Dent.*, 3, 184, 1994.
44. Mundorff, S. A. et al., Cariogenic potential of foods, *Caries Res.*, 24, 344, 1990.
45. Bibby, B. J. et al., Protective effect of milk against *in vitro* caries, *J. Dent. Res.*, 59 (10), 1565, 1980.
46. Edgar, W. M. and Geddes, D. A. M., Plaque acidity models for cariogenicity testing — some theoretical and practical observations, *J. Dent. Res.*, 65, 1498, 1986.
47. Jensen, M. E., Evaluation of the acidogenic and antacid properties of cheeses by telemetric monitoring of human dental plaque pH, in *Foods, Nutrition and Dental Health*, Hefferren, J. J., Ayer, W. A., Koehler, H. M., and McEnery, C. T., Eds., Vol. 4, American Dental Assoc., Chicago, IL, pp. 31–47, 1984.

48. Schachtele, C. F. and Harlander, S. K., Will the diets of the future be less cariogenic? *J. Can. Dent. Assoc.*, 3, 213, 1984.
49. Jensen, M. E. and Schachtele, C. F., The acidogenic potential of reference foods and snacks at interproximal sites in the human dentition, *J. Dent. Res.*, 62 (8), 889, 1983.
50. Higham, S. M. and Edgar, W. M., Effects of parafilm and cheese chewing on human dental plaque pH and metabolism, *Caries Res.*, 23, 42, 1989.
51. Jensen, M. E. and Wefel, J. S., Effects of processed cheese on human plaque pH and demineralization and remineralization, *Am. J. Dent.*, 3 (5), 217, 1990.
52. Linke, H. A. B. and Riba, H. K., Oral clearance and acid production of dairy products during interaction with sweet foods, *Ann. Nutr. Metab.*, 45, 202, 2001.
53. Dodds, M. W. J. and Edgar, W. M., The relationship between plaque pH, plaque acid anion profiles, and oral carbohydrate retention after ingestion of several "reference foods" by human subjects, *J. Dent. Res.*, 67 (5), 861, 1988.
54. Silva, M. F. et al., Effects of cheese on experimental caries in human subjects, *Caries Res.*, 20, 263, 1986.
55. Thomson, M. E., Effects of cheese, breadcrumbs, and a breadcrumb and cheese mixture on microhardness of bovine dental enamel intraoral experiments, *Caries Res.*, 22, 246, 1988.
56. Thomson, M. E., Effect of fruit juice, with or without 1% added whey mineral, on bovine dental enamel in intraoral experiments, *Caries Res.*, 24 (5), 334, 1990.
57. Drummond, B. K., Chandler, N. P., and Meldrum, A. M., Comparison of the cariogenicity of some processed cheeses, *Eur. J. Paediatr. Dent.*, 3, 188, 2002.
58. Gedalia, I. et al., Tooth enamel softening with a cola type drink and rehardening with hard cheese or stimulated saliva *in situ*, *J. Oral Rehabil.*, 18 (6), 501, 1991.
59. Featherstone, J. D. B. and Zero, D. T., An *in situ* model for simultaneous assessment of inhibition of demineralization and enhancement of remineralization, *J. Dent. Res.*, 71 (spec. 55), 804, 1992.
60. Reynolds, E. C., Riley, P. F., and Storey, E., Phosphoprotein inhibition of hydroxyapatite dissolution, *Calcif. Tissue Int.*, 34 (suppl.), 2, 52, 1982.
61. Reynolds, E. C., The prevention of sub-surface demineralization of bovine enamel and change in plaque composition by casein in an intra-oral model, *J. Dent. Res.*, 66 (6), 1120, 1987.
62. McDougall, W. A., Effect of milk on enamel demineralization and remineralization *in vitro*, *Caries Res.*, 11, 166, 1977.
63. Gedalia, I. et al., Enamel softening with Coca-Cola and rehardening with milk or saliva, *Am. J. Dent.*, 4 (3), 120, 1991.
64. Papas, A. S. et al., Relationship of diet to root caries, *Am. J. Clin. Nutr.*, 61, 423, 1995.
65. Rugg-Gunn, A. J. et al., Relationship between dietary habits and caries increment assessed over two years in 405 English adolescent school children, *Arch. Oral Biol.*, 29, 983, 1984.
66. Holund, U., Relationship between diet-related behavior and caries in a group of 14-year-old Danish children, *Commun. Dent. Oral Epidemiol.*, 15, 184, 1987.
67. Freeman, L. et al., Relationships between DEF, demographic and behavioral variables among multiracial preschool children, ASDC, *J. Dent. Child*, 56 (3), 205, 1989.
68. Petti, S., Simonetti, R., and Simonetti D'Arca, A., The effect of milk and sucrose consumption on caries in 6- to 11-year old Italian schoolchildren, *Eur. J. Epidemiol.*, 13, 659, 1997.
69. Papas, A. S. et al., Dietary models for root caries, *Am. J. Clin. Nutr.*, 61, 417, 1995.
70. Gedalia, I. et al., Dental caries protection with hard cheese consumption, *Am. J. Dent.*, 7, 331, 1994.
71. Silva, M. F. et al., Effects of water-soluble components of cheese on experimental caries in humans, *J. Dent. Res.*, 66 (1), 38, 1987.
72. Jenkins, G. N. and Hargreaves, J. A., Effect of eating cheese on Ca and P concentrations of whole mouth saliva and plaque, *Caries Res.*, 23, 159, 1989.
73. Brudevold, F. et al., Effects of some salts of calcium, sodium, potassium, and strontium on intra-oral enamel de-mineralization, *J. Dent. Res.*, 64 (1), 24, 1985.
74. Reynolds, E.-C. et al., Anticariogenicity of calcium phosphate complexes of tryptic casein phosphopeptides in the rat, *J. Dent. Res.*, 74, 1272, 1995.
75. Aimutis, W. R., Bioactive properties of milk proteins with particular focus on anticariogenesis, *J. Nutr.*, 134, 989s, 2004.

76. Walker, G. et al., Increased remineralization of tooth enamel by milk containing added casein phosphopeptide–amorphous calcium phosphate, *J. Dairy Res.*, 73, 74, 2006.
77. Grenby, T. H. et al., Dental caries protective agents in milk and milk products: investigations *in vitro*, *J. Dent.*, 29, 83, 2001.
78. Nesser, J. R. et al., *In vitro* modulation of oral bacterial adherence to saliva-coated hydroxyapatite beads by milk casein-derivatives, *Oral. Microbiol. Immunol.*, 9, 193, 1994.
79. Vacca-Smith, A. M. and Bowen, W. H., The effect of milk and kappa casein on Streptococcal glucosyltransferase, *Caries Res.*, 29, 498, 1995.
80. Guggenheim, B. et al., Powdered milk micellar casein prevents oral colonization of *Streptococcus sobrinus* and dental caries in rats: a basis for the caries-protective effect of dairy products, *Caries Res.*, 33, 446, 1999.
81. Lewinstein, I., Ofek, L., and Gedalia, I., Enamel rehardening by soft cheeses, *Am. J. Dent.*, 6, 46, 1993.
82. Moynihan, P. J., Ferrier, S., and Jenkins, G. N., The cariostatic potential of cheese: cooked cheese-containing meals increase plaque calcium concentration, *Br. Dent. J.*, 187, 664, 1999.
83. Marques, A. P. F. and Messer, L. B., Nutrient intake and dental caries in the primary dentition, *Pediatr. Dent.*, 14, 314, 1992.
84. Stralfors, A., Inhibition of hamster caries by cocoa, the effect of whole and defatted cocoa, and the absence of activity in cocoa fat, *Arch. Oral Biol.*, 11, 149, 1966.
85. Paolino, V. J. and Kashket, S., Inhibition of cocoa extracts of biosynthesis of extracellular polysaccharide by human oral bacteria, *Arch. Oral Biol.*, 30 (4), 359, 1985.
86. Levine, R. S., Milk, flavoured milk products, and caries, *Br. Dent. J.*, 191, 20, 2001.
87. American Academy of Pediatric Dentistry, Diet and dental health, AAPD Fast Facts 2002 to 2003.
88. American Dental Association, ADA statement on early childhood caries, www.ada.org/prof/resources/positions/statements/caries.asp.
89. Bowen, W. H., Response to Seow: biological mechanisms of early childhood caries, *Commun. Dent. Oral Epidemiol.*, 26, 28, 1998.
90. Lopez, L. et al., Topical antimicrobial therapy in the prevention of early childhood caries, *Pediatr. Dent.*, 21, 9, 1999.
91. The American Dietetic Association, Position of The American Dietetic Association: the impact of fluoride on health, *J. Am. Diet. Assoc.*, 105, 1620, 2005.
92. Marshall, T. A. et al., Associations between intakes of fluoride from beverages during infancy and dental fluorosis of primary teeth, *J. Am. Coll. Nutr.*, 23, 108, 2004.
93. World Health Organization, Diet, Nutrition and the Prevention of Chronic Diseases, Report of a Joint WHO/FAO Expert Consultation, WHO Technical Report Series 916, World Health Organization, Geneva, 2003.
94. Banoczy, J. et al., Anticariogenic effect of fluoridated milk and water in rats, *Acta Physiol. Hungarica*, 76 (4), 341, 1990.
95. Stosser, L., Kneist, S., and Grosser, W., The effects of non-fluoridated and fluoridated milk on experimental caries in rats, *Adv. Dent. Res.*, 9 (2), 122, 1995.
96. Toth, Z. et al., The effect of fluoridated milk on human dental enamel in an *in vitro* demineralization model, *Caries Res.*, 31, 212, 1997.
97. Arnold, W. H. et al., Volumetric assessment and quantitative element analysis of the effect of fluoridated milk on enamel demineralization, *Arch. Oral. Biol.*, 48, 467, 2003.
98. Ivancakova, R. et al., Effect of fluoridated milk on progression of root surface lesions *in vitro* under pH cycling conditions, *Caries Res.*, 37, 166, 2003.
99. Petersson, L. G. et al., Fluoride concentrations in saliva and dental plaque in young children after intake of fluoridated milk, *Caries Res.*, 36, 40, 2002.
100. Bian, J. Y. et al., Effect of fluoridated milk on caries in primary teeth: 21-month results, *Commun. Dent. Oral Epidemiol.*, 31, 241, 2003.
101. Pakhomov, G. N. et al., Dental caries-reducing effects of milk fluoridation project in Bulgaria, *J. Public Health Dent.*, 55 (4), 234, 1995.
102. Krall, E. A., Calcium and oral health, in *Nutrition and Bone Health*, Weaver, C. M., Heaney, R.P., Eds., Humana Press Inc., Totowa, NJ, 2006, chap. 20.
103. Krall, E. A., The oral effects of osteoporosis, *Nutr. Clin. Care*, 4, 22, 2001.

104. Neiva, R. F. et al., Effects of specific nutrients on periodontal disease onset, progression and treatment, *J. Clin. Periodontol.*, 30, 579, 2003.
105. Enwonwu, C. O., Interface of malnutrition and periodontal diseases, *Am. J. Clin. Nutr.*, 61, 430, 1995.
106. Krall, E. A., Garcia, R. I., and Dawson-Hughes, B., Increased risk of tooth loss is related to bone loss at the whole body, hip and spine, *Calcif., Tissue Int.*, 59, 433, 1996.
107. Krall, E. A. et al., Calcium and vitamin D supplements reduce tooth loss in the elderly, *Am. J. Med.*, 111, 452, 2001.
108. Nishida, M. et al., Calcium and the risk for periodontal disease, *J. Periodontol.*, 71, 1057, 2000.
109. Dietrich, T. et al., Association between serum concentrations of 25-hydroxyvitamin D3 and periodontal disease in the U.S. population, *Am. J. Clin. Nutr.*, 80, 108, 2004.
110. Al-Zahrani, M. S., Increased intake of dairy products is related to lower periodontitis prevalence, *J. Periodontol.*, 77, 289, 2006.
111. Krall, E. A. et al., Tooth loss and skeletal bone density in healthy postmenopausal women, *Osteoporosis Int.*, 4, 104, 1994.
112. Taguchi, A. et al., Relationship between dental panoramic radiographic findings and biochemical markers of bone turnover, *J. Bone Mineral. Res.*, 18, 1689, 2003.

7 Dairy Foods and a Healthy Weight

7.1 INTRODUCTION

Overweight and obesity are becoming a global epidemic [1,2]. In the United States, overweight and obesity have risen dramatically during the past 20 years, and are now considered a great public health concern [3–5]. Two-thirds (66.3%) of adults 20 years of age and older are overweight (body mass index or BMI of 25 to 29.9 kg/m^2) or obese (BMI of 30 kg/m^2 or higher) [5]. Among children and adolescents aged 2 through 19 years, 17.1% are overweight [5]. A recent report indicates that if current trends continue, nearly half of the children in North and South America will be overweight by 2010 [2].

People who are overweight or obese are at increased risk of premature death, coronary heart disease, type 2 diabetes, hypertension, stroke, gallbladder disease, osteoarthritis, respiratory problems, and some types of cancer (e.g., endometrial, colon, kidney, postmenopausal breast cancer) [3,6–8]. According to the U.S. Surgeon General's report, "Call to Action to Prevent and Decrease Overweight and Obesity," health problems resulting from overweight and obesity could reverse many of the recent health gains in this country [3].

Overweight and obesity are the end result of a positive energy balance, or excess calorie intake relative to energy expenditure. However, multiple factors — both genetic and environmental (e.g., dietary) — are involved in the development of overweight and obesity [3,4]. To reverse the trend toward obesity, most Americans need to consume fewer calories, increase their physical activity, and make wiser food choices [4]. Researchers recognize that small shifts in energy balance over time influence body weight. For example, consuming an excess of 10 kcal/day can increase weight by one pound over a year [9]. Likewise, achieving a small negative energy balance over time can lead to weight loss.

Emerging scientific evidence indicates that small beneficial shifts in body weight and body fatness may be achieved by increasing calcium intake, and particularly the consumption of dairy products, the major dietary source of calcium. This relationship was first observed several decades ago [10,11]. During the course of a clinical trial, of the antihypertensive effect of calcium conducted in the 1980s in obese hypertensive African Americans, Zemel and colleagues [11] observed that increasing dietary calcium (i.e., from ~400 to ~1000 mg/day) by consuming 2 servings a day of yogurt while maintaining similar energy intakes for 1 year decreased body fat by nearly 11 pounds. This finding demonstrates that consuming recommended amounts of dairy foods can impact energy metabolism. Some individuals eliminate dairy products from their diet, believing them to be fattening; this approach to prevent or treat overweight may be counterproductive. Americans' low intake of calcium and dairy products may be a contributing factor to the obesity epidemic. Many Americans fail to meet calcium recommendations largely because of their low intake of dairy products [12,13] (see Chapter 5).

Research on the role of dairy products and calcium in both the prevention and treatment of overweight or obesity is discussed in several reviews [14–26]. Emerging scientific evidence indicates that consuming 3 to 4 servings a day of dairy foods high in calcium and a good source of protein (i.e., milk, cheese, yogurt) in an energy-reduced diet may help obese and overweight adults lose more body weight and body fat than reducing energy alone. In addition, consumption of adequate amounts of dairy foods without energy restriction appears to decrease body fat and enhance lean body mass without weight loss; moreover, intake of recommended servings of dairy foods may help children and adolescents achieve a healthy body composition. This chapter reviews observational studies and randomized clinical trials in humans, as well as experimental animal and *in vitro* studies, related to the role of dairy foods and calcium in a healthy body weight. Potential mechanisms by which dairy products and dietary calcium may regulate body weight and body fat are also discussed.

7.2 DAIRY PRODUCTS AND A HEALTHY WEIGHT IN ADULTS

The goal for adults is to achieve and maintain a body weight that optimizes their health [4]. For obese adults, even modest weight loss (e.g., 5% to 10% of body weight) has health benefits, and the prevention of further weight gain is important.

7.2.1 Observational Studies

Observational and epidemiological studies are useful for generating hypotheses or critical questions. However, for several reasons (presence of confounding factors, biases, difficulty in accurately quantifying dietary intakes of individuals consuming self-selected diets, and the like), these types of studies cannot establish a cause-and-effect relationship.

Several observational studies have directly examined the impact of increased dairy food or calcium intake on changes in body weight or body fat [10,11,27–36]. Overall, these studies have shown a fairly consistent inverse association between dairy product or calcium intake and body weight or fat across various study designs and data bases, such as the National Health and Nutrition Examination Survey (NHANES III) [11], the Quebec Family Study [30], the Heritage Study [31], the Coronary Artery Risk Development in Young Adults (CARDIA) study [29], and the Tehran Lipid and Glucose Study [33,35]. This inverse association has been shown in young and older adults, in women and men, and in African American and white adults. Reviewed below are some of these cross-sectional and prospective studies.

In an analysis of NHANES III data, dietary calcium intake (mainly from dairy foods) was inversely associated with body fat in women [11]. After controlling for factors such as energy intake, activity level, age, and race or ethnicity, the risk of obesity was 84% lower in women who consumed the highest amount of dairy foods (3½ servings/day) compared to those who consumed the lowest amount of dairy foods (1 serving/day) (Table 7.1). A similar, although less strong, association was observed in men [11].

The Quebec Family study, a cross-sectional study of 235 men and 235 women aged 20 to 65, found that women who had a daily calcium intake of <600 mg had significantly greater body weight, percentage of body fat, fat mass, BMI, waist circumference, and abdominal fat, after controlling for confounding factors (e.g., age, other dietary variables, socioeconomic status) than women who consumed more than 600 mg calcium/day [30]. Although a trend for these associations was also found in men, it was not significant after considering confounding factors. Dairy foods provided about 62% of the calcium in the women's diets and about 60% in the men's diets.

Findings from a cross-sectional study of adults enrolled in the Heritage Family Study found that the association between energy-adjusted calcium intake and body composition was significantly different between males and females, and between African Americans and whites [31]. In this study of 362 men (109 African Americans and 253 whites) and 462 women (201 blacks and 261 whites) aged 17 to 65, high vs. low calcium intake was associated with significantly lower BMI, percent body fat, and abdominal fatness in African American men (1025 mg/day vs. 517 mg/day calcium)

TABLE 17.1
Effects of Dietary Calcium and Dairy Intake on the Risk of Being in the Highest Quartile of Body Fat for Women

Quartile of Calcium and Dairy Consumption	Calcium Intake (mg/day; mean ± SEM)	Dairy Consumption (servings/month) mean ± SEM	Odds Ratio of being in the Highest Body Fat Quartile
1	255+20	14.4+1.9	1.00[a]
2	484+13	38+1.3	0.75 (0.13, 4.22)[b]
3	773+28	57.2+1.0	0.40 (0.04, 3.90)[b]
4	1346+113	102.8+3.6	0.16 (0.03, 0.88)[b]

[a] Model is controlled for race/ethnicity and activity level, with age and caloric intake as continuous covariates.
[b] 95% Confidence interval in parentheses.

Source: From Zemel. M. B. et al., *FASEB J.*, 14, 1132, 2000. With permission.

and white women (1494 mg/day vs. 642 mg/day calcium). In white men, a high calcium intake (1637 mg/day) was significantly associated with a lower percent body fat. In African American women, an adequate vs. low calcium intake (1171 mg/day vs. 568 mg/day) was associated with a tendency toward higher BMI and waist circumference and a significantly higher fat-free mass. The researchers concluded that a low intake of dietary calcium may be associated with higher body fat, especially in men and white women [31]. Other cross-sectional studies have demonstrated an inverse association between dietary calcium intake and adiposity in African American women [27,28].

A study in Portugal found that the association between milk intake and obesity varied according to gender and menopausal status [34]. In this large cross-sectional study, milk intake was inversely associated with BMI in men and premenopausal women, but not in postmenopausal women. The researchers suggest that hormonal status in women may influence the effect of milk (calcium) on BMI, however, an explanation for the findings awaits additional study [34].

An inverse association between dairy food consumption and BMI in Iranian adults has been demonstrated in cross-sectional studies [33,35]. When researchers assessed the relationship between dairy consumption and BMI in a group of 462 urban residents of Tehran who participated in the Tehran Lipid and Glucose Study, they found that increased consumption of dairy products was associated with a lower BMI, even after controlling for confounding factors [33]. High dairy intake was associated with a low risk of enlarged waist circumference in Tehranian adults participating in a cross-sectional study to evaluate the relation between dairy consumption and metabolic syndrome, one aspect of which is abdominal obesity [35]. Dairy consumption was inversely associated with the risk of metabolic syndrome in this study.

To learn more about the mechanism by which calcium or dairy products may influence body weight, Melanson and colleagues [32], in a cross-sectional study, measured calcium intake and fat oxidation in 35 nonobese, healthy adults (21 males, 14 females; 31 ± 6 years; BMI 23.7 ± 2.9) during a 24-hour stay in a whole-room calorimeter. Fat oxidation was measured during sleep and light physical activity. Habitual calcium intake was determined from 4-day food diaries completed by a trained dietitian. Acute calcium intake was determined from measured food intake during the calorimeter stay. Calcium from dairy was calculated from whole calcium-containing foods (milk, cheese, etc.).

Simple correlations were run between calcium intake measures and fat oxidation, and multiple regression models were used to adjust for factors known to confound the relationship with fat oxidation (e.g., fat mass, fat-free mass, energy balance, acute fat intake, and habitual fat intake.)

Acute total and dairy calcium intakes (but not habitual intake) were positively correlated with 24-hours fat oxidation before and after adjustment for confounding factors. Both current calcium and dairy calcium intakes were positively associated with fat oxidation during sleep, but not during walk/step exercise. The researchers say that the data support the hypothesis that high dietary calcium promotes lipolysis (fat breakdown), which may protect against fat mass accumulation. The stronger relationship between acute calcium intake and fat oxidation indicates that this effect may be mediated quickly. Alternatively, it may reflect a reduced reliability of the retrospective dietary data for chronic calcium intake. There was little data to demonstrate that dairy calcium had a stronger effect, although its effect may only be apparent in a resting state [32]. In a follow-up randomized, crossover trial discussed below [37], these investigators demonstrated that a high intake of dairy foods specifically increased fat oxidation during conditions of energy deficit.

In addition to cross-sectional studies, a number of longitudinal prospective investigations have been conducted to assess the relationship between dairy food or calcium intake and body weight or body fat. Pereira and colleagues [29] examined the associations between dairy food intake and major components of the insulin resistance syndrome (IRS), including obesity, in 3157 black and white adults aged 18 to 30 years participating in the CARDIA study, a 10-year population-based prospective study. After adjusting for confounding lifestyle and dietary factors, overweight participants who consumed the most dairy products had a 72% lower incidence of IRS than those who consumed few dairy products [29]. Further, the cumulative incidence of obesity in those who were overweight at the start of the study was significantly reduced from 64.8% in those who consumed the least amount of dairy foods to 45.1% in the highest dairy food group (Figure 7.1). Increased dairy food intake was equally beneficial for African Americans and Caucasians, and both reduced fat and full-fat versions of dairy were effective. The beneficial association between dairy food intake and reduced incidence of IRS was not explained by any specific nutrient(s) (e.g., calcium) in dairy foods or by lifestyle factors (physical activity, smoking, or alcohol intake). This finding indicates that the antiobesity effect of dairy foods may be explained by other dairy components in addition to calcium. The researchers concluded that dietary patterns characterized by

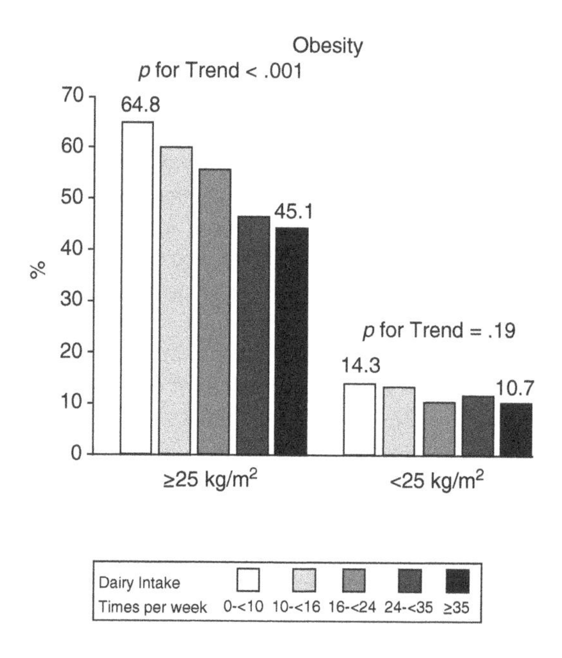

FIGURE 7.1 Ten-year cumulative incidence of obesity by categories of total dairy intake with stratification by baseline overweight status. (From Pereira, M. A. et al., *JAMA*, 287, 2081, 2002. With permission.)

increased dairy consumption have a strong inverse association with IRS (which includes obesity) among overweight adults, and may reduce the risk of type 2 diabetes mellitus and cardiovascular disease [29]. Some other recent prospective studies in adults indicate that healthful dietary patterns, including increased intake of reduced-fat dairy foods, were associated with smaller gains in body weight or BMI and waist circumference over time [38–40].

Liu and colleagues [36] examined the associations between dairy, calcium, and vitamin D intake and the prevalence of metabolic syndrome in over 10,000 women aged 45 years and older participating in the Women's Health Study. In age- and calorie-adjusted analyses, higher intakes of total, dietary, and supplemental calcium were significantly and inversely associated with the prevalence of metabolic syndrome. After further adjustments, the odds ratios of having the metabolic syndrome for each increasing quintile of total calcium intake were 1.00, 0.82, 0.84, 0.70, and 0.64. Similarly, a strong relationship between intakes of dairy products and metabolic syndrome was also observed. After adjusting for lifestyle and dietary factors, the multivariable odd ratios comparing the highest with the lowest intake categories were 0.66 for total dairy products and 0.85 for total milk intake. Furthermore, both high-fat and low-fat dairy foods were associated with a lower prevalence of metabolic syndrome. Dietary vitamin D was inversely associated with prevalence of metabolic syndrome, but was not independent of total calcium intake. Specifically, the abdominal obesity (measured by waist circumference) component of metabolic syndrome was significantly reduced in those with higher calcium intakes, and the number of women with BMI$\geq$30 was reduced. These results indicate that dairy product and calcium consumption may be associated with a lower prevalence of the metabolic syndrome (of which obesity is a feature) in middle-aged and older women.

In other longitudinal, observational studies, the association between dairy food or calcium intake and body weight or fatness appears to be affected by other factors (e.g., level or calcium consumed, body fatness). Dietary calcium intake had no significant effect on body weight or weight change in a longitudinal study in 898 women in Scotland aged 45 to 54 years at baseline (premenopausal) [41]. This study examined whether energy intake or energy expenditure, use of hormone replacement therapy, or intake of dietary calcium was associated with a 5- to 7-year weight change in women. Differences in physical activity, baseline weight, and smoking significantly predicted changes in weight. The researchers suggest that the lack of association between dietary calcium and body weight in this study may have been due to the high usual calcium intake of the women. The average calcium intake was more than 1000 mg/day, and that of the lowest quartile was 800 mg/day [41]. Without a broader range of calcium intakes above and below the threshold at which calcium may affect body weight, it is difficult to draw conclusions about calcium and body weight from this study.

Researchers in The Netherlands followed a group of men and women from age 13 to age 36 who participated in the Amsterdam Growth and Health Longitudinal Study to determine whether dietary calcium intake was related to BMI and body fatness [42]. Over the course of the study, average calcium intake was 1269 mg/day for men and 1148 mg/day for women, which met the recommended calcium intake of 1000 to 1200 mg/day for adults in The Netherlands. For men, a higher intake of dietary calcium was associated with significantly lower body fat when adjusted for age. The magnitude of this association increased with age. In addition, older men had considerably higher BMI and body fat than younger men, which led the researchers to suggest that the effect of dietary calcium was stronger in subjects with a larger fat mass [42]. For women, a significantly lower skin-fold thickness was found in the group consuming the highest dietary calcium intake ($>$1200 mg/day) than the group consuming less than 800 mg/day, when adjusted for age. No differences in BMI or body fatness were observed between the middle and highest groups of calcium intake. This observation led the researchers to suggest that a low calcium intake may increase the risk of developing obesity, but above a threshold level (i.e., 800 mg calcium/day in this study), an increased intake of calcium does not confer additional benefit [42]. The researchers also suggested that the dietary recall method used in this study was less accurate than methods employed in some intervention studies that report an antiobesity effect of calcium.

A 12-year prospective study of more than 19,000 men aged 40 to 75 years who were enrolled in the Health Professionals Follow-up Study found that neither calcium (dietary or supplemental) nor dairy foods was associated with changes in body weight [43]. In this study, participants self-reported their dairy and calcium intake (i.e., by a food frequency questionnaire), as well as their weight at the beginning and at the end of the 12-year period. With any self-reporting, the chance for measurement error is greater compared to trained assessments. The researchers acknowledge that a limitation of this study was that the components of any weight change in the subjects were unknown because body composition was not measured [43]. Additionally, participants in this study followed their normal, not energy-restricted, diets. That is, this study was not designed to examine the association between dairy food/calcium intake and weight loss. In addition, most of the study subjects were already at a healthy weight (mean BMI of ~25). The findings of this study are consistent with those of other investigations that demonstrate that calcium or dairy food intake is not associated with excessive weight gain.

7.2.2 Secondary Analyses of Studies

The concept that dairy products and dietary calcium may beneficially modulate body weight and fat in humans has also been examined via secondary analyses of other observational and clinical trials originally conducted with skeletal or blood pressure end points [11,15,26,44–48]. Davies and colleagues [44] and Heaney, et al. [15,45] analyzed data from nine studies, including three controlled trials and six observational studies in which body weight was assessed as a secondary outcome. Overall, increased calcium intake was consistently associated with reduced body weight, body fat, and/or weight gain. The aggregate effect was that each 300-mg (~1 dairy serving) increase in daily calcium intake was associated with a decreased weight gain of 0.11 to 0.16 kg/year in middle-aged and older women [15]. Although in this work calcium intake explained only a relatively small fraction of the variability in weight or weight gain, data analyzed by Heaney [45] led this researcher to estimate that ensuring population-wide calcium intakes at currently recommended intakes could reduce the prevalence of obesity (or weight gain) by 60% to 80%.

A secondary analysis of a 2-year study originally designed to examine the effects of exercise on bone measures in young, normal-weight women aged 18 to 31 years found that dietary calcium's effect on body weight and fat was dependent on energy intake [46]. In this study, calcium, but not energy intake, predicted changes in body weight and fat in women when energy intakes were below the mean of the cohort (1876 kcal/day), whereas in those who consumed higher energy intakes (>1876 kcal/day), energy intake alone predicted changes in body weight and fat. In addition, the effects of calcium appeared to be specific to dairy calcium, because dairy calcium, but not nondairy calcium, predicted changes in body weight and fat [46]. The findings of this study indicate that it is unlikely that dairy products or dietary calcium will have an effect on body weight or composition independent of higher energy intake. That is, the effect of dairy food or calcium intake on weight loss in adults seems to be greatest in the context of a diet moderately reduced in energy. Very high or very low energy intakes may alter biochemistry in a way that overrides the effect of dairy foods or calcium intake on energy metabolism.

Increased calcium intake did not significantly affect body weight or fat loss in a secondary analysis of three separate 25-week randomized controlled trials originally conducted for the purpose of determining the effects of calcium on bone during weight loss [47]. In this study, 100 premenopausal and postmenopausal women were given a calcium supplement (1000 mg/day) or a placebo for 25 weeks and counseled to follow a moderately energy-restricted diet. Although no significant effects of calcium on weight or fat were observed, the researchers point out that the magnitude and direction of the differences for group means are consistent with a small beneficial effect of calcium [47]. In another randomized controlled trial originally designed to examine bone health outcomes, researchers in New Zealand found no significant effects of calcium on body weight or composition in normal-weight postmenopausal women who received a calcium supplement (1000 mg/day) or a placebo [48]. However, when data were analyzed for those with baseline calcium intakes of <600 mg/day, there was a trend towards greater weight loss in those who consumed the supplemental calcium. It is important to recognize that secondary analyses of studies not designed to examine changes in body weight or body composition may fail to find an effect of dairy products or calcium intake due to a variety of factors, such as an insufficient number of subjects, high baseline dairy food or calcium intake, normal body weight, and no energy restriction.

7.2.3 Randomized Clinical Trials

Randomized controlled trials (clinical trials) in humans are considered to be the "gold standard" for evaluating a dietary hypothesis and providing evidence of causality between diet and a clinical end point. Discussed below are randomized controlled trials that have examined the effect of calcium or dairy foods on body weight and composition in adults, as well as clinical studies designed to determine potential mechanisms.

7.2.3.1 Weight Loss and Body Composition Studies

Randomized clinical trials have been conducted to specifically evaluate the effects of dairy products or calcium on body weight/fat loss as the primary outcome under caloric restriction in obese and overweight adults or changes in body composition under caloric maintenance in obese and normal weight adults [49–56].

In a 16-week controlled weight loss study in England, 45 obese adults (BMI >27 kg/m^2) were randomly assigned to one of three iso-energetic diets: a conventional balanced diet, a milk-only diet, or a milk plus one designated food daily diet [49]. Those who consumed the iso-energetic milk-only diet lost significantly more weight (9.4 kg) than did those who consumed the milk plus one food diet (7.0 kg) or the conventional diet (1.7 kg) [49]. The authors speculated that it may have been the novelty (with better compliance) of the milk-only diet that contributed to its success. This study was published before the hypothesis that dairy food consumption impacts weight and body composition was proposed.

In the United States, a 6-month randomized controlled clinical trial in 32 young obese adults on a calorie-reduced diet (500 kcal/day deficit) found that increasing dairy product or dietary calcium intake from inadequate to adequate levels enhanced the effectiveness of a calorie-reduced diet in increasing body weight and fat losses [50]. In this study, the adults were maintained on balanced calorie-reduced diets and randomly assigned to one of three groups: a low-calcium, low-dairy food control group (0 to 1 serving of dairy foods/day and 400 to 500 mg calcium/day); an adequate-calcium group (control diet supplemented with 800 mg calcium/day); or an adequate-dairy group (3 to 4 servings of milk, yogurt, and/or cheese a day, total calcium intake of 1200 to 1300 mg/day) [50]. Adults in the control group lost 6.4% of their body weight over the 6 months, and this loss was increased to 8.6% on the high-calcium diet and 11% on the adequate-dairy food diet [50]. Fat loss followed a similar trend, with the adequate-dairy food and adequate-calcium diets increasing fat loss relative to the low-calcium diet by 64% and 38%, respectively (Figure 7.2) [50]. An unexpected finding was a marked change in the distribution of body fat. On the low-dairy food, low-calcium diet, fat loss from the trunk (abdominal) region represented 19% of the total fat lost, and this was increased to 50% of the fat lost on the adequate-calcium diet and 66% on the adequate-dairy food diet (Figure 7.2) [50]. Based on the findings, the researchers concluded that "a high-calcium diet and a high-dairy diet enhanced the efficacy of an energy-restricted diet in weight control, with a significantly greater effect of dairy vs. a nondairy (supplemental) source of calcium. Furthermore, both diets had a particularly beneficial effect on central obesity" [50].

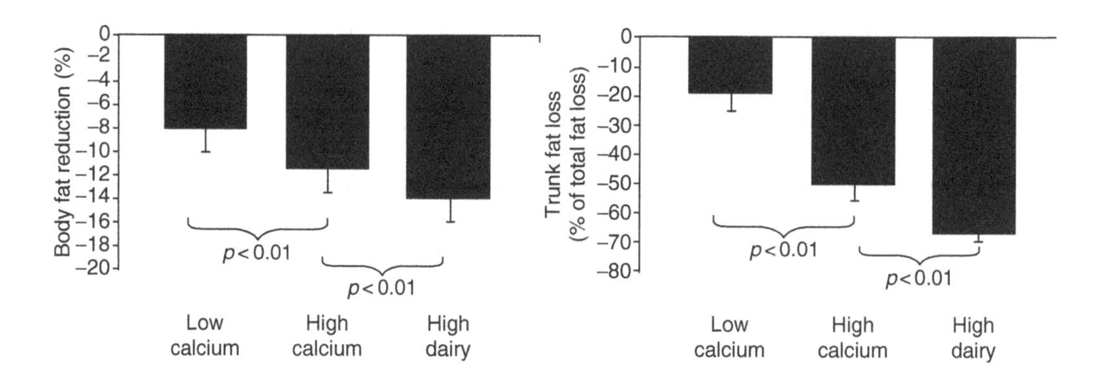

FIGURE 7.2 Effects of high-calcium and high-dairy diets on body fat and trunk fat reduction. (From Zemel, M. B. et al., *Obes. Res.*, 12, 582, 2004. With permission.)

The above findings are supported by a follow-up clinical trial which investigated the effect of substituting yogurt for other foods in a calorie-reduced diet on weight and body fat loss in obese adults [51]. In this study, 34 obese adults were placed on a balanced 500-calorie-deficit diet and randomly assigned to a yogurt diet (three 6-ounce servings/day of fat-free yogurt, for a total calcium intake of 1100 mg/day) or a control diet (0 to 1 serving of dairy products a day, 400 to 500 mg of calcium) for 12 weeks [51]. Both groups lost weight, but the yogurt group lost 22% more body weight than the control group (Figure 7.3). Additionally, the yogurt group lost 61% more fat and 81% more abdominal fat than the control group. Similarly to the previous clinical trial, which used a mixture of milk, cheese, and yogurt as dairy sources [50], this study found that the percentage of fat lost from the trunk was markedly higher in the yogurt group compared to the control group [51]. Further, in the yogurt study, there was a significant 31% reduction in the loss of lean tissue mass during calorie restriction compared to the control group [51].

According to findings from a multicenter trial of overweight and obese adults consuming a calorie-reduced diet, an adequate-dairy food diet (i.e., 3 servings a day of milk, cheese, or yogurt)

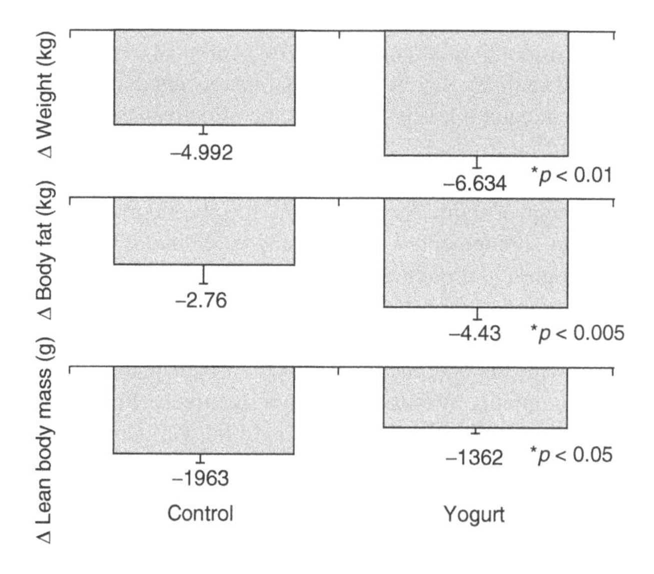

FIGURE 7.3 Effect of yogurt intake on body weight and body composition. (From Zemel, M. B. et al., *Int. J. Obes.*, 29, 391, 2005. With permission.)

resulted in significantly greater losses in body fat, trunk fat, and waist circumference compared to groups receiving a low-calcium control diet or an elemental calcium-rich diet [52]. The design of this multicenter study was similar to the previous clinical trial, which used a mixture of dairy products [50]. That is, adults consuming calorie-reduced (−500 kcal/day) diets were randomized to receive low-calcium, adequatecalcium, or adequate-dairy food diets [52]. The duration of this multicenter trial was 12 weeks compared to the 24 weeks in the previous study [50,52]. In addition, in contrast to the previous clinical trial [50], the elemental calcium-rich diet had no significant effect on weight loss or body composition compared to the low-calcium control diet [52]. However, the adequate-dairy food diet resulted in a nonsignificant trend of greater body weight loss and significantly greater body fat loss compared to the low-calcium and high-calcium diets [52]. These findings indicate that dairy-rich diets increase weight loss by targeting the fat compartment during energy restriction.

Zemel and colleagues [53] examined the effects of a diet with recommended servings of dairy foods on body fatness and body composition in obese African American adults in two separate, randomized clinical trials, one for weight loss and the other for weight maintenance. In both 6-month studies, participants were randomly chosen to follow one of two diets, a low-dairy diet (0 to 1 serving of dairy foods/day; 500 mg of calcium/day) or an adequate-dairy food diet (3 servings/day of milk, yogurt, or cheese; 1200 to 1300 mg calcium/day). In the weight-loss study involving 29 obese African American adults, inclusion of 3 daily servings of dairy foods into a balanced calorie-reduced diet (−500 kcal/day) with no change in dietary macronutrients resulted in an approximately twofold greater body weight and fat loss compared to the low-dairy/low-calcium diet (Figure 7.4). In addition, the adequate-dairy food diet produced greater trunk fat loss and markedly reduced loss of lean mass compared with the low-dairy food, low-calcium diet (Figure 7.5) [53]. There was also a significantly greater increase of circulating glycerol levels, indicating an increase in lipolysis. A significant reduction in circulating insulin levels in the adequate-dairy food/calcium group vs. the low-dairy/low-calcium group was observed [53]. This study supports other investigations indicating that dairy foods accelerate loss of body weight and total and central adipose tissue mass secondary to calorie restriction in obese adults.

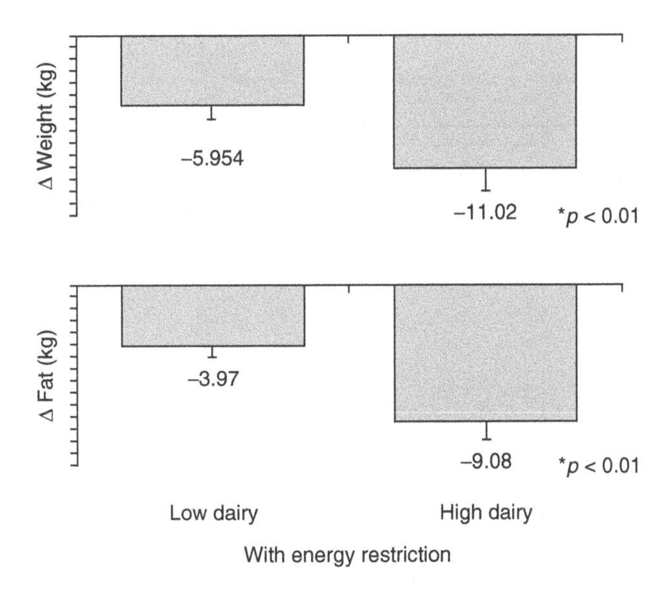

FIGURE 7.4 Effect of dairy intake on body weight and fat loss after weight loss. (From Zemel, M. B. et al., *Obes. Res.*, 13, 1218, 2005. With permission.)

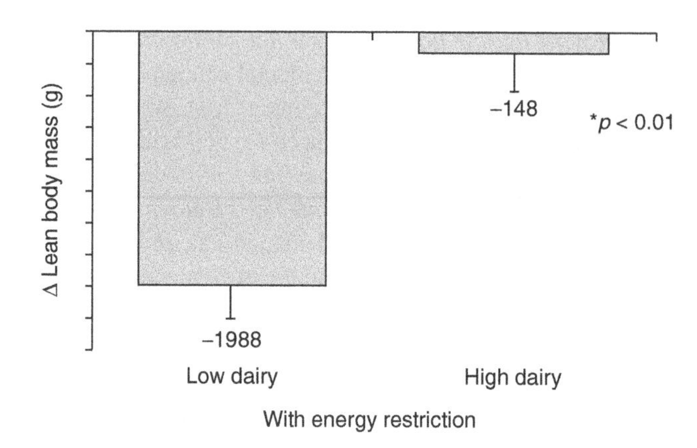

FIGURE 7.5 Effect of dairy intake on lean body mass after weight loss. (From Zemel, M. B. et al., *Obes. Res.*, 13, 1218, 2005. With permission.)

In the weight maintenance study, 34 obese African American adults were placed on a diet to maintain their current weight and were randomly assigned to either the low-dairy food or adequate-dairy food diet [53]. As expected, there was no change in body weight for both groups. However, in the group consuming 3 servings of dairy foods a day, there was a 5.4% reduction in total body fat, a 4.6% decrease in trunk fat, and a 2.2% increase in lean body mass, whereas there were no significant changes in the low-dairy group (Figure 7.6). In addition, insulin levels and blood pressure decreased, and circulating glycerol levels significantly increased in the adequate-dairy food group [53]. This weight maintenance study indicates that consuming 3 servings of dairy foods a day results in significant reductions in total and central adiposity in obese adults without weight loss or caloric restriction.

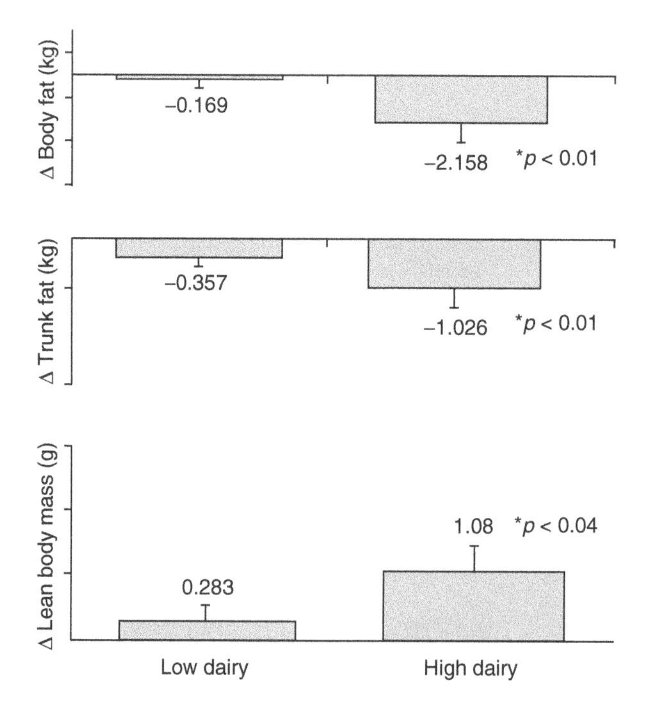

FIGURE 7.6 Effect of dairy intake on body composition without calorie restriction. (From Zemel, M. B. et al., *Obes. Res.*, 13, 1218, 2005. With permission.)

In contrast to the above findings, other randomized clinical trials have reported no significant enhancements in body weight or fat loss under energy restriction in obese adults consuming moderate- vs. high-dairy diets [54], or in overweight and obese subjects consuming low- versus adequate-dairy food diets under conditions of calorie restriction and exercise [55]. In a clinical trial, 70 obese adults consuming an energy-reduced diet (500 kcal/day deficit) were randomly assigned to one of three diets: a "moderate-dairy" diet that included 2 servings of dairy foods each day; a "high-dairy" diet that included 4 servings of dairy products a day (at least two of which were fluid milk); and a "high-dairy/high-fiber/low-glycemic index" diet that included 4 servings of dairy products a day [54]. The participants prepared their own food, kept a food diary daily, and met with a dietitian weekly for the first half of the study and biweekly thereafter. They were instructed to exercise (e.g., brisk walking, treadmill, or exercise bike) at least 30 minutes four times a week. After 48 weeks, the participants in all three groups experienced significant weight and body fat loss [54]. While all groups lost similar amounts of weight and body fat, the participants in the high-dairy group who most closely followed the prescribed diet and exercise plan consumed 4 daily servings of dairy and about 100 to 150 kcal more each day. Even with the higher calorie intake, they lost the same amount of weight as the participants who consumed 2 dairy servings a day and fewer calories [54]. The researchers point out that previous studies have demonstrated that the weight loss effect may be strongest when dairy and calcium intakes are increased from inadequate (1 serving or less) to adequate (3 servings each day), indicating the possibility of a threshold effect. They add that their study did not have enough subjects with calcium intakes less than 600 mg/day to evaluate the possibility of a threshold effect [54]. Nonetheless, among adherent subjects, comparable weight and fat losses were achieved with a lesser degree of energy restriction (i.e., while consuming a significantly greater number of calories).

Researchers at the University of Vermont compared weight and body fat loss in 44 overweight and obese adults who participated in a 12-month clinical trial in which they were randomly assigned to consume a calorie-reduced diet (500 kcal/day deficit) low in dairy (1 serving of dairy/day, 400 to 500 mg calcium/day) or adequate in dairy (3 to 4 servings of milk, yogurt, or cheese a day, 1200 to 1400 mg calcium/day) [55]. During the study, all participants were encouraged to expend at least 1000 kcal/week in physical activity (e.g., walking). Although all participants lost body weight, there were no statistically significant differences between the groups. The researchers [55] suggest that significantly more subjects would have been needed to achieve statistically significant differences in this study, especially considering the higher weight loss in the low-dairy calcium group compared to that found in the study by Zemel and colleagues [50]. The slightly larger calorie deficit in this study than in previous trials may also have contributed to the findings. The findings of this study [55], as well as those of the clinical trial discussed above [54], demonstrate that including 3 to 4 servings of dairy products as part of a weight-loss diet does not adversely affect weight-loss efforts.

Additional support for the finding that adults can increase intake of calcium-rich dairy foods without threat of weight gain comes from a study reported by Gunther and coworkers [56]. In this randomized 1-year clinical trial, 135 healthy, normal-weight young women (ages 18 to 30) were randomly assigned to one of three groups: a control group consuming their habitual dairy food intake (800 mg calcium); a medium-dairy food (1000 to 1100 mg calcium) group; or a high-dairy food (1300 to 1400 mg calcium) group [56]. The two dairy-food groups were instructed to substitute low-fat dairy products for other foods to achieve the desired calcium levels and to maintain caloric intake. Results showed no significant differences between groups in body weight, BMI, and fat mass or lean mass. Throughout the intervention, the medium- and high-dairy food groups had slightly higher, but not statistically significant, average calorie intakes than the control group [56]. The researchers state that "results from this study show that dairy products do not promote gains in body weight or fat mass in young, healthy women" [56]. Unlike several other randomized controlled trials which involved overweight or obese subjects who consumed energy-restricted diets, this study involved normal-weight participants who consumed diets to maintain their weight [56]. Thus, the ability to observe significant weight or body fat loss appears to be dependent on initial body fat levels. This is similar to the observed effects of dairy foods on blood pressure, in that the effect of dairy food consumption on reducing blood pressure is most discernable in subjects with moderately elevated or high blood pressure.

7.2.3.2 Substrate Oxidation/Energy Expenditure Studies

In addition to the above randomized clinical trials that focused on weight loss and body composition, some clinical trials have been conducted to examine the effects of increased dairy food or calcium consumption on fat oxidation, energy expenditure, and the thermic effects of food [37,57–59]. These studies provide insight into plausible mechanisms by which calcium/dairy intake may benefit weight management.

One potential mechanism may relate to macronutrient oxidation. Melanson and colleagues [37] evaluated the effect of low- and high-calcium dairy-based diets on macronutrient (carbohydrate, protein, fat) oxidation in a randomized controlled clinical trial involving 19 overweight adults. The study included four 7-day experimental periods carried out in random order. Each participant consumed a low-dairy (1 serving of 2% milk, low-fat cheese, or yogurt, ~500 mg calcium/day) and a high-dairy diet (3 to 4 servings of 2% milk, low-fat cheese, or yogurt, ~1400 mg calcium/day) separated by a week on their usual diet. On day seven of the low-dairy or high-dairy diet, participants were studied in a room calorimeter which measured energy expenditure and macronutrient oxidation under conditions of energy balance (maintained weight) and acute energy deficit. The energy deficit (600 cal) was produced by a combination of calorie reduction (100 cal) and exercise (500 cal) [37]. Under conditions of energy balance, diet had no effect on the respiratory quotient or 24-hour macronutrient oxidation, whereas under conditions of energy deficit, 24-hour fat oxidation was significantly increased when participants consumed the high-dairy (~3 to 4 servings/day) diet compared to the low-dairy diet (Figure 7.7). Although the researchers were unable to determine whether the increase in fat utilization was due to the energy deficit itself or the exercise, they believe that exercise promoted the increase in fat oxidation after the participants consumed the high-dairy diet [37]. The dairy-based high-calcium diet also induced about a 10% reduction in circulating 1,25-$(OH)_2D$, the active form of vitamin D, which has been shown to promote fat breakdown in adipocytes (see below, under mechanism). The researchers speculate that "if lipolysis was increased in response to the decline in 1,25-OH_2D, then fat oxidation would be increased during exercise due to both the increased availability and use of FFA (free fatty acids) during exercise" [37]. Additional research is needed to confirm this hypothesis.

In another randomized clinical trial, researchers at Purdue University evaluated whether increased dairy calcium intake altered whole-body fat oxidation after a meal and if such an effect was due to changes in parathyroid hormone (PTH) concentrations [57]. Nineteen normal-weight women aged 18 to 30 years were randomly assigned to a low-calcium (<800 mg/day) control group or a high-dairy calcium (1000 to 1400 mg/day) group. Participants in the high-calcium group were instructed to substitute calcium-rich dairy products (particularly nonfat and low-fat milk) for other foods. Whole-body fat oxidation after a low- and high-calcium liquid meal was measured by respiratory gas exchange both at baseline and after 1 year. Additionally, fasting blood levels of PTH were determined at baseline and after 1 year. The findings showed that adequate dairy food consumption over 1 year resulted in a greater increase in postprandial fat oxidation after both a high- and low-calcium liquid meal challenge compared to a low dietary calcium intake [57]. Furthermore, the 1-year change in PTH levels correlated with the 1-year change in fat oxidation when the 1-year change in total body fat mass or group assignment was controlled. The researchers concluded that their results "suggest that women who increase their dairy calcium over a prolonged period, while total energy intake is controlled for, will oxidize higher amounts of fat, potentially through suppression of serum PTH" [57]. The increased fat oxidation in the intervention group did not translate into measurable body weight loss or prevention

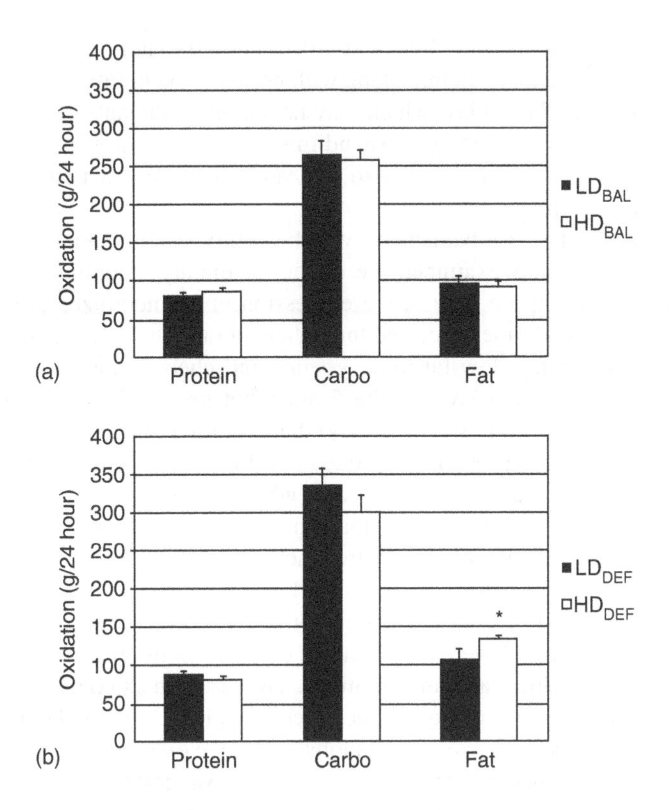

FIGURE 7.7 Effect of low (LD)- and high (HD)-calcium dairy-based diets on macronutrient oxidation in subjects in energy balance (a) and acute energy deficit (b). Mean (SE). *$p < 0.025$. (From Melanson, E. L. et al., *Obes. Res.*, 13, 2102, 2005.)

of weight gain. However, this study utilized normal-weight subjects and was not designed for weight loss, as participants were not instructed to restrict calories. The investigators recommended that additional research be conducted to better understand how alterations in fat oxidation might affect body weight and/or body fat [57].

Fat excretion may contribute to the beneficial effect of dairy food or calcium intake on body weight, according to a randomized crossover study in ten moderately-overweight adults [58]. In this study, participants were instructed to follow all three of the following diets (not energy-restricted) for 1 week in randomly-assigned order: a low-calcium/normal-protein (500 mg of calcium, 15% of energy from protein) diet; a high-calcium/normal-protein (1800 mg of calcium, 15% of energy from protein) diet; and a high-calcium/high-protein (1800 mg calcium, 23% of energy from protein) diet. Calcium intake was increased by increasing the consumption of low-fat dairy products. After 1 week, calcium had no effect on 24-hour energy expenditure or fat oxidation. However, fecal fat excretion significantly increased ~2.5-fold (i.e., from 5.9 to 14.2 g/day) and fecal energy excretion significantly increased by 55% during the high-calcium/normal-protein diet compared to the other two diets [58]. The researchers speculated that the differences in fecal fat excretion between the high-calcium, normal-protein and high-calcium, high-protein diet groups may be due to greater calcium binding to dietary protein in the upper gastrointestinal tract in the high-calcium, higher-protein diet group rather than calcium binding to dietary fat and being excreted, as was observed in the high-calcium, normal-protein diet group. Thus, with higher dietary protein, a reduced formation of calcium fatty acid soaps could occur, leading to less fecal fat excretion. The researchers also suggested that the preferential binding of calcium to phosphorylated proteins, such as casein found in dairy products, could lead to less calcium binding to dietary fat and could affect bile acid utilization, ultimately influencing fat absorption. The short-term increase in dietary calcium along with normal protein intake increased fecal energy excretion by approximately 84 cal/day, which may help explain the antiobesity effect of calcium. However, this small increase in energy expenditure required a large intake of calcium (i.e., 1800 mg/day). The findings of this study also indicate that an interaction with dietary protein level may be important [58].

To learn more about the mechanism by which dietary calcium may lower body weight, researchers in The Netherlands examined the effects of dietary calcium intake on energy and substrate metabolism and adipose tissue gene expression in a randomized crossover study [59]. Twelve healthy, normal-weight men received three diets in random order: a high-dairy food/high-calcium (1259 mg calcium/day, low-fat milk, yogurt, and cheese) diet; a low-dairy food/high-calcium diet at the same calcium level as the former, but provided by calcium carbonate; and low-dairy food/low-calcium (349 mg calcium/day) diet. All three diets provided the same amount of calories and proportion of carbohydrate, protein and fat, and were designed to maintain body weight. Each diet was fed for a 7-day period, after which 24-hour energy expenditure, substrate metabolism, and fat biopsy specimens were obtained. Neither 24-hour energy expenditure nor fat oxidation was significantly affected by dietary treatment. In addition, expression of genes involved in the lipolytic and lipogenic pathways did not differ significantly between dietary treatments. Blood levels of 1,25-$(OH)_2D$ decreased under both of the high-calcium diets and increased under the low-calcium diet, and were significantly different between the high-dairy food/high-calcium and low-dairy food/low-calcium conditions. The researchers concluded that, while changing dietary calcium for 7 days leads to significant changes in 1,25-$(OH)_2D$, there is no apparent influence on substrate metabolism, energy metabolism, or gene expression in proteins related to fat metabolism. In their discussion of the results, the researchers suggest that there are several possible reasons why their findings did not reach significance. For example, 7 days may have been too short a time to adapt to a high-calcium diet. In addition, the calcium content of participants' usual diets (average of 1027 mg calcium/day) was near the recommended levels, so moving them from an adequate intake to a depleted intake, rather than from depletion to adequacy, may have influenced the results [59]. Other research findings also demonstrated that a calorie deficit was needed to stimulate increased fat oxidation [37].

7.3 EXPERIMENTAL ANIMAL STUDIES

The effect of dairy food/calcium intake on weight gain, weight loss, and body fat alterations has been examined in experimental animal studies [11,22,60–62]. Several of these studies have been carried out in transgenic mice which overexpress the *agouti* gene in adipose tissue under the control of the aP2 promoter and are susceptible to adult-onset diet-induced obesity [11,22,60]. These mice provide a good model for human diet-induced weight gain or loss.

Zemel and colleagues [11] evaluated the effects of diets high in sucrose and fat containing graded levels of calcium from dairy (nonfat dry milk) or calcium carbonate on body weight and body fat gain in aP2 transgenic mice. The mice were randomly assigned to one of the following diet groups (all with increased levels of fat and sucrose to promote adiposity) for 6 weeks: a baseline group, receiving a low-calcium diet (0.4% calcium by weight); a "high-calcium" group, which received supplemental calcium carbonate to increase dietary calcium to 1.2% by weight; a "medium-dairy" group, which received nonfat dry milk to replace 25% of the protein and a calcium intake of 1.2%; and a "high-dairy" group which received nonfat dry milk to replace 50% of the protein and increase dietary calcium to 2.4% of the diet [11]. The groups all consumed the same energy intake. Mice on the baseline low-calcium diet gained about 7.5 g during the 6-week study. However, compared to a low-calcium control diet (0.4%), weight gain was reduced by 26% and 29% in the animals consuming "medium-calcium" diets (1.2% wt/wt) from either calcium

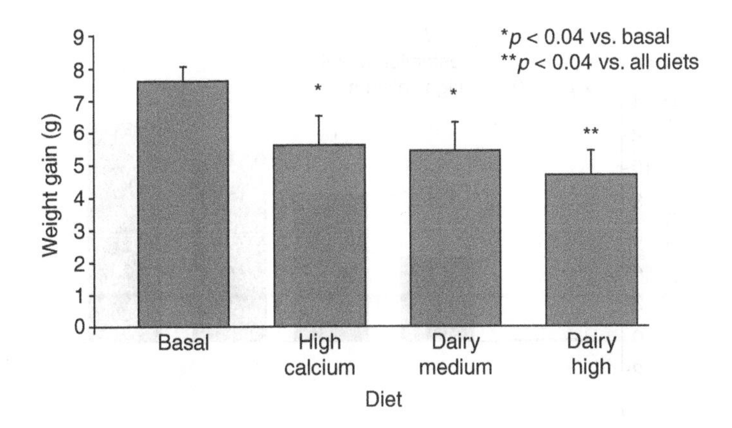

FIGURE 7.8 Effects of calcium and dairy products on 6-week weight gain in transgenic mice expressing *agouti* in adipose tissue under the control of the aP2 promoter. (From Zemel, M. B. et al., *FASEB J.*, 14, 1132, 2000. With permission.)

carbonate or from dairy (25% protein), respectively, without changes in food intake [11]. On a "high-calcium" diet containing 2.4% calcium derived from dairy (50% of total dietary protein), body weight was reduced further by 39% compared with the baseline group (Figure 7.8). These results indicate that a "high-dairy" diet is associated with less weight gain, even when energy intake is not restricted. Total fat pad mass was reduced 36% by all three elevated calcium diets, whereas the reduction in abdominal fat pad mass was greater on the "medium-dairy" and "high-dairy" diets than on the higher calcium carbonate diets [11].

In another similarly-designed study, researchers evaluated the effects of graded levels of calcium from dairy foods (nonfat dry milk) or calcium carbonate on body weight and lipid metabolism in aP2-*agouti* transgenic mice fed an energy-restricted diet [60]. A low-calcium (0.4% wt/wt) diet fed *ad libitum* resulted in ~100% increase in adipocyte calcium levels, a 29% increase in body weight, and a doubling of total fat pad mass, whereas the higher-calcium diets resulted in a 50% reduction in adipocyte calcium levels. Restricted feeding of the low-calcium control diet had no effect on adipocyte calcium levels, but did result in an 11% decrease in body weight. However, markedly greater body weight reductions of 19%, 25%, and 29% were observed in the high-calcium (calcium carbonate), medium-dairy food (1.2% calcium) and high-dairy food (2.4% calcium) diets (Figure 7.9) [60]. All three higher-calcium diets caused a significant reduction in total fat pad mass measured in four areas of the trunk. Significantly greater decreases in total fat pad mass were observed in mice on the "medium-dairy" and "high-dairy" diets than in those on the "high-calcium" diet from supplements (Figure 7.9). The "medium-dairy" and "high-dairy" diets resulted in a 60% and 69% further reduction of fat pad mass, respectively, than that from the high-calcium diet [60].

The above studies in transgenic mice made obese show that, compared to a calcium carbonate supplement, the use of dairy products as a calcium source is more effective in inhibiting diet-induced weight gain and accelerating weight and fat loss during energy restriction [60]. However, a greater challenge than losing weight is long-term weight maintenance after short-term weight loss. To investigate the effect of dietary calcium content and source in regulating fat metabolism during weight regain after weight loss, Sun and Zemel [61] conducted a three-phase study in aP2-*agouti* transgenic mice.

In Phase 1 (obesity induction), a group of 60 mice was fed a low-calcium (0.4%), high-sucrose and high-fat diet for 6 weeks to induce weight gain. In Phase II (weight loss), mice were fed an energy-restricted (70% of basal), high-calcium diet (basal diet plus calcium-fortified cereal) for 6 weeks to promote body weight and fat loss. In Phase III (refeeding after energy restriction), mice had free access to one of five diets: (i) low-calcium diet described in Phase I; (ii) a high-calcium cereal diet described in Phase II; (iii) a nonfat dry milk plus high-calcium cereal diet; and

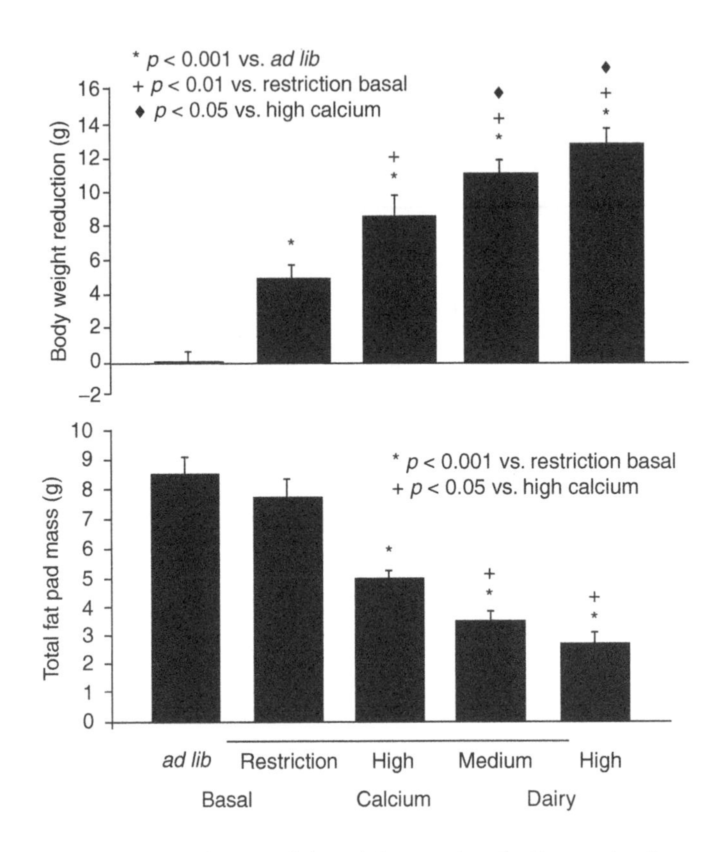

FIGURE 7.9 Calcium and dairy accelerate weight and fat mass loss in diet-restricted transgenic obese mice. (From Shi, H. et al., *FASEB J.*, 15, 291, 2001. With permission.)

(iv) a yogurt-based high-calcium diet, cereal control diet (basic diet plus calcium-free cereal). The amount of food consumed by the mice during refeeding after energy restriction did not differ between groups, but the amount of weight gain and fat pad weight differed substantially by diet (Figure 7.10) [61]. For example, mice fed the two low-calcium diets regained 27% more weight than they had lost and exhibited nearly a fivefold increase in fat pad mass. In contrast, mice refed high-calcium diets regained only half the weight they had lost. The dairy-containing high-calcium diets were more effective in preventing fat gain than the high-calcium cereal. The yogurt or the cereal plus milk diets prevented 85% of the fat gain, whereas the high-calcium cereal diet prevented 55% of the fat gain [61].

Findings from the above studies using aP2-*agouti* transgenic mice indicate that calcium and, to a greater degree, dairy-based products, including nonfat dried milk and freeze-dried yogurt, reduce the rate of weight and fat gain in mice fed an obesity-promoting diet (i.e., high-fat, high-sugar, low-calcium) and accelerate the loss of body weight and fat in mice fed energy-restricted diets [11,60]. In addition, a high-dairy diet effectively slows the rate of weight and fat regain during refeeding after weight loss [61].

Studies in other animal models (e.g., Zucker lean and obese rats, Wistar rats, and Spontaneous Hypertensive rats) have also demonstrated that increased calcium intake reduces body weight and fat content [22]. For example, Papakonstantinou and colleagues [62] fed male Wistar rats a control diet (25% of calories as fat, 14% of calories as protein from casein, 0.4% calcium by weight) or a high-calcium diet (25% of calories as fat, 7% of calories as protein from nonfat dry milk, 7% of calories as protein from casein, 2.4% calcium by weight) for 85 days to investigate the influence of a high calcium, high-dairy protein diet on body fat content and to explore potential

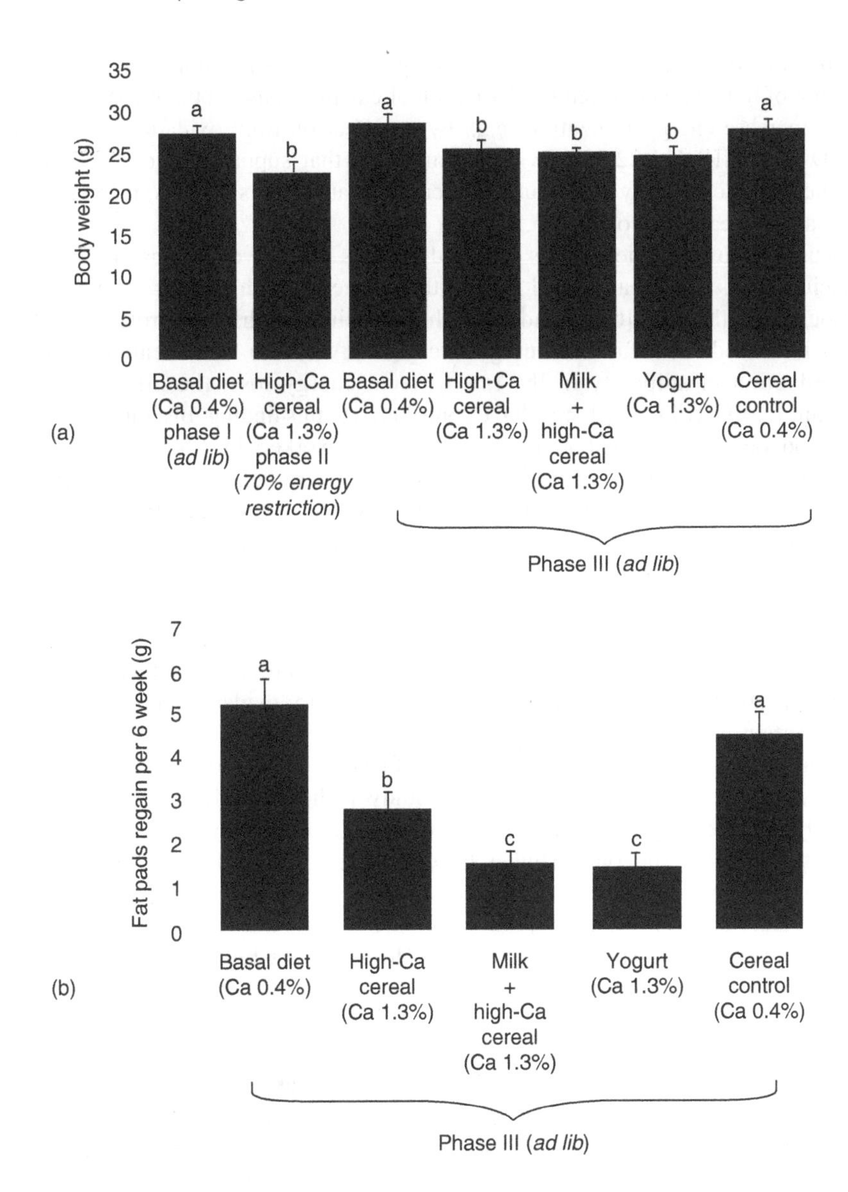

FIGURE 7.10 Effect of dietary calcium and dairy on body weight (a) and fat mass regain (b) in aP2 transgenic mice. Values are means ±SEM. ($n = 5$ for Phase 1 and Phase II, $n = 8$ for Phase III.) (From Sun, X. and Zemel, M. B., *J. Nutr.*, 134, 3054, 2004. With permission.)

mechanisms. Rats fed the high-calcium, high-dairy protein diet gained significantly less weight than the controls and had 29% less carcass fat.

7.4 POTENTIAL MECHANISMS

Experimental animal, *in vitro*, and human studies have sought to determine potential mechanisms to explain the effect of dietary calcium and the augmented effect of dairy product consumption on a healthy body weight and body composition [14,16–18,21–23,63]. It is likely that multiple mechanisms underlie the ability of calcium and dairy products to regulate energy metabolism.

The balance between available energy and energy utilization influences body weight and body fat [23]. Dairy foods and dietary calcium have been proposed to influence this balance. Increased consumption of dairy foods and dietary calcium may reduce energy availability (e.g., by decreasing the absorption of fatty acids through the formation of calcium soaps in the intestine and increasing satiety) and increase energy utilization (e.g., by an effect on lipid oxidation and the hormones, $1,25(OH)_2D$ and PTH) [11,22,23]. Evidence indicates that suppression of these hormones by increased dietary calcium may contribute to decreased fatty acid synthesis, increased lipolysis in adipocytes, and increased fat oxidation.

As discussed above, studies in rats [62] and humans [58] have demonstrated that increasing dietary calcium leads to a greater fecal fat loss than achieved with a lower calcium intake. Papakonstantinou and colleagues [62] found that a high-calcium, high-dairy protein diet fed to male Wistar rats increased fecal fat and energy excretion. Although the researchers attributed the observed reduction in adiposity in the rats to fecal energy loss, the high-calcium diet also reduced serum $1,25(OH)_2D$, which may have contributed to this finding. In a randomized, crossover trial in ten moderately overweight adults, Jacobsen and coworkers [58] found that a high-calcium, normal-protein diet substantially increased fecal fat and energy excretion. However, the level of calcium (1800 mg/day) that produced these results was above the calcium level (1200 mg/day) currently recommended or used in clinical trials of calcium and obesity. While increased dietary calcium increases fecal fat losses, the contribution of this effect to overall energy balance is unclear, but provides a plausible mechanism [18,22].

Another mechanism whereby calcium or dairy products may influence available energy is through the effect on satiety [23]. The few studies investigating this subject have focused on dairy products, rather than calcium *per se*. Some preliminary evidence indicates a satiety effect of milk and certain whey-derived peptides [64]. Although protein is claimed to be more satiating than either carbohydrate or fat, whether the source of protein (i.e., dairy, meat, wheat, soy) contributes to its satiety is controversial [65,66]. A study in healthy older adults found that they compensated for the energy contained in 3 daily servings of milk by reducing food intake from other sources [67]. However, other studies have failed to demonstrate this compensatory effect [68,69]. When the satiating power of semisolid and liquid yogurts was compared with that of fruit beverages and dairy drinks in 32 healthy adults, the two yogurts were more satiating (lower hunger, higher fullness ratings) than the two beverages. However, the higher satiety ratings following yogurt consumption did not suppress energy intake at the next meal [69]. A randomized, crossover study in 24 young adults found that intake of meals containing dairy products increased levels of cholecystokinin (a hormone associated with meal-induced satiety) more than nondairy product meals; however, the nondairy product meals were more satiating than the dairy product meals, as determined by subjective measures of appetite and satiety relative to test meal conditions [70]. Clearly, more research is needed to establish the role of dairy products and calcium on satiety.

Most of the research examining the antiobesity effect of dairy products and calcium has focused on their impact on energy utilization, specifically fat oxidation and dietary calcium-induced hormonal changes. As described above, randomized clinical trials of dairy interventions [37,57] and a cross-sectional study using self-selected intakes [32] examined the effect of dairy or calcium intake on fat oxidation. The cross-sectional study of normal-weight adults showed that higher self-selected acute intakes of total and dairy calcium, but not habitual intakes, were associated with higher rates of whole body fat oxidation over a 24-hour period [32]. In contrast, a 1-year randomized, intervention trial in normal weight adults conducted by Gunther and coworkers [57] found that a long-term, habitual increase in dairy calcium, corrected for energy intake, increased fat oxidation. In another randomized, controlled trial which examined the effect of low- and high-calcium dairy-based diets on fat oxidation in overweight adults, the high-dairy diet (3 to 4 servings/day) increased 24-hour fat oxidation under conditions of energy deficit, but not energy balance (Figure 7.7) [37]. These studies indicate that dairy food intake increases overall body fat oxidation. Human studies that show an increase in body fat loss with or without caloric reduction, but with adequate dairy consumption (3 servings/day) vs. low dairy food intake provide indirect support for this mechanism.

The ability of dietary calcium to regulate, at least acutely, levels of the hormones 1,25$(OH)_2D$ and PTH and their ability to influence adipocyte fatty acid metabolism is the mechanism most often cited to explain calcium's effect on energy utilization [23]. *In vitro* studies in human fat cells (adipocytes) and animal studies (e.g., in *agouti* mice) provide evidence supporting this mechanism [11,16,17,22,23,60,71–73]. Regulation of adipocyte lipid metabolism by intracellular ionic calcium provides the key framework for dietary calcium's effect on adiposity. Both PTH [73] and 1,25 $(OH)_2D$ [11,71] influence adipocyte intracellular ionic calcium levels. A low intake of dietary calcium increases the production of 1,25 $(OH)_2D$, which stimulates the influx of calcium across the adipocyte membrane. The rise in intracellular ionic calcium leads to a coordinated decrease in lipolysis (fat breakdown) and utilization with a subsequent increase in fat storage (i.e., increased *de novo* lipogenesis) via increased expression and activity of the enzyme, fatty acid synthase (FAS) (Figure 7.11) [11,20]. That is, the response to a low calcium intake is an increase in intracellular ionic calcium, which leads to stimulation of lipogenic gene expression and lipogenesis and suppression of lipolysis, resulting in adipocyte lipid filling and increased adiposity [22].

Conversely, a high calcium intake exerts an antiobesity effect by suppressing the production of 1,25 $(OH)_2D$, which reduces the influx of ionic calcium into the adipocyte. This decrease in intracellular ionic calcium leads to increased lipolysis and utilization of energy and inhibition of fat storage [22,71]. This framework for the plausible mechanism by which dietary calcium regulates body weight is derived from studies in cultured human adipocytes and the *agouti* mouse model. However, a direct effect of calcium or calcitrophic hormones (i.e., 1,25 $(OH)_2D$ and PTH) has yet to be determined using *in vivo* techniques [22]. Nevertheless, a potential role for these hormones in human obesity is indicated by other findings [22,23]. For example, polymorphisms in the nuclear vitamin D receptor (nVDR) gene are associated with increased risk of obesity in humans, and alterations of the vitamin D endocrine system have been shown in obese humans [22]. In addition, serum levels of PTH have been shown to be positively associated with BMI and body fat mass in humans [23,57,74].

Although both PTH and 1,25 $(OH)_2D$ influence adipocyte intracellular ionic calcium, research findings indicate a key role for 1,25 $(OH)_2D$ in lipid metabolism [22]. Membrane (nongenomic)

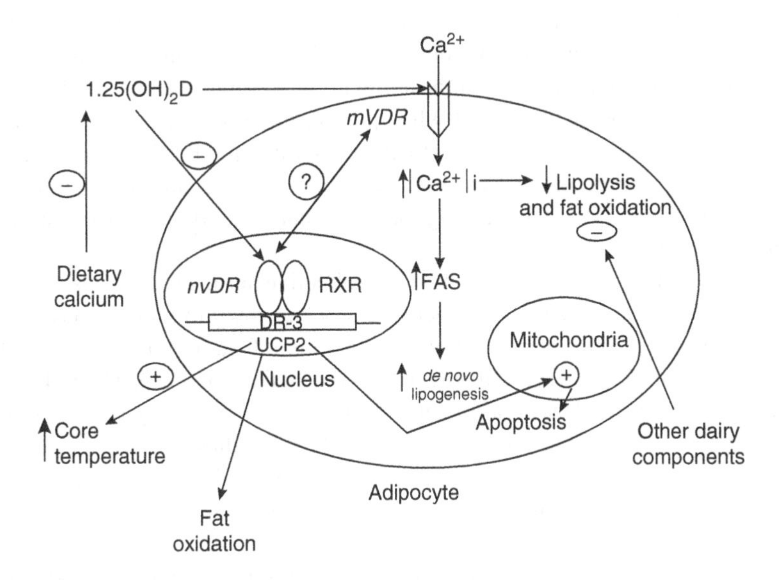

FIGURE 7.11 Proposed mechanisms of dietary calcium and dairy modulation of adiposity. (From Zemel, M., *Am. J. Clin. Nutr.*, 79, 907s, 2004. With permission.)

vitamin D receptors in human adipocytes have been shown to transduce a rapid intracellular ionic calcium response to 1,25 $(OH)_2D$ [21,71]. As a result, treatment of human adipocytes with 1,25 $(OH)_2D$ leads to a coordinated activation of FAS expression and activity and suppression of lipolysis, leading to an expansion of adipocyte lipid storage [11,21,60]. In addition, 1,25 $(OH)_2D$ may inhibit the expression of uncoupling protein 2 (UCP2) [72]. Feeding a high-calcium diet to mice suppresses 1,25$(OH)_2D$ levels, which, in turn, increases adipose tissue UCP2 expression and attenuates the decline in thermogenesis which occurs with energy restriction [22,72]. That is, a high-calcium diet may affect energy partitioning by suppressing 1,25 $(OH)_2D$-mediated inhibition of adipocyte UCP2 expression. However, the role of UCP2 in thermogenesis in unclear and may be mediated by other, as-yet-unidentified mechanisms [22]. Furthermore, it is unknown whether dairy products or dietary calcium influence thermogenesis in humans. In addition to regulating adipocyte metabolism via a nongenomic membrane receptor and by influencing the expression of UCP2, 1,25 $(OH)_2D$ may also modulate adiposity by its effect on apoptosis (programmed cell death) [61]. A study in mice found that adipocyte apoptosis was significantly impaired in association with increased 1,25 $(OH)_2D$ in response to a low-calcium diet, whereas adipocyte apoptosis markedly increased in mice fed high-dairy food and/or high-calcium diets [61]. The above theoretical framework provides a plausible mechanism for calcium's effect on adiposity.

Findings from experimental animal and human studies demonstrating that dairy sources of calcium attenuate weight and fat gain and accelerate fat loss to a greater degree than do calcium from supplements [11,50,60] indicate that dairy products may contain components in addition to calcium that alter energy metabolism. Likely candidates for this additional bioactivity reside in the whey fraction of milk. Whey is a rich source of bioactive components [75,76], such as proteins, that may act independently or synergistically with calcium to contribute to the antiobesity effect of dairy products [17,19].

Whey proteins have been shown to exhibit strong angiotensin-converting enzyme (ACE)-inhibitory activity [17]. This enzyme is necessary for the cleavage of angiotensin I to form angiotensin II. Although angiotensin II is generally considered in relation to its role in blood pressure regulation, it also exerts potent local effects on adipocyte lipogenesis. Additionally, the high concentration of leucine and other branched chain amino acids in dairy protein, especially whey protein, may contribute to the beneficial effect of dairy by repartitioning dietary energy from adipose tissue to skeletal muscle [17,77,78]. Researchers found that intake of leucine and other branched chain amino acids in dairy protein, especially whey protein, during fasting or energy restriction stimulated muscle protein synthesis, thereby sparing lean tissue during weight loss [77,78]. Further support for the benefit of whey protein in weight management is provided by a study in Wistar rats [79]. In this study, weight gain and tissue lipid levels were reduced to a greater degree in rats fed a high-protein diet based on whey protein, compared to a similar diet with red meat as the protein source [79]. This finding indicates that whey protein promotes a less-positive energy balance than red meat.

Although conjugated linoleic acid (CLA), a collective term used to describe one or more isomers of linoleic acid (an essential fatty acid), has been shown to reduce body fat and increase lean body mass in some experimental animal studies, the effects in humans are conflicting [23]. Dairy foods such as milk, cheese, and yogurt are the major source of CLA. Because CLA is associated with fat, dairy foods with a higher milk fat content generally contain more CLA than do lower-fat products. As pointed out by Teegarden [23], studies in mice that demonstrated an enhanced effect of dairy products on body weight used nonfat dry milk, which does not contain CLA. Recent investigations in humans generally have found no effect of CLA on body weight, body fat mass, or fat-free mass [80–82]. Therefore, it is unlikely that CLA in dairy products contributes to their antiobesity effect. Identification of components in dairy products that may be responsible for their augmented antiobesity effect compared to calcium alone is an area of ongoing research.

7.5 DAIRY PRODUCTS AND WEIGHT/BODY COMPOSITION IN CHILDREN AND ADOLESCENTS

For overweight children and adolescents, the goal is to slow the rate of weight gain while achieving normal growth and development [4]. Maintaining a healthy weight throughout childhood may reduce the risk of becoming an overweight or obese adult [4,83]. Relatively little research has explicitly examined the relationship between dairy foods or calcium and body weight or body fat in children and adolescents. Further, only a few of these studies include overweight children or adolescents or minority youth, who are at high risk for overweight [84]. In general, findings from studies in children and adolescents indicate either a beneficial or neutral effect of dairy foods or calcium on body weight or body composition.

7.5.1 Observational Studies

Observational studies, both cross-sectional and prospective analyses, have investigated the relationship between milk, overall dairy foods, or calcium intake in relation to BMI, weight, or indices of obesity in children and adolescents. Reviewed below are several cross-sectional analyses. Some of these analyses have focused on different ethnic groups to understand the influence of race on the connection between diet and obesity.

A cross-sectional study in southern Italy investigated the relationship between frequency of milk consumption and body weight and BMI in 884 school children aged 5 to 11 years [85]. The frequency of milk consumption was categorized as poor ($\leq$1/week), moderate (>1 but $\leq$5 to 6/week), regular (1/day), and high ($\geq$2/day). When taking into account other factors influencing body weight (e.g., age, birth weight, parental overweight/obesity, parental education, and physical activity), parental overweight/obesity and frequency of milk consumption were the only significant predictors of BMI. Milk consumption was significantly and inversely associated with a lower BMI in whole milk consumers when adjusted for age and the frequency of consuming other foods. The researchers note that this is the first report showing a significant inverse association between frequency of milk consumption and BMI in children [85].

In a cross-sectional study in New Zealand, researchers evaluated dietary calcium intakes, anthropometric measures, and bone health in 50 prepubertal children (aged 3 to 10 years) who had a history of avoiding milk consumption [86]. The milk-avoiding cohort was compared to 200 milk-drinking control children. Dietary calcium intakes of milk-avoiders were low, and few children consumed substitute calcium-rich drinks or mineral supplements. The milk-avoiders were shorter, had smaller skeletons, and poor bone health (e.g., lower total body bone mineral) than did the control children of the same age and sex from the same community. Moreover, milk-avoiders had higher BMIs than did the milk-drinking control children. These data indicate that in growing children, long-term avoidance of cow's milk is associated with small stature, poor bone health, and may be related to increased risk of obesity [86]. In a cross-sectional study in the United States that examined the relationship between ready-to-eat cereal consumption and BMI in 603 children aged 4 to 12 years, children in the highest tertile of cereal intake (8 or more servings over 14 days) with milk had lower mean BMIs than those in the lowest tertile of intake (3 or fewer servings over 14 days) [87]. Furthermore, calcium intakes were higher for the high-cereal consumers who also had the more appropriate body weight [87].

In contrast, BMI was not associated with consumption of milk, regular soft drinks, regular or diet fruit drinks, or noncitrus juices in a descriptive and multivariate regression analysis of data from children ages 6 to 19 participating in the U.S. Department of Agriculture's Continuing Survey of Food Intakes, 1994 to 1996, 1998 [88]. However, unlike these findings for the entire population, there was a negative association in girls of BMI with milk consumption and a positive association with diet carbonated beverages, but these relationships were weak. Total beverage consumption and beverage choices were strongly related to age, race, and gender [88].

A cross-sectional analysis of baseline data from an ongoing longitudinal study in Hawaii (i.e., a Kaiser-Permanente study) including 323 Asian and Caucasian young adolescents aged 9 to 14 years demonstrated that total calcium intake was associated with statistically lower body fat and lower body weight (borderline significance) after adjusting for confounding factors [89]. Calcium from dairy food sources had a stronger association than total calcium intake in relation to iliac skinfold thickness, but nondairy calcium was not associated with weight or iliac skinfold thickness. One serving of milk was associated with a 0.78-mm reduction in iliac skinfold thickness, whereas soda intake was significantly associated with higher body weight. The researchers suggest that soda consumption could promote weight gain by increasing energy intake or by replacing milk in the diet. A significant interaction between Asian ethnicity and dairy intake was noted. The findings of this study led the researchers to conclude that decreasing soda and increasing dairy food consumption may help Asians maintain body fat and weight during adolescence [89].

Low intake of dairy products was significantly associated with increased risk of obesity in a cross-sectional study of 1701 children from 3rd to 7th grade in nine schools located in three geographical regions in Chile [90]. Likewise, in an analysis of baseline cross-sectional data from a cohort of 16,882 U.S. adolescents aged 9 to 14 years participating in the Longitudinal Growing Up Today Study, researchers found that overweight participants consumed fewer dairy products than nonoverweight youths [91]. In an observational case-control study of 53 prepubertal Puerto Rican children aged 7 to 10 years, daily frequency of dairy product intake was inversely associated with obesity [92].

In another cross-sectional analysis of data from 3044 Portuguese children (1503 girls and 1541 boys) aged 7 to 9 years, an inverse association was found between calcium intake and BMI in girls, but not in boys, even after adjusting for age, energy intake, parental education, and physical activity [93]. Calcium intake explained only a small percentage of the variability in BMI, which is not surprising given the multitude of factors that relate to body weight gain. As a result of this study's findings, the researchers called for more controlled trials to assess the effects of dietary calcium on body mass in each gender [93].

Several prospective longitudinal studies tracking children throughout childhood (some into adolescent period) report a relationship between dairy intake and BMI, body weight, and body fat.

In a longitudinal study of 53 healthy preschool children in Tennessee, Carruth and Skinner [94] demonstrated that more servings of dairy foods and higher mean calcium intake during the first 5 years of life were associated with lower body fat at 70 months. In a follow-up study in these same children, Skinner and colleagues [95] showed that the inverse relationship between calcium and percentage of body fat continued at 8 years of age. This finding indicates that dairy and calcium intake in the first few years of life are significant inverse determinants of body fat at age 8 [95]. The researchers recommend that children be strongly encouraged to regularly include calcium-rich foods and beverages in their diets, specifically skim, 1% or 2% fat milk, and other low-fat dairy products [95]. Similar findings were reported by Fisher and colleagues [96]. In their study, girls followed from ages 5 to 9 years who met calcium recommendations had higher energy intakes, but not higher BMIs, than girls who failed to meet calcium recommendations [96].

Longitudinal data from the Framingham Children's Study found that higher intakes of total calcium early in life were associated with a decreased gain of body fat in early adolescence and that increasing servings of dairy foods was more strongly correlated to reduced body fat than dietary calcium per se [97]. Moore and colleagues [97] used prospective data from 99 children to determine whether dairy intake in early childhood (3.0 to 5.9 years old) related to changes in the level of body fat from the preschool years to early adolescence (10 to 13 years old). Dietary intake was assessed by using multiple sets of 3-day diet records collected throughout each year, an annual food frequency questionnaire, and dietary interviews. Children were classified into tertiles of dairy intake. Anthropometry measurements were obtained at each annual clinic visit, including height and weight (used to estimate yearly BMIs), and triceps, subscapular, suprailiac, and abdominal skinfolds. Yearly change in body fat was estimated by calculating the slope for these anthropometry measures from age 5 to 13 [97]. Children in the highest tertile of dairy food servings had higher intakes of energy, percent calories from saturated fat and protein, and energy-adjusted intakes of calcium, magnesium, vitamin A, and vitamin D compared with children in lower gender-specific tertiles of dairy food intake. Children in the lowest tertile of dairy food servings per day had statistically greater gains in BMI and the sum of four skinfolds from childhood to early adolescence than did children in the upper two tertiles of dairy intake [97]. This study provides evidence that dairy food intake does not have an adverse impact on body fat change in developing children and indicates that low levels of dairy food intake during preschool years may be associated with a greater gain of body fat throughout childhood [97]. The researchers suggested that low levels of dairy food intake should be avoided and that higher intake levels may be more beneficial when they are not accompanied by excessively high intakes of calories or fat.

A longitudinal study of young children (average age of 8 years) demonstrated that milk-avoiders had low calcium intakes, were shorter in stature with elevated BMIs, and had poor skeletons compared with a reference population of milk drinkers [98]. Over 2 years of follow-up, the milk-avoiders remained significantly shorter than the reference population, and had elevated BMIs despite modest increases in milk consumption and calcium intake from all sources [98].

Other longitudinal studies have found no association between calcium or dairy intake and body fat in children [99–101]. An investigation of low-income preschool children aged 2 to 5 years in North Dakota found no association between milk intake and weight change [99]. Longitudinal data from MIT's Growth and Development Study, which is a longitudinal prospective study in 196 non-obese premenarcheal girls aged 8 to 12 years followed until 4 years postmenarche (~age 18), revealed no relationship between BMI z-scores or percent body fat and dairy or calcium consumption over time [100]. The researchers stated that the results refute the idea that dairy foods should be reduced during adolescence to avoid excess body weight or body fat accumulation [100]. In a 3-year longitudinal observational study of 5388 boys and 6943 girls, ages 9 to 14 years, enrolled in the Growing Up Today Study (i.e., children of participants in the Nurses' Health Study II), Berkey and colleagues [101] found that children who drank the most milk gained more weight, but this was due to the higher calorie intake. Children who drank more than 3 servings of milk a day (the current recommended intake is 3 servings/day) experienced gains in BMI greater than those who drank smaller amounts [101]. Quantities of 1% milk in boys and skim milk in girls were significantly associated with BMI gain, as was total dietary calcium. However, when adjusted for total calorie intake, these associations were no longer statistically significant. The researchers concluded that calorie intake was the most important predictor of weight gain in this study [101]. That is, increased energy intake may mask the potentially beneficial effect of dairy on body weight or body fat. It is important to note that children in this study self-reported their weight and completed a food frequency questionnaire to provide information on their food intake during the previous year [101]. Use of these methods requires caution in the interpretation of results.

When researchers assessed the relationship between dairy food or calcium intake at baseline and over 1 year on measures of weight and body fatness in 342 nonobese children aged 4 to 10 years with normal or elevated blood cholesterol levels, they found that factors such as age and blood cholesterol levels influenced these relationships [102]. Three 24-hour dietary recalls were employed to determine dietary intake, and BMI and the sum of skinfolds and trunk skinfold measurements were used to assess obesity at baseline, 3, 6, and 12 months. Calcium intake (after adjusting for age, sex, energy intake, and percentage of energy from fat) was inversely associated with BMI, sum of skinfolds, and trunk skinfolds at baseline and over 1-year in the 7- to 10-year-old children who had normal blood cholesterol levels. In addition, a higher intake of dairy foods was associated with lower measures of obesity in the 7- to 10-year-old children with normal blood cholesterol. However, dairy food or calcium intake was not associated with measures of obesity in children with high cholesterol levels or in the 4- to 6-year-old children with normal blood cholesterol [102]. Skinfold measures in the older children with high blood cholesterol tended to decrease (non-significantly) with increasing calcium intake until ~963 mg/day and were consistently lower at dairy intakes of >3.8 servings/day. The researchers speculated that these older children with high blood cholesterol may be more resistant to the positive effects of calcium or experience a threshold effect at higher intakes of calcium or dairy foods. They also suggested that older children without risk of metabolic syndrome may benefit the most from increased calcium intake [102].

Huang and McCory [84], in a review of studies (observational and clinical) examining the relationship between dairy intake and obesity in children and adolescents, also note that potentially confounding factors may influence the outcome of these studies. For example, it is unknown if the effects of dairy on body weight are independent of overall energy intakes, or other eating patterns. They point out that inconsistencies in studies may be explained by failure to control for potentially confounding variables, as well as the difficulty in accurately measuring dietary intake. These researchers concluded that future research on the relationship between dairy or calcium intake and body weight or fat in children and adolescents can be enhanced by carefully defining dairy consumption and improving the quality of dietary intake data [84].

7.5.2 Clinical Trials

Few clinical trials have been conducted to specifically investigate the effect of consumption of dairy foods or calcium on body composition changes in children and adolescents. For the most part, these types of studies were primarily designed to assess the effects of dairy foods or calcium on bone health and used calcium supplements or a form of calcium derived from milk, with only some studies using dairy products [84]. In clinical trials in children and adolescents that have used dairy products as the intervention, either a neutral or a beneficial effect of dairy food intake on body weight or body composition has been reported [26,84,103–108].

Chan and colleagues [103], in a randomized controlled study, investigated the effect of calcium supplementation with dairy products on bone and body composition in 48 pubertal girls aged 9 to 13 years in Utah. Increasing calcium intake from 728 mg/day to 1437 mg/day with dairy foods for a year had no effect on body weight gain or fatness. The additional intake of dairy foods increased the rate of bone mineralization and the girls' nutrient intake (e.g., calcium, phosphorus, vitamin D, protein) [103]. Similar findings have been reported by Cadogan and coworkers [104]. In this clinical trial of 80 healthy white girls (average age of 12.2 years) in New Zealand, subjects were randomized into milk or control groups stratified by pubertal stage to investigate the effect on milk on total body mineral acquisition, height, weight, and lean body mass. The milk group consumed an additional two cups of whole or reduced fat milk a day for 18 months, while the control group followed their habitual diet, which included about ¾ cup of milk per day. Bone mineral content and bone mineral density increased more for the milk group as compared to the control group, yet there were no significant differences in changes in height, weight, lean body mass, and fat body mass. However, a trend toward greater gain in lean body mass with a concomitant reduction in percent body fat was observed in the milk group. The researchers concluded that increased milk consumption may positively impact body composition based on the lean and body fat mass changes in this study cohort [104].

Another randomized clinical trial examined the effects of increasing milk consumption on bone density and body composition in 28 boys aged 13 to 17 years during a 12-week resistance-training program [106]. In addition to their usual diet, the boys were randomly assigned to consume 3 additional servings a day of 1% fluid milk or juice not fortified with calcium. The milk group had significantly higher intakes of protein, fat, vitamins A and D, riboflavin, calcium, phosphorus, and magnesium, and lower intakes of carbohydrate and vitamin C. The milk group consumed, on average, approximately 250 cal less per day; however, this difference in energy intake was not statistically significant. All subjects experienced significant changes in height, sum of seven skinfold measurements, body mass, lean body mass, fat mass, whole-body bone mineral content, bone mineral density, and maximal strength in the squat and bench press. The milk group had a significantly greater increase in bone mineral density compared to the juice group. Additionally, there was a trend for those in the milk group to lose more body fat, but it was not statistically significant. The researchers suggested that increasing the intake of milk in physically-active adolescent boys may enhance bone health and potentially have a beneficial effect on body fat [106].

A 2-year pilot study conducted in Omaha, Nebraska demonstrated that pubertal girls can increase their calcium intake, primarily from dairy foods, without increasing their body weight or body fat [105]. In this secondary analysis, data was obtained from a subsample of 59 9-year old girls enrolled in a 4-year clinical trial to test the effect of increasing dietary calcium to 1500 mg/day on bone mass. The girls were randomly assigned to a calcium-rich diet supplying at least 1500 mg calcium a day (approximately three-quarters from dairy foods) or their usual diet. Girls in the calcium-rich diet group had a mean calcium intake of 1656 ± 191 mg/day, while girls consuming their usual diets had an average calcium intake of 961 ± 268 mg/day [105]. Although the girls in the treatment group consumed approximately 150 more calories per day (a nonsignificant increase), they did not have greater increases in body weight, BMI, or fat or lean mass compared to the control group. Over the 2-year period, girls on the calcium-rich diet significantly increased the nutritional quality of their diets due to increased intake of essential nutrients. Researchers concluded that calcium-rich diets, primarily from dairy foods, do not cause excessive weight gain in pubertal girls while contributing positively to overall nutrition [105]. Similar findings are reported by Merrilees and colleagues [107] based on a 3-year study of adolescent girls aged 15 to 18 years in New Zealand.

A randomized, double-blind, placebo-controlled intervention study in 110 Danish girls aged 12 years old found that habitual dietary calcium intake, but not modest calcium supplementation (500 mg a day as calcium carbonate), influenced body weight and body fat [108]. This study represents a secondary analysis of data originally designed to evaluate the effect of calcium supplementation on bone accumulation and had the statistical power to detect a change in body weight of 3% or more. Two groups of girls were selected on the basis of habitual dietary calcium — those with a calcium intake of 1000 to 1304 mg/day and those with a calcium intake of <713 mg/day — to receive either the calcium supplement or placebo. At baseline, a higher habitual intake of dietary calcium primarily from dairy foods was significantly associated with a lower percentage of body fat. However, adding calcium supplements to the diet had no effect on height, body weight, or percentage of body fat over the year [108]. The researchers suggested that the effect of calcium on body weight may be exerted only if consumed as part of a meal. An alternative explanation is that the effect may be due to other ingredients in dairy products and calcium may be just a marker for a high dairy intake.

7.6 SUMMARY

The high prevalence of overweight and obesity, with their associated health and financial burden, creates the urgency for preventative actions [3]. Although consuming excess energy (i.e., too many calories) in relation to energy expenditure is the major determinant of overweight and obesity, a growing body of scientific evidence indicates that Americans' low intake of dairy foods, the major source of calcium, may be a contributing factor to this public health problem [14,15,18,19,21–23]. Research findings from observational studies and randomized controlled clinical trials in humans, along with experimental animal and cellular studies, provide substantial evidence that adequate intake of dairy products or calcium contributes to regulation of body weight and fat mass. This research also demonstrates that consuming recommended intakes of dairy products (milk, yogurt, cheese) does not lead to weight gain.

Support for a role of dairy products and/or calcium in a healthy weight in adults comes from observational studies, both cross-sectional and longitudinal. Although these types of studies do not prove a cause-and-effect relationship, they demonstrate that consumption of dairy products and/or calcium is associated with either a beneficial effect or no effect on body weight and fat mass [11,29,30]. As reviewed by Teegarden [23], there are a number of issues to consider when examining the results of these epidemiological studies. For example, findings of a link between high dairy intake and reduced body weight/fat mass may be explained not only by calcium, but by other components in dairy foods as well. Further, a high calcium intake may be a surrogate for a healthy lifestyle, or vice versa. Inconsistencies in the findings may be explained by failure to consider energy intake. The weight benefits of dairy foods or calcium appear to be strongest in the context of a diet moderately reduced in energy [46]. That is, high energy intake may obscure any effect of dairy food or calcium intake on body weight or body fat. Additionally, high energy restriction may override the effects of dairy foods or calcium on body weight or body fat loss. Consumption of dairy foods or calcium may only have an effect under specific circumstances, such as during modest weight loss, in obese or overweight individuals, or in those who are low-dairy food consumers (i.e., calcium-deficient). In addition, there appears to be a threshold effect, such that if an individual is already consuming adequate dairy food or calcium intake, increasing consumption is unlikely to confer any additional weight or fat loss benefit [23]. Studies may also need to be of sufficient duration before an effect on body weight or composition is observed. Other factors such as gender, menopausal status, and race and ethnicity may influence the findings. It is important to appreciate that a number of the observational studies are secondary analyses of studies with other end points, such as skeletal health or blood pressure. These studies may not have adequate power to observe differences in body weight or fat due to changes in dairy food or calcium intake.

Randomized clinical trials (considered the "gold standard" of study designs) in adults provide the most compelling evidence of the beneficial role of dairy foods and calcium in a healthy weight. In these clinical trials of overweight or obese adults (males, females, whites, African Americans) following reduced-calorie diets, increasing consumption of dairy foods from inadequate (1 serving or less/day) to adequate (3 servings/day) enhances body weight and body fat losses, reduces abdominal (trunk) obesity, and minimizes loss of lean body tissue [50,51,53]. Moreover, dairy sources of calcium appear to exert a greater antiobesity effect than does calcium alone [50]. In addition, consuming 3 servings of dairy foods a day as part of a weight maintenance diet has been shown to improve body composition (i.e., reduce total body and trunk fat and increase lean body mass) and metabolic profile in overweight adults [53].

Although a few randomized clinical trials in adults fail to support the above weight- or fat-loss benefits of dairy products or calcium, these studies demonstrate that 3 servings/day of dairy products can be included in weight reduction or weight maintenance diets without promoting body weight or fat mass gain [54–56]. These studies indicate that the antiobesity effect of calcium or dairy products depends on total energy intake and appears to be strongest in the presence of a modestly energy-reduced diet, in individuals whose dairy intake or calcium is initially low, and in those who are overweight or obese.

Experimental animal studies, especially in transgenic mice which over-express the *agouti* gene and are susceptible to adult-onset diet-induced obesity, demonstrate that increasing dairy food and calcium intake reduces body weight and body fat during energy restriction and helps prevent weight and fat regain after weight loss [11,17,60,61]. Moreover, dairy foods exert markedly greater effects than calcium in attenuating weight and fat gain and accelerating fat loss than an equivalent amount of supplemental calcium [11,60].

The mechanism(s) to explain the antiobesity effect of calcium and the augmented effect of dairy foods has been explored in experimental animal, *in vitro*, and human studies. The balance between available energy and energy utilization influences body weight and body fat [4]. Dairy food and dietary calcium intake has been proposed to influence this balance. Specifically, increased consumption of dairy foods or calcium may reduce the availability of energy (e.g., by decreasing the absorption of fatty acids and increasing satiety) and increase energy utilization (e.g., by increasing lipid oxidation or by its effect on hormonal control of fat metabolism). Most of the research has focused on the effect of dairy products and calcium on energy utilization. Randomized clinical trials [37,57] and a cross-sectional study [32] in adults indicate that increased dairy calcium increases fat oxidation.

The ability of dietary calcium to regulate the hormones $1,25(OH)_2D$ and PTH is the mechanism most often cited to explain dietary calcium's effect on energy utilization [16,17,22,71–73]. Studies using the *agouti* mouse model and cultured human adipocytes provide the following key framework to explain the effect of calcium on energy utilization. A low intake of dietary calcium increases secretion of PTH and the production of $1,25(OH)_2D$ which increases intracellular ionic calcium in adipocytes, leading to a coordinated decrease in lipolysis and increase in lipogenesis, resulting in increased adipocyte lipid filling and increased adiposity [22]. In addition, $1,25(OH)_2D$ exerts a genomic effect on UCP2 expression, thereby suppressing adipocyte apoptosis. A high calcium intake exerts an antiobesity effect by suppressing the production of PTH and $1,25(OH)_2D$, which reduces adipocyte intracellular ionic calcium and, in turn, leads to increased lipolysis and utilization of energy and inhibition of fat storage [22]. The decrease in $1,25(OH)_2D$ also results in increased adipocyte apoptosis. Findings demonstrating that dairy sources of calcium have a greater beneficial effect on body weight and composition than calcium from supplements [11,21,60] indicate that dairy products contain other components in addition to calcium that influence energy metabolism. This augmented antiobesity effect of dairy products is attributed in large part to bioactive compounds in the whey fraction of dairy foods (e.g., ACE inhibitors and branched chain amino acids such as leucine).

While the goal for overweight or obese adults is to reduce body weight, the goal for overweight children and adolescents is to achieve normal growth and development with a healthy body composition [4]. Relatively little research has explicitly examined the relation between dairy foods or calcium and body weight or body fat in children and adolescents [84]. Many of the studies in children and adolescents are primarily designed to examine the effect of dairy foods or calcium on bone health. Nevertheless, findings to date indicate that increasing calcium-rich foods such as dairy products or calcium has no adverse effect on children's weight or body composition, and, in fact, may play a role in promoting a healthy body composition or preventing an unhealthy weight gain. Similar to studies in adults, a number of confounding factors such as energy intake, age, metabolic syndrome, and the quality of dietary intake data influence the findings of studies examining the association between consumption of calcium or dairy products and children's or adolescents' weight and body composition.

Additional research is needed to clarify the antiobesity effects of dairy products and calcium and to understand the underlying mechanism(s). However, substantial data indicates that consuming 3 servings of dairy products (e.g., milk, yogurt, cheese) a day markedly accelerates weight and fat loss secondary to caloric restriction and results in significant reductions in body fat mass in the absence of caloric restriction in overweight adults [22]. In children, consuming 3 servings of dairy products a day may help prevent the development of overweight and have a favorable effect on body composition. Although these dairy food- or calcium-induced beneficial effects on body weight or body fat mass are likely to be modest, they may substantially contribute to weight changes over time, leading to a significant decrease in the incidence of obesity [23,44,45,109]. This is one more reason why health professionals are encouraging adults and children to consume 3 servings of dairy foods a day [22–24,45]. As stated by one researcher, "if current recommendations for calcium intake were met through food sources in the promotion of optimal bone health, this might also help to reduce the incidence and development of overweight and obesity" [22]. The cause of overweight and obesity is multifactorial and successful prevention or treatment depends on multiple actions. Emerging scientific research indicates that consuming recommended intakes of dairy products and calcium is one of these actions.

REFERENCES

1. World Health Organization, Obesity: preventing and managing the global epidemic, WHO Technical Report Series No. 894, World Health Organization, Geneva, 2000.
2. Wang, Y. and Lobstein, T., Worldwide trends in childhood overweight and obesity, *Int. J. Pediatr. Obes.*, 1, 11, 2006.
3. U.S. Department of Health and Human Services, Public Health Service, Office of the Surgeon General, *The Surgeon General's Call to Action to Prevent and Decrease Overweight and Obesity*, U.S. Government Printing Office, Washington, D.C., 2000, www.surgeongeneral.gov/library.
4. U.S. Department of Health and Human Services and U.S. Department of Agriculture, *Dietary Guidelines for Americans, 2005*, 6th ed., U.S. Government Printing Office, Washington, D.C., January 2005, www.healthierus.gov/dietaryguidelines.
5. Ogden, C. L. et al., Prevalence of overweight and obesity in the United States, 1999–2004, *JAMA*, 295, 1549, 2006.
6. Flegal, K. M. et al., Excess deaths associated with underweight, overweight, and obesity, *JAMA*, 293, 1861, 2004.
7. Poirier, P. et al., Obesity and cardiovascular disease: pathophysiology, evaluation, and effect of weight loss, *Circulation*, 113, 898, 2006.
8. Olshansky, S. J. et al., A potential decline in life expectancy in the United States in the 21st century, *N. Engl. J. Med.*, 352, 1138, 2005.
9. Shepard, T. Y. et al., Occasional physical inactivity combined with a high-fat diet may be important in the development and maintenance of obesity in human subjects, *Am. J. Clin. Nutr.*, 73, 703, 2001.
10. McCarron, D. A. et al., Blood pressure and nutrient intake in the United States, *Science*, 224, 1392, 1984.
11. Zemel, M. B. et al., Regulation of adiposity by dietary calcium, *FASEB J.*, 14, 1132, 2000.
12. Moshfegh, A., Goldman, J., and Cleveland, L., *What We Eat in America, NHANES 2001–2002: Usual Nutrient Intakes from Food Compared to Dietary Reference Intakes*, U.S. Department of Agriculture, Agricultural Research Service, 2005, www.ars.usda.gov/foodsurvey.
13. Cook, A. J. and Friday, J. E., *Pyramid Servings Intakes in the United States, 1999–2002, 1 Day*, CNRG Table Set 3.0, USDA Agricultural Research Service, Community Nutrition Research Group, Beltsville, MD, March 2005, www.barc.usda.gov/bhnrc/cnrg.
14. Zemel, M. B., Calcium modulation of hypertension and obesity: mechanisms and implications, *J. Am. Coll. Nutr.*, 20, 428s, 2001.
15. Heaney, R. P., Davies, K. M., and Barger-Lux, M. J., Calcium and weight: clinical studies, *J. Am. Coll. Nutr.*, 21, 152s, 2002.
16. Zemel, M. B., Regulation of adiposity and obesity risk by dietary calcium: mechanisms and implications, *J. Am. Coll. Nutr.*, 21, 146s, 2002.
17. Zemel, M. B., Role of dietary calcium and dairy products in modulating adiposity, *Lipids*, 38, 139, 2003.
18. Parikh, S. J. and Yanovski, J. A., Calcium intake and adiposity, *Am. J. Clin. Nutr.*, 77, 281, 2003.
19. Teegarden, D. and Zemel, M. B., Dairy product components and weight regulation: symposium overview, *J. Nutr.*, 133, 243s, 2003.
20. Zemel, M. B. and Miller, S. L., Dietary calcium and dairy modulation of adiposity and obesity risk, *Nutr. Rev.*, 62, 125, 2004.
21. Zemel, M. B., Role of calcium and dairy products in energy partitioning and weight management, *Am. J. Clin. Nutr.*, 79, 907s, 2004.
22. Zemel, M. B., The role of dairy foods in weight management, *J. Am. Coll. Nutr.*, 24, 537s, 2005.
23. Teegarden, D., The influence of dairy product consumption on body composition, *J. Nutr.*, 135, 2749, 2005.
24. Schrager, S., Dietary calcium intake and obesity, *J. Am. Board Fam. Pract.*, 18, 205, 2005.
25. Tremblay, A. and Joanisse, D. R., Calcium intake, body composition and plasma lipid–lipoprotein concentrations in adults, *Aust. J. Dairy Technol.*, 60, 66, 2005.
26. Barr, S. I., Increased dairy product or calcium intake: is body weight or composition affected in humans? *J. Nutr.*, 133, 245s, 2003.

27. Lovejoy, J. C. et al., Ethnic differences in dietary intakes, physical activity, and energy expenditure in middle-aged, premenopausal women: the healthy transitions study, *Am. J. Clin. Nutr.*, 74, 90, 2001.
28. Buchowski, M. S. et al., Dietary calcium intake in lactose maldigesting intolerant and tolerant African American women, *J. Am. Coll. Nutr.*, 21, 47, 2002.
29. Pereira, M. A. et al., Dairy consumption, obesity, and the insulin resistance syndrome in young adults: the CARDIA study, *JAMA*, 287, 2081, 2002.
30. Jacqmain, M. et al., Calcium intake, body composition, and lipoprotein–lipid concentrations in adults, *Am. J. Clin. Nutr.*, 77, 1448, 2003.
31. Loos, R. et al., Calcium intake and body composition in the HERITAGE Family Study, *Obes. Res.*, 11, 597, 2003.
32. Melanson, E. L. et al., Relation between calcium intake and fat oxidation in adult humans, *Int. J. Obes.*, 27, 196, 2003.
33. Mirmiran, P., Esmaillzadeh, A., and Azizi, F., Dairy consumption and body mass index: an inverse relationship, *Int. J. Obes.*, 29, 115, 2005.
34. Marques-Vidal, P., Goncalves, A., and Dias, C. M., Milk intake is inversely related to obesity in men and in young women: data from the Portuguese Health Interview Survey 1998–1999, *Int. J. Obes.*, 30, 88, 2006.
35. Azadbakht, L. et al., Dairy consumption is inversely associated with the prevalence of metabolic syndrome in Tehranian adults, *Am. J. Clin. Nutr.*, 82, 523, 2005.
36. Liu, S. et al., Dietary calcium, vitamin D, and the prevalence of metabolic syndrome in middle-aged and older women, *Diabetes Care*, 28, 2926, 2005.
37. Melanson, E. L. et al., Effect of low- and high-calcium dairy-based diets on macronutrient oxidation in humans, *Obes. Res.*, 13, 2102, 2005.
38. Drapeau, V. et al., Modifications in food-group consumption are related to long-term body-weight changes, *Am. J. Clin. Nutr.*, 80, 29, 2004.
39. Newby, P. K. et al., Dietary patterns and changes in body mass index and waist circumference in adults, *Am. J. Clin. Nutr.*, 77, 1417, 2003.
40. Newby, P. K. et al., Food patterns measured by factor analysis and anthropometric changes in adults, *Am. J. Clin. Nutr.*, 80, 504, 2004.
41. Macdonald, H. M. et al., Longitudinal changes in weight in perimenopausal and early postmenopausal women: effects of dietary energy intake, energy expenditure, dietary calcium intake and hormone replacement therapy, *Int. J. Obes.*, 27, 669, 2003.
42. Boon, N. et al., The relation between calcium intake and body composition in a Dutch population, The Amsterdam Growth and Health Longitudinal Study, *Am. J. Epidemiol.*, 162, 27, 2005.
43. Rajpathak, S. N. et al., Calcium and dairy intakes in relation to long-term weight gain in U.S. men, *Am. J. Clin. Nutr.*, 83, 559, 2006.
44. Davies, K. M. et al., Calcium intake and body weight, *J. Clin. Endocrinol. Metab.*, 85, 4635, 2000.
45. Heaney, R. P., Normalizing calcium intake: projected population effects for body weight, *J. Nutr.*, 133, 268s, 2003.
46. Lin, Y. C. et al., Dairy calcium is related to changes in body composition during a two-year exercise intervention in young women, *J. Am. Coll. Nutr.*, 19, 754, 2000.
47. Shapses, S. A., Heshka, S., and Heymsfield, S. B., Effect of calcium supplementation on weight and fat loss in women, *J. Clin. Endocrinol. Metab.*, 89, 632, 2004.
48. Reid, I. R. et al., Effects of calcium supplementation on body weight and blood pressure in normal older women: a randomized controlled trial, *J. Clin. Endocrinol. Metab.*, 90, 3824, 2005.
49. Summerbell, C. D. et al., Randomized controlled trial of novel, simple, and well supervised weight reducing diets in outpatients, *Br. Med. J.*, 317, 1487, 1998.
50. Zemel, M. B. et al., Calcium and dairy acceleration of weight and fat loss during energy restriction in obese adults, *Obes. Res.*, 12, 582, 2004.
51. Zemel, M. B. et al., Dairy augmentation of total and central fat loss in obese subjects, *Int. J. Obes.*, 29, 341, 2005.
52. Zemel, M. B. et al., Role of dairy products in modulating weight and fat loss: a multi-center trial, *FASEB J.*, 18, A845, (Abst. # 566.5), 2004.
53. Zemel, M. B. et al., Effects of calcium and dairy on body composition and weight loss in African American adults, *Obes. Res.*, 13, 1218, 2005.

54. Thompson, W. G. et al., Effect of energy-reduced diets high in dairy products and fiber on weight loss in obese adults, *Obes. Res.*, 13, 1344, 2005.
55. Harvey-Berino, J. et al., The impact of calcium and dairy product consumption on weight loss, *Obes. Res.*, 13, 1720, 2005.
56. Gunther, C. W. et al., Dairy products do not lead to alterations in body weight and fat mass in young women in a one year intervention, *Am. J. Clin. Nutr.*, 81, 751, 2005.
57. Gunther, C. W. et al., Fat oxidation and its relation to serum parathyroid hormone in young women enrolled in a 1-y dairy calcium intervention, *Am. J. Clin. Nutr.*, 82, 1228, 2005.
58. Jacobsen, R. et al., Effect of short-term high dietary calcium intake on 24-h energy expenditure, fat oxidation, and fecal fat excretion, *Int. J. Obes.*, 29, 292, 2005.
59. Boon, N. et al., Effects of 3 diets with various calcium contents on 24-h energy expenditure, fat oxidation, and adipose tissue message RNA expression of lipid metabolism-related proteins, *Am. J. Clin. Nutr.*, 82, 1244, 2005.
60. Shi, H., DiRienzo, D., and Zemel, M. B., Effects of dietary calcium on adipocyte lipid metabolism and body weight regulation in energy-restricted aP2-*agouti* transgenic mice, *FASEB J.*, 15, 291, 2001.
61. Sun, X. and Zemel, M. B., Calcium and dairy products inhibit weight and fat regain during ad libitum consumption following energy restriction in Ap2-*agouti* transgenic mice, *J. Nutr.*, 34, 3054, 2004.
62. Papakonstantinou, E. et al., High dietary calcium reduces body fat content, digestibility of fat, and serum vitamin D in rats, *Obes. Res.*, 11, 387, 2003.
63. Zemel, M., Calcium modulation of adiposity, *Obes. Res.*, 11, 375, 2003.
64. Hall, W. L. et al., Casein and whey exert different effects on plasma amino acid profiles, gastro-intestinal hormone secretion, and appetite, *Br. J. Nutr.*, 89, 239, 2003.
65. Anderson, G. H. and Moore, S. E., Dietary proteins in the regulation of food intake and body weight in humans, *J. Nutr.*, 134, 974s, 2004.
66. Noakes, M., Bowen, J., and Clifton, P., Dairy foods or fractions for appetite and weight control, *Aust. J. Dairy Technol.*, 60, 152, 2005.
67. Barr, S. I. et al., Effects of increased consumption of fluid milk on energy and nutrient intake, body weight, and cardiovascular risk factors in healthy older adults, *J. Am. Diet. Assoc.*, 100, 810, 2000.
68. Almiron-Roig, E. and Drewnowski, A., Hunger, thirst, and energy intakes following consumption of caloric beverages, *Physiol. Behav.*, 79, 767, 2003.
69. Tsuchiya, A. et al., Higher satiety ratings following yogurt consumption relative to fruit drink or dairy fruit drinks, *J. Am. Diet. Assoc.*, 106, 550, 2006.
70. Schneeman, B. O., Burton-Freeman, B., and Davis, P., Incorporating dairy foods into low and high fat diets increases the postprandial cholecystokinin response in men and women, *J. Nutr.*, 133, 4124, 2003.
71. Shi, H. et al., 1α,25-Dihydroxyvitamin D_3 modulates human adipocyte metabolism via non-genomic action, *FASEB J.*, 14, 2751, 2001.
72. Shi, H. et al., 1-25-Dihydroxyvitamin D_3 inhibits uncoupling protein 2 expression in human adipocytes, *FASEB J.*, 16, 1808, 2002.
73. Xue, B., Mechanism of intracellular calcium inhibition of lipolysis in human adipocytes, *FASEB J.*, 15, 2527, 2001.
74. Parikh, S. J. et al., The relationship between obesity and serum 1,25-dihydroxyvitamin D concentration in healthy adults, *J. Clin. Endocrinol. Metab.*, 89, 1196, 2004.
75. Shah, N. P., Effects of milk-derived bioactives: an overview, *Br. J. Nutr.*, 84, 3s, 2000.
76. Ha, E. and Zemel, M. B., Functional properties of whey, whey components, and essential amino acids: mechanisms underlying health benefits for active people, *J. Nutr. Biochem.*, 14, 251, 2003.
77. Layman, D. K., The role of leucine in weight loss diets and glucose homeostasis, *J. Nutr.*, 133, 261s, 2003.
78. Layman, D. K. and Baum, J. I., Dietary protein impact on glycemic control during weight loss, *J. Nutr.*, 134, 968s, 2004.
79. Belobrajdic, D. P., McIntosh, G. H., and Owens, J. A., A high-whey-protein diet reduces body weight gain and alters insulin sensitivity relative to red meat in Wistar rats, *J. Nutr.*, 134, 1454, 2004.
80. Larsen, T. M. et al., Conjugated linoleic acid supplementation for 1 year does not prevent weight or body fat regain, *Am. J. Clin. Nutr.*, 83, 606, 2006.

81. Kamphuis, M. M. et al., The effect of conjugated linoleic acid supplementation after weight loss on body weight regain, body composition, and resting metabolic rate in overweight subjects, *Int. J. Obes. Relat. Metab. Disord.*, 27, 840, 2003.
82. Whigham, L. D. et al., Safety profile of conjugated linoleic acid in a 12-month trial in obese humans, *Food Chem. Toxicol.*, 42, 1701, 2004.
83. Freedman, D. S. et al., The relation of childhood BMI to adult adiposity: the Bogalusa Heart Study, *Pediatrics*, 115, 22, 2005.
84. Huang, T. and McCrory, M., Dairy intake, obesity, and metabolic syndrome in children and adolescents, *Nutr. Rev.*, 63, 71, 2005.
85. Barba, G. et al., Inverse association between body mass and frequency of milk consumption in children, *Br. J. Nutr.*, 93, 15, 2005.
86. Black, R. E. et al., Children who avoid drinking cow milk have low dietary calcium intakes and poor bone health, *Am. J. Clin. Nutr.*, 76, 675, 2002.
87. Albertson, A. M. et al., Ready-to-eat cereal consumption: its relationship with BMI and nutrient intake of children aged 4 to 12 years, *J. Am. Diet. Assoc.*, 103, 1613, 2003.
88. Forshee, R. A. and Storey, M. L., Total beverage consumption and beverage choices among children and adolescents, *Int. J. Food Sci. Nutr.*, 54, 297, 2003.
89. Novotny, R. et al., Dairy intake is associated with lower body fat and soda intake with greater weight in adolescent girls, *J. Nutr.*, 134, 1905, 2004.
90. Olivares, S. et al., Nutritional status, food consumption and physical activity among Chilean school children: a descriptive study, *Eur. J. Clin. Nutr.*, 58, 1278, 2004.
91. Rockett, H. R., Cross-sectional measurements of nutrient intake among adolescents in 1996, *Prev. Med.*, 33, 27, 2001.
92. Tanasescu, M. et al., Biobehavioral factors are associated with obesity in Puerto Rican children, *J. Nutr.*, 130, 1734, 2000.
93. Moreira, P. et al., Dietary calcium and body mass index in Portuguese children, *Eur. J. Clin. Nutr.*, 59, 861, 2005.
94. Carruth, B. R. and Skinner, J. D., The role of dietary calcium and other nutrients in moderating body fat in preschool children, *Int. J. Obes.*, 25, 559, 2001.
95. Skinner, J. D. et al., Longitudinal calcium intake is negatively related to children's body fat indexes, *J. Am. Diet. Assoc.*, 103, 1626, 2003.
96. Fisher, J. O. et al., Meeting calcium recommendations during middle childhood reflects mother–daughter beverage choices and predicts bone mineral status, *Am. J. Clin. Nutr.*, 79, 698, 2004.
97. Moore, L. L., Bradlee, M. L., Goo, D. and Singer, M. R., Low airy intake in early childhood predicts excess body fat gain, *Obesity*, 14, 1010–1018, 2006.
98. Rockell, J. E. B. et al., Two-year changes in bone and body composition in young children with a history of prolonged milk avoidance, *Osteop. Int.*, 16, 1016, 2005.
99. Newby, P. K. et al., Beverage consumption is not associated with changes in weight and body mass index among low-income preschool children in North Dakota, *J. Am. Diet. Assoc.*, 104, 1086, 2004.
100. Phillips, S. M. et al., Dairy food consumption and body weight and fatness studied longitudinally over the adolescent period, *Int. J. Obes.*, 27, 1106, 2003.
101. Berkey, C. S. et al., Milk, dairy fat, dietary calcium, and weight gain, *Arch. Pediatr. Adolesc. Med.*, 159, 543, 2005.
102. Dixon, L. B. et al., Calcium and dairy intake and measures of obesity in hyper- and normocholesterolemic children, *Obes. Res.*, 13, 1727, 2005.
103. Chan, G., Hoffman, K., and McMurry, M., Effects of dairy products on bone and body composition in pubertal girls, *J. Pediatr.*, 126, 551, 1995.
104. Cadogan, J. et al., Milk intake and bone mineral acquisition in adolescent girls: randomized, controlled intervention trial, *Br. Med. J.*, 315, 1255, 1997.
105. Lappe, J. M. et al., Girls on a high-calcium diet gain weight at the same rate as girls on a normal diet: a pilot study, *J. Am. Diet. Assoc.*, 104, 1361, 2004.
106. Volek, J. S. et al., Increasing fluid milk favorably affects bone mineral density response to resistance training in adolescent boys, *J. Am. Diet. Assoc.*, 103, 1353, 2003.

107. Merrilees, M. J. et al., Effects of dairy food supplements on bone mineral density in teenage girls, *Eur. J. Nutr.*, 39, 256, 2000.
108. Lorenzen, J. K. et al., Calcium supplementation for 1 year does not reduce body weight or fat mass in young girls, *Am. J. Clin. Nutr.*, 83, 18, 2006.
109. McCarron, D. A. and Heaney, R. P., Estimated health care savings associated with adequate dairy food intake, *Am. J. Hypertens.*, 17, 88, 2004.

8 Lactose Digestion

8.1 INTRODUCTION

Dairy products are an important source of calcium, high-quality protein, potassium, phosphorus, riboflavin, and many other nutrients. Dairy foods are an important contributor of nutrients to the diets of children and adults in the United States, Canada, and Europe — as well as in other countries. It has been estimated that up to 75% of the world's adult population (approximately 25% of American adults) have a genetically controlled limited ability to digest lactose, the principle carbohydrate in milk and other dairy foods [1]. This condition is called lactase nonpersistence. Limited digestion of lactose can lead to unpleasant gastrointestinal symptoms of varying severity, termed lactose intolerance. However, limited digestion of lactose does not necessarily produce the symptoms of intolerance. Widely publicized incidence figures, based on artificial dietary conditions, greatly overestimate the percentage of those who are lactose maldigesters and the practical significance of their sensitivity. Prevalence estimates are based on studies that employed a 50 g test dose of lactose — the amount contained in a quart of milk — rather than on an amount usually consumed (12 g) in an 8-ounce serving.

All young mammals and human infants (except those with a congenital defect) are born with high levels of the enzyme "lactase" which enables them to digest lactose in their mother's milk. Lactase activity declines after weaning in most racial/ethnic groups except most Caucasian North Americans, northern Europeans, and some Africans and Middle Easterners [2].

Some have attempted to explain this phenomenon in terms of genetics and evolution. In this culture-historical hypothesis, the selection of a genetic trait (lactase persistence) is influenced by the cultural environment (dairying) [3]. An analysis supports the hypothesis that lactase persistence is an adaptation to dairying [4]. A complementary hypothesis, the "dairy barrier" hypothesis, is supported by an analysis showing that the frequency of lactose nonpersistence is greater in parts of the world where extremes of hot or cold and the historical presence of deadly cattle disease (prior to 1900) prevented successful dairying [5].

The pediatricians Czerny, Finkelstein and Jacobi first described intolerance to milk in 1901 when they noticed the association between diarrhea and carbohydrate ingestion [6]. In 1901, the famed biochemist Lafayette B. Mendel published a series of nine papers demonstrating that in most mammals the lactase enzyme reached maximal activity soon after birth; lactase activity then decreased gradually, reaching a low level after weaning. In 1921, John Howland, in his address to the American Pediatric Society, proposed that milk intolerance in infants and children was due to the lack of the enzyme necessary to hydrolyze lactose. It was not until the mid 1960 s that lactose intolerance again attracted the interest of researchers. It was reported that 70% of Black adults, but only 6% to 12% of Caucasian adults studied in Baltimore, were intolerant to the amount of lactose in a quart of milk [7]. As studies were conducted in many populations around the world, it soon became apparent that a marked reduction of lactase activity in early childhood was common.

Scientific investigations from many different disciplines, including biochemistry, cultural anthropology, genetics, and nutrition have added to our knowledge about lactose digestion. As a result of these studies, we have learned that the ability to digest lactose in adults is most common in northern Europeans and white American ethnic groups; that the trait is genetically transmitted; that the activity of the enzyme cannot be "induced" by continued exposure to lactose, and that adaptation in the colon may improve tolerance to continued milk intake [8].

Several well-controlled studies have demonstrated that the majority of those who maldigest lactose do not experience symptoms after consuming moderate amounts of lactose in foods [8]. Many studies have failed to recognize that cultural and psychosomatic factors as well as biologic mechanisms affect milk tolerance [2,9]. To properly compare and interpret research results, it is important to carefully define the terms used. For this reason, a definition of terms is included at the end of the chapter.

Persons who consume less milk and other dairy foods as a result of experiencing lactose intolerance generally have lower intakes of calcium and other nutrients supplied by milk, such as vitamin D, riboflavin, potassium, phosphorus and magnesium. An inadequate calcium and dairy food intake increases the risk of osteoporosis, hypertension, obesity, and colon cancer [10]. Recognizing that hypertension, stroke, colon cancer, and obesity disproportionately affect African Americans, and that these conditions are exacerbated by a low calcium and dairy food intake, a Consensus Report of the National Medical Association recommends that "African Americans should get 3 to 4 servings of low-fat dairy a day" [11]. A review of lactose intolerance among African Americans concludes that African Americans should not avoid dairy products due to concerns about lactose intolerance and should follow the dietary recommendations of the 2005 *Dietary Guidelines for Americans* and the National Medical Association [12]. Research into the factors involved in lactose digestion has fostered the development of strategies that allow those with low lactase activity to consume dairy products comfortably — so that lactose maldigestion need not be a barrier to attaining good health [13,14].

In this chapter, we will review the current literature on the subject to provide a clear understanding of the biologic mechanisms involved in lactose maldigestion and how individuals can best avoid the unpleasant symptoms which often accompany this condition. Since lactose maldigestion in a majority of non-Caucasian children in this country and developing countries has implications for public health and nutrition policy, we will also review recommendations for including milk in food aid programs and for the treatment of diarrheal disease and malnutrition in children.

8.2 PHYSIOLOGY OF LACTOSE DIGESTION

Lactose, or milk sugar, is the principle carbohydrate in human and animal milk. Human milk contains an average of 7% lactose, while whole cow's milk contains 4.8%. Lactose is a disaccharide made up of equal portions of two monosaccharides, glucose and galactose (Figure 8.1). A unique intestinal enzyme, lactase, a beta-galactosidase, is needed to hydrolyze lactose. It breaks the chemical bond between glucose and galactose, freeing them for absorption [15]. Lactase is one of five disaccharidases located on the brush border of the intestinal epithelium. Activity of the

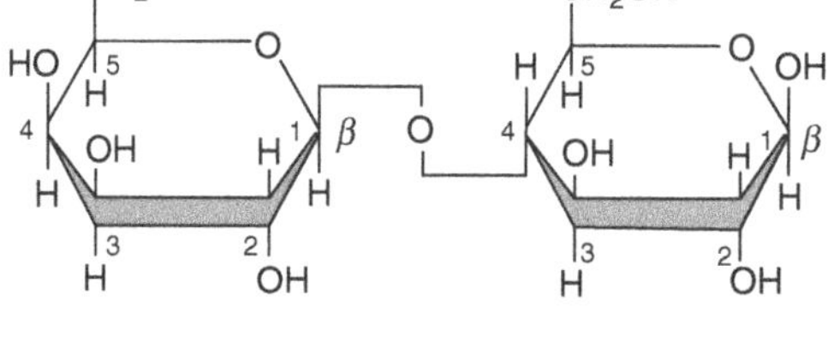

FIGURE 8.1 Chemical structure of lactose (βform). O-β-D-galactopyranosyl-(1→4)-βD-glucopyranose (From Lehninger, A. L., *Lehninger: Principles of Biochemistry*, Worth Publishers, New York, 1982, 285. With permission.)

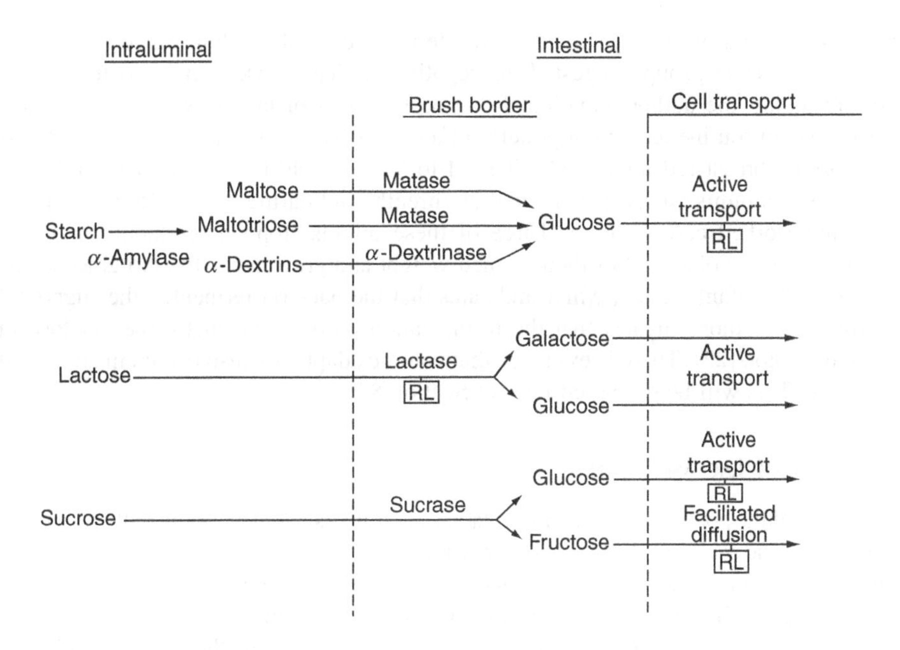

FIGURE 8.2 Schematic diagram of absorption of dietary carbohydrate at the level of the intestinal brush border. RL indicates the rate-limiting step in overall digestion and absorption of the sugar. (From Saavedra, J. M. and Perman, J. A., *Ann. Rev. Nutr.*, 9, 475, 1989. With permission.)

lactase enzyme is highest in the proximal ileum and very low in the first portion of the duodenum and in the terminal ileum [16].

Of all the dietary sugars, lactose is hydrolyzed the most slowly [15]. The hydrolysis of lactose occurs at only half the rate of sucrose hydrolysis. The rate at which lactose is assimilated is dependent on the rate of the hydrolysis. The relative slowness with which lactose is broken down, accompanied by a lack of reserve of the enzyme, helps explain why many people are vulnerable to lactose maldigestion (Figure 8.2) [15]. It has been suggested that a faster-than-normal rate of gastric emptying in persons with low lactase activity may also contribute to symptoms of intolerance after milk ingestion [17].

8.2.1 Course of Development of Lactase

In contrast to the other disaccharidases, lactase appears very late in fetal development. It is estimated that at 35 to 38 weeks of gestation lactase levels are approximately 70% of their full-term level [18]. Most studies of lactase development have been conducted in stillborn infants. Because premature infants who survive even for a short time have lactase levels above those of stillborn infants of the same gestational age, it was speculated that feeding might influence the infant's lactase level after birth [15]. The first study to directly measure lactose digestion and absorption, lactase activity, and small-intestinal surface area in preterm infants found that feeding directly influenced small intestinal mucosal growth, but that changes in lactose absorption were primarily related to lactase activity, not mucosal growth [19]. Lactase activity was correlated with gestational age at birth [19].

It is interesting to note that both preterm and term infants in the first few months of life do not completely hydrolyze the lactose in their mother's milk, as indicated by high breath hydrogen concentrations, though they tolerate and thrive on human milk and formulas that contain lactose [20,21,22]. Kien and colleagues at The Ohio State University measured lactose digestion in 14 preterm infants (26 to 31weeks gestation) [20]. They found that these infants digested $<85\%$ of lactose consumed, and an average of 35% was fermented by the colon. Since previous studies conducted by the same group suggested no negative clinical consequences to feeding lactose-containing formulas, the authors concluded that replacement of lactose with other sugars might not be necessary for routine feeding of preterm infants. Lifshitz et al. evaluated lactose digestion in 17 white, normal, breast-fed infants who were 4 to 5 weeks old [22]. Five of the infants (29%) produced large amounts of hydrogen in their breath, indicating that colonic bacteria were fermenting unabsorbed carbohydrate. Three of these infants stopped producing high levels of hydrogen as they grew older; all of them gained weight and grew normally. No glucose appeared in the stools of the infants tested, which indicates that the bacteria fermented the sugars released from lactose. The authors suggest that the fermentation products of unabsorbed lactose may be absorbed in the colon [22]. There is evidence that colonic adaptation also occurs in adults with low lactase activity. This will be discussed later in Section 8.7.

8.2.2 Decline of Lactase Expression

The age of onset of the postweaning decline in lactase activity is variable, but usually occurs by 3 to 5 years of age [23]. The decline in lactase activity is not due to a decline or absence of lactose in the diet. Many studies have documented that continued lactose consumption does not maintain or enhance lactase activity [2,24]. Instead, researchers have concluded that human adult-onset lactase decline is controlled by a single autosomal recessive gene [25]. Researchers using the sucrase/lactase ratio and the lactase/maltase ratio measured in intestinal biopsies, found a trimodal distribution (low, intermediate, and high) of lactase expression. Subjects with a homozygous recessive inheritance pattern had low levels of lactase expression; those who were heterozygous had intermediate levels; those who had a homozygous dominant pattern had high lactase activity [25]. Heterozygotes are more prone to experience lactose intolerance than homozygotes, particularly under conditions of stress or mild pathology [26].

8.2.3 Molecular Regulation

The lactase gene is located on chromosome 2. Differences in the structure of the gene itself, however, are not responsible for differences in lactase expression. Lactase messenger RNA (mRNA) in humans, rats and rabbits changes coordinately with the amount of enzyme activity — suggesting control of lactase expression at the level of gene transcription. It is now generally agreed that lactase nonpersistent individuals have lower levels of lactase mRNA [26].

Researchers in Italy examined lactase activity, biosynthesis, and the levels of mRNA in jejunal mucosa of lactase persistent and nonpersistent adults. They concluded that both transcriptional and posttranscriptional factors cause the decline of intestinal lactase [27]. Biosynthesis of prolactase (the precursor of lactase) correlated well with lactase mRNA levels, indicating transcriptional control. A high rate of biosynthesis was the main factor distinguishing those with lactase persistence; the rate was five times higher than in those with nonpersistence. These Italian researchers found that posttranscriptional factors (e.g., the routing of prolactase from the endoplasmic reticulum to the brush border membrane, the speed of processing during this routing, or the breakdown of lactase) also influenced lactase levels to some degree. However, they observed wide variability of mRNA level, lactase sysnthesis, and activity in both lactase-persistent and lactase-nonpersistent individuals. With such a variety of factors responsible for the decrease in intestinal lactase, it is not surprising, say these researchers, that the time of onset of adult-type hypolactasia can vary widely among various population groups [27]. The Caco-2 cell line derived from a human colon adenocarcinoma, which expresses hydrolases such as lactase and sucrase-isomaltase, has also been used to study the regulation of lactase expression. Studies using Caco-2 cells have demonstrated that biosynthesis of lactase is preceded by a large increase in messenger RNA levels, supporting studies indicating transcriptional control [28,29].

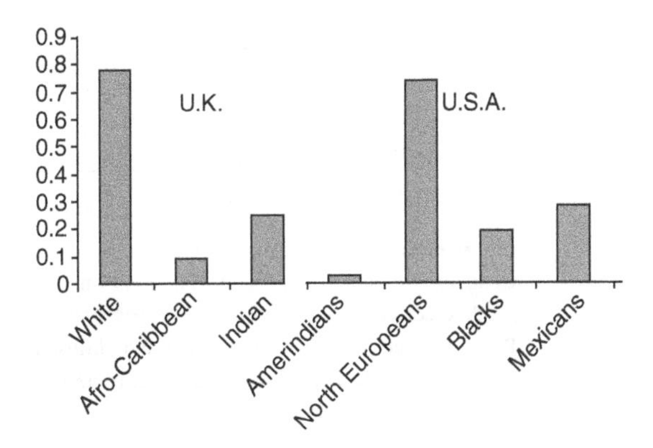

FIGURE 8.3 Pathophysiologic events following lactose maldigestion. VFA indicates volatile fatty acids. (From Saavedra, J. M. and Perman, J. A., *Ann. Rev. Nutr.*, 9, 475, 1989. With permission.)

Studies have shown that the decrease in lactase activity is determined by the age of the tissue, not the age of the host. Therefore the pattern for expression is apparently imprinted in the tissue of intestinal epithelium. Several mechanisms for controlling lactase expression have been hypothesized and are currently under investigation, including regulation by corticoid or thyroid hormones. One promising line of research involves a nuclear factor (NF-LPH1), which binds specifically to the lactase promoter and may be an important regulator of gene transcription [30].

The genetic variants associated with lactase persistence were identified in 2002 [31]. Subsequently, researchers at Stanford University used human intestinal Caco-2 cells to demonstrate that the DNA sequence surrounding the single nucleotide genetic variant in the region of C/T_{-13910} (nonpersistent/persistent) performed a functional role in differentially enhancing lactase promoter activity and in specifying lactase persistence/nonpersistence phenotypes [23]. Researchers in Austria who classified 258 postmenopausal women by genotype found that 24% of this study population had the CC genotype and genetic lactase deficiency — a proportion consistent with the frequency of lactose malabsorption detected with the breath hydrogen test in this geographical area [32]. Bone mineral density, fracture incidence and milk consumption were lowest in the CC genotype and highest in the TT genotype, with the TC genotype being intermediate between the two [32]. Figure 8.3 illustrates the frequency of distribution of genetic lactase persistence in populations of different ancestry in the United States and the United Kingdom.

8.2.4 Types of Lactase Deficiency

The absence or decline of intestinal lactase can be described as being *congenital, primary or secondary* (Table 8.1) [33]. Congenital lactase deficiency, or alactasia, is an extremely rare condition in which detectable levels of lactase are absent at birth. An infant with congenital lactase deficiency will have severe diarrheal illness beginning a few days after birth. In addition to measuring breath hydrogen production in these infants, other more aggressive diagnostic procedures, such as an intestinal biopsy to measure lactase activity or an intestinal perfusion study, may be required to rule out other diagnoses [34]. In congenital lactase deficiency the histology of the small bowel is normal, as is the level of other disaccharidases. Symptoms will resolve if the infant is put on a lactose-free diet. According to a position paper by the American Academy of Pediatrics, soy protein-based formulas (lactose-free) are appropriate for infants with this form of hereditary lactase deficiency [35]. Persons with this disorder are unable to tolerate even small amounts of lactose, and will need to follow a lactose-free diet for the rest of their lives [36]. It is not known whether colonic adaptation might allow a measure of tolerance in these individuals.

TABLE 8.1
Lactase Deficiency

Lactase Deficiency	
Type	**Pathogenesis**
Congenial	Enzyme activity absent from birth
Primary	Genetically predetermined reduction of enzyme activity during childhood or adolescence
Secondary	Reduced to enzyme activity in response to diffuse intestinal insult — giardiasis rotavirus, topical sprue, celiac disease, bacterial overgrowth, Crohn's disease, intestinal resection

Source: From Rusynyk, A. R. and Still, C. D., *JAOA*, 101 (4), S10–S12, 2001. With permission.

In primary lactase deficiency, decline of lactase activity occurs at variable periods after weaning, depending on racial/ethnic background. In the United States, some degree of lactose maldigestion occurs in an estimated 15% (6% to 19%) of Caucasians, 53% of Mexican Americans, 62% to 100% of Native Americans, 80% of African Americans, and 90% of Asian Americans [2,37]. Although the standard lactose tolerance test is effective for determining genetic differences in lactase expression among populations, it tends to overestimate the number of individuals who are intolerant to more physiologic amounts of lactose. This was borne out by a nationally-representative survey of African American adults of whom only 24% considered themselves to be lactose intolerant [11]. African Americans surveyed who consumed a medium-to-high amount of dairy foods per day (more than 1 serving) were less likely to experience symptoms [11]. Lactase deficiency is seldom total, and whether symptoms of intolerance are experienced depends on the level of lactase activity remaining, the amount of lactose consumed, the adaptation of intestinal flora, and the irritability of the colon. Symptoms such as bloating, cramping, diarrhea, or flatulence will develop in about one-third to one-fifth of individuals with lactase nonpersistence [33]. Primary lactase deficiency or lactase nonpersistence is genetically determined and is inherited as an autosomal recessive trait. In contrast, lactase persistence is inherited as an autosomal dominant characteristic [2,15].

The prevalence of lactose maldigestion is projected to increase in the future, when based on U.S. Department of Commerce population projections for increases in ethnic populations genetically predisposed to this condition [38]. However, it is interesting to note that as those who have the ability to digest lactose intermarry with those from a racial/ethnic group that typically does not digest lactose, the rate of maldigestion falls [39]. For example, though African Americans have an expected rate of lactose maldigestion near 100%, the prevalence has decreased to 70% due to intermixing with white Americans [39]. The ability of Native Americans to digest lactose has also increased over time. As the United States becomes a more "blended" population, it remains to be seen how the opposing forces of population increases in ethnic populations and the trend of intermarriage will impact the prevalence of lactose maldigestion.

A large number of studies have been conducted around the world to examine the incidence of lactase nonpersistence [2]. Many studies have included wide age ranges of subjects, spanning from the early teens into the seventies, making it difficult to establish a precise relationship between age and prevalence. It appears that the primary reduction in lactase activity occurs in early childhood and is thought not to progress throughout life [2,25].

Few studies have evaluated lactose malabsorption and intolerance in the elderly. A study comparing lactose tolerance between adult (20 to 40 years) and elderly (> 65 years) Asian-Americans found no significant differences in breath hydrogen production, flatulence, or fecal beta-galactosidase activity between the adult and elderly subjects who were fed a challenge dose of 0.5 g lactose/kg body weight [40]. Similarly, the frequency of lactose maldigestion did not differ significantly among different age groups of northern Indians [41]. However, the results of an Italian study demonstrated that the prevalence of lactose malabsorption increases significantly after the age of 74 years [42]. The researchers evaluated lactose malabsorption and prevalence of intolerance symptoms in 84 healthy adults aged 23 to 94 years grouped into three age ranges, <65 years, 65 to 74 years, and >75 years. They found that as age increased, the prevalence of lactose malabsorption, as measured by the breath hydrogen test, also increased — but the prevalence of intolerance symptoms reported by malabsorbers decreased with age. They conclude that lactose malabsorption is one of the age-related changes occurring in the gut, but that the lower prevalence of intolerance symptoms in lactose malabsorbers allows the elderly to maintain an adequate dairy intake and protect them from nutritional deficiencies. The authors say the elderly should be encouraged to consume dairy foods, since they have a reduced capacity to absorb calcium and a reduced ability to adapt to a low calcium intake [42].

In general, individuals with primary lactase deficiency do not need to avoid foods containing lactose. By using the management strategies outlined later in this chapter, a variety of dairy foods may be comfortably included in the diet.

Secondary lactase deficiency is a temporary condition, caused by any environmental factors that injure the intestinal mucosa where lactase is expressed. It can occur at any age. The most important causes of secondary lactase deficiency are infectious diarrhea, the parasites giardia and ascaria, inflammatory bowel disease such as Crohn's disease, celiac disease, gastrointestinal surgery, radiation treatment, and certain medications such as aspirin, nonsteroidal antiinflammatory drugs, and antibiotics. Secondary lactase deficiency is reversed when the causative factor is corrected [33].

When diarrhea is of infectious origin, loss of lactase activity may persist for a long time if the diarrhea is recurrent. In severe protein-calorie malnutrition, such as kwashiorkor, lactase activity is reduced along with all other enzyme activity. Lactose tolerance increases quickly as nutritional status improves. In children who developed a lactase deficiency secondary to cancer chemotherapy treatments, yogurt proved a useful dietary supplement [43].

Medical nutrition therapy for secondary lactose intolerance involves restricting or eliminating lactose-containing foods depending upon the tolerance of the patient [44]. Since tolerance varies between patients, the diet is administered on a trial-and-error basis. Consultation with a nutrition professional will help prevent nutritional deficiencies during treatment of the underlying disease. Patients may need to temporarily restrict all lactose-containing foods, or use lactose-hydrolyzed products or enzyme supplements.

However, a low-lactose diet may not always improve symptoms of patients who malabsorb lactose secondary to Irritable Bowel Syndrome or Inflammatory Bowel Disease. The prevalence of lactose maldigestion among white Northern European patients with Irritable Bowel Syndrome (IBS) is approximately 25% [45] — much higher than the 5% or 6% prevalence of lactose malabsorption reported in the general healthy north European population. The symptoms experienced by patients with lactose intolerance are very similar to those of IBS. Researchers from the United Kingdom studied 122 IBS patients to determine whether identifying and treating lactose maldigestion in these patients would be clinically advantageous [46]. Twenty-seven percent (33 patients) of the IBS patients studied malabsorbed lactose according to the breath hydrogen test. However, when these patients were treated with a low lactose diet (<1 g/day) for 21 days, only 39% reported an improvement in their symptoms — and that improvement was small. Therefore, the researchers concluded there was little advantage in separating those with lactose malabsorption from others with IBS.

A commentary on dairy sensitivity in patients with IBD, states that patients with either ulcerative colitis or Crohn's disease often avoid dairy products more than they need to because they have incorrect perceptions, and receive arbitrary advice from physicians and authors of popular diet books [47]. Since dairy products are an important source of calcium and other nutrients, the author recommends testing IBD patients for lactose malabsorption using the breath hydrogen test before recommending the elimination of dairy foods or the use of lactose-reduced products. In a study of 161 IBD patients, those with diagnosed lactose maldigestion (29%) did not have significantly different gastrointestinal symptoms or improvement/worsening of their condition than those who digested lactose. Most of the patients felt, however, that identifying lactose maldigestion helped them to gain awareness of food-symptom relationships [48].

If secondary lactose intolerance is severe, patients may need to check ingredient labels and avoid products with the following ingredients: milk, lactose, milk solids, whey, curds, skim milk powder, and skim milk solids. Manufacturers of candy, confections and bakery products, such as pancakes, waffles and toaster pastries use lactose as an ingredient. Its limited sweetness, solubility, crystallization and browning properties make it ideal for use in these products. Other nondairy foods that may contain lactose include shakes and instant breakfast mixes, coffee whiteners, commercial breakfast and baby cereals, cake mixes, mayonnaise, salad dressings, luncheon meats, sausage, and frankfurters [49]. Medication and vitamin labels should be checked as well, since some contain lactose as a carrier. Some dairy foods, such as Cheddar cheese and other aged natural cheeses, have a relatively low lactose content. A table listing the lactose content of a variety of dairy foods is included at the end of the chapter.

8.2.5 Lactose Maldigestion

It is estimated that of the lactose that remains unhydrolyzed in the small intestine, approximately 1% is absorbed by passive diffusion into the bloodstream and is then excreted into the urine unmetabolized [15]. As the remainder of unabsorbed lactose reaches the jejunum, it exerts an osmotic effect, causing water and sodium to be secreted into the intestinal lumen. Transit of the contents of the small bowel accelerates. Significant amounts of lactose may then enter the colon, where it is fermented by colonic bacteria. The majority of the undigested lactose reaching the colon is metabolized to short chain organic acids, and hydrogen, methane, and carbon dioxide gases. Some of the organic acids are absorbed into the bloodstream, while some may be excreted in the feces, resulting in acidic stools [15].

8.3 SYMPTOMS

Lactose intolerance refers to gastrointestinal symptoms associated with the incomplete digestion of lactose. The presence of fermentation products in the colon may produce a variety of symptoms including abdominal discomfort, cramps or distention; nausea; flatulence; or diarrhea [15,50]. The clinical response to a given dose of lactose is highly variable in lactase nonpersistent persons, and may be partly explained by the number of colonic bacteria available to ferment lactose [51]. A study conducted among 43 healthy Chinese adults with lactose maldigestion demonstrated an inverse association between the metabolic capacity of colonic bacteria available to ferment lactose and total symptom score after consumption of a challenge dose of 25 g of lactose in water [51]. Symptoms resulting from lactose maldigestion may be more pronounced in women than in men, according to a study conducted in Germany [52]. The women in the study, who were diagnosed as maldigesters by a breath hydrogen test, had lower breath hydrogen concentrations after ingestion of 50 g of lactose and complained of more abdominal pain, gas, and distension than did their male counterparts.

Individuals with an allergy to cow's milk protein may experience symptoms similar to those of lactose intolerance. Therefore, it is important to make the distinction between these two very different milk sensitivities (Table 8.2).

In milk allergy, gastrointestinal symptoms may predominate, but other symptoms involving the respiratory tract and skin, such as rhinitis and atopic dermatitis, are also common. Cow's milk

TABLE 8.2
Comparison and Contrast of Cow's Milk Allergy and Lactose Intolerance

	Milk Allergy	Lactose Intolerance
Cause	Abnormal immune response to ingestion of cow's milk protein	Low intestinal levels of the lactase enzyme that digests lactose (milk sugar)
Age of Onset Symptoms	Usually in infancy; abdominal pain, vomiting, diarrhea, nasal congestion, skin rash	Early/late childhood; abdominal gas, bloating, cramps, diarrhea
Diagnosis	Food elimination and challenge; RAST blood test	Breath hydrogen test
Dairy Food Use/Avoidance	Eliminate cow's milk protein from the diet for a time	No need to eliminate dairy foods; experiment with varying amounts/types of dairy foods to improve tolerance

allergy usually occurs within the first 4 months of life in bottle-fed infants, though it may in rare instances be first detected in adolescence or adulthood. The incidence of cow's milk allergy as determined by double-blind studies is quite low — in the range of 1% to 3% of infants and children in the first 2 years of life [53]. Most children with milk allergy outgrow it by age 2 to 3 years as a result of maturation of the gastrointestinal and immune system, and should be monitored regularly by a multidisciplinary team that includes a dietitian and allergy nurse specialist [54,55]. This is the reverse of the time-course of lactose intolerance, which may begin to appear at this age in some individuals [2].

8.4 DIAGNOSIS

Most lactose intolerance is either self-diagnosed by the patient or diagnosed by a physician using subjective evaluation tools (i.e., description of symptoms, elimination diets) rather than objective testing methods [56,49]. In a convenience sample of 159 adults with self-reported lactose intolerance living in Vancouver Canada, 54% had self-diagnosed their lactose intolerance, but of the 42% who were diagnosed by a physician, only 10% had been diagnosed using a valid test — and none had been diagnosed with the breath hydrogen test, considered the "gold standard" for diagnosing lactose maldigestion [56]. This approach is unsatisfactory primarily because it is highly inaccurate. Several double-blinded studies have shown that many patients who believe they are intolerant to milk and milk products continue to report symptoms when lactose is removed from the diet [57–61]. In addition, exclusion diets usually involve removing only dairy products from the diet and have several drawbacks, whether used by a physician or for self-diagnosis. First, excluding dairy foods from the diet for an arbitrary amount of time could result in nutritional shortcomings. In the Vancouver Canada survey, only about 11% of the women and 12% of the men with self-reported lactose intolerance met their Adequate Intake recommendation for calcium from food sources [56]. Second, if all foods containing lactose are not removed from the diet, symptoms may continue, leading the client to believe lactose was not the cause of the symptoms. Or the reverse could be true; removal of lactose from the diet may happen to coincide with resolution of the symptoms from a totally unrelated cause, thus perpetuating unnecessary dietary restrictions. In addition, self-diagnosis could delay treatment for another more serious gastrointestinal problem. If symptoms are chronic, a physician should be consulted, and an objective test for lactose maldigestion conducted. Physicians need to be educated in the use of valid diagnostic tools and how to counsel patients to use dietary strategies that make avoidance of dairy foods unnecessary [56].

Both direct and indirect methods are available to diagnose lactase deficiency (Table 8.3). It is possible to directly assay the lactase activity in the small bowel by taking an intestinal biopsy. Researchers have used this method to identify populations with primary lactase deficiency. The procedure is invasive and time-consuming, and may not yield accurate results when intestinal injury is involved. This is because intestinal lesions may affect only a small area that may be missed during the biopsy. Symptoms of intolerance do not correlate as well with mucosal lactase activity as they do with the breath hydrogen test, an indirect measure of lactose maldigestion [15].

Indirect methods for diagnosing lactose maldigestion include the lactose tolerance test, a stool acidity test, and the breath hydrogen (H_2) test. The lactose tolerance test, which measures the rise in blood glucose after a dose of lactose, is performed in a manner similar to that of the glucose tolerance test used for the diagnosis of diabetes mellitus. A relatively large dose of lactose is required to separate digesters from maldigesters. Typically, an aqueous solution of 50 g of lactose is consumed. In persons who weigh more than 25 kg, a dose of 100 g may be required [34]. Blood is drawn before lactose ingestion, then at intervals of 30, 60, 90, and 120 minutes thereafter [49]. Failure of blood glucose to rise 20 mg/dl from baseline, in the presence of symptoms, indicates lactase deficiency. Even though the lactose tolerance test (actually, a test for lactose maldigestion) is positive, smaller amounts of lactose may be tolerated [36]. This method is mildly invasive, since several blood samplings are involved, and results correlate poorly with actual mucosal lactase levels. Since the rate of gastric emptying slows the rate at which glucose enters the bloodstream, individuals with delayed gastric emptying will have a false-positive test [36]. Results will be questionable if used with diabetic patients or those with malabsorption syndromes.

Testing stool samples for acidity and reducing sugars has been used for years to assess whether infants and young children are absorbing lactose. The test, however, requires the presence of lactose in the diet and availability of fresh stool. The test is not sensitive enough to exclude lactose intolerance, but can be used to confirm the results of another test [49].

The breath hydrogen (H_2) test has become the "gold standard" or method of choice for diagnosing lactose maldigestion. The test is noninvasive, inexpensive, and can easily be performed on children and adults. The results of this test are reported to correlate well with lactase activity in mucosal biopsy specimens [62]. When lactose or any other dietary sugar is not completely absorbed, the unabsorbed portion is fermented by colonic bacteria, forming hydrogen (as well as methane in some individuals and CO_2), some of which is absorbed into the portal circulation and exhaled in breath [15].

Test protocol requires the patient to report after an overnight fast, where a baseline breath sample is taken. Historically, the patients were given a 20% aqueous solution of 2 g of lactose per kg of body weight (10 to 50 g) to drink. Fifty grams of lactose is the amount contained in one quart of milk. The solution may be diluted to 10% in infants younger than 6 months or in adults when severe lactose intolerance is suspected. Breath samples are taken every 30 minutes for 3 hours;

TABLE 8.3
Diagnostic Tests for Lactose Intolerance

Test	Result
Breath hydrogen	Rise in breath hydrogen >20 ppm
Stool pH	Acid pH (<6.0)
Small-bowel biopsy	Disaccharidase assay (<13 IU/g of mucosal protein)
Lactose absorption (fecal-reducing substances)	+ to++++

Key: + = minimal; ++++ = significant.

Source: From Rusynyk A. R. and Still, C. D., *JAOA*, 101 (4), S10–S12, 2001. With permission.

samples are collected in test tubes, and hydrogen in breath is analyzed by gas chromatography. An increase in breath hydrogen of >10 to 20 ppm above the baseline value indicates fermentation of unabsorbed carbohydrate, and is positive for lactose maldigestion [49]. The sensitivity of the breath hydrogen test to diagnose lactose maldigestion was demonstrated to be greatly reduced when the duration of the test was shortened 3 hours to 1 hour, as may often be done in clinical practice [63].

Few data are available concerning what breath hydrogen response accurately identifies lactose malabsorption. Even though a rise in breath hydrogen of 10 ppm above baseline indicates the presence of incompletely absorbed lactose in the colon (more than can be accounted for by variability of the technique), many investigators recommend that a rise of 20 ppm be used as the criterion for judging lactose digestion as "abnormal" [34]. This criterion is often used because it correlates with less than a 20 mg/dl rise in blood glucose following a 50 g dose of aqueous lactose. However, this rationale has been questioned, because using the >20 ppm criterion unnecessarily limits the sensitivity of the breath hydrogen test to that of the lactose tolerance test, especially when the dose of lactose given is less than 50 g [64]. Hydrogen production is proportional to the lactose dose. Therefore, when the dose of lactose given is small (10 to 12 g), the criterion of >10 ppm above baseline is diagnostic of lactose maldigestion. Patients with a breath hydrogen rise of only 10 ppm are less likely to experience intolerance symptoms than those with a higher rise [65]. The lactose dose used for the test may also be administered in the form of milk, infant formula or yogurt (not with active cultures), and the lactose doses in the range of usual intakes (10 to 12 g) can be used, since the test can determine the maldigestion of as little as 2 g of carbohydrate [15].

When the hydrogen breath test is used for research purposes, many investigators collect samples for 8 hours. This increases the sensitivity of the test when lower doses of lactose are administered. Researchers in Italy have proposed a new criterion for determining lactose malabsorption requiring a hydrogen breath excretion greater than 15 ppm at 5, 6, and 7 hours after lactose challenge [66]. This method diagnosed lactose malabsorption in roughly 25% more patients than did a more traditional approach [66]. A small percentage of people do not have colonic flora that ferment lactose, which can lead to false negative results. This situation is uncommon and may be the result of the use of an antibiotic before the test [49]. Smoking prior to the test may lead to a false-positive result [15].

The breath hydrogen test is also useful in diagnosing an underlying condition, such as bacterial overgrowth, which can cause secondary lactose intolerance. The bacterial overgrowth in the small bowel can be treated with antibiotic therapy and the secondary lactose maldigestion is managed with a lactose-controlled diet [49]. Lactose maldigestion eventually resolves with the treatment of the underlying condition. In children less than 5 years of age, an abnormal breath hydrogen test indicates an abnormal intestinal mucosa and lactose maldigestion secondary to another problem [67].

Now that the genetic variant responsible for lactase nonpersistence has been identified, researchers are evaluating whether genetic testing could replace other traditional diagnostic methods [68,69,70]. Genotyping for the DNA variant associated with adult hypolactasia demonstrate an excellent correlation between both the hydrogen breath test [68,69] and rise in blood glucose following a lactose challenge [70]. Genetic testing may soon complement other indirect methods for identifying individuals at risk for both lactose malabsorption and osteoporosis [32].

8.5 RELATIONSHIP BETWEEN LACTOSE MALDIGESTION, INTOLERANCE, AND MILK INTOLERANCE

8.5.1 Dose Dependence

Controlled studies have shown that consuming one cup of milk (240 ml) or its lactose equivalent (12 g) at a time produces little or no intolerance symptoms in adults with primary lactase deficiency. The vast majority of those with low lactase levels can tolerate ingestion of 12 g of lactose, particularly if consumed with a meal or other foods [71,72]. Hertzler et al. found that individuals with lactase nonpersistence could tolerate up to 6 g of lactose under fasting conditions when consumed in water [73]. When the lactose dose is 50 vs. 12 g, a much higher percentage of those with hypolactasia experience intolerance symptoms. Newcomer first illustrated this phenomenon in a group of American Indians studied in 1978. Less than 20% of the subjects experienced symptoms when the lactose dose was between 0 and 18 g. However, 88% were symptomatic to a dose of 50 g [74].

Therefore, the term lactose intolerance should only be used when referring to the symptomatic response to a defined lactose load. For example, an individual might be tolerant to 12 g of lactose, but be intolerant to 24 g. Determination of the presence and severity of symptoms is somewhat subjective, and may be influenced by factors other than the presence of lactose. Lactose maldigestion, on the other hand, is determined by an objective test, such as the breath hydrogen test. Both the objective determination of maldigestion and the subjective determination of intolerance are needed to develop a dietary strategy. Those with limited lactose digestion may or may not experience intolerance symptoms.

8.5.2 Milk Intolerance

Milk intolerance due to lactose is characterized by at least one clinical sign of intolerance experienced a few hours after ingestion of a known quantity of milk or milk-containing products. When the prevalence of milk intolerance is being evaluated rather than lactose maldigestion, several factors — such as the amount and form in which lactose is given, whether it is consumed with a meal, and whether the study is double-blinded — may influence the results.

Several studies have demonstrated poor correlation between objectively measured lactose maldigestion and self-reported milk intolerance. Johnson et al. evaluated the relationship between maldigestion and intolerance in 164 African American adolescents and adults [59]. Objective testing with the breath hydrogen test revealed that 50% of the subjects maldigested and were intolerant to 25 g of lactose, the amount in 2 cups of milk (480 ml); 86% of this group experienced symptoms of lactose intolerance. Eight percent of the subjects were maldigesters, but tolerant; 15% were digesters but intolerant; and 27% were digesters and tolerant (Table 8.4). This study exemplifies the complex relationship between lactose maldigestion, lactose intolerance and milk intolerance.

It is important that studies evaluating lactose tolerance (or other food tolerance) be double blind. This means that neither the subject nor the investigator knows whether the test solution contains lactose or a placebo. Unblinded studies may overestimate intolerance due to expectations of the subjects or the researcher. Lactose is often given in water for tolerance testing, and can easily

TABLE 8.4
Outcome of Lactose-Tolerance Breath-Hydrogen Study in 164 Volunteers; All Volunteers Claimed to Be Intolerant of a Cup (240 mL) of Milk

Group	Classification	Symptoms[a]	*n* (%)
1	Maldigesters, intolerant	+	82 (50)
2	Maldigesters, tolerant	–	13(8)
3	Digesters, intolerant	+	25(15)
4	Digesters, tolerant	–	44 (27)
Total			164(100)

[a] Symptoms: abdominal fullness, cramps, flatulence, borborygmi, nausea, vomiting, diarrhea.

Source: From Johnson, A. O. et al., *Am. J. Clin. Nutr.*, 57, 399, 1993. With permission.

be distinguished from a solution of glucose and galactose. When different levels of lactose are tested in milk, it is important to give the same volume of milk. When tolerance to milk is compared to that of lactose-hydrolyzed milk, an artificial sweetener should be added to the milk so that subjects cannot distinguish a taste difference between products. Subjects who are aware that the solution they are drinking contains lactose or that the volumes are being increased sometimes experience symptoms they would not have otherwise. Newcomer estimates that if all the studies evaluating tolerance were blinded, the percentage of subjects intolerant to 12 g of lactose would be only 10% to 15% [75]. Results of recent double-blind, randomized, crossover trials indicate that most individuals with primary lactase deficiency can tolerate one cup (240 ml) of milk with a meal or two cups (480 ml) if consumed in divided doses with breakfast and dinner [57,58]. Subsequently, the same investigators found that women with limited lactose digestion can eat a dairy-rich diet that includes milk, yogurt and cheese, supplying about 1500 mg of calcium per day, without major impediment [76] (Table 8.5).

Suarez et al. measured gastrointestinal symptoms in 30 subjects who described themselves as intolerant to very small amounts of milk, such as the amount used on cereal or in coffee [57]. Of the 30 subjects, 21 (70%) were lactose maldigesters based on breath hydrogen concentrations after intake of 15 g of lactose, whereas 9 (30%) were lactose digesters. Both groups then participated in a randomized, double-blind, crossover trial in which they received either one cup of 2% milk (lactose-containing) or lactose-hydrolyzed milk every day with breakfast for 1 week. Since hydrolysis of the milk increases the sweetness, aspartame was added to the regular milk so that the sensory characteristics of the two milks were indistinguishable. The symptoms reported by both maldigesting and digesting subjects after consumption of one cup of milk (240 ml) were minimal,

TABLE 8.5
Many Individuals Who Describe Themselves as "Lactose Intolerant" (LI) Can Digest Lactose; Most Who Are Diagnosed as Lactose Maldigesters Can Tolerate the Amount of Lactose in a Serving or More of Milk and Other Dairy Foods

Study	Subject	Lactose Dose (g) Breath Hydrogen Test (g)	Lactose Digesters (%)	Lactose Maldigesters (%)	Milk Products Tested	Results
Suarez et al. 1995	30 self-described, LI racially mixed adults	15	30	70	One cup of milk (12 g lactose) with breakfast	All tolerant
Suarez et al. 1997	49 self-described, LI racially mixed adults	15	30	69	Two cups of milk/day consumed in divided doses with breakfast and dinner	All tolerant
Suarez et al. 1998	62 female racially mixed adults	15	50	50	One cup of milk at breakfast, 1 ounce of cheese and 8 ounces of yogurt at lunch, 1 cup milk and 1 ounce of cheese at dinner	All tolerant increased flatus frequency rated "trivial" in maldi-gesters

and were not significantly different than those reported after consumption of lactose-free milk. The researchers concluded that lactose-digestive aids are not necessary when lactose intake is limited to the equivalent of 240 ml of milk or less a day [57].

The same researchers conducted a similar trial to test tolerance to two cups of milk daily (i.e., the average amount usually consumed) [58]. A secondary goal of the study was to determine whether psychological factors play a role in a subject's perception of intolerance (this will be discussed in more detail in the next section). Two groups of lactose maldigesters (confirmed by a breath hydrogen test to 15 g of lactose) participated in the study: those who believed they were markedly intolerant to lactose (symptomatic) and those who believed that lactose did not induce symptoms (asymptomatic). Participants received either one cup of 2% milk (lactose-containing) or one cup of lactose-hydrolyzed milk with breakfast and another at dinner for 1 week. After a 7-day washout period, study participants switched to the opposite treatment. Both symptomatic and asymptomatic lactose maldigesters reported only minimal symptoms following intake of regular or lactose-free milk. These findings indicate that most self-described lactose intolerant subjects can readily tolerate 2 cups of milk daily if this milk is ingested in divided doses with breakfast and dinner [58].

In a subsequent randomized, double-blind, crossover design study, Suarez and colleagues at the University of Minnesota tested whether lactose maldigesting pre- and postmenopausal women could tolerate a dairy-rich diet providing approximately 1500 mg of calcium/day [76]. The intake of dairy products was spread out over the day, and a variety of dairy products were used. The participants (50% maldigesters and 50% digesters per the breath hydrogen test) were randomly assigned to one of two dietary regimens for 1 week, then switched to the other: (1) 240 ml of 1% fat milk with breakfast and dinner, plus 1 serving (30 g) of a hard cheese at lunch and dinner, and 8 ounces of low-fat, strawberry flavored yogurt at lunch, or (2) a similar regimen using lactose-hydrolyzed milk and yogurt. The dairy products provided about 1300 mg of calcium per day; it was assumed that the remainder of the diet would provide about 200 mg of calcium daily. Lactose maldigesters who consumed the dairy-rich diet experienced a significantly greater frequency of small flatus, but no differences in bloating, abdominal pain, nausea, fullness or diarrhea, than when they consumed lactose-hydrolyzed products.

The above findings indicate that primary lactase deficiency need not be an obstacle to meeting calcium needs with milk and milk products. It has been confirmed with double-blind trials that lactose maldigesters can tolerate the amount of lactose in approximately 3 to 4 servings of milk and milk products, which provides the amount of calcium recommended by an expert panel of the National Institutes of Health (i.e., 1000 to 1500 mg) or the National Academy of Sciences for American adults (i.e., 1000 to 1200 mg) [77,78].

8.5.3 Subjective Factors Affecting Lactose Tolerance

Some individuals, whether or not they are able to digest lactose, experience intolerance symptoms to whatever placebo is used in double-blind studies. This phenomenon complicates the diagnostic process, making it difficult for clinicians to accurately assess their patient's condition. Tolerance to milk is sometimes affected by factors unrelated to its lactose content, such as psychological factors or cultural attitudes toward milk.

A discussion of studies observing this phenomenon may help illustrate the complexity of the problem. Haverberg et al., in a double-blind trial, evaluated tolerance to 240 and 480 ml of a lactose-free and lactose-containing chocolate dairy drink in a group of 110 healthy Boston teenagers, 14 to 19 years of age [60]. Theoretically, symptoms due to lactose should occur only in those with limited lactose digestion in response to a lactose-containing beverage. However, 40% of those identified as lactose digesters per a breath hydrogen test, and 31% of maldigesters reported symptoms after consuming the lactose-free beverage or after both the lactose-containing and the lactose-free beverage. Suspecting that perhaps the large number of false-positive results were because too much emphasis had been placed on reporting symptoms, the researchers conducted a follow-up study in a similar population of high school students using a simplified questionnaire that placed less emphasis on possible symptoms [60]. This time, 29% of the lactose digesters reported symptoms that apparently were due to an unidentified cause other than lactose. One criticism of these studies is that since chocolate has been shown to improve tolerance to lactose, the addition of chocolate to the dairy drinks (used to make the drinks similar in taste) may have affected the level of symptoms reported. Healthy elderly lactose digesters and maldigesters following a similar protocol to that of Haverberg, reported symptoms with the same degree of frequency to a lactose-containing drink as to a lactose-free drink [61]. The authors concluded that the symptoms were either psychosomatic or were the result of other physiologic causes.

Johnson et al. tested for milk tolerance a subgroup of 45 African American subjects who had confirmed lactose maldigestion and intolerance to 25 g of aqueous lactose [59]. Subjects were given either 315 ml of lactose-containing milk or lactose-hydrolyzed milk alternately on three different days in a double-blind test. One third of the subjects experienced symptoms of intolerance to both types of milk, indicating that their symptoms were not due to lactose. The authors conclude that social and cultural habits and attitudes also affect tolerance to milk drinking.

Two studies by Suarez et al. discussed earlier also illustrate this phenomenon [57,58]. In a study testing tolerance to 1 cup of milk served with breakfast, the researchers recruited subjects who reported severe lactose intolerance and who said they consistently experienced symptoms after consuming less than 240 ml of milk. Surprisingly, approximately one third (9/30) of the subjects who claimed intolerance were able to digest lactose per the breath hydrogen test. The authors concluded that people who identify themselves as severely lactose-intolerant may mistakenly attribute a variety of abdominal symptoms to lactose intolerance [57].

Similarly, in a second study designed to test tolerance to 2 cups of milk, approximately a third (31%) of recruited subjects (of mixed ethnic background) who claimed severe intolerance were able to digest lactose as measured by the breath hydrogen test [58]. This group was not included in the subsequent milk trial, but was included with the other subjects in a psychological assessment, using the Minnesota Multiphasic Personality Inventory. The lactase deficient subjects who complained of symptoms demonstrated a high level of psychasthenia (incapacity to resist irrational phobias, obsessions, and compulsions), but no correlations with any clinical psychological conditions (e.g., depression, hypochondriasis, paranoia) in response to the personality inventory. However, since these individuals also failed to respond candidly to the test (they tended to exaggerate, minimize or conceal information), the researchers question the validity of these findings.

One researcher says lactose intolerance may be a self-fulfilling prophecy [79]. Individuals who experience symptoms after a generous serving of milk may avoid future milk consumption — even though a smaller amount of milk may be tolerated. Thus, a learned aversion for milk develops. Avoiding milk may become a food practice passed down to the children and perpetuated for years, resulting in poor bone health for the entire family.

These studies further emphasize the need for objective testing for those complaining of gastrointestinal symptoms after drinking milk, since it appears that a significant portion of the population misattribute their symptoms to lactose.

8.5.4 Lactose Tolerance during Pregnancy

Pregnant women need to consume at least 3 servings of Milk Group foods to obtain the 1000 mg of calcium/day recommended by the National Academy of Sciences for pregnant women [77]. Women with limited lactose digestion may be encouraged to discover that their tolerance to lactose-containing milk and milk products may improve during pregnancy.

For example, Villar and colleagues demonstrated that 44% of women who maldigested 360 ml of milk (18 g of lactose) before the 15th week of gestation were able to digest that amount of lactose by the end of their pregnancy [80]. Average breath hydrogen (an indication that undigested lactose is being metabolized by colonic bacteria) decreased by more than half over this time period.

Some researchers hypothesize that slower intestinal transit time during pregnancy improves tolerance to lactose [81,82]. For example, investigators compared lactose maldigestion and symptoms of intolerance between pregnant African American women and nonpregnant controls [81]. The pregnant women reported fewer symptoms than the nonpregnant women after drinking 8 ounces of 1% milk, although their ability to digest lactose did not change. The authors suggest that the improved tolerance was most likely due to slower intestinal transit time. They explain that because the rise in breath hydrogen in response to ingested lactose occurs approximately an hour later in pregnant vs. nonpregnant women, breath hydrogen should be measured over a longer time period. This may be why earlier studies showed improved digestion. A longitudinal study utilized an 8-hour breath hydrogen test to evaluate lactose digestion in a group of African American women in early pregnancy (prior to 16 weeks), late pregnancy (30 to 35 weeks), and 8 weeks postpartum, compared to a control group of nonpregnant African American women [83]. Women in early pregnancy had a significantly lower prevalence of lactose maldigestion (66.2%) than the control women (80.2%), but there was no significant change in prevalence from early pregnancy to late pregnancy, to 8 weeks postpartum. However the maldigesting pregnant women reported fewer symptoms after consuming 1 cup (240 ml) of 1% milk than did the nonpregnant control women [83]. Whether actual digestion improves or not, it is clear from these studies that women may enjoy improved tolerance to milk and milk products while they are pregnant.

8.6 LONG-TERM CONSEQUENCES OF LACTOSE MALDIGESTION

8.6.1 Lactose Digestion and Calcium/Nutrient Absorption

Studies conducted in the 1970s and 1980s in both animals and humans failed to provide any evidence that the maldigestion of lactose impaired the absorption of any other nutrient [2]. Nutrients studied include protein, fat, vitamins A and C, calcium, magnesium, copper, manganese, and zinc. In a review of this information, Leichter concluded that "if the unabsorbed lactose has some effect on the absorption of other nutrients it is doubtful whether this effect has significant nutritional consequences in healthy lactose-intolerant adults who consume milk and milk products in moderate amounts" [84].

Because some portion of the lactose consumed passes undigested into the colon, those with limited lactose digestion obtain slightly less energy from milk and milk products than do lactose digesters. Part of the unabsorbed lactose is converted by fermentation into volatile fatty acids (primarily acetate) which are a source of energy and may help maintain the health of intestinal cells [2]. The small amount of energy lost seems to be of no practical significance.

While the presence of lactose stimulates the intestinal absorption of calcium in laboratory animals [85] and in human infants [86], there is no evidence that it improves calcium absorption in adults [87]. Conversely, limited digestion and absorption of lactose does not appear to decrease calcium absorption. A review of research in this area concludes "the bulk of the evidence indicates a favorable or neutral effect of lactose on Ca absorption in both lactose digesters and maldigesters" [2].

Tremaine and colleagues investigated how lactose might influence the absorption of calcium from milk in adults with and without lactase deficiency [88]. Using a double-isotope method, the researchers compared calcium absorption between lactose-containing milk and hydrolyzed milk in both lactase-deficient and -sufficient adults. The subjects with lactase deficiency absorbed calcium equally well from lactose-containing or lactose-hydrolyzed milk. Mean calcium absorption was greater in lactase-deficient subjects, presumably due to a habitually lower calcium intake. Decreased calcium intake is known to cause an increase in fractional calcium absorption, although calcium intake was not verified by diet history in this study. Horowitz et al. found no relationship between lactose and calcium absorption when an oral dose of 5 μ Ci of radioactive calcium chloride (20 mg of calcium) was measured in serum an hour later in 46 postmenopausal women with osteoporosis [89]. Roughly half of all subjects, whether or not they were lactose maldigesters, had below normal absorption of calcium. Griessen and colleagues also studied what influence lactase deficiency might have on calcium absorption [90]. Using a double-isotope technique, they compared calcium absorption in young adult lactase-deficient and -sufficient males from two commercial milks, one containing lactose and the other containing glucose. They then compared absorption between lactose-containing milk and water. Results demonstrated that all subjects absorbed calcium equally well from milk and from water. Glucose, when substituted for lactose in milk, did not improve calcium absorption. Lactase-deficient subjects absorbed calcium from the lactose-containing milk better than did the lactase-sufficient subjects. The authors did not attribute the increase to lower calcium status of the lactase-deficient group, since calcium intake of all subjects was normalized prior to the beginning of the study. Avoidance of dairy foods, rather than calcium malabsorption, is most likely the cause of increased risk of osteoporosis in lactase-deficient individuals [90].

8.6.2 Effect on Milk Consumption and Nutritional Status

Lactose maldigestion and the symptoms of intolerance that may occur is a factor that may influence milk consumption. Data from most studies, but not all [91], suggest that individuals with primary lactose deficiency consume less milk than those who digest lactose normally [32,38,61,84,92, 93,94]. For example, in a study conducted at the University of Connecticut, subjects with a history of milk intolerance consumed significantly less milk than the control subjects. The adult subjects consumed an 8-ounce serving (240 ml) of milk less than one to three times per month, while the lactose-tolerant control group consumed an average of 1 to 2 servings of milk per day [92]. Finkenstedt et al. observed that lactose maldigestion affected milk intake in middle-aged women. The daily intake of calcium from milk was significantly lower in those women with osteoporosis (125 mg/day) vs. controls (252 mg/day), more of whom were lactose maldigesters [95]. Similarly, Kudlacek et al. found that calcium intake from milk was highest in subjects without lactose malabsorption (212 mg/day) and significantly decreased in those with moderate (188 mg/d) and severe (167 mg/day) lactose malabsorption [93]. In a study comparing dietary calcium intake between lactose tolerant and intolerant (to 25 g lactose) maldigesting African American premenopausal women, 45% of the dietary calcium in the diet of lactose tolerant women came from milk and other dairy foods, whereas only 12% of dietary calcium in the diets of the lactose intolerant women came from these foods (Figure 8.4) [94]. Total average calcium intake in the lactose maldigesting intolerant women was significantly lower than in the lactose tolerant women (388 mg/day vs. 763 mg/day) [94]. Postmenopausal women with the CC genotype (lactose maldigesters) obtained a 55% lower intake of calcium from fresh milk than did women with the TT genotype (lactose digesters), though there were no significant differences in the amount of calcium obtained from yogurt or other foods between genotypic groups (Figure 8.5) [32].

Interestingly, decreased milk intake as a result of lactose intolerance is not always a deliberate, conscious decision. Horowitz et al. found that even though only 5% of the lactose maldigesters he studied reported a history of milk intolerance, they drank significantly less milk (<1 cup/day) than those who digested milk normally (2 cups/day) [89]. Newcomer observed a similar phenomenon [96]. Subjects diagnosed as lactose maldigesters by the breath hydrogen test were not aware of milk intolerance, yet their intake of milk and calcium was significantly lower than that of lactose digesting subjects. He suggested that perhaps these subjects had decreased their milk intake during childhood as a result of lactose intolerance, but were unaware they had done so [96].

Several studies demonstrate that a low calcium intake and/or low milk intake results in a low intake of other milk-related nutrients such as riboflavin, vitamin A, phosphorus, vitamin B_{12}, magnesium, and potassium in both adults and teenagers [97,98,99]. It was observed, "a diet

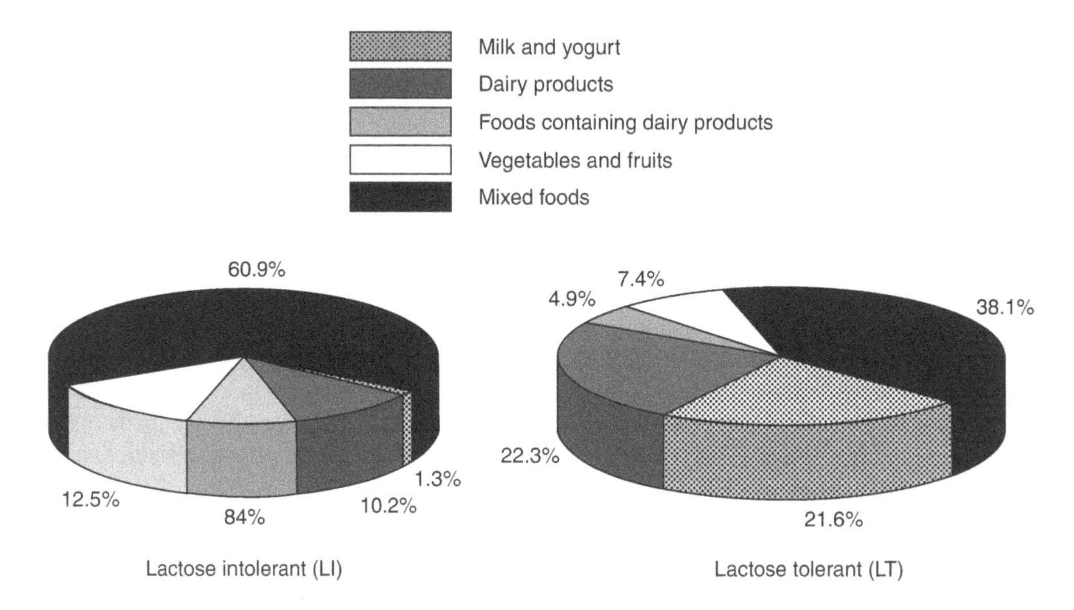

FIGURE 8.4 Percentage contributions of calcium sources in diet of African American women according to self-reported food intake. (From Buchowski, M. S., *J. Am. College Nutr.*, 21 (1), 47–54, 2002. With permission.)

which consistently excludes or limits dairy foods will not only provide less calcium, but may also limit those nutrients that track with calcium in foods" [99].

Those with limited lactose digestion do not necessarily dislike the taste of milk and other dairy foods, [100,32] so should utilize available strategies to maintain dairy food intake and nutritional integrity of the diet. Teens with lactose maldigestion should especially be encouraged to maintain

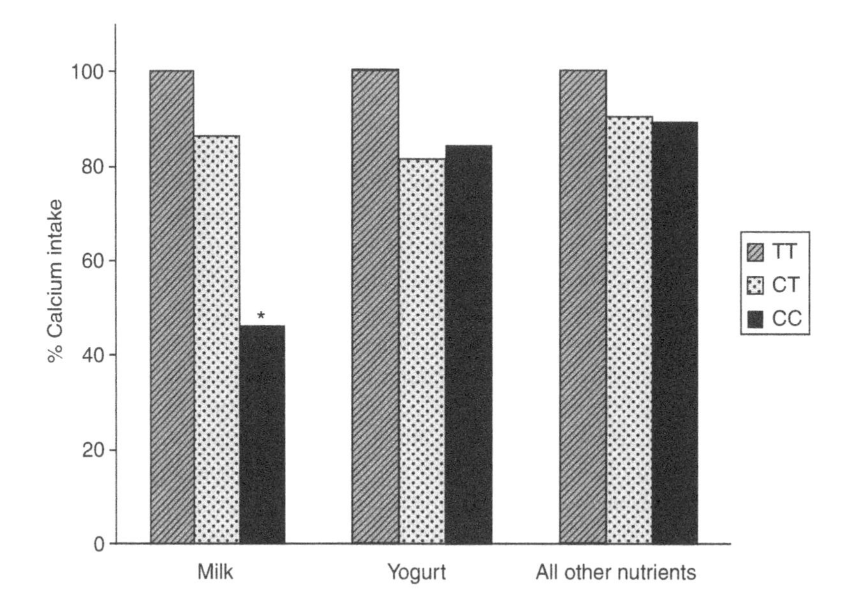

FIGURE 8.5 Calcium intake per day from milk, yogurt, and all other nutrients according to LCT genotypes expressed as percentage of TT genotypes. Individuals with genotype CC (dark bars) had significantly lower calcium intake from milk ($*p = 0.004$) compared with TT (dashed bars), and TC (shaded bars) genotypes. (From Obermayer-Pietsch, B. M. et al., *J. Bone Min. Res.*, 19 (1), 42, 2004. With permission.)

calcium and dairy food intake, since maximizing bone mass attained before age 30 is the most effective way to prevent osteoporosis later in life [101].

8.6.3 Risk of Osteoporosis/Chronic Disease

The medical literature over the last two to three decades implicates low calcium and dairy food intake in the etiology of several chronic diseases including obesity, hypertension, type 2 diabetes, osteoporosis, and some cancers [102,103,104,11]. Drawing on data from prospective longitudinal studies and randomized controlled trials, researchers conservatively estimated that increasing dairy food intake to the recommended 3 to 4 servings per day could result in health care cost savings of approximately $26 billion the first year or $200 billion over 5 years [103].

Lactose maldigestion, when accompanied by low calcium intake, has been suggested as a risk factor for osteoporosis, and should not be overlooked as a contributing factor to this disease [32,95,105,106]. Studies conducted in the 1970s and 1980s reported a higher prevalence of lactase maldigestion among women with osteoporosis than in those without metabolic bone disease [89,95,96]. More recent research links lactose intolerance (report of symptoms) with low dairy food/calcium intake and low bone density in perimenopausal and postmenopausal women [107,108] and with increased osteoporotic fractures in both women and men [109,110]. Postmenopausal women with a genetic predisposition to lactose maldigestion (CC genotype) had significantly lower bone mineral density at the spine and three areas of the hip as well as significantly higher fracture incidence than the other genotypes (TT and TC) (Figure 8.6 and Figure 8.7) [32]. Enattah et al. also studied the relationship between molecularly defined lactose maldigestion and self-reported lactose intolerance on bone mineral density and fractures in two groups of Finnish postmenopausal women (453 women aged 62 to 78 years and 52 women with osteoporotic fractures

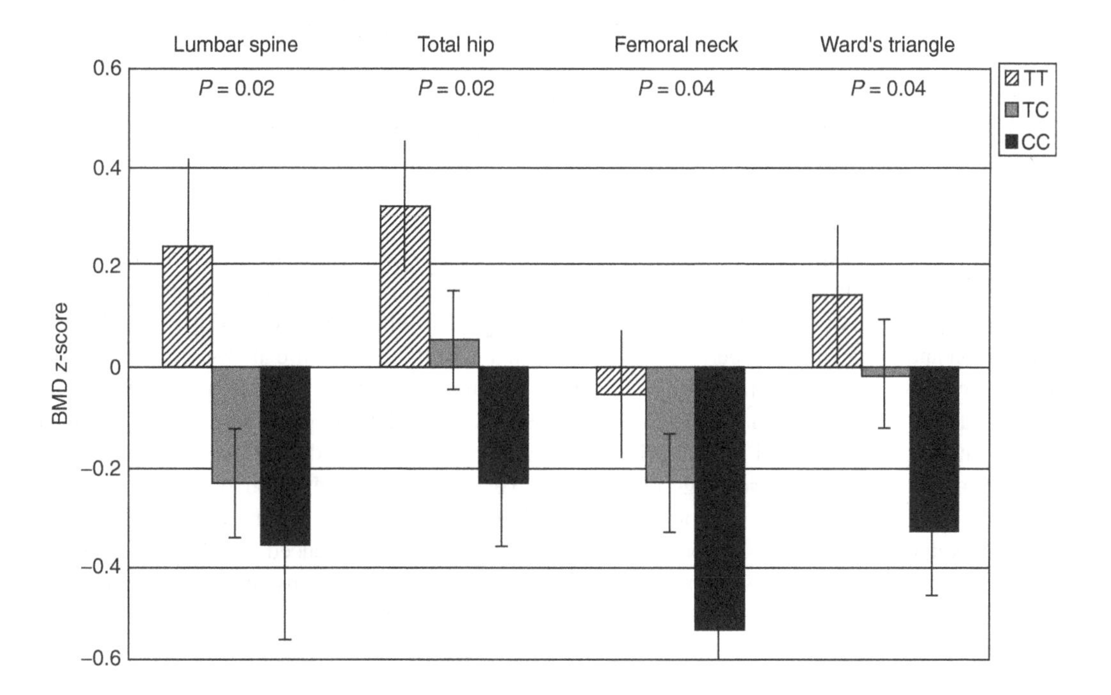

FIGURE 8.6. Age-adjusted measurements of BMD expressed as Z-scores at the lumbar spine, the total hip, femoral neck, and Ward's triangle according to LCT genotypes in 258 postmenopausal women. Individuals with genotype CC (dark bars) had significantly lower BMD Z-scores than the other genotypes. (From Obermayer-Pietsch, B. M. et al., *J. Bone Min. Res.*, 19 (1), 42, 2004. With permission.)

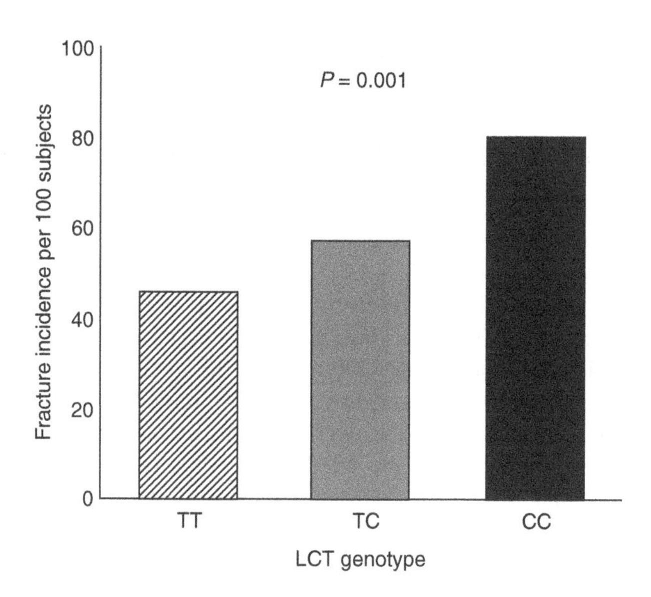

FIGURE 8.7 Fracture incidences per 100 subjects in postmenopausal women according to LCT genotypes. Individuals with genotype CC (dark bars) had significantly higher nonvertebral fracture incidence ($*p = 0.001$) than TC (shaded bars) and TT (dashed bars) genotypes, showing an increasing gene-dose effect towards these genotypes. (From Obermayer-Pietsch, B. M. et al., *J. Bone Min. Res.*, 19 (1), 42, 2004. With permission)

aged 69 to 85 years), but with different results [111]. They found the frequency of the CC_{-13910} genotype for 52 women with osteoporosis was similar to that of the control women (23.1% vs. 15%). Calcium intake from dairy products and bone mineral density of the heel was similar among genotypes. Those with self-reported lactose intolerance consumed less dairy foods, but were frequent users of calcium supplements. Results may have differed between these studies because of the different bone sites measured (hip and spine vs. heel). Fracture risk appears to depend on the severity of lactose malabsorption and the degree to which it limits calcium and dairy food intake [93].

The Joint National Committee on Detection, Evaluation, and Treatment of High Blood Pressure, National Institutes of Health, National Heart, Lung and Blood Institute (NHLBI), recommends an adequate intake of calcium, potassium, and magnesium as part of the dairy-rich DASH (Dietary Approaches to Stop Hypertension) diet along with other lifestyle modifications for the prevention and treatment of hypertension [112]. Milk and milk products are an important source of all three of these minerals, contributing 72% of the calcium, 18% of the potassium, and 15% of the magnesium to the U.S. food supply [113]. These recommendations came after a clinical trial investigating DASH, funded by the NHLBI, found that a diet including 3 servings of low-fat dairy products and 8 to 10 servings of fruits and vegetables lowered blood pressure in people with or without existing hypertension [114]. In the DASH trial, African Americans who consumed 3 servings/day of dairy foods as part of the combination diet experienced a reduction of blood pressure twice that of Caucasian participants, but without any symptoms of lactose intolerance [115]. Recognizing that some of the minority participants may be lactose intolerant, DASH nutritionists designed the meal plans using simple dietary strategies to minimize any symptoms [116]. The eating plan for the DASH diet, which is low in fat, and high in dietary fiber, potassium, calcium, and magnesium, is included in the 2005 *Dietary Guidelines for Americans* as a health-promoting alternative to the U.S. Department of Agriculture (USDA) dietary pattern. Based on collective observations from a variety of studies, including the DASH trials, researchers estimate that consuming a healthful diet containing 3 to 4 servings of dairy foods/day would lead to a 40%

reduction in the prevalence of mild to moderate hypertension and result in first year health care cost savings of $14 billion, with cumulative savings of $70 billion at 5 years [103]. For more detailed information on this topic, see Chapter 3 on Dairy Foods and Hypertension.

Dairy foods' beneficial role in regulating body fat and weight loss has been demonstrated in African Americans and in whites [102,117,118]. Interestingly, one of the first observations of a beneficial relationship between dairy foods and body fat was during the course of a clinical trial of the antihypertensive effect of calcium in obese African American males [119]. Increasing calcium intake ~400 mg to ~1000 mg/day by feeding 2 cups of yogurt/day for 1 year reduced body fat by nearly 11 pounds and lowered circulating insulin levels without an accompanying decrease in caloric intake [119]. Research from *in vitro* and experimental animal studies indicates that dietary calcium and other dairy components (e.g., protein, branched chain amino acids, bioactives) may regulate energy metabolism and obesity risk — and that dairy foods have a greater beneficial effect on body weight/fat than calcium alone [102]. In a recent analysis, researchers conservatively estimate that consuming 3 to 4 servings/day of milk, cheese, or yogurt could reduce the incidence of obesity by 5% a year, resulting in health care cost savings of $2.5 billion in the first year and more than $37.5 billion at 5 years [103]. See Chapter 7 on Dairy Foods and a Healthy Weight for further information.

Epidemiological studies, animal studies, and *in vitro* studies using human cancer cells indicate that several nutrients/components in milk and milk products may be protective against cancer [120,121,122,123]. The potentially anticarcinogenic agents include calcium, vitamin D, protein, vitamin A, beta-carotene, lactic acid bacteria, and components of milk fat, such as sphingolipids, conjugated linoleic acid (CLA), butyric acid, and ether lipids. A consensus report of the National Medical Association recommends that the American public as a whole and African Americans in particular consume 3 to 4 servings/day of low-fat milk, cheese, and/or yogurt to help reduce the risk of certain chronic diseases including colon cancer [11]. Based on a review of the science, researchers conservatively estimated that consuming 3 to 4 servings of dairy foods/day could reduce the risk of colorectal cancer by 5% annually after three years, resulting in health care cost savings of $0.75 billion over five years [103]. For further information, see Chapter 4 on Dairy Foods and Cancer.

8.7 STRATEGIES FOR DIETARY MANAGEMENT OF PRIMARY LACTOSE MALDIGESTION

Several strategies are available for managing primary lactose maldigestion without compromising nutritional status or health [1,38,124]. Total elimination of dairy foods is unnecessary and not recommended [2,125]. Milk and other dairy foods contribute high quality protein to the diet and contribute 72% of the calcium, 26% of the riboflavin, 16% of the vitamin A, 20% of the vitamin B_{12}, 18% of the potassium, 16.5% of the zinc, 15% of the magnesium, and 19% of the protein available for consumption in the United States [113]. Recognizing the important nutritional contribution of dairy foods, the 2005 *Dietary Guidelines for Americans* recommend that those with lactose intolerance who are looking for alternatives to milk consider foods within the milk group first, such as lactose-free milk, yogurt, and cheese [126].

Several factors influence an individual's tolerance to dairy foods, including the amount of lactose, the type of dairy food, whether the lactose-containing food is eaten with a meal, whether the food has been fermented or hydrolyzed with an enzyme preparation, and colonic adaptation [127,33].

8.7.1 Amount of Lactose

As discussed earlier, most of those with limited lactose digestion can tolerate the amount of lactose contained in an 8 ounce (240 ml) serving of milk. Few individuals may need to consume smaller amounts (i.e., 4 ounces or 120 ml) at a time. A meta-analysis of 21 studies measuring lactose intolerance symptoms of lactose maldigesters after consuming either a product with the amount of lactose commonly found in a meal or a lactose-free placebo confirmed that in doses below 12 g of lactose (the amount in 1 cup of milk), maldigesters had no noticeable symptoms [128]. The blinded studies reviewed showed no significant differences in symptoms after the ingestion of 1 serving of dairy foods (i.e., 1 cup of milk) as compared with 1 cup of lactose-free (lactose hydrolyzed) milk or a serving of yogurt.

Milk is also better tolerated when it is consumed with a meal [71]. Psyllium fiber, when added to aqueous lactose or milk, reduces hydrogen production and symptoms of intolerance [129]. This finding led to further studies that demonstrated similar alterations in breath hydrogen kinetics when lactose was consumed with a meal [71,130]. When lactose-containing foods are consumed with other solid foods, gastric emptying is delayed, both reducing and delaying peak hydrogen production. Martini and Savaiano found that only 3 out of 12 subjects experienced symptoms following a 19 g lactose load (equivalent to 1.6 glasses or 384 ml of milk) consumed with a breakfast meal [71]. This amounted to a three-fold reduction in both severity and incidence of symptoms when compared to aqueous lactose. Delayed gastric emptying allows more time for any endogenous lactase enzyme present to digest dietary lactose. It also reduces the amount of undigested lactose that reaches the colon at any one time.

8.7.2 Type of Dairy Food

People with limited lactose digestion tolerate some types of dairy foods better than others. Some studies have shown that whole milk is better tolerated than lower fat milks [132,133]; owever, not all studies have confirmed this [134]. The fat content of milk influences milk tolerance, presumably by slowing gastric emptying. When 11 lactose-maldigesting and intolerant subjects were given 50 g of lactose as whole milk, they experienced a significantly lower rise in blood glucose and decreased severity of symptoms, as compared to the same amount of lactose in either skim milk or an aqueous solution [131]. Dehkordi et al. examined digestion (rather than tolerance) of various milks as measured by breath hydrogen production [132]. They found that absolute hydrogen production of maldigesters was lower for 18 g of lactose in whole milk than for skim milk, but the differences were not significant and neither milk completely alleviated lactose malabsorption (breath hydrogen <20 ppm). Only consumption of whole milk (18 g of lactose) with cornflakes significantly improved lactose digestion when compared to whole, skim, chocolate, or commercial milk containing *L. acidophilus* and *Bifidobacterium*. In this study breath hydrogen was collected for only 5 hours; however, some investigators believe that an 8-hour collection provides more accurate results. Vesa reported no differences in symptoms among free-living maldigesting subjects who consumed either fat-free or full-fat milk (8% fat). This group then conducted a more comprehensive study to determine whether raising the energy content of milk slows gastric emptying and improves tolerance [135]. Gastric emptying in 11 lactose maldigesting adults was significantly longer after ingestion of the high-energy milk (18 g of lactose) than after the half-skimmed milk; symptoms were not significantly improved, though there was a trend toward improved lactose digestion. The authors conclude that the positive effect was not strong enough to recommend high-energy milk to lactose maldigesters as a way to improve tolerance. The same group also found that increasing the viscosity of high-energy milk formulas with rice starch did not affect the rate of gastric emptying or improve milk tolerance [136].

Chocolate milk appears to be better tolerated than unflavored milk by lactose maldigesters [137], which can be explained by reduced breath hydrogen production when compared to skim milk [134]. The addition of cocoa to 250 ml of milk formula significantly reduced the breath hydrogen response and symptoms of bloating and cramping in 37 lactose maldigesters [137]. A randomized crossover study of 27 symptomatic, maldigesting adults found that 12 g of lactose present in 100 g of milk chocolate was well tolerated [138]. Gastrointestinal complaints were minor and did not differ significantly from those after eating lactose-free chocolate. While the mechanism for cocoa's affect on lactose tolerance is unclear, researchers propose three possible mechanisms: (1) cocoa might stimulate lactase activity, (2) cocoa might reduce the number of gas-producing bacteria in the colon, or (3) cocoa might slow gastric emptying [137]. These possible mechanisms need further study.

Some dairy foods, such as hard cheeses, cottage cheese, ice cream, and yogurt contain a lower amount of lactose per serving relative to milk, and therefore cause fewer symptoms (Table 8.6). For example, Cheddar cheese contains very little lactose. During the cheese-making process, the whey is removed from the curds. Since 94% of the lactose remains primarily with the whey portion, the finished cheese has a relatively low lactose content.

8.7.3 Fermented Milk Products

Lactose (milk sugar) is a fermentable substrate. It can be fermented outside the body to produce cheeses, yogurts and acidified milks — or it can be fermented by the colonic microflora [139]. Several lines of evidence demonstrate that the appropriate strain of lactic acid bacteria, in adequate amounts, can alleviate the symptoms of lactose intolerance. Probiotics — living microorganisms that when consumed in sufficient amounts provide health benefits beyond basic nutrition — are emerging as important dietary ingredients in functional foods [140].

Yogurt containing lactic acid bacteria and up to 20 g of lactose is well tolerated by a majority of lactase deficient individuals [141]. Improved lactose digestion with yogurt appears to be partly the result of its reduced lactose content, but is primarily due to autodigestion within the intestine by the microbial beta-galactosidase enzyme [142]. Three related factors appear to be important to the survival and expression of microbial enzyme activity from yogurt: (1) the buffering of stomach acid by yogurt, (2) protection by the intact microbial cell against degradation by stomach acid or enzymes, and (3) action of digestive enzymes and bile acids on the microbial cell which releases beta-galactosidase activity [141]. In yogurt-making, the starter cultures *Lactobacillus bulgaricus* and *Streptococcus thermophilus* are incubated with fresh milk to which milk solids have been added. Both of these organisms synthesize the beta-galactosidase enzyme. The action of the beta-galactosidase present in these two organisms reduces the level of lactose in the concentrated milk. During the fermentation process the pH falls to about 4.6. (Beta-galactosidase is rapidly destroyed at pH <3.0.). Further lactase activity is inhibited by the combination of low pH and low temperature during storage. When yogurt is eaten, the casein, lactate, and calcium phosphate in the yogurt act as buffers to the stomach acid, allowing the microbes (and the enzyme activity) to reach the duodenum intact [127]. The buffering capacity of yogurt was found to be almost three times that of whole milk, presumably due to the proteins in the added milk solids [143]. Kolars et al. demonstrated that lactase activity in the duodenum after yogurt ingestion is enough to digest 50 to 100% of a 20 g lactose load [142]. A number of variables may influence the delivery of beta-galactosidase to the duodenum, including gastric acid secretion, rate of gastric emptying, quantity of yogurt ingested, pancreatic and intestinal digestive enzyme activity, and lipid emulsification by bile acids [143]. There is some evidence that after the intact bacteria reach the intestinal tract they are disrupted by bile acids, releasing the enzyme to digest lactose. Pochart et al. confirmed the earlier finding of Kolars et al. that beta-galactosidase activity in yogurt survives passage through the stomach (Figure 8.8) [144]. In addition they found that minimal lactose hydrolysis occurred in the duodenum after yogurt ingestion, indicating that digestion probably occurs further along the intestinal tract as bacterial (yogurt) lactase activity is stimulated by the progressively increasing pH.

Kolars et al. used the breath hydrogen technique to determine whether lactose in yogurt is better absorbed by lactose maldigesters than is lactose in milk [142]. The total area under the breath hydrogen curve was significantly lower for 440 g of yogurt (18 g of lactose) than for milk or a lactose solution containing a similar amount of lactose. Hydrogen production after ingestion of yogurt was only about one-third that of milk. A smaller amount of yogurt (270 g) containing 11 g of

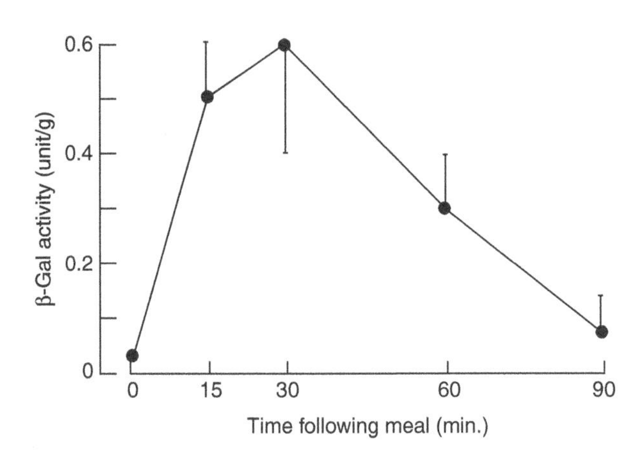

FIGURE 8.8 Beta-galactosidase activity in duodenal samples after ingestion of fresh yogurt. Results for the mean for seven subjects. Bars represent the SEM. (From Pochart, P., DeWitt, O., Desjeux, J., and Bourlioux, P., *Am. J. Clin. Nutr.*, 49, 828, 1989. With permission.)

lactose — an amount closer to that typically consumed — produced only a negligible amount of hydrogen. Symptoms of diarrhea or flatulence were experienced by 80% of the subjects when they consumed 18 g of lactose in milk, but these same subjects were symptom-free after consuming the same amount of lactose in yogurt.

Studies in adults and children demonstrate that the semisolid nature of yogurt, which slows its gastric emptying, may be an important factor in its improved tolerance. Researchers at Johns Hopkins School of Medicine in Boston tested whether yogurt was better tolerated than milk in 14 lactose-malabsorbing children (mean age 9.5 years) [145]. The children experienced significantly fewer symptoms after consumption of 8 ounces of yogurt containing active cultures than after consuming milk. Since the children experienced improved tolerance to both yogurt with live active cultures and pasteurized yogurt (which decreased bacterial activity), the authors suggest that yogurt's osmolality, energy density, and delayed transit time played a greater role in improving tolerance than did its ability to "autodigest" lactose. Researchers in France reached a similar conclusion when three yogurts containing different bacterial cultures and lactase activity were equally digested and tolerated by 15 lactase-deficient adults [146].

Although consuming yogurt (when compared with milk) reduces the occurrence and severity of symptoms associated with lactose maldigestion, lactase activity varies considerably between brands of active-culture yogurt [147]. In addition, if yogurt is pasteurized after the addition of active cultures (which is sometimes done to extend shelf-life of the product), it loses much of its ability to hydrolyze lactose in the gut [100,148]. Furthermore, eating yogurt may not assist the digestion of lactose from other dairy foods eaten with it as part of a meal [149]. Ingestion of yogurt over eight days provided no additional benefit [148].

Some people find flavored yogurts more acceptable than plain [100]. When lactose digestion was compared between milk, flavored, and plain yogurt in 16 lactase-deficient subjects, flavored yogurt produced a breath hydrogen level slightly higher than did plain yogurt, but lower than did milk [150]. Although only the hydrogen production from the plain yogurt was statistically significantly lower than that of milk, none of the subjects experienced any symptoms after eating either variety of yogurt, while three reported symptoms after drinking milk [150]. It is unclear how the addition of fruit, sweeteners and flavorings might reduce the beta-galactosidase activity in flavored yogurts. Frozen yogurt that has been pasteurized prior to freezing (typical commercial practice) lacks beta-galactosidase activity. Lactose maldigestion and tolerance have been found to be similar between frozen yogurt, ice milk, and ice cream. However, lactase-deficient persons may tolerate significant amounts of these products, presumably due to their slower gastric transit time owing to their high solids and/or fat content [150].

Kefir, a fermented milk made by inoculation and incubation with kefir grains, has been demonstrated to improve lactose tolerance [151]. Kefir grains are a mass of bacteria, yeasts, polysaccharides, and other products of bacterial metabolism, together with milk protein — and contain a larger range of microorganisms in its starter culture than does yogurt. Researchers from The Ohio State University, using a randomized block protocol, compared breath hydrogen excretion and lactose intolerance symptoms between test meals of 2% milk, plain and flavored yogurt, and plain and flavored kefir in 15 healthy adults with lactose maldigestion [151]. Breath hydrogen over 8 hours was significantly lower for plain and flavored yogurt and for plain kefir when compared to milk. Hydrogen excretion for kefir had an intermediate response — all yogurts and kefirs similarly reduced intolerance symptoms. Since this is the first study to evaluate lactose digestion from kefir, further studies about cell counts and bile sensitivity are needed to identify and explain the mechanism for improving lactose tolerance [151].

Consuming dairy products with appropriate strains and levels of lactic acid bacteria is a good way for lactose maldigesting individuals to make dairy foods and their accompanying nutrients and health benefits part of a healthy lifestyle [140].

8.7.4 Unfermented Milk with Bacterial Cultures

Whether nonfermented dairy products containing bacterial starter cultures — such as sweet acidophilus milk or yogurt milk — have the potential to improve lactose tolerance is controversial [152].

Acidophilus milk is a nonfermented beverage made by adding viable *L. acidophilus* strains to cold milk, then refrigerating to prevent further growth of the organism. It has an advantage over yogurt in that it does not have a tart taste. Yogurt milk is prepared in a manner similar to acidophilus milk, except that *Streptococcus thermophilus* and *Lactobacillus bulgaricus* is added to the fresh milk.

Several studies conducted in the 1980s found that acidophilus milk or capsules containing high concentrations of mixed lactic acid bacteria or *Bifidobacteria bifidum* did not improve lactose digestion or alleviate symptoms in lactose maldigesting subjects [153–156]. It has since been learned that certain factors — such as insufficient concentration of the culture, extended storage, use of frozen concentration starter culture, level of lactic acid, and use of inappropriate substrates for culture growth — contribute to the ineffectiveness of these unfermented products [152,157]. The strain of *L. acidophilus* used in studies of lactose maldigestion is of critical importance, since beta-galactosidase activity, bile sensitivity, and acid tolerance vary considerably among strains.

For example, acidophilus milk (prepared with three different strains of *L. acidophilus* in two different concentrations) and yogurt milk (prepared with two concentrations of *S. thermophilus* and *L. bulgaricus)* were evaluated on the basis of beta-galactosidase activity, bile tolerance, and ability to digest lactose in ten lactose-maldigesting adults [158]. Only yogurt milk and acidophilus milk prepared with the highest concentration (10^8 cfu/ml) of starter cultures were effective in significantly decreasing breath hydrogen concentrations in the subjects. Only the most bile-tolerant strain of *L. acidophilus* was effective in this regard. This characteristic appears to be important for the release of beta-galactosidase within the intestinal tract. Furthermore, subjects who normally experienced symptoms after ingestion of 20 g of lactose reported fewer symptoms following consumption of 400 ml of yogurt milk containing 10^8 cfu/ml than with 400 ml of acidophilus milk containing the same cell concentration. The researchers conclude that consumption of nonfermented yogurt milk containing high concentrations of yogurt cultures was able to reduce breath hydrogen concentrations threefold. This is similar to the effect of fermented yogurt, which reduces gas production by three- to fourfold, when compared to milk [158]. Montes et al. tested digestibility and tolerance of unfermented milks among 20 children with limited lactose digestion [159]. They found that consumption of 250 ml of low-fat milk inoculated with 10^{10} cells of

Lactobacillus acidophilus improved tolerance, while consumption of the same amount of milk inoculated with a commercial yogurt starter culture containing 10^8 cells of *Lactobacillus lactis* and 10^{10} cells of *Streptococcus thermophilus* improved both digestion and tolerance, compared to regular milk.

More recently, researchers at Purdue University tested four strains of *L. acidophilus* with varying degrees of lactose transport, beta-galactosidase activity, and bile acid sensitivity on lactose digestion and tolerance in a group of lactose maldigesting adults [157]. Acidophilus milk prepared with the bacterial strain with the greatest bile and acid tolerance was the most effective in improving lactose digestion and tolerance. Further studies are needed, however, to determine the extent of the importance of these factors.

Bifidobacteria may have potential for use in products designed to improve lactose digestion because they contain a relatively high level of beta-galactosidase activity and are stable under normal storage conditions. A study conducted among 15 lactose-maldigesting adults showed that unfermented milk containing *Bifidobacteria longum* that was grown in a lactose-containing medium had the greatest beta-galactosidase activity and significantly improved lactose digestion (per breath hydrogen) and symptoms of flatulence, compared to other bifido strains or regular low-fat milk [160].

8.7.5 Enzyme Preparations

Lactose-hydrolyzed milk or commercial oral enzyme replacement therapy has proven beneficial in adults and children and is recommended as a strategy for improving lactose tolerance [2,15,124,161,162]. Oral enzyme replacement in tablet form offers the advantage of allowing a more liberal use of lactose-containing dairy foods. This may prove a useful therapy even for young children, making specialized nutritional management unnecessary [163]. Beta-galactosidases extracted from yeast (*Kluyveromyces lactis*) or fungi (*Aspergillus niger* or *Aspergillus oryzae*) have been found effective [72,164,165,166]. These enzymes, as well as the final products of their addition to food, have been classified as Generally Recognized as Safe (GRAS) by the U.S. Food and Drug Administration (FDA) under the broad classification of carbohydrases [167].

The addition of *Kluyveromyces lactis* to milk 10 hours or 5 minutes prior to consumption was evaluated in a double-blind, placebo-controlled trial among 11 male and 19 female symptomatic lactose malabsorbing adults [166]. Results showed that beta-galactosidase obtained from *K. lactis* in two different concentrations (3000 or 6000 U) both significantly reduced breath hydrogen production and the symptom score when compared to the placebo, with slightly better improvement when the lactase enzyme was added to milk 10 hours prior to consumption rather than at mealtime. Although purchasing lactose-free milk may be more practical than adding exogenous lactase enzymes to milk, prehydrolyzing milk at mealtime or prior to mealtime is useful when away from home or when lactose-free milk is not available.

Lactose-reduced milk is prepared at a processing plant by adding the liquid enzyme to previously pasteurized milk and holding for 24 hours. When the appropriate level of reduction has been reached, usually 70%, the milk is pasteurized again to stop lactose hydrolysis [168]. Milk that has 99.9% of its lactose hydrolyzed, labeled "lactose free", is now available on the market [169]. A milk labeled "lactose-reduced" must contain at least 70% less lactose than regular milk [170]. In addition to lactose-reduced milk, a variety of other lactose-reduced dairy products are now on the market.

Lactose-hydrolyzed milk and an oral enzyme tablet taken with milk were evaluated along with milk, acidophilus milk, and yogurt for their effectiveness in facilitating lactose digestion and for their acceptability [155]. Acidophilus milk induced the greatest rise in breath hydrogen production, followed by whole milk, whole milk plus a lactase tablet, hydrolyzed-lactose milk, and yogurt, respectively. Even though yogurt was the most effective at reducing breath hydrogen production compared to exogenous lactase products, the study subjects did not like it as well as milk.

Acceptability of hydrolyzed-lactose milk did not differ significantly from yogurt. While some found yogurt unacceptable because of its tart taste, others gave hydrolyzed-lactose milk a lower rating due to its sweetness [155]. When lactose is hydrolyzed into glucose and galactose, the free glucose makes the product taste slightly sweeter. Children have found lactose-hydrolyzed milk quite acceptable for this reason [171]. At least a 50% reduction of lactose content in milk is adequate to relieve symptoms of lactose intolerance in a majority of lactose maldigesters [172]. Those more sensitive to lactose (e.g., those with secondary lactose intolerance) may need lactose-free milk or additional lactase tablets to relieve symptoms.

Controlled clinical trials among lactose maldigesters have helped put the practical significance of this condition into perspective, and have fostered the development of several simple strategies listed below that allow those with low lactase activity to consume dairy foods without experiencing unpleasant symptoms. Health professionals can help individuals with lactase deficiency understand that even if they have experienced symptoms after consuming a generous serving of milk in the past, avoiding milk will only perpetuate their intolerance, as the colonic bacteria will not be adapted to efficiently ferment lactose [79].

Management Strategies for Those with Lactose Intolerance

1. Drink milk in servings of one cup or less.
2. Drink milk with a meal or with other food.
3. Try whole or chocolate milk.
4. Try natural aged cheese. Much of the lactose is removed during processing.
5. Try yogurt with active cultures.
6. Use milk and other dairy foods that are lactose-reduced or lactose-free.
7. Prepare lactose-reduced milk at home using an enzyme preparation.
8. Use an oral lactase supplement with your first bite or sip of dairy foods.

8.7.6 Colonic Adaptation

Although continued exposure to lactose does not induce the intestinal synthesis of the lactase enzyme, there is evidence that adaptation to lactose occurs in the colon. This phenomenon was first noted in the 1950s when supplemental milk feeding programs for preschool and school-aged children were initiated as part of global relief efforts. When milk was first introduced, it was sometimes associated with complaints of diarrhea and gastrointestinal discomfort. However, these complaints soon stopped as the program continued. This phenomenon was initially explained as a child's psychological reaction to an unfamiliar food. An early clinical trial, however, demonstrated that continued lactose intake increases the amount of lactose tolerated without symptoms, and without change in intestinal lactase activity [173].

Clinical trials have demonstrated that the colonic flora of persons with limited lactase digestion adapts to continued milk intakes. Twenty-five African American adolescents and young adults, who were confirmed lactose maldigesters and intolerant to the amount of lactose in one glass of milk (12 g), were given gradually increasing amounts of lactose in milk (beginning at 5 g) over a period of time until their maximum level of tolerance was determined [174]. Of the 22 subjects who completed the study, 77% tolerated >12 g of lactose (the amount in 8 ounces or 240 ml of milk) without disturbing symptoms. All individuals were able to adapt to >7 g of lactose, the amount in 150 ml of milk. Objective testing of breath hydrogen production revealed that a majority of the subjects continued to maldigest the lactose dose they tolerated. In a controlled feeding study conducted at Purdue University, 17 adolescent African American girls, 14 of whom were diagnosed as having lactose maldigestion, consumed a dairy-rich diet that provided 1200 mg of calcium and 33 g of lactose per day for 21 days [175]. Among the maldigesters, there was a significant decrease in the amount of hydrogen produced on day 21 when compared to day 1 of the study, indicating colonic adaptation (Figure 8.9). Dairy foods were consumed at each meal and often at snack times. The diet was well tolerated by all subjects throughout the study, with minimal or nonexistent symptoms reported during the lactose challenges. The researchers concluded that lactose maldigestion should not be a restricting factor in developing adequate calcium diets in this population.

Hertzler and Savaiano conducted a two-part blinded, controlled crossover trial to determine the effect of continued lactose feeding on: (1) the ability of fecal bacteria to metabolize lactose, and (2) the symptomatic response to lactose [176]. Results from the first part of the study indicated that lactose feeding altered the ability of fecal bacteria to metabolize lactose. Fecal beta-galactosidase began to rise within 48 hours of beginning lactose feeding, and by 10 days had peaked at three times the control value. In part two of the study, subjects were given 0.6 g/kg body weight per day of lactose in water divided between breakfast, lunch, and dinner. This amount was increased by 0.2 g/kg increments every other day, up to a maximum of 1.0 g/kg per day. Subjects increased their intake of lactose over a 10-day period from an average of 42 to 70 g per day (equivalent to the amount of lactose in 800 to 1500 ml of milk). Symptoms in the lactose group were not significantly different from the control group (fed dextrose), and did not increase from the beginning to the end of the lactose feeding period, even though the lactose dose was nearly doubled. In fact, a breath hydrogen test, administered at the end of the study, indicated that the subjects had no increase in breath hydrogen. The authors conclude that adaptation of the colonic flora offers a simpler and less expensive solution for subjects who wish to consume large amounts of lactose-containing foods on a regular basis.

A double-blind study conducted by researchers in France among severely intolerant (all experienced diarrhea) Asian subjects, also demonstrated metabolic adaptation and reduction of symptoms (except diarrhea) to lactose in water feeding (17 g twice daily) over 13 days [177]. The control group (fed sucrose) also reported fewer symptoms, though they did not demonstrate biochemical adaptation (e.g., increased fecal beta-galactosidase activity, lower pH, and decreased breath hydrogen), as did the group fed lactose. The authors suggest that improved clinical tolerance may sometimes be the result of becoming familiar with the test procedures.

The mechanism by which adaptation occurs is not completely understood; however, the following mechanisms have been proposed: (1) The presence of unhydrolyzed lactose in the colon stimulates organic acid production which lowers the pH, inhibiting further fermentation and hydrogen production, (2) undigested lactose may alter the composition of colonic bacteria

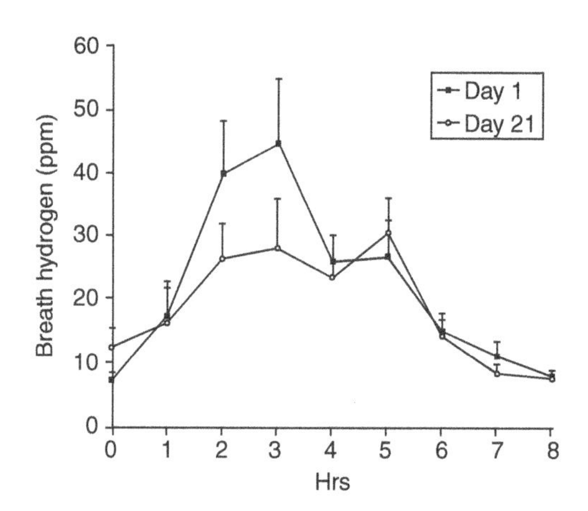

FIGURE 8.9 A comparison of the amount of total hydrogen produced over 8 hours at the time of experiment 1 and experiment 2, after the subjects had been on a controlled high-lactose diet for 21 days. Hydrogen production was measured in parts per milion (ppm). Data points represent the mean hydrogen production per hour + SEM, $n = 14$. $^*P < .03$. (From Pribila, B. A., *J. Am. Diet. Assoc.*, 100, 524, 2000. With permission.)

by reducing the number of gas-forming bacteria in favor of nongas-producing organisms, or (3) lactose in the colon stimulates colonic bacterial fermentation and the removal of end products [174].

Theoretically, a reduction in breath hydrogen after continued lactose feeding could be either the result of decreased absolute hydrogen production or increased hydrogen consumption by colonic bacteria. Using a technique that distinguishes production from consumption, Hertzler et al. established that lactose feeding decreased absolute hydrogen production, possibly by stimulating the proliferation of bacterial species such as bifidobacteria, which ferment lactose without producing hydrogen [178]. Jiang and Savaiano, simulating lactose adaptation *in vitro*, found that supplementation of the culture medium with *Lactobacillus acidophilus* enhanced lactose utilization, during the first day [160]. They conclude that *L. acidophilus* may enhance lactose fermentation in the colon during the early period of lactose feeding before adaptation is established.

8.8 TREATMENT OF MALNUTRITION/DIARRHEAL DISEASE IN CHILDREN

Diarrheal illness and accompanying dehydration accounts for a large proportion of childhood illness and expense, as well as preventable childhood deaths in the United States [179]. The use of oral rehydration solutions to treat diarrheal illness has reduced children's death rates worldwide. After appropriate rehydration therapy, data support the use of lactose-containing milks during diarrhea, especially if given with carbohydrates [179]. Diarrhea caused by most common organisms is self-limiting, and rarely persists for more than 4 to 5 days. Even during acute infectious enteritis, the gut retains a significant capacity to assimilate nutrients [180]. During this phase, the goal of nutritional management is to maintain hydration status and prevent starvation in the malnourished infant; the number and character of stools should not guide management [180]. According to current recommendations, when diarrhea is not accompanied by dehydration (as is usually the case), age-appropriate feeding is the only therapy required [179]. Nonweaned infants should receive breast milk or regular infant formula. Formula should not be diluted if diarrhea is mild. If diluted formula is used, it is important to increase the concentration rapidly if diarrhea does not worsen. Weaned infants and children should be fed their regular nutritionally balanced diet, emphasizing complex carbohydrates (i.e., rice, wheat, potatoes), meats, and regular milk or formula [179].

A meta-analysis of 29 randomized clinical trials evaluating the use of nonhuman milks or formulas in the dietary management of acute diarrhea in children found that those who continued to receive lactose-containing milk diets had a treatment failure rate of about 10%. The authors conclude, "the vast majority of young children with acute diarrhea can safely continue to receive undiluted, nonhuman milk" [181].

A lactose-free infant formula may be needed if stool output increases on a milk-based diet [179]. Infants or children with secondary lactose intolerance due to gastrointestinal diseases leading to villus atrophy such as Crohn's disease or protein-sensitive enteropathy may benefit from a protein-hydrolyzed formula [182].

Children with severe protein energy malnutrition (PEM) commonly have reduced activity of intestinal lactase due to nutritional injury and infection [124]. Milk has been used extensively along with other protein sources in refeeding programs aimed at reversing PEM. A study involving 20 Guatemalan preschool children with PEM demonstrated that lactose-hydrolyzed milk offered no advantages over lactose-containing milk in recovery from PEM [183]. The group receiving intact lactose experienced more diarrhea, but recovery was satisfactory in both groups during the 45-day refeeding period, with no differences in rates of growth, body protein repletion, restoration of energy reserves or intestinal function. A study of malnourished Senegalese children age 6 to 36 months demonstrated that fermented milk may also be useful in the treatment of malnourished children with acute diarrhea and sugar intolerance [184].

8.9 RECOMMENDATIONS FOR FEEDING PROGRAMS

The American Academy of Pediatrics stated the following position in 1978, which was reaffirmed in 1990: "On the basis of present evidence it would be inappropriate to discourage supplemental milk feeding programs targeted at children on the basis of primary lactose intolerance" [125].

8.9.1 INTERNATIONAL

Milk can provide an inexpensive source of carbohydrate, protein and calcium to children in countries where protein-calorie malnutrition is prevalent. In Gambia, West Africa, for example, growth failure and undernutrition is common, as is lactose maldigestion after the second year of life. In a study involving Gambian children, lactose maldigestion was not associated with growth failure. Consumption of cow's milk was common among the children and was rarely associated with any adverse effects [185]. The authors recommend that cow's milk be given to Gambian children after weaning as a means of supplementing their diet.

As discussed in the section on adaptation, children who receive milk as part of a supplemental feeding program usually tolerate it quite well. Powdered fermented milk might also be a viable option for providing supplemental milk to children in countries where there is a high prevalence of lactase deficiency [186]. When 25 Gabonese lactase-deficient children consumed 150 ml of powdered fermented milk formula containing 10.5 g lactose, breath hydrogen production was reduced to normal levels and symptoms of intolerance were reduced by one-third, when compared to a regular milk formula. Since this product may be purchased in dry powdered form, it has advantages for use in developing countries where refrigeration may not be available.

8.9.2 UNITED STATES

Supplemental feeding programs in the United States, such as the National School Lunch Program (NSLP), the National School Breakfast Program (NSBP), and the Women, Infants and Children Supplemental Food Program (WIC), serve clients with a variety of ethnic backgrounds. While many schools serve populations where lactose maldigestion is common, milk is not contraindicated, and dairy products are included as part of the standard meal plan. Nearly all children with low lactase activity can tolerate the 8 ounces of milk required in the school meal pattern, especially since it is served with a meal.

After the age of eight, milk intake decreases in some student populations, increasing the chance of clinical consequences [187]. Therefore, it may be beneficial for schools serving such populations to make available a selection of dairy foods, such as aged cheese, yogurt, whole milk, and chocolate milk. Yogurt was approved for use in school meals as a meat alternate [188].

Under the Child Nutrition and WIC Reauthorization Act of 2004, "Lunches served by schools participating in the school lunch program shall offer students fluid milk in variety of fat contents and may offer students flavored and unflavored fluid milk and lactose-free fluid milk"[189]. For students who cannot consume fluid milk because of a medical or other special dietary need, a school may substitute a nondairy beverage that is nutritionally equivalent to fluid milk and meets nutritional standards established by the Secretary of Agriculture, including fortification of calcium, protein, vitamin A, and vitamin D to levels found in cow's milk. The substitution must be requested by a written statement of a medical authority or by a student's parent or legal guardian. Any additional costs of substitute foods must be born by the school. However, schools could offer lactose-free milk instead of instituting a specific substitute beverage policy [189].

Cultural food values, rather than lactose intolerance, is the main factor affecting acceptance of dairy products among WIC participants, according to a review of WIC food packages conducted by a panel of researchers at The Pennsylvania State University [190]. Nevertheless, the panel felt there are valid scientific reasons for accommodating food preferences — whether they have a biological or cultural basis. The Institute of Medicine conducted a scientific review of the supplemental foods available for the Special Supplemental Nutrition Program for Women, Infants, and Children (WIC) and issued a final report, WIC Food Packages: Time for a Change, on April 25, 2005 [190]. The recommendations in the IOM report for the amount of milk to be provided in WIC food packages are consistent with the 2005 *Dietary Guidelines for Americans*. To accommodate cultural food preferences as well as persons with lactose maldigestion, the IOM report proposes that allowed foods include fat-reduced yogurt as a partial substitute for fluid milk for women and children, calcium-set tofu and calcium- and vitamin D-fortified soy beverage as partial milk substitutes for women. The Secretary shall promulgate a final rule updating the prescribed supplemental foods available through the program not later than 18 months after the date of receiving the IOM review [190].

8.10 FUTURE RESEARCH NEEDS

Active areas of research currently include the genetic regulation of lactase gene expression in the human intestine [30] and studies aimed at identifying strains of bacterial cultures in fermented and nonfermented dairy foods that will aid the hydrolysis of lactose *in vivo* most effectively [140]. Knowledge of bacterial cultures will lead to the development of new, more effective products [140]. A further understanding of how the colon adapts to continued milk intakes is important; this will allow development of protocols for encouraging milk intake in those with lactase nonpersistence. Research is needed to identify behavioral strategies to encourage dairy food consumption among those who maldigest lactose. More can be done to educate practitioners and the public about appropriate diagnosis and treatment strategies available for those with lactose intolerance [56].

8.11 CONCLUSION

Lactose intolerance, whether real or perceived, causes individuals to reduce or eliminate milk and milk products from their diets. Tolerance to dairy foods can be improved by following the simple strategies outlined in this chapter. Research has shown that current calcium recommendations can be met through the strategic use of dairy foods by most people who have low lactase levels. A low intake of milk and milk products has been shown to increase the risk of osteoporosis, hypertension, obesity, and some forms of cancer. Overcoming the barrier of lactose intolerance by using the simple dietary strategies that follow could have an important positive effect on overall health, and is one way to contribute toward reducing existing health disparities. Health professionals should be prepared to counsel patients with lactose maldigestion about the strategies they can employ so that dairy avoidance will seldom be necessary.

Future research will extend our knowledge in the areas of genetics and in the development of new dairy products that will be well tolerated by those with low lactase activity. Nearly all children and most adults should be encouraged to benefit from the nutritional value of milk — even if lactose intolerance limits the quantities of milk they can consume at one time, or the forms in which they may enjoy dairy products.

GLOSSARY OF TERMS

Lactase Beta-galactosidase, an enzyme of the hydrolase class that catalyzes the hydrolysis (digestion) of lactose, a disaccharide, into its monosaccharide components of glucose and galactose. Lactase is present on the brush border of the intestinal mucosa where such digestion takes place.

Lactase nonpersistence Refers to the decrease in lactase activity that occurs after weaning. This characteristic is transmitted as an autosomal-recessive trait.

Lactase persistence Refers to the retention of significant intestinal lactase into adulthood. This characteristic is transmitted as an autosomal-dominant trait.

Low lactase activity or hypolactasia Low levels of the intestinal enzyme, lactase, in the brush border membrane. Low lactase activity (lactase deficiency) can be measured directly by small bowel biopsy, or indirectly using the lactose tolerance test or the breath hydrogen test.
Lactose A disaccharide which yields upon hydrolysis the monosaccharides glucose and galactose. Since milk is the sole natural source of lactose, it is commonly referred to as *milk sugar*.
Lactose intolerance The clinical signs and symptoms, which include bloating, flatulence, abdominal pain, and diarrhea, following consumption of a dose of lactose greater than the body's ability to digest and absorb. "Tolerance" and "intolerance" are not synonymous with "digestion" and "maldigestion" and should be used only in reference to a defined dose of lactose delivered in a specific vehicle (i.e., the subject was intolerant to 50 g of lactose in aqueous solution).
Congenital lactase deficiency A rare genetic abnormality in which the enzyme lactase is very low or absent at birth.
Primary lactase deficiency The normal developmental decrease in lactase activity beyond the age of weaning.

TABLE 8.6
Lactose Content of Dairy Products

Product	Lactose (g)
Milk (1 cup)	
Whole	9 to 12
2%	9 to 13
1%	12 to 13
Skim	11 to 14
Chocolate	10 to 12
Buttermilk	9 to 12
Evaporated	24 to 28
Sweetened condensed	31 to 50
[a]Lactaid (lactose-reduced low-fat milk)	3
Goat's milk	11 to 12
Acidophilus, skim	11
Yogurt, low-fat (1 cup)	4 to 17
Cheese (1 oz)	
Cottage (1/2 cup)	0.7 to 4
Cheddar, sharp	0.4 to 0.6
Swiss	0.5 to 1
Mozzarella, part skim, low moisture	0.08 to 0.09
American, pasteurized, processed	0.5 to 4
Ricotta (1/2 cup)	0.3 to 6
Cream	0.1 to 0.8
Butter (1 pat)	0.04 to 0.05
Cream (1 tbsp)	
Light	0.6
Whipping	0.4 to 0.5
Sour	0.4 to 0.5
Ice Cream (1/2 cup)	2 to 6
Ice Milk (1/2 cup)	5
Sherbet (1/2 cup)	0.6 to 2

[a] Bowes & Church's *Food Values of Portions Commonly Used*, Jean A. Pennington, 1989.

Source: Scrimshaw, N.S. and Murray, E. B., *Am. J. Clin. Nut.*, (suppl. 48), 4, 1988. With permission.

Secondary lactase deficiency Temporary low levels of the lactase enzyme due to an underlying disease or medical condition affecting the gastrointestinal tract, such as gastroenteritis, tropical sprue, recovery from gastrointestinal surgery, radiation therapy, or certain drugs.
Lactose maldigestion Reduced digestion of lactose due to low lactase activity.
Milk intolerance due to lactose One or more clinical signs of abdominal pain, bloating, flatulence, or diarrhea experienced a few hours after ingestion of a known quantity of milk or milk-containing products in a person with proven lactose maldigestion. (Table 8.6).

REFERENCES

1. National Digestive Diseases Information Clearinghouse (NDDIC), *Lactose Intolerance*, NIH Publication No. 03-2751, Bethesda, MD: National Digestive Diseases Information Clearinghouse, March 2003.
2. Scrimshaw, N. S. and Murray, E. B., The acceptability of milk and milk products in populations with a high prevalence of lactose intolerance, *Am. J. Clin. Nutr.*, 48 (suppl. 4), 1988.
3. Johnson, J. D., Kretchmer, N., and Simoons, F. J., Lactose malabsorption: its biology and history, in *Advances in Pediatrics*, Schulman, I., Ed., 21, Yearbook Medical Publishers, Chicago, p. 197, 1974.
4. Holden, C. and Mace, R., Phylogenetic analysis of the evolution of lactose digestion in adults, *Hum. Biol.*, 69 (5), 605, 1997.
5. Bloom, G. and Sherman, P. W., Dairying barriers affect the distribution of lactose malabsorption, *Evol. Hum. Behav.*, 26 (4), 301, 2005.
6. Kretchmer, N., The significance of lactose intolerance: an overview, in *Lactose Digestion: Clinical and Nutritional Implications*, Paige, D. M. and Bayless, T. M., Eds., The Johns Hopkins University Press, Baltimore and London, 1981, chap. 1.
7. Bayless, T. M. and Rosensweig, N. S., A racial difference in incidence of lactase deficiency, *J. Am. Med. Assoc.*, 197, 968, 1966.
8. Vesa, T. H., Marteau, P., and Korpela, R., Lactose Intolerance, *J. Am. Coll. Nutr.*, 19 (2), 154S, 2000.
9. Suarez, F. and Levitt, M. D., Abdominal symptoms and lactose: the discrepancy between patients' claims and the results of blinded trials, *Am. J. Clin. Nutr.*, 64, 251, 1996.
10. Heaney, R. P., Calcium intake and the prevention of chronic discasc: from osteoporosis to premenstrual syndrome, in *Frontiers in Nutrition*, Wilson, T. and Temple, N., Eds., Humana Press, Totowa, NJ, 2000.
11. Wooten, W. J. and Price, W., Consensus report of the National Medical Association: the role of dairy and dairy nutrients in the diet of African Americans, *J. Natl Med. Assoc.*, 96 (suppl. 12), 2002.
12. Byers, K. G. and Savaiano, D. A., The myth of increased lactose intolerance among African Americans, *J. Am. Coll. Nutr.*, 24 (6), 569S, 2005.
13. McBean, L. D. and Miller, G. D., Allaying fears and fallacies about lactose intolerance, *J. Am. Diet. Assoc.*, 98 (6), 671, 1998.
14. Jarvis, J. K. and Miller, G. D., Overcoming the barrier of lactose intolerance to reduce health disparities, *J. Natl Med. Assoc.*, 94, 55, 2002.
15. Saavedra, J. M. and Perman, J. A., Current concepts in lactose malabsorption and intolerance, *Ann. Rev. Nutr.*, 9, 475, 1989.
16. Torun, B., Solomons, N. W., and Viteri, F. E., Lactose malabsorption and lactose intolerance: implications for general milk consumption, *Archivos Latinoamericanos De Nutricion*, 29 (4), 446, 1979.
17. Troncon, L. E. et al., Gastric emptying of lactose and glucose–galactose in patients with low intestinal lactase activity, *Arquivos De Gastroenterologia*, 20 (1), 8, 1983.
18. Grand, R. J., Watkins, J. B., and Torti, F. T., Development of the human gastrointestinal tract: a review, *Gastroenterology*, 70, 790, 1976.
19. Shulman, R. J., Wong, W. W., and Smith, E. O., Influence of changes in lactase activity and small-intestinal mucosal growth on lactose digestion and absorption in preterm infants, *Am. J. Clin. Nutr.*, 81 (2), 472, 2005.
20. Kien, C. L., McClead, R. E., and Leandro, C., *In vivo* lactose digestion in preterm infants, *Am. J. Clin. Nutr.*, 64, 700, 1996.

21. MacLean, W. C. Jr. and Fink, B. B., Lactose malabsorption by premature infants: magnitude and clinical significance, *J. Ped.*, 97, 383, 1980.
22. Lifschitz, C. H., Smith, E. O., and Garza, C., Delayed complete functional lactase sufficiency in breast-fed infants, *J. Ped. Gastroenterol. Nutr.*, 2 (3), 478, 1983.
23. Olds, L. C. and Sibley, E., Lactase persistence DNA variant enhances lactase promoter activity *in vitro:* functional role as a *cis* regulatory element, *Hum. Mol. Genet.*, 12 (18), 2333, 2003.
24. Gilat, T., Russo, S., Gelman-Malachi, E., and Aldor, T. A., Lactase in man: a non-adaptable enzyme, *Gastroenterology*, 62, 1125, 1972.
25. Lee, M.-F. and Krasinski, S. D., Human adult-onset lactase decline: an update, *Nutr. Rev.*, 56 (1), 1, 1998.
26. Swallow, D. M., Genetics of lactase persistence and lactose intolerance, *Annu. Rev. Genet.*, 37, 197, 2003.
27. Rossi, M. et al., Lactase persistence versus decline in human adults: multifactorial events are involved in down-regulation after weaning, *Gastroenterology*, 112, 1506, 1997.
28. Hauri, H.-P., Sander, B., and Naim, H., Induction of lactase biosynthesis in the human intestinal epithelial cell line Caco-2, *Eur. J. Biochem.*, 219, 539, 1994.
29. Van Beers, E. et al., Lactase and sucrase-isomaltase gene expression during Caco-2 cell differentiation, *J. Biochem.*, 308, 769, 1995.
30. Rings, E. H. H. M. et al., Origin, gene expression, localization, and function, *Nutr. Res.*, 14 (5), 775, 1994.
31. Enattah, N. S. et al., Identification of a variant associated with adult-type hypolactasia, *Nature Genet.*, 30, 233, 2002.
32. Obermayer-Pietsch, B. M. et al., Genetic predisposition for adult lactose intolerance and relation to diet, bone density, and bone fractures, *J. Bone Miner. Res.*, 19, 42, 2004.
33. Rusynyk, R. A. and Still, C. D., Lactose intolerance, *JAOA*, 101 (4), S10, 2001.
34. Solomons, N. W., Diagnosis and screening techniques for lactose maldigestion: advantages of the hydrogen breath test, in *Lactose Digestion: Clinical and Nutritional Implications*, Paige, D. M. and Bayless, T. M., Eds., The Johns Hopkins University Press, Baltimore and London, p. 105, 1981, chap. 8.
35. American Academy of Pediatrics, Committee on Nutrition, Soy protein-based formulas: recommendations for use in infant feeding, *Pediatrics*, 101 (1), 148, 1998.
36. Aurisicchio, L. N. and Pitchumoni, C. S., Lactose intolerance: recognizing the link between diet and discomfort, *Postgrad. Med.*, 95 (1), 113, 1994.
37. Sahi, T., Genetics and epidemiology of adult-type hypolactasia, *Scand. J. Gastroenterol.*, 29 (suppl. 202), 7, 1994.
38. Jackson, K. A. and Savaiano, D. A., Lactose maldigestion, calcium intake and osteoporosis in African-, Asian-, and Hispanic-Americans, *J. Am. Coll. Nutr.*, 20 (2), 198S, 2001.
39. American Academy of Pediatrics, Practical significance of lactose intolerance in children: supplement, *Pediatrics*, 86 (4), 643, 1990.
40. Suarez, F. L. and Savaiano, D. A., Lactose digestion and tolerance in adult and elderly Asian-Americans, *Am. J. Clin. Nutr.*, 59, 1021, 1994.
41. Rana, S. V. et al., Lactose maldigestion in different age groups of north Indians, *Trop. Gastroenterol.*, 25 (1), 18, 2004.
42. Di Stefano, M. et al., Lactose malabsorption and intolerance in the elderly, *Scand. J. Gastroenterol.*, 12, 1274, 2001.
43. Pettoello-Mantovani, M. et al., Prospective study of lactose absorption during cancer chemotherapy: feasibility of a yogurt-supplemented diet in lactose malabsorbers, *J. Ped. Gastroenterol. Nutr.*, 20, 189, 1995.
44. American Dietic Association/Dietitians of Canada, *Manual of Clinical Dietetics,* 2000.
45. Enck, P. et al., Prevalence of lactose malabsorption among patients with functional bowel disorders, *Z. Gastroenterol.*, 28, 239, 1990.
46. Parker, T. J. et al., Irritable bowel syndrome: is the search for lactose intolerance justified? *Eur. J. Gastroenterol. Hepatol.*, 13, 219, 2001.
47. Mishkin, S., Dairy sensitivity, lactose malabsorption, and elimination diets in inflammatory bowel disease, *Am. J. Clin. Nutr.*, 65, 564, 1997.

48. Tolliver, B. A. et al., Does lactose maldigestion really play a role in the irritable bowel? *J. Clin. Gastroenterol.*, 23 (1), 15, 1996.
49. Montes, R. G. and Perman, J. A., Lactose intolerance: pinpointing the sources of nonspecific gastrointestinal symptoms, *Postgrad. Med.*, 89 (8), 175, 1991.
50. Martens, R. A. and Martens, S., *The Milk Sugar Dilemma: Living with Lactose Intolerance*, Medi-Ed Press, Lansing, MI, 1987.
51. Zhong, Y. et al., The role of colonic microbiota in lactose intolerance, *Dig. Dis. Sci.*, 49 (1), 78, 2004.
52. Krause, J., Kaltbeitzer, I., and Erckenbrecht, J. F., Lactose malabsorption produces more symptoms in women than in men, (Abstr.), *Gastroenterology*, 110 (suppl.), A339, 1996.
53. Husby, S., Halken, S., and Host, A., Food allergy, in *Nutrition and Immunology*, Klurfeld, D., Ed., Plenum Press, New York, p. 25, 1993.
54. Bock, S. A., Prospective appraisal of complaints of adverse reactions to foods in children during the first 3 years of life, *Pediatrics*, 79, 683, 1987.
55. Thong, B. Y. and Hourihane, J. O., Monitoring of IgE-mediated food allergy in childhood, *Acta Paediatr.*, 93 (6), 759, 2004.
56. Lovelace, H. Y. and Barr, S. I., Diagnosis, symptoms, and calcium intakes of individuals with self-reported lactose intolerance, *J. Am. Coll. Nutr.*, 24 (1), 51, 2005.
57. Suarez, F. L., Savaiano, D. A., and Levitt, M. D., A comparison of symptoms with self-reported severe lactose intolerance after drinking milk or lactose-hydrolyzed milk, *N. Engl. J. Med.*, 333, 1, 1995.
58. Suarez, F. L., Savaiano, D., Arbisi, P., and Levitt, M. D., Tolerance to the daily ingestion of two cups of milk by individuals claiming lactose intolerance, *Am. J. Clin. Nutr.*, 65, 1502, 1997.
59. Johnson, A. O. et al., Correlation of lactose maldigestion, lactose tolerance, and milk intolerance, *Am. J. Clin. Nutr.*, 57, 399, 1993.
60. Haverberg, L., Kwon, P. H., and Scrimshaw, N. S., Comparative tolerance of adolescents of differing ethnic backgrounds to lactose-containing and lactose-free dairy drinks, I. Initial experience with a double-blind procedure, *Am. J. Clin. Nutr.*, 33, 17, 1980.
61. Rorick, M. H. and Scrimshaw, N. S., Comparative tolerance of elderly from differing ethnic backgrounds to lactose-containing and lactose-free dairy drinks: a double-blind study, *J. Gerontol.*, 34 (2), 191, 1979.
62. Barr, R. G., Watkins, R. B., and Perman, J. A., Mucosal function and breath hydrogen excretion: comparative studies in the clinical evaluation of children with nonspecific abdominal complaints, *Pediatrics*, 68 (4), 526, 1981.
63. Casellas, F. and Malagelada, J. R., Applicability of short hydrogen breath test for screening of lactose malabsorption, *Dig. Dis. Sci.*, 48 (7), 1333, 2003.
64. Barr, R. G., Limitations of the hydrogen breath test and other techniques for predicting incomplete lactose absorption, in *Lactose Digestion: Clinical and Nutritional Implications*, Paige, D. M. and Bayless, T. M., Eds., The Johns Hopkins University Press, Baltimore and London, 1981, chap. 9.
65. Bayless, T. M., Lactose malabsorption, milk intolerance, and symptom awareness in adults, in *Lactose Digestion: Clinical and Nutritional Implications*, Paige, D. M. and Bayless, T. M., Eds., The Johns Hopkins University Press, Baltimore and London, 1981, chap. 10.
66. Distefano, M. et al., Hydrogen breath test in the diagnosis of lactose malabsorption: accuracy of new versus conventional criteria, *J. Lab. Clin. Med.*, 144 (6), 313, 2004.
67. Buller, H. A. and Grand, R. J., Lactose intolerance, *Ann. Rev. Med.*, 41, 141, 1990.
68. Hogenauer, C. et al., Evaluation of a new DNA test compared with the lactose hydrogen breath test for the diagnosis of lactase non-persistence, *Eur. J. Gastroenterol. Hepatol.*, 17 (3), 371, 2005.
69. Buning, C. et al., Introducing genetic testing for adult-type hypolactasia, *Digestion*, 71 (4), 245, 2005.
70. Ridefelt, P. and Hakansson, L. D., Lactose intolerance: lactose tolerance test versus genotyping, *Scan. J. Gastroenterol.*, 40 (7), 822, 2005.
71. Martini, M. C. and Savaianno, D. A., Reduced intolerance symptoms from lactose consumed during a meal, *Am. J. Clin. Nutr.*, 47, 57, 1988.
72. Villako, K. and Maaroos, H., Clinical picture of hypolactasia and lactose intolerance, *Scand. J. Gastroenterol.*, 29 (suppl. 202), 36, 1994.

73. Hertzler, F. R., Huynh, B.-C.L., and Savaianno, D. A., How much lactose is low lactose?, *J. Am. Diet. Assoc.*, 96, 243, 1996.
74. Newcomer, A. D., McGill, D. B., Thomas, P. J., and Hoffman, A. F., Tolerance to lactose among lactase-deficient American Indians, *Gastroenterol.*, 74, 44, 1978.
75. Newcomer, A., Immediate sympotomatic and long-term nutritional consequences of hypolactasia, in *Lactose digestion: Clinical and nutritional implications*, Paige, D. M. and Bayless, T. M., Eds., The Johns Hopkins University Press, Baltimore and London, 1981, chap. 11.
76. Suarez, F. L. et al., Lactose maldigesters tolerate ingestion of a dairy-rich diet containing approximately 1500 mg calcium/day, *Am. J.Clin. Nutr.*, 68 (5), 1118, 1998.
77. Food and Nutrition Board/Institute of Medicine, *Dietary Reference Intakes for Calcium, Phosphorus, Magnesium, Vitamin D, and Fluoride, Uncorrected Proofs*, National Academy Press, Washington, D.C., 1997.
78. U.S. Department of Health and Human Services, Public Health Service, National Institutes of Health, *Consensus Development Conference Statement. Optimal Calcium Intake*, June 6–8; 12 (4), 1, 1994.
79. Savaiano, D., Lactose intolerance: a self-fulfilling prophecy leading to osteoporosis? *Nutr. Rev.*, 61 (6), 221, 2003.
80. Villar, J. et al., Improved lactose digestion during pregnancy: a case of physiologic adaptation? *Obstet. Gynecol.*, 71 (5), 697, 1988.
81. Szilagyi, A. et al., Lactose handling by women with lactose malabsorption is improved during pregnancy, *Clin. Investeg. Med.*, 19 (6), 416, 1996.
82. Paige, D. M. et al., Lactose intolerance in pregnant African American women, *J. Am. Coll. Nutr.*, 16 5 (Abstract 69), 488, 1997.
83. Paige, D. M. et al., Lactose digestion in pregnant African Americans, *Public Health Nutrition*, 6 (8), 801–807, 2003.
84. Leichter, J., Effects of lactose on the absorption of other nutrients: implications in lactose-intolerant adults, in *Lactose Digestion: Clinical and Nutritional Implications*, Paige, D. M. and Bayless, T. M., Eds., The John Hopkins University Press, Baltimore and London, 1981, chap. 13.
85. Buchowski, M. S. and Miller, D. D., Lactose, calcium source, and age affect calcium bioavailability in rats, *J. Nutr.*, 121, 1746, 1991.
86. Ziegler, E. E. and Foman, S. J., Lactose enhances mineral absorption in infancy, *J. Ped. Gastroenterol. Nutr.*, 2, 288, 1983.
87. Miller, D. D., Calcium in the diet: food sources, recommended intakes, and nutritional bioavailability, *Adv. Food Nutr. Res.*, 33, 103, 1989.
88. Tremaine, W. J. et al., Calcium absorption from milk in lactase-deficient and lactase-sufficient adults, *Dig. Dis. Sci.*, 31 (4), 376, 1986.
89. Horowitz, M. et al., Lactose and calcium absorption in postmenopausal osteoporosis, *Arch. Inter. Med.*, 147, 534, 1987.
90. Griessen, M. et al., Calcium absorption from milk in lactase-deficient subjects, *Am. J. Clin. Nutr.*, 49, 377, 1989.
91. Garza, C. and Scrimshaw, N. S., Relationship of lactose intolerance to milk intolerance in young children, *Am. J. Clin. Nutr.*, 29, 192, 1976.
92. Rosado, J. L., Allen, L. H., and Solomons, N. W., Milk consumption, symptom response, and lactose digestion in milk intolerance, *Am. J. Clin. Nutr.*, 45, 1457, 1987.
93. Kudlacek, S. et al., Lactose intolerance: a risk factor for reduced bone mineral density and vertebral fractures? *J. Gastroenterol.*, 37, 1014, 2002.
94. Buchowski, M. S., Semenya, J., and Johnson, A. O., Dietary calcium intake in lactose maldigesting intolerant and tolerant African American women, *J. Am. Coll. Nutr.*, 21 (1), 47, 2002.
95. Finkenstedt, G. et al., Lactose absorption, milk consumption, and fasting blood glucose concentrations in women with idiopathic osteoporosis, *Br. Med. J.*, 292 (6514), 161, 1986.
96. Newcomer, A. D., Hodgson, S. F., and McGill, D. B., Lactase deficiency: prevalence in osteoporosis, *Ann. Int. Med.*, 89, 218, 1978.
97. Barger-Lux, M. J. et al., Nutritional correlates of low calcium intake, *Clin. Appl. Nutr.*, 2 (4), 39, 1992.

98. Fleming, K. and Heimbach, J. R., Availability and consumption of calcium in the U.S.: levels and sources, *J. Nutr.*, 124 (suppl. 8), 1426S, 1994.
99. Karanja, N. et al., Impact of increasing calcium in the diet on nutrient consumption, plasma lipids, and lipoproteins in humans, *Am. J. Clin. Nutr.*, 59, 900, 1994.
100. Varela-Moreairas, G. et al., Effects of yogurt and fermented-then-pasteurized milk on lactose absorption in an institutionalized elderly group, *J. Am. Coll. Nutr.*, 11 (2), 168, 1992.
101. U.S. Department of Health and Human Services, *Bone Health and Osteoporosis: A Report of the U.S. Surgeon General*, U.S. Department of Health and Human Services, Office of the Surgeon General, Rockville, MD, 2004, www.surgcongeneral.gov/library.
102. Zemel, M. B., Role of calcium and dairy products in energy partitioning and weight management, *Am. J. Clin. Nutr.*, 79 (5), 907S, 2004.
103. McCarron, D. A. and Heaney, R. P., Estimated healthcare savings associated with adequate dairy food intake, *Am. J. Hypertens.*, 17, 88, 2004.
104. Barger-Lux, M. J. and Heaney, R. P., The role of calcium intake in preventing bone fragility, hypertension, and certain cancers, *J. Nutr.*, 124, 1406s, 1994.
105. Wheadon, M. et al., Lactose malabsorption and calcium intake as a risk factor for osteoporosis in elderly New Zealand women, *N. Zealand Med. J.*, 104 (921), 417, 1991.
106. Jackson, K. A. and Savaiano, D. A., Lactose maldigestion, calcium intake and osteoporosis in African-, Asian-, and Hispanic-Americans, *J. Am. Coll. Nutr.*, 20 (2), 198S, 2001.
107. Honkanen, R. et al., Does lactose intolerance predispose to low bone density? A population-based study of perimenopausal finnish women, *Bone*, 19 (1), 23, 1996.
108. Corazza, G. R. et al., Lactose intolerance and bone mass in postmenopausal Italian women, *Br. J. Nutr.*, 73, 479, 1995.
109. Honkanen, R. et al., Lactose intolerance associated with fractures of weight-bearing bones in Finnish women aged 38–57 years, *Bone*, 21 (6), 473, 1997.
110. Laroche, M. et al., Lactose intolerance and osteoporosis in men, *Expansion Scientifique Francaise*, 62 (11), 766, 1995.
111. Enattah, N. et al., Genetically defined adult-type hypolactasia and self-reported lactose intolerance as risk factors of osteoporosis in Finnish postmenopausal women, *Eur. J. Clin. Nutr.*, 59, 1105, 2005.
112. The 7th Report of the Joint National Committee on Detection, Evaluation, and Treatment of High Blood Pressure (JNC-VII), *Hypertension*, 42, 1206, 2003.
113. USDA Center for Nutrition Policy and Promotion, *Nutrient Content of the U.S. Food Supply 1909–2000*, Home Economics Research Report, No. 56. November, 2004, www.usda.gov/cnpp/foodsupp.pdf.
114. Appel, I. J. et al., A clinical trial of the effects of dietary patterns on blood pressure, *N. Engl. J. Med.*, 336, 1117, 1997.
115. Svetkey, L. P. et al., Effects of dietary patterns on blood pressure: subgroup analysis of the dietary approaches to stop hypertension (DASH) randomized clinical trial, *Arch. Inter. Med.*, 159 (3), 285, 1999.
116. Vogt, T. M. et al., Dietary approaches to stop hypertension: rationale, design, and methods. DASH collaborative research group, *J. Am. Diet. Assoc.*, 99 (suppl. 8), S12, 1999.
117. Zemel, M. B. et al., Calcium and dairy acceleration of weight and fat loss during energy restriction in obese adults, *Obesity Res.*, 12, 582, 2004.
118. Zemel, M. B. et al., Effects of calcium and dairy on body composition and weight loss in African American adults, *Obesity Res.*, 13 (7), 1218, 2005.
119. Zemel, M. B. et al., Regulation of adiposity by dietary calcium, *FASEB J.*, 14, 1132, 2000.
120. Parodi, P. W., Cow's milk components with anti-cancer potential, *Austr. J. Dairy Technol.*, 56, 65, 2001.
121. Parodi, P. W., Cow's milk fat components as potential anticarcinogenic agents, *J. Nutr.*, 127, 1055, 1997.
122. Parodi, P. W., Anti-cancer agents in milkfat, *Austr. J. Dairy Technol.*, 58, 114, 2003.
123. Parodi, P. W., A role for milk proteins in cancer prevention, *Austr. J. Dairy Technol.*, 53, 37, 1998.
124. Dobler, M. L., *Lactose Intolerance-Revised Edition*, The American Dietetic Association, Chicago, 1991.

125. The American Academy of Pediatrics, Committee on Nutrition, Practical significance of lactose intolerance in children: supplement, *Pediatrics*, 86 (4), 643, 1978.
126. U.S. Department of Health and Human Services and U.S. Department of Agriculture, *Dietary Guidelines for Americans*, 2005, 6th ed., Washington, D.C., U.S. Government Printing Office, January, 2005, www.healthieurs.gov/dietaryguidelines.
127. Savaiano, D. A. and Kotz, C., Recent advances in the management of lactose intolerance, *Cont. Nutr.*, 13 (9,10), 1988.
128. Savaianno, D. A., Boushey, C. J., and McCabe, G. P., Lactose intolerance symptoms assessed by meta-analysis: a grain of truth that leads to exaggeration, *J. Nutr.*, 136, 1107, 2006.
129. Nguyen, K. N. et al., Effect of fiber on breath hydrogen response and symptoms after oral lactose in lactose malabsorbers, *Am. J. Clin. Nutr.*, 35, 1347, 1982.
130. Solomons, N. W., Guerrero, A., and Torun, R., Dietary manipulation of postprandial colonic lactose fermentation: I. Effect of solid foods in a meal, *Am. J. Clin. Nutr.*, 41, 199, 1985.
131. Leichter, J., Comparison of whole milk and skim milk with aqueous lactose solution in lactose tolerance testing, *Am. J. Clin. Nutr.*, 26, 393, 1973.
132. Dehkordi, N. et al., Lactose malabsorption as influenced by chocolate milk, skim, milk, sucrose, whole milk, and lactic cultures, *J. Am. Diet. Assoc.*, 95, 484, 1995.
133. Vesa, T. H., Lember, M., and Korpela, R., Milk fat does not affect the symptoms of lactose intolerance, *Eur. J. Clin. Nutr.*, 51, 633, 1997.
134. Vesa, T. H. et al., Raising milk energy content retards gastric emptying of lactose in lactose-intolerant humans with little effect on lactose digestion, *J. Nutr.*, 127, 2316, 1997.
135. Vesa, T. H. et al., Effects of milk viscosity on gastric emptying and lactose intolerance in lactose maldigesters, *Am. J. Clin. Nutr.*, 66, 123, 1997.
136. Chong, M. L. and Hardy, C. M., Cocoa feeding and human lactose intolerance, *Am. J. Clin. Nutr.*, 49, 840, 1989.
137. Jarvinen, R. M. K., Loukaskorpi, M., and Uusitupa, M. I. J., Tolerance of symptomatic lactose malabsorbers to lactose in milk chocolate, *Eur. J. Clin. Nutr.*, 57, 701, 2003.
138. Solomons, N. W., Fermentation, fermented foods and lactose intolerance, *Eur. J. Clin. Nutr.*, 56 (suppl. 4), S50, 2002.
139. Kopp-Hoolihan, L., Prophylactic and therapeutic uses of probiotics: a review, *J. Am. Diet. Assoc.*, 101 (2), 229, 2001.
140. Savaiano, D. A. and Levitt, M. D., Milk intolerance and microbe-containing dairy foods, *J. Dairy Sci.*, 70, 397, 1987.
141. Kolars, J. C. et al., Yogurt — an autodigesting source of lactose, *N. Engl. J. Med.*, 310, 1, 1984.
142. Martini, M. C. et al., Lactose digestion by yogurt beta-galactosidase: influence of pH and microbial cell integrity, *Am. J. Clin. Nutr.*, 45, 432, 1987.
143. Pochart, P. et al., Viable starter culture, beta-galactosidase activity, and lactose in duodenum after yogurt ingestion in lactase-deficient humans, *Am. J. Clin. Nutr.*, 49, 828, 1989.
144. Shermack, M. A. et al., Effect of yogurt on symptoms and kinetics of hydrogen production in lactose-malabsorbing children, *Am. J. Clin. Nutr.*, 62, 1003, 1995.
145. Vesa, T. H. et al., Digestion and tolerance of lactose from yogurt and different semi-solid fermented dairy products containing Lactobacillus acidophilus and bifidobacteria in lactose maldigesters — Is bacterial lactase important? *Eur. J. Clin. Nutr.*, 50, 730, 1996.
146. Wytock, D. H. and DiPalma, J. A., All yogurts are not created equal, *Am. J. Clin. Nutr.*, 47, 454, 1988.
147. Lerebours, E. et al., Yogurt and fermented-then-pasteurized milk: effects of short-term and long-term ingestion on lactose absorption and mucosal lactase activity in lactase-deficient subjects, *Am. J. Clin. Nutr.*, 49, 823, 1989.
148. Martini, M. S., Kukeilka, D., and Savaiano, D. A., Lactose digestion from yogurt: influence of a meal and additional lactose, *Am. J. Clin. Nutr.*, 53, 1253, 1991.
149. Martini, M. C., Smith, D. E., and Savaiano, D. A., Lactose digestion from flavored and frozen yogurts, ice milk, and ice cream by lactase-deficient persons, *Am. J. Clin. Nutr.*, 46, 636, 1987.
150. Hertzler, S. R. and Clancy, S. M., Kefir improves lactose digestion and tolerance in adults with lactose maldigestion, *J. Am. Diet. Assoc.*, 103, 582, 2003.

151. Gilliland, S. E., Acidophilus milk products: a review of potential benefits to consumers, *J. Dairy Sci.*, 72, 2483, 1989.
152. Payne, D. L. et al., Effectiveness of milk products in dietary management of lactose malabsorption, *Am. J. Clin. Nutr.*, 34, 2711, 1981.
153. Savaiano, D. A. et al., Lactose malabsorption from yogurt, pasteurized yogurt, sweet acidophilus milk, and cultured milk in lactase-deficient individuals, *Am. J. Clin. Nutr.*, 40, 1219, 1984.
154. Onwulata, C. I., Rao, D. R., and Vankineni, P., Relative efficiency of yogurt, sweet acidophilus milk, hydrolyzed-lactose milk, and a commercial lactase tablet in alleviating lactose maldigestion, *Am. J. Clin. Nutr.*, 49, 1233, 1989.
155. Hove, H., Nordgaard-Andersen, I., and Mortensen, P. B., Effect of lactic acid bacteria on the intestinal production of lactate and short-chain fatty acids, and the absorption of lactose, *Am. J. Clin. Nutr.*, 59, 74, 1994.
156. Mustapha, A., Jiang, T., and Savaiano, D. A., Improvement of lactose digestion by humans following ingestion of unfermented acidophilus milk: influence of bile sensitivity, lactose transport, and acid tolerance of lactobacillus acidophilus, *J. Dairy Sci.*, 80, 1537, 1997.
157. Lin, M., Savaiano, D., and Harlander, S., Influence of nonfermented dairy products containing bacterial starter cultures on lactose maldigestion in humans, *J. Dairy Sci.*, 74, 87, 1991.
158. Montes, R. G. et al., Effect of milks inoculated with Lactobacillus acidophilus or a yogurt starter culture in lactose-maldigesting children, *J. Dairy Sci.*, 78, 1657, 1995.
159. Jiang, T., Mustapha, A., and Savaiano, D. A., Improvement of lactose digestion in humans by ingestion of unfermented milk containing Bifidobacterium longum, *J. Dairy Sci.*, 79, 750, 1996.
160. Solomons, N. W., Guerrero, A., and Torun, B., Dietary manipulation of postprandial colonic lactose fermentation: II. addition of exogenous, microbial beta-galactosidases at mealtime, *Am. J. Clin. Nutr.*, 41, 209, 1985.
161. Sinden, A. A. and Sutphen, J. L., Dietary treatment of lactose intolerance in infants and children, *J. Am. Dietetic Assoc.*, 91, 1567, 1991.
162. Medow, M. S. et al., Beta-galactosidase tablets in the treatment of lactose intolerance in pediatrics, *Am. J. Dis. Child.*, 144, 1261, 1990.
163. Corazza, G. R. et al., Beta-galactosidase from aspergillus niger in adult lactose malabsorption: a double-blind crossover study, *Alimen. Pharmacol. Therapeut.*, 6 (1), 61, 1992.
164. DiPalma, J. A. and Collins, M. S., Enzyme replacement for lactose malabsorption using a beta-D-galactosidase, *J. Clin. Gastroenterol.*, 11 (3), 290, 1989.
165. Montalto, M. et al., Effect of exogenous beta-galactosidase in patients with lactose malabsorption and intolerance: a crossover double-blind placebo-controlled study, *Eur. J. Clin. Nutr.*, 59, 489, 2005.
166. Food and Drug Administration/HHS, Direct food substances generally recognized as safe, *21 CFR*, 184.1, 1992.
167. Holsinger, V. H. and Kligerman, A. E., Applications of lactase in dairy foods and other foods containing lactose, *Food Technol.*, 45 (1), 92, 1991.
168. Gannett News Service, Missing enzyme means body can't handle lactose: alternative products lack lactose, *St. Cloud Times*, Dec. 5, 1993.
169. Food and Drug Administration, HHS, Code of Federal Regulations, 21 CFR, 184.1388, April 1, 1993.
170. Nielson, O. H. et al., Calcium absorption and acceptance of low-lactose milk among children with primary lactase deficiency, *J. Ped. Gastroenterol. Nutr.*, 3 (2), 219, 1984.
171. Brand, J. C. and Holt, S., Relative effectiveness of milks with reduced amounts of lactose in alleviating milk intolerance, *Am. J. Clin. Nutr.*, 54, 148, 1991.
172. Reddy, V. and Pershad, J., Lactase deficiency in Indians, *Am. J. Clin. Nutr.*, 25, 114, 1972.
173. Johnson, A. O. et al., Adaptation of lactose maldigesters to continued milk intakes, *Am. J. Clin. Nutr.*, 58, 879, 1993.
174. Pribila, B. A. et al., Improved lactose digestion and intolerance among African–American adolescent girls fed a dairy-rich diet, *J. Am. Diet. Assoc.*, 100, 524, 2000.
175. Hertzler, S. R. and Savaiano, D. A., Colonic adaptation to daily lactose feeding in lactose maldigesters reduces lactose intolerance, *Am. J. Clin. Nutr.*, 64, 232, 1996.

176. Briet, R. et al., Improved clinical tolerance to chronic lactose ingestion in subjects with lactose intolerance: a placebo effect? *Gut*, 41, 632, 1997.
177. Hertzler, S. R., Savaiano, D. A., and Levitt, M. D., Fecal hydrogen production and consumption measurements, *Dig. Dis. Sci.*, 42 (2), 348, 1997.
178. Committee on Nutrition, American Academy of Pediatrics, Oral therapy for acute diarrhea, in *Pediatric Nutrition Handbook*, Kleinman, R. E., Ed., 5th ed., The American Academy of Pediatrics, Elk Grove Village, 2004, chap. 28.
179. Heird, W. C. and Cooper, A., Cooper, nutrition in infants and children, In *Modern Nutrition in Health and Disease*, Shils, M. E. and Young, V. R., Eds., Lea and Febiger, Philadelphia, p. 958, 1988.
180. Brown, K. H., Peerson, J. M., and Fontaine, O., Use of nonhuman milks in the dietary management of young children with acute diarrhea: a meta-analysis of clinical trials, *Pediatrics*, 93 (1), 17, 1994.
181. Lifschitz, F. et al., The response to dietary treatment of patients with chronic post-infectious diarrhea and lactose intolerance, *J. Am. Coll. Nutr.*, 9 (3), 231, 1990.
182. Solomons, N. W. et al., The effect of dietary lactose on the early recovery from protein-energy malnutrition, *Am. J. Clin. Nutr.*, 40 (3), 591, 1984.
183. Beau, J. P., Fontaine, O., and Garenne, M., Management of malnourished children with acute diarrhoea and sugar intolerance, *J. Trop. Peds.*, 35 (6), 281, 1989.
184. Erinoso, H. O. et al., Is cow's milk suitable for the dietary supplementation of rural Gambian children? 1. Prevalence of lactose maldigestion, *Ann. Trop. Peds.*, 12, 359, 1992.
185. Gendrel, D. et al., Feeding lactose-intolerant children with a powdered fermented milk, *J. Ped. Gastroenterol. Nutr.*, 10 (1), 44, 1990.
186. Paige, D. M., Lactose malabsorption in children: prevalence, symptoms and nutritional considerations, in *Lactose Digestion: Clinical and Nutritional Implications*, Paige, D. M. and Bayless, T. M., Eds., The Johns Hopkins University Press, Baltimore, 1981, chap. 14.
187. Department of Agriculture/Food and Consumer Service, National School Lunch Program, School Breakfast Program, Summer Food Service Program for Children and Child and Adult Care Food Program: Meat Alternates Used in the Child Nutrition Programs, *Federal Register*, 7 CFR Parts 210, 220, 225, and 226, Vol. 62, No. 44, March 6, 1997.
188. Child Nutrition and WIC Reauthorization Act of 2004, Public Law 108–265, 108th Congress, Amendments to Richard B. Russell National School Lunch Act, Section 102, http://thomas.loc.gov.
189. USDA, Food and Nutrition Service, Notice of solicitation of comments, Special supplemental food program for women, infants, and children (WIC): accommodation of cultural food preferences in the WIC program, Federal Register, 59(120) FR 32406, June 23, 1994.
190. National Academy of Sciences, Institute of Medicine, WIC Food Packages: Time for a Change, April 2005, http://www.fns.usda.gov/oane/menu/Published/WIC/WIC.htm.

9 Contribution of Dairy Foods to Health throughout the Life Cycle

9.1 INTRODUCTION

Adequate amounts of milk and milk products are needed throughout the life cycle to promote bone health, to help reduce the risk of chronic diseases such as osteoporosis, hypertension, and some cancers, and to contribute to overall nutritional status. The need for calcium and other nutrients supplied by dairy foods is influenced by age and life stage due to changes in physiological need, hormonal status, the absorption and retention of nutrients, and other factors. However, many population groups in the United States, particularly adolescent and adult females and older Americans, consume significantly less calcium and fewer servings of Milk Group foods than recommended. Psychosocial and environmental factors influence the intake of milk and milk products differently throughout life, so that no one educational approach to improve consumption is relevant for all ages. In this chapter we will discuss the benefits of milk and milk products at each stage of the life cycle, as well as important issues and concerns unique to each life stage group from infancy to old age. Although this chapter focuses primarily on the role of dairy foods and health, the information should be viewed in the context of the total diet and life-style of the individual.

9.2 INFANCY

9.2.1 Characteristics

The infant period is characterized by rapid growth and development. Infant growth rates are highly variable and are influenced by genetic, hormonal, nutritional, and environmental factors. Over the first year, the average infant generally triples his birth weight and gains about 50% in length, and approximately 30% in head circumference [1]. The infant grows about an inch in length and adds about 2.2 pounds per month for the first 6 months. During the second 6 months, growth velocity slows to about 0.5 inches in length and about 1 pound per month [1]. As the infant grows, his body composition changes; for example, the percentage of water decreases and the proportions of fat and protein increase. About 3.2% of the infant's body weight is composed of minerals (mostly bone). Between 5 and 9 months the first deciduous teeth erupt and, by 1 year of age, most infants have four to eight teeth [1]. Occurring simultaneously with physical development is neurological, cognitive, language, and psychosocial development.

9.2.2 Recommendations for Feeding

The infant's first food is human milk or iron-fortified infant formula. The American Academy of Pediatrics (AAP) strongly recommends human milk as the exclusive nutrient source for feeding full-term infants during the first 6 months after birth and supports its continuation, with the addition of solid foods, at least through the first year — as long as mutually desired by mother and child [2]. This recommendation stems from the acknowledged benefits of human milk to the infant (improved nutrition, gastrointestinal function, host defense, neurological development, and psychological

TABLE 9.1
Calcium Recommendations for Infancy

Age	Calcium (mg/d)
Birth to 6 months	210
6 to 12 months	270

Source: From Dietary Reference Intakes, National Academy of Sciences, 1997.

well-being), to the mother (faster shrinking of the uterus and postpartum weight loss, possible reduction in premenopausal breast cancer, ovarian cancer, and osteoporosis), as well as to society (saves health care costs, conserves natural resources, reduces environmental waste) [3]. The American Dietetic Association (ADA) supports breast-feeding as optimal infant nutrition and health protection for the first 6 to 12 months of life and encourages nutrition professionals to promote breast-feeding as the norm for infant feeding [4].

Adequate amounts of calcium in the diet of infants are needed for skeletal growth and for the development of teeth. Table 9.1 presents the 1997 Calcium Recommendations for Infancy from the Food and Nutrition Board of the National Academy of Sciences (NAS) [5]. The NAS recommendations are Adequate Intakes (AI), and for infancy are based on the amount of calcium supplied by human milk. Recommended intakes for children 6 to 12 months were based on expected intakes from human milk and solid food.

9.2.2.1 Standard Cow's Milk-Based Formulas

Standard iron-fortified cow's milk-based formula is an appropriate substitute when breast-feeding is not used or is stopped before 1 year of age [6]. Commercial cow's milk-based infant formulas have been tested extensively, and can provide adequate nutrition for the healthy infant when used exclusively for the first 4 to 6 months of life [6]. Their nutrient composition, however, can differ substantially from human milk and from each other — and may change over time, so it is important to check the label. While human milk serves as a model for the composition of infant formulas, these formulas are not identical to the composition of human milk, which contains hormones, immunologic agents, and enzymes [6]. Standards for the nutrient composition of infant formula are governed by the Infant Formula Act of 1980, revised in 1986 [7,8]. Since calcium is absorbed more efficiently from human milk, cow's milk-based formulas are formulated to contain approximately 40% more calcium. Soy formulas are considered a safe and nutritionally equivalent alternative to cow's milk formula for term infants, including those with hereditary or transient lactase deficiency, for parents seeking a vegetarian diet for their infant, or for infants with documented IgE-mediated allergy to cow's milk. However, soy formulas may be allergenic to some infants who are allergic to cow milk protein. Soy infant formula is not recommended for (1) preterm infants with birth weights less than 1800 g, (2) to prevent colic or allergy, or (3) for infants with cow milk protein-induced enterocolitis or enteropathy. Protein hydrolysate formulas are available for preterm infants or for infants who are allergic to cow's milk or soy protein [6].

9.2.2.2 Cow's Milk

Full-fat cow's milk, fat-free (skim) milk, 1% (low-fat) to 2% (reduced-fat) milk, goat's milk, evaporated milk, and other "milks" not formulated to meet an infant's nutritional needs are not recommended for use during the first 12 months of life (Table 9.2) [9]. There are several reasons for this recommendation. Since cow's milk contains a low concentration and bioavailability of iron when compared to human milk, feeding cow's milk to infants increases the risk of iron deficiency anemia and possible increased intestinal blood loss in infants with milk sensitivity. Cow's milk also

TABLE 9.2
Human Milk, Cow Milk, and Goat Milk

	g/100 mL			mg/100 mL Source			Source		Osmolality (m Osm/kg of H_2O) and General Cumments
	Pro	Fast	CHO	Na/K	Ca/P	Fe	CHO	Fat	
Human milk (Mature) (20 kcal/30 mL)	0.9	3.9	6.7	12−25/40− −55	20−25/12−14	<0.1	Lactose glucose oligosaccarhides	Human milk fat	(260 to 300) Whey:casein ratio is 60:40.
Evaporated whole milk (43 kcal/30 mL)	7.0	8.0	10.7	113/322	278/216	0.2	Lactose	Butterfat	Milk is diluted and dextrose added to make a 20 calorie per oz formula.
Skim milk (11 kcal/30 mL)	3.5	0.2	5.0	53/171	128/104	Trace	Lactose	Butterfat	(279) Trace Definition essential fatty acids. Not recommended for children <2 y.
2% Milk (15 kcal/30 mL)	3.4	2.0	5.0	51/159	125/98	Trace	Lactose	Trace Butterfat	(279) Deficient in essential fatty acids. Not recommended for children <2 y.
Whole milk (19 kcal/30 mL)	3.3	3.4	4.8	50/156	123/96	Trace	Lactose	Butterfat	(279) Whey:casein ratio is 18:82. Not recommended for infants <1 y.
Goat milk (21 kcal/30 mL)	3.7	4.3	4.6	51/210	138/114	Trace	Lactose	Butterfat	(267) Fat more readily digested than fat in cow milk. Used rarely for intolerance to cow milk. Not appropriate for use in infancy, as it is inadequate in folate and other essential nutrients.

increases the risk of deficiency of essential fatty acids, vitamin E, and zinc, since concentrations of these nutrients are lower than in human milk. In addition, fat-free, low-fat, and reduced-fat milk may cause the infant to consume excessive amounts of protein as the infant consumes an increased volume of milk to satisfy caloric needs. Excessive protein intake (as well as higher sodium, potassium, and chloride in cow's milk) increases the renal solute load and risks overtaxing the kidneys, particularly if the infant becomes dehydrated [6].

9.2.2.3 Cow's Milk Allergy

Cow's milk hypersensitivity involves a reaction to milk protein by the infant's immune system. It is a complex disorder, in which most major cow's milk proteins (more than 30 identified so far) have been implicated in allergic responses, including both casein and whey proteins [10]. It develops in 2.2% to 2.8% of infants, of whom 85% outgrow the reactivity by 4 years of age [11]. Symptoms may involve the gastrointestinal and respiratory systems, and the skin. Infants typically exhibit diarrhea, vomiting, and failure to thrive.

An IgE-mediated hypersensitivity to cow's milk is diagnosed based on a combination of history, physical examination, and a demonstration of food-specific IgE to the suspected food [12]. Symptoms associated with eating certain foods can stem from several factors other than food hypersensitivity (allergy). To avoid diagnostic errors and unnecessary dietary restriction, it is important to use a process that excludes subject bias to confirm food allergy [11]. If milk allergy is suspected in children older than 1 year, either a skin prick test or a blood test (Radioallergosorbent Test or RAST) which estimates the amount of antigen-specific IgE antibodies in the serum, should be conducted. If the skin prick test is positive, milk should be excluded from the diet for about 2 weeks, followed by a double-blind challenge with the offending food. If the RAST is positive, a food challenge is not generally required to confirm hypersensitivity [11].

Infants who have confirmed cow's milk sensitivity should be fed a substitute hypoallergenic formula (e.g., protein hydrolysate) until they are 1 year of age or older [11]. Soy protein-based formulas are no less allergenic than cow milk protein-based formulas, according to the AAP. However, the AAP says most infants with documented IgE-associated mediated allergy to cow's milk will tolerate a soy protein-based formula [6]. Appropriate nutrition counseling will be needed for older infants to ensure the elimination of all food sources of the antigen and to ensure the nutritional adequacy of the diet. A rechallenge with milk in a controlled setting will determine whether symptoms persist. When cow's milk allergy is diagnosed in infancy, controlled rechallenges are recommended every 6 to 12 months, to avoid unnecessarily prolonging a milk-free diet [13]. The rate of remission of cow's milk allergy is about 50% per year [11].

Experts agree that eliminating allergenic foods from the maternal diet during pregnancy is unlikely to prevent food allergies in the infant. The following recommendations from the AAP may help delay or prevent some cow's milk allergy in infants at high risk of atopic disease (e.g., parents or siblings have allergies): (1) breast-feed exclusively for the first 4 to 6 months of life or use a protein hydrolyzed formula, (2) delay introduction of solid foods until after 6 months of age, (3) delay introduction of cow's milk until 1 year of age (eggs until 2 years; peanuts, nuts, and fish until 3 years) [14]. Soy formulas should not be considered hypoallergenic or be used to prevent food allergy (including cow's milk allergy) in infants [11,15]. Recent studies indicate that feeding a partially-hydrolyzed whey formula (or exclusive breast-feeding) decreases the risk of food (including cow's milk) allergy in high risk infants for up to 5 years [16,17]. A study in laboratory rats found that feeding a partially-hydrolyzed whey formula suppressed an immune response to cow's milk protein [18]. The authors suggest that selected peptides in cow's milk protein may induce oral tolerance.

Whether eliminating cow's milk or other allergenic foods from the diet of the mother during lactation will help prevent milk (or other food) allergy in infants remains controversial, since study results conflict [19]. A review by Zeiger states that, "More definitive randomized studies with both food challenges and immunologic confirmation are mandatory before maternal lactation diets can be recommended as effective in the prevention of atopic disease" [15].

9.2.3 Introduction of Solid Foods

By 4 to 6 months of age the infant is developmentally ready for the introduction of solid foods to complement the liquid diet. By this time the extrusion reflex (tongue pushes food out of the mouth) has disappeared, pureed solids can be swallowed, and the infant can sit with support [20]. In 2001, the World Health Organization revised its recommendations for the timing of introduction of complementary foods based on a scientific review of available evidence in both developed and developing countries; they now recommend exclusive breast-feeding for 6 months [21]. The AAP recommends that complementary foods can be introduced at 4 to 6 months, particularly in developed countries such as the United States where there is a low risk for contaminated or low nutrient-dense foods. They state, "There is no evidence for harm when safe, nutritious complementary foods are introduced after 4 months when the infant is developmentally ready" [20]. Despite these recommendations, data from the National Health and Nutrition Examination Survey (NHANES III) 1988 to 1994 indicates that more than half of nonbreast-fed and about 30% of breast-fed infants 2 to 3 months old are being fed infant cereal [20].

The introduction of complementary foods during late infancy is an opportunity for care givers to expose young children to a wide variety of foods and beverages which may form the basis for lifelong healthful eating habits [22]. Solid single foods, such as iron-fortified infant cereals, strained fruits and vegetables, and meats should be introduced one at a time for 1 week, before trying a different food, so that possible allergic reactions can be identified. There is no evidence to support introducing foods in a particular order [20]. In all cases, single foods should be introduced before mixtures. Although human milk or infant formula is still the mainstay of the infant's diet, cow's milk, yogurt, and cheese may be introduced at 6 months [23]. Fruit juice should be limited to 4 to 6 ounces per day after the age of 6 months, since excess fruit juice intake can lead to diarrhea [20]. A resource for guidance on complementary feeding is the Start Healthy Feeding Guidelines for Infants and Toddlers. Developed by a panel of experts in pediatric nutrition, it provides parents and care givers practical guidance about how to feed infants and toddlers to ensure normal growth and lay the groundwork for later healthy eating habits [24].

As the infant's eye-hand coordination develops and the first teeth erupt, he develops the ability to chew and can begin to feed himself. By 7 months he will begin to finger-feed soft foods [25]. Cheese cubes/slices and cottage cheese are among the foods appropriate for self-feeding (Table 9.3).

The addition of yogurt to the diet with its lactic acid bacteria may have a beneficial effect on an infant's intestinal microflora. In a study conducted among 39 healthy infants aged 10 to 18 months, the daily ingestion of 125 g of yogurt or milk fermented with yogurt cultures (*Lactobacillus casei*), significantly reduced the activity of harmful intestinal enzymes [26]. The authors suggest that feeding of these foods may prove useful in preventing infectious disease, stimulating the immune system, and in protecting the infant from exposure to some carcinogens.

9.2.4 Vitamin D and Rickets

Vitamin D is essential to a healthy skeleton throughout life. Vitamin D promotes the intestinal absorption of calcium as well as acting directly on bone mineralization. The vitamin D deficiency disease, rickets, results in soft and deformed bones, bowed legs, and knock-knees [27]. Infants and young children are most vulnerable to vitamin D deficiency because of their rapid growth and bone formation. Although it was thought that rickets was a problem of the early 1900s and no longer an issue in the United States due to widespread fortification of milk with vitamin D, it is again becoming a health concern [28]. Studies among Asian children and African American toddlers

TABLE 9.3
Some Appropriate Foods for Infant Self-Feeding

Fruits	Soft, fresh or canned, unsweetened, such as bananas, peeled apples, apricots, peaches, or pears
Vegetables	Tender pieces of cooked vegetables such as carrots, potatoes, green beans, summer squash, yellow squash, sweet potatoes
Dairy	Cubes or slices of milk cheese, cottage cheese
Meat, Poultry, Fish	Small, tender pieces of cooked chicken, turkey, or white flaky fish without bones; ground meat such as meat balls, pieces of hamburger patty or meatloaf
Bread/Cereals/Other	Toast, plain unsalted crackers, teething biscuits, individual cereal pieces, plain wafer cookies

suggest that low dietary calcium intakes also contribute to the development of vitamin D deficiency and rickets by increasing the catabolism of vitamin D [29].

Vitamin D is synthesized in the skin when exposed to sunlight and is also obtained from foods. Only a few foods, such as egg yolks, butter, fatty fish (e.g., salmon), and liver naturally contain vitamin D. Human milk contains very little vitamin D (0.5 μg), and rickets can occur in deeply pigmented breastfed infants or in those not exposed to sunlight [30]. One liter of standard infant formula contains 10 μg (400 IU) of vitamin D. The Dietary Reference Intake Report (DRI) from the NAS recommends at least 5 μg (200 IU) of vitamin D daily for infants, children, and adults, but does not deem the amount of vitamin D in infant formula to be excessive [5].

Adequate sunlight exposure is difficult to determine. Therefore, the AAP recommends a supplement of 200 IU of vitamin D for the following: (1) all breast-fed infants unless they are weaned to at least 500 mL/d of vitamin D-fortified formula or milk, (2) all nonbreast-fed infants who are ingesting less than 500 mL/d of vitamin D-fortified formula or milk, (3) children and adolescents who do not get regular sun exposure, do not consume at least 500 mL/day of vitamin D-fortified milk, or do not take a multivitamin supplement containing at least 200 IU of vitamin D [30]. Others recommend that the current vitamin-D supplementation guidelines be extended to all infants, regardless of feeding volume or source, or at least to all infants born to dark-skinned mothers [31]. After age 1, the recommended amount of vitamin D may be supplied by two 8-ounce servings of vitamin D-fortified cow's milk, which is voluntarily fortified to a level of 100 IU per 8-ounce serving.

9.3 TODDLER AND PRESCHOOL YEARS

9.3.1 CHARACTERISTICS

During the toddler (12 to 15 months) and preschool years (ages 3 to 5), the rate of growth gradually decelerates from the rapid growth in height and weight seen in infancy. During the second and third year of life, height increases about 12 cm (5 inches) and weight increases about 2.5 kg (5 to 6 pounds) per year. From 3 to 5 years of age, the child gains about 2 kg (4.5 pounds) and grows about 6 to 8 cm (2.5 to 3.5 inches) in height per year. Appetite decreases in proportion to decreases in growth rates and at times the child's food intake from meal to meal appears to be erratic and unpredictable, yet total daily energy intake remains fairly constant [32]. Motor skills are becoming fine-tuned. At 12 months (or before), a toddler is able to pick up and release a piece of food and hand-feed himself, and by age 2 he is able to handle a spoon and fork [33]. At 15 months, the child can drink from a cup, though not without spilling. Children between the ages of 2 and 5 are often resistant to consuming new foods (food neophobia). Parents can facilitate children's acceptance of new foods through repeated exposures (between 5 and 10 repetitions), and trust that children can learn to like new foods and can self-regulate their energy intake [32].

Social, intellectual, and emotional growth is rapid. Speech develops, so that by the time a child is 3 years of age he can use short sentences and hold a brief conversation. During the second year, the child begins to imitate parents, siblings, and playmates. As the child becomes increasingly aware that he will become a larger child and eventually an adult, he begins to emulate role models.

There are no comprehensive guidelines for feeding toddlers, but experts agree they do not have the innate ability to choose a balanced diet for themselves [32]. It is therefore the responsibility of care givers to provide toddlers with small, frequent feedings of a variety of foods to meet nutrient and energy needs [34]. Milk (whole and 2%) and American cheese are among the top ten table foods most frequently fed to toddlers and provide abundant amounts of a wide range of nutrients, including calcium, riboflavin, vitamin B_{12}, magnesium, phosphorus, vitamin A, and vitamin D (if vitamin-D fortified) [34]. However, almost half the foods toddlers eat most often are not important sources of nutrients (i.e., peeled apples, white bread, graham crackers). Care givers should be informed about more nutrient-dense foods, such as milk products (milk, cheese, and yogurt), fortified cereal, and fruit, to feed to this age group [34].

9.3.2 Contribution of Milk Group Foods

Milk and milk products provide the majority of calcium and several other vitamins and minerals in the diets of toddlers. Milk is the leading contributor among toddler's (12 to 54 months) diets of all minerals (calcium, phosphorus, zinc, magnesium) except iron and sodium, according to the Feeding Infants and Toddlers Study (FITS), which is the first study to provide national estimates of the sources of nutrients in the diets of more than 3000 U.S. infants and toddlers [35]. In addition, milk was the number one source of vitamins A, B_6, B_{12}, D, thiamine, riboflavin, and potassium in the diets of toddlers in this nationally-representative sample [35].

Calcium is needed throughout childhood to maintain existing bone and for bone growth. In children 1 to 2 years of age, milk and milk products contribute about 77% of the calcium in their diet (milk 63.9%; cheese 9.7%; yogurt 3.1%), and another 2.4% is contributed by infant formula [35]. Data are not available for older preschoolers. According to FITS, the average calcium intake of both Hispanic and non-Hispanic toddlers (12 to 24 months) was 976 mg/day and 935 mg/day, respectively — well above the recommendation for this age group (500 mg calcium/day) [36].

9.3.3 Calcium/Dairy Recommendations and Consumption

Milk and milk products provide calcium, protein, phosphorus, and vitamin D needed for maximum skeletal growth. Few studies have measured the accretion of calcium into bone in the toddler age group. However, it is estimated that about 100 mg of calcium per day is retained in the skeleton of children 2 to 3 years old [5]. Total calcium retention for weight is relatively low in toddlers compared with other age groups [23]. The NAS recommends 500 mg of calcium (expressed as Adequate Intakes) per day for children ages one to three and 800 mg per day for children ages 4 to 8 [5]. The NAS chose to develop separate recommendations for children ages one to three. Although calcium balance data was not available for this age group, the committee chose an estimate of net calcium retention to establish what they felt was a reasonable recommendation. They acknowledge the need for more information to more precisely estimate calcium needs [5]. Approximately 94% of children ages 1 to 3 exceed the NAS calcium recommendations, and about 69% of children ages 4 to 8 do so [37]. The median usual calcium intake for children ages 1 to 3 is 932 mg/day and for children ages 4 to 8 years is 929 mg/day [37].

It is important for young children to develop dietary practices that will promote adequate calcium intake later in life; 2 or 3 years of age (after the infant is no longer taking human milk or formula) is a good time for pediatricians to first assess calcium intake [23]. In a 2006 report,

Optimizing Bone Health and Calcium Intakes of Infants, Children, and Adolescents, the AAP recommends three age-appropriate sized servings of milk or equivalent amounts of cheese or yogurt for children ages 1 to 3 years — and 3 adult-sized servings of milk or milk equivalents for children ages 4 to 8 years (Table 9.4) [23]. The report (Table 9.5) does not define an age-appropriate

TABLE 9.4
Food Guide for Children Ages 7 to 13 Years

Eat the Five Food Group Way!™

Food Group, Health Benefits, and Nutrients[a]	MyPyramid.gov Total Daily Portions	→ Translating Portions Into Daily Servings[b]	Food	Common Serving Size
Grain group[c] Provides energy and aids digestion *Key nutrients:* Carbohydrate Fiber	Ages 7-10 = 5-6 ounces Ages 11-13 = 6-7 ounces	→ 5-6 Servings → 6-7 Servings	Bread Tortilla, roll, muffin Bagel, hamburger bun Rice, pasta, cooked cereal, grits Ready-to-eat cereal Pancake, waffle	1 Slice 1 1/2 1/2 Cup 1 ounces (Flakes or round) 1 (4" Diameter)
Vegetable group Helps you see in the dark *Key nutrients:* Vitamin A Fiber	Ages 7-10 = 2-2 1/2 cups Ages 11-13 = 2 1/2-3 cups	→ 4-5 Servings → 5-6 Servings	Cooked vegetables Chopped, raw vegetables Raw, leafy vegetables Vegetable juice	1/2 Cup 1/2 Cup 1 Cup 3/4 Cup
Fruit group Heals cuts and bruises *Key nutrients:* Vitamin C Potassium	Ages 7-10 = 1 1/2 cups Ages 11-13 = 1 1/2-2 cups	→ 3 Servings → 3-4 Servings	Apple, banana, orange, pear Grapefruit Cantaloupe Raisins, dried fruit Chopped fruit 100% fruit juice	1 Medium 1/2 Fruit 1/4 Fruit 1/4 Cup 1/2 Cup 3/4 Cup
Milk group Builds strong bones and teeth *Key nutrients:* Calcium Vitamin D	Ages 7-10 = 3 cups Ages 11-13 = 3 cups	→ 3 Servings → 3 Servings	Milk Yogurt Cheese Pudding Frozen yogurt	1 Cup (8 oz) 8 ounces container 1-1/2 to 2 oz 1/2 Cup 1/2 Cup
Meat group Builds strong muscles *Key nutrients:* Protein Iron	Ages 7-10 = 5 ounces Ages 11-13 = 5-6 ounces	→ 2 Servings → 2 Servings	Cooked lean meat, poultry, fish Egg Peanut butter Cooked dried peas or beans Nuts, seeds	2-3 ounces 1 (1 ounces) 2 Tbsp (1 oz) 1/2 Cup 1/3 Cup
"Others" Category	See MyPyramid.gov for information on "Oils" and "Discretionary Calories"	Active children can consume "Others" in moderation, as long as they eat the recommended amounts from the Five Food Groups.	Fats, oils, spreads Candy Cookies Cake Chips Soft drinks	1Tsp to1 tbsp 1 ounces 2 Small 1/16 of Cake 1 ounces 12 ounces

[a] All of the Five Food Groups provide many nutrients. Listed here are some of the most important ones.

[b] These are minimum recommended number of servings. Some people will need more or less servings, depending on their gender, size, activity level and growth.

[c] At least half of the daily servings should come from whole grains.

TABLE 9.5
Calcium and Dairy Food Recommendations for Young Children

Age	Adequate Calcium Intake (mglday)[a]	Servings of Dairy per day[b]
1 to 3 Years	500	3[c]

[a] Institute of Medicine, Food and Nutrition Board, *Dietary Reference Intakes for Calcium, Phosphorus, Magnesiin, Vitamin D, and Flouride*, Washington, D.C., National Academy Press, 1997.
[b] American Academy of Pediatrics, Optimizing bone health and calcium intakes of infants, children, and adolescents, *Pediatrics*, 117 (2), 578–585, February, 2006.
[c] Age-appropriate servings.

serving size for children ages 1 to 3. However, the AAP's Pediatric Nutrition Handbook suggests the following serving sizes for milk and milk products for children 2 to 3 years of age: 4 ounces of milk or yogurt, and ½ to ¾ ounces of cheese [32]. Another food guide suggests that serving sizes from milk, yogurt, and cheese for children ages 1 to 3 slowly increase from 4 ounces of milk/yogurt and ½ ounce of cheese at age 1, to 5 ounces of milk/yogurt and ½ ounce of cheese at age 2, to 6 ounces of milk/yogurt and ¾ of an ounce of cheese at age 3 [33]. Both guides recommend a total of 16 to 24 ounces of milk/milk products per day for this age group.

Nationally representative data on average portions consumed by toddlers indicates that children ages 19 to 24 months consume on average 6 ounces of fluid milk, about 4 ounces of yogurt, and 1 ounce of cheese per eating occasion [38].

9.3.4 Strategies to Improve Intake

9.3.4.1 Snacks

Because children in this age group have a small stomach capacity, they do best when fed four to six times a day. Snacks should be treated as minimeals that are planned to contribute to the daily nutrient intake [32]. Foods chosen for snacks should come mainly from the Five Food Groups and include milk, fruits, vegetables, meats, and whole grains.

A telephone survey of mothers and care givers of more than 600 toddlers found that morning snacks provided 124 to 156 kcals and afternoon snacks provided from 139 to 170 kcals [39]. Foods typically eaten at morning snacks for all locations (home, day-care, and away from home) were water, whole cow's milk, crackers, and 100% fruit juice. Most frequently consumed beverages and foods for afternoon snacks eaten at home or day-care were water, whole cow's milk, fruit-flavored drinks, 100% apple juice, crackers, or nonbaby food cookies. Morning snacks consumed at home had a significantly higher nutrient density for potassium, calcium, phosphorus, magnesium, vitamins B_6, B_{12}, C, D, and K, and riboflavin than snacks consumed at day-care or other away-from-home eating locations [39]. Nutrient density of afternoon snacks did not differ by location.

Milk, yogurt, and cheese are excellent, nutrient-dense snack choices and will help young children meet daily calcium requirements. If a child dislikes white milk, offer a flavored milk, such as chocolate milk, to encourage milk consumption. Flavored milk has a similar sugar content to orange juice, and contains all the same nutrients as white milk.

9.3.4.2 Parental Role Modeling

Children begin to acquire their adult food preferences during the preschool years. Parental role models can have a profound impact on a child's food preferences and eating patterns. Young children will not choose a well-balanced diet unassisted. Parents must provide the child with a variety of nutritious foods and model patterns of food acceptance [32]. A child will become more positive toward a food the more often it is presented. A parent may need to offer a food eight or ten times before the child will accept it [40]. The care giver feeding style can also impact food choices of young children. An authoritative feeding style — in which the adults choose which foods are offered, and the child determines which foods are eaten — has been positively associated with attempts to get the child to eat dairy foods, fruits, and vegetables and with reported child-consumption of dairy foods and vegetables [41]. Parents can encourage adequate intake of Milk Group foods both by serving milk, yogurt, and cheese at meal and snack time, and by consuming these foods themselves. Since the child begins to emulate role models at this stage of life, it is important for the preschooler to see his parents, preschool teachers, and other children enjoying these foods.

9.3.5 Nutritional Concerns

9.3.5.1 Eating Away from Home

Although eating food away from home is often thought to be a problem primarily for older children, a large survey of more than 600 parents and care givers of toddlers (15 to 24 months) found that about half had one or more eating occasions away from home (other than day-care) in a 24-hour period [39]. When the nutrient density of lunches consumed away from home (other than day-care) were analyzed, they were considered to be less healthful. In contrast, day-care lunches provided higher intakes of nutrients such as calcium, phosphorus, vitamin D, and magnesium — nutrients associated with milk and other dairy foods — than did lunches consumed at home or away [39]. The food item most frequently consumed by toddlers away from home (other than day-care) was French fries (35% of toddlers). In addition, 16% of toddlers consumed carbonated beverages at away lunches, whereas only 3% of toddlers consumed carbonated beverages at home or at day-care. The authors say the higher frequency of consuming carbonated soda and fruit-flavored drinks at lunches eaten away from home (other than day-care) may displace milk from toddlers' diets [39].

According to a position of the ADA, eating away from home may be one of several factors contributing to the increasing overweight among 2-to 5-year-old children, and to their over-consumption of energy-dense, nutrient-poor foods [42]. The paper acknowledges that most children do not meet recommendations for fruit, grain, and dairy intakes, and encourages the use of the U.S. Department of Agriculture's (USDA's) Food Guide Pyramid for Young Children ages 2 to 6 as a tool to encourage adequate intakes of nutrient dense foods [43].

9.3.5.2 Low-Fat Diets

Fat-modified foods, including nonfat and low-fat milks, are not recommended for children between the ages of 1 and 2 [32]. Children of this age need foods with high caloric density for growth. Failure to thrive has been reported in preschool children whose overzealous parents have offered their children very low-fat, restrictive diets in the misguided hope of preventing adult obesity and/or cardiovascular disease [44].

The 2005 *Dietary Guidelines for Americans* recommends that children ages 2 to 5 years consume between 30% to 35% of their calories from fat, and children aged 4 to 18 years should have a fat intake from 25% to 35% of calories [45]. Health Canada determined that there was no scientific evidence that a fat-restricted diet during childhood had any demonstrated value either while the child was young or later in adulthood. Long-standing guidelines from Health Canada recommend that children should not be required to adhere to adult fat recommendations (30% of calories) until linear growth has ceased in later adolescence [46].

Instead of focusing on fat restriction, parents and care givers of young children should emphasize foods that will provide the energy and variety of nutrients needed for growth and development — which is the top priority for children's nutrition.

9.3.5.3 Excessive Fruit Juice Consumption

While 100% fruit juice can be a nutritious and appropriate food for preschoolers, it may have a negative nutritional impact if it replaces milk in the diet [32]. Smith and Lifshitz reported that toddlers (14 to 27 months) with growth failure consumed large amounts of 100% fruit juice, primarily apple juice [47]. The 100% fruit juice displaced other calorie- and nutrient-dense foods from the diet, such as milk, whole grains, fruits, and vegetables. The result was an inadequate intake of calories, protein, fat, calcium, vitamin D, iron, and zinc. All of the parents perceived fruit juice as being a healthy food choice because it was "natural," and it was readily accepted by the children because of the sweet taste. One mother gave her child skim milk after weaning because she felt the child was getting too heavy. When the child refused the skim milk, she offered juice as a "healthy" substitute. When juice consumption was discontinued and replaced by whole milk and increased amounts of solid foods (three meals and two or three snacks), the dietary intakes of calcium, vitamin D, iron, and zinc increased to recommended levels in these children. It was reported that excess fruit juice consumption is associated with short stature and obesity in preschool children [48], though these results have been challenged [49,50]. A longitudinal study of children ages 1 to 5 found that beverages with added sugar and fruit juice (to a lesser extent) decreased the diet quality of young children [51]. A higher dairy intake predicted overall diet quality and was an important source of calcium and vitamin D for this age group [51].

The AAP recommends that intake of fruit juice should be limited to 4 to 6 ounces per day in children 1 to 6 years old and children should be encouraged to eat whole fruits to meet their recommended fruit intake [52]. The 2005 Dietary Guidelines Advisory Committee report states that no more than one-third of the total recommended fruit group intakes come from fruit juice, with the rest coming from whole fruit, in order to meet requirements for vitamin C, folate, and potassium [53].

9.3.5.4 Lead Toxicity

Lead toxicity, which comes from exposure to high levels of lead in the environment (lead-based paint, newspaper ink dust, automobile emissions), is the number one environmental health threat to infants and children [33]. It can impair growth and results in lowered IQ and learning disabilities. Blood lead levels in the general population have decreased dramatically since the 1970s due to regulatory and voluntary bans on the use of lead in gasoline, household paint, food and drink cans, and plumbing. Data from the NHANES collected during 1999 to 2002 indicated that blood lead levels continued to decrease in all age groups and racial/ethnic populations [54]. During 1999 to 2002, the overall prevalence of elevated blood lead levels for the U.S. population aged >1 year was 0.7%. Blood lead levels in non-Hispanic black children remained higher than in non-Hispanic white or Mexican American children, although the proportion of blood lead levels at or above the toxic level (>10 mcg/dL) in this population decreased by 72% since 1991 to 1994. Approximately 310,000 children aged 1 to 5 years remain at risk for exposure to harmful lead levels [54]. Elevated blood lead levels in children 1 to 5 years are more likely to be higher among lower income minorities living in older urban housing.

Some nutrients, including calcium and iron, influence the body's handling of lead and protect against toxicity by decreasing lead's absorption into the bloodstream [33,55]. Deficiencies of calcium, phosphorus, iron, and zinc make children more susceptible to lead intoxication.

Also, lead is absorbed more rapidly in the fasting state. All children with blood lead levels between 15 μg/dl and 19 μg/dl should receive nutritional and environmental counseling [56]. The Centers for Disease Control (CDC) no longer recommends that all children from 6 to 36 months of age have a blood test for lead, but only recommends universal screening in areas where at least 27% of the housing was built before 1950 and in populations in which 12% or more of 1- and 2-year-old children have elevated blood lead levels [57]. They recommend more frequent screening for children who live in environments with higher exposure to lead (e.g., old houses). Dietary recommendations to prevent and treat lead toxicity are as follows: (1) evaluate and treat iron deficiency, (2) eat three meals and a midmorning and midafternoon snack daily, and (3) give 4 to 6 ounces of milk or yogurt with meals and snacks. The molar excess of calcium in milk is high enough to inhibit lead absorption. Milk also contains phosphorus, which further decreases lead absorption [58]. A balanced diet that includes a variety of foods, including adequate amounts of meat and dairy, will help decrease the risk of lead toxicity in young children [58].

9.4 SCHOOL-AGED CHILD

9.4.1 Characteristics

Children between 7 and 12 years of age enjoy slow but steady growth, with an increase in appetite and food intake. Since they spend much of their day in school, they eat fewer times a day than preschool children, but after-school snacks are almost universal. Elementary schoolchildren often take responsibility for preparing their own breakfast, packing their own lunch and finding snacks after school. Occasionally they assume responsibility for grocery shopping and preparing the evening meal. Although children at this age make their own eating decisions, parents still influence family food habits, attitudes, and expectations [33].

Peers and the media begin to have a stronger influence on food attitudes and choices [33,32]. A report of the Institute of Medicine, *Food Marketing to Children and Youth: Threat or Opportunity?* provides a comprehensive review of the scientific evidence on the influence of food marketing on diets and diet-related health of children and youth, and finds that some of the current food and beverage marketing practices put children's long-term health at risk. The report provides recommendations for different segments of society to guide the development of effective marketing and advertising strategies that promote healthier foods, beverages, and meal options to children and youth [59].

9.4.2 Importance of Milk Group Foods

9.4.2.1 Bone Growth and Fracture Prevention

Bone growth begins to accelerate in the midgrade school years, making this an important time for building optimal bone mass (Figure 9.1). Maintaining an adequate calcium and vitamin D intake during childhood and adolescence, along with physical activity, is necessary to achieve an optimal peak bone mass. This is considered the best way to prevent osteoporosis later in life [60,23]. Calcium absorption efficiency is about 28% in prepubertal children and increases to 34% in early puberty, giving this age group the greatest potential for bone mass development [61]. Many other nutrients important for children's bone health are abundant in milk and milk products. A study evaluating the effect of longitudinal nutrient intakes of children from ages 2 to 8 on bone mineral content/density at age 8 found that higher intakes of energy, calcium, phosphorus, protein, magnesium, and zinc were correlated with significantly greater bone mineral density at age 8 [62]. Several retrospective studies have associated higher milk intake in early life with higher bone density and/or osteoporosis risk in later years [63,64]. For more details on these studies, see Chapter 5.

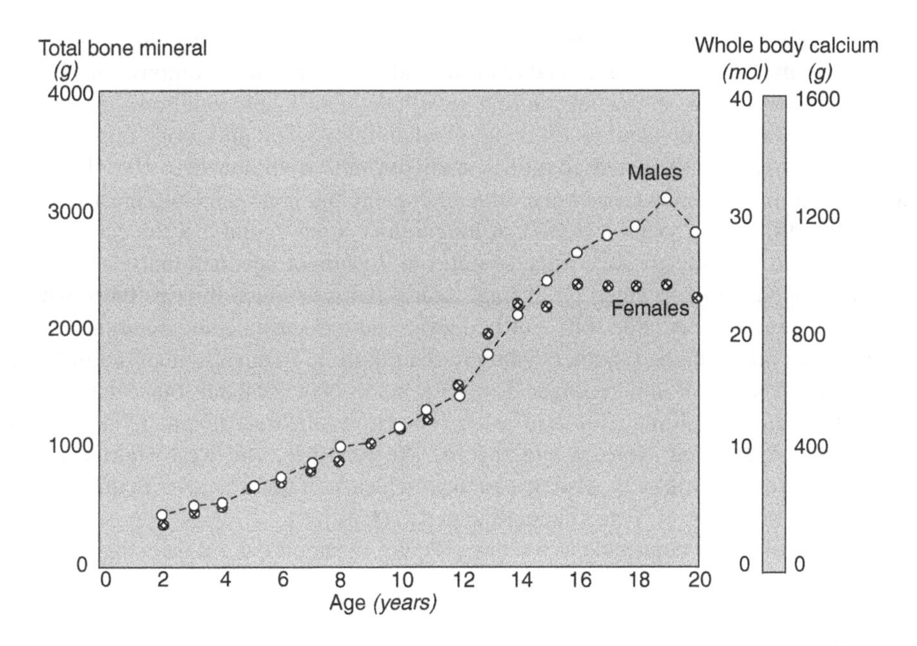

FIGURE 9.1 Accumulation of total bone mineral and whole body calcium in boys and girls as a function of age. (From FAO Food, Nutrition and Agriculture Division, *Food, Nutrition and Agriculture: Calcium Throughout Life*, 20, 14, 1997. With permission.)

The NAS recommends 800 mg of calcium for children ages 4 to 8 and 1300 mg of calcium for preadolescents and adolescents ages 9 to 18 (Table 9.6) [5]. This translates into a daily consumption of 3 or 4 servings of milk or milk equivalents (yogurt and cheese) as recommended by the AAP [23].

Most U.S. children older than 8 years fail to achieve their recommended amount of calcium [23,37,5]. Among children ages 9 to 13 years, 94% of girls and 72% of boys do not have a usual calcium intake that meets or exceeds the AI level of 1300 mg per day [5,37]. Boys and girls ages 6 to 11 are consuming an average of 2.2 and 1.9 servings of milk, cheese, or yogurt, respectively — which is about 1 serving short of what is recommended [65].

TABLE 9.6
Calcium and Dairy Food Recommendations for School-Aged Children

Age	Adequate Calcium Intake (mg/day)[a]	Servings of Dairy per Day[b]
4 to 8 Years	800	3[c]
9 to 18 Years	1300	4

[a] Institute of Medicine, Food and Nutrition Board, *Dietary Reference Intakes for Calcium, Phosphorus, Magnesim, Vitamin D, and Flouride,* Washington, D.C., National Academy Press, 1997.

[b] American Academy of Pediatrics, Optimizing bone health and calcium intakes of infants, children, and adolescents, *Pediatrics,* 117 (2), 578–585, February, 2006.

[c] One serving equals 8 ounces of milk or yogurt, 1 ounce of cheese.

Studies in children and adolescents demonstrate that (1) increasing consumption of dairy foods has a beneficial effect on bone health, and (2) low intake of dairy foods compromises bone health and increases the risk for bone fractures during growth. When Chinese children ages 9 to 10 years consumed milk powder equivalent to 1300 mg of calcium for 18 months, bone mineral density of the hip and spine significantly increased [66]. A study of Chinese children ages 10 to 12 years found that increasing milk intake increases bone mineral content and bone mineral density, particularly when milk is fortified with vitamin D [67]. A longitudinal study found that the calcium intake of girls from age 5 to 9 predicted bone mineral status at 9 years of age, and that girls who met the calcium recommendation consumed on average nearly twice as much milk as those who did not meet the calcium recommendation [68]. Further, girls who met the calcium recommendation were served milk more often and had mothers who drank milk more frequently than did girls with low calcium intakes. A study of children ages 3 to 10 years in New Zealand found that those with a history of chronically avoiding milk had a lower average dietary calcium intake, lower bone mineral density of the total skeleton and specific skeletal sites, and were shorter and heavier than children who drank milk [69]. Also, the annual incidence of arm fractures in the milk avoiders was higher (3.5%) than the expected annual incidence (1%) [69].

Low bone density may contribute to fracture risk during childhood. An investigation found that significantly more children ages 3 to 13 years who avoided milk for prolonged periods experienced bone fractures (especially forearm fractures) compared to a group of children born at the same time from the same city [70]. Nearly one in three of the milk avoiders experienced a bone fracture before 8 years of age, most often from a minor trip or fall. Previously, these researchers showed that bone density was 3% to 5% lower at different skeletal sites in girls ages 3 to 15 years with a recent forearm fracture compared to those who had never broken a bone — and the older girls with forearm fracture reported lower current and past calcium intakes than did the controls [71]. Interestingly, a new report documents a significant increase in the number of distal forearm (wrist) fractures in U.S. children and adolescents over the past 30 years [72]. Although the specific cause of this increase was not explored, the researchers suggest that the decline in milk consumption and dramatic increase in soft drink intake in recent decades is likely a contributing factor [72]. However, more research is needed to better understand what factors may be associated with the increase in fractures among children and adolescents.

9.4.2.2 Prevention of Dental Caries

Although the prevalence of dental caries in children is declining, 21.9% of children ages 6 to 17 years had untreated dental caries in 1999 to 2002 [73].

Dental caries in children can be prevented by increasing tooth resistance (e.g., fluoride), changing the oral environment (e.g., dietary intervention), and by reducing oral microorganisms with proper oral hygiene. Diet plays an important role in dental caries risk. Fermentable carbohydrates (e.g., sugar, starches) in a food are cariogenic, while cheese and milk may protect against tooth decay [74–76]. Components in cheese or milk such as protein (casein and whey), lipids, calcium, and phosphorus may be responsible for the caries-protective effects of these foods. Milk, particularly casein, has been demonstrated to decrease the adherence of cavity-causing bacteria to the teeth [77]. A review of cheese and dental caries discusses the evidence that cheese may protect against tooth decay by several mechanisms, including the buffering of acid, stimulation of saliva, reduction of bacterial adhesion to tooth surfaces, reduction of enamel demineralization, and/or the promotion of remineralization by casein and ionizable calcium and phosphorus [74].

Minor milk protein and protein-associated components (proteose-peptone fractions 3 and 5) have been found to strongly adhere to the tooth surface and reduce the extent of demineralization by acid buffer solutions [78]. Bioactive peptides that result from the digestion of casein have also been investigated for their anticariogenic properties. Two such bioactive peptides, caseinophosphopeptides (CPP) and glycomacropeptide (GMP) have been patented for use in common personal hygiene products to prevent dental caries. Both have demonstrated the ability to inhibit demineralization and promote remineralization of tooth enamel [79]. In addition, various bacterial strains of probiotics used in dairy foods are under investigation for their ability to reduce cariogenic bacteria [80].

Although, more research is needed on the carcinogenicity of chocolate milk, it will contribute less to dental caries than sucrose alone or snack foods such as potato chips, cookies, and raisins. There is evidence that its cocoa content, milk fat, calcium, and phosphorus may contribute to this favorable effect [81]. In addition, since chocolate milk and other flavored milk are liquid and clear the mouth rapidly, they are less likely to cause dental caries than sticky carbohydrate foods [82]. Evidence indicates that flavored milk, including chocolate milk, when consumed in moderation, has a low cariogenic potential [83].

To reduce the incidence of dental caries, children should limit their intake of sugar-containing foods to mealtimes, should eat plenty of noncariogenic foods, such as cheese, fresh fruits, or vegetables, and practice good oral hygiene. Since eating frequency increases caries risk, the AAP suggests limiting eating occasions to three meals and a few snacks per day [84].

9.4.2.3 Achieving Nutrient Adequacy

Milk and milk products are a major contributor of calcium and are a leading source of many other nutrients in children's diets, including protein, phosphorus, potassium, riboflavin, vitamin A, vitamin B_{12}, niacin, and vitamin D (if fortified) [85]. An analysis of dietary sources of nutrients in the diets of U.S. children reported that milk was the number one source of calcium, magnesium, and protein, and a major source of zinc, vitamin A, and folate [86]. The authors found that milk and milk products (milk, cheese, and ice cream/sherbet/frozen yogurt) supplied 69.7% of the calcium in the diets of children ages 6 to 11 (Table 9.7). Because milk and milk products are nutrient-dense foods, their intake improves the overall nutritional quality of children's diets [85,87,88]. When school-aged children included milk as part of their noon meal, intakes of calcium, vitamins A and E, and zinc increased [89]. There is growing recognition of the importance of nutrition for cognitive and physical development of children. A study of single-parent, rural African American families found that in female 6- to 9-year-old children, higher milk intake was related to better cognitive outcomes, including applied problem score, passage comprehension, calculation, synonym/antonym identification, and quantitative concept scores [90]. However, more prospective studies are needed on larger samples of children from various ethnic groups to confirm these findings.

Moreover, intake of dairy foods has been shown to increase the nutritional quality of the diets of children and adolescents without adverse effects on body weight/fat [91,92].

9.4.3 Strategies to Improve Dairy Consumption

Many children fail to consume the recommended amount of calcium and servings of Milk Group foods. The 2005 *Dietary Guidelines for Americans* recommends 2 to 3 cups per day of fat-free or low-fat milk or equivalent milk products (i.e., cheese, yogurt) for children age 2 and older depending on their level of activity [45]. *MyPyramid for Kids* was developed to give age-appropriate food guidance to children ages 6 to 11 years [93]. Children are encouraged to eat more whole grains, fruits, vegetables, lean meats, and low-fat or fat-free milk, and other calcium-rich milk products. Web site materials include an interactive online game, lesson plans for grades one to six, and colorful posters and flyers, worksheets, and tip for families — encouraging children, teachers, and parents to work together to make healthier food choices and be active every day.

The National Institute of Child Health Development (NICHD) has sponsored a publicly funded campaign called "Milk Matters." The goal of this campaign is to educate pediatricians, other health care professionals, children and adolescents 11 to 15 years, and their parents about the benefits of consuming more calcium-rich foods, particularly milk. The campaign recommends 3 cups of

TABLE 9.7
Contribution of Milk Group Foods to Children's Diets (Ages 2 to 5 and 6 to 11)

	Ages 2 to 5				Ages 6 to 11			
Milk Group Foods	**Milk (%)**	**Cheese (%)**	**Ice Cream (%)**	**Total (%)**	**Milk (%)**	**Cheese (%)**	**Ice Cream (%)**	**Total (%)**
Energy	15.4	3.3	2.6	21.3	12.4	3.4	2.8	18.6
Fat	19.0	7.1	3.3	29.4	15.0	7.0	3.1	25.1
Carbohydrate	10.2	—[a]	2.8	13.0	8.2	—[a]	3.3	11.5
Protein	25.0	5.8	1.1	31.9	20.5	6.3	1.2	28.0
Calcium	58.9	10.8	2.5	72.2	53.6	13.2	2.9	69.7
Magnesium	27.8	1.7	1.3	30.8	24.2	2.0	1.6	27.8
Vitamin A	22.4	4.3	2.0	28.7	19.9	4.9	2.2	27.0
Zinc	21.1	5.3	1.5	27.9	16.7	5.5	1.6	23.8
Folate	9.4	—[a]	—[a]	9.4	8.1	—[a]	—[a]	8.1
Carotene	3.9	1.4	—[a]	5.3	3.0	1.3	—[a]	4.3

[a] Not a significant source in this age group.

Source: From Subar, A. F. et. al., *Pediatrics*, 102, 4, 913, 1999. With permission.

low-fat or fat-free milk every day. Educational materials are available on the National Institute of Child Health Development (NICHD) Web site [94].

In addition to using the educational materials above, here are some important ways parents, teachers, and health professionals can encourage children to consume the recommended amounts of milk and milk products.

9.4.3.1 Parental Role Modeling

Children's eating patterns are strongly influenced by adults as well as by the marketplace [86]. Parents serve as role models for their children's eating behavior and in this age group a parent's persistence in encouraging milk consumption has a positive influence on their children's milk intake. In an analysis of USDA 1994 to 95 Continuing Survey of Food Intakes by Individuals (CSFII) data, researchers found that the amount of milk consumed by the mothers of children ages 5 to 17 was the strongest predictor of the children's milk intake [95]. Children's milk intake increased by 1 g for every 0.64 g of milk consumed by their mothers. The authors suggest that the influence of parental role modeling should be considered when designing nutrition intervention programs designed to increase children's milk intake.

By making dairy foods readily available at family mealtimes and as snacks and consuming these foods themselves, mothers can play a positive role in shaping children's dietary habits, including their intake of dairy products [96–98]. A 5-year prospective study of 192 mothers and their young daughters found that mothers' consumption of milk and how frequently they made milk available to their daughters at meals and snacks was positively related to their daughters' milk consumption, calcium intake, and bone health [68].

A nationally representative survey of children and their parents revealed that most parents of boys ages 5 to 8 increasingly agreed that "milk is absolutely essential to a child's growth," and "I try to make sure everyone in my household has milk every day" [98]. These parental attitudes corresponded with an 8% yearly increase in milk consumption in this age group. However, fewer parents of boys 9 to 12 years old felt that milk was "absolutely essential" to their child's growth, and they increasingly agreed that, "It's less important for older children to drink milk," and that "It's hard to get my older children to drink milk." Consequently, boys of this age felt less compelled to drink milk, and their consumption decreased by 6% yearly. Other factors, such as problems with away-from-home portability and school milk quality, also influenced this decline.

The pattern is similar for girls. Although girls' milk consumption remains fairly steady between the ages of 6 and 11, the stage is being set for a dramatic decline in consumption during their teenage years. Fewer parents say that they "Encourage my kids to drink milk at school," and "Insist kids drink at least one glass of milk at mealtime" as their girls get older. Unfortunately, parents set the stage for girls' weight concerns. As girls approach age 11, more and more parents say, "I'm concerned about the calories in milk for members of my household." This is matched by girls who increasingly say more frequently as they age that "Drinking milk will make me fat" [98]. This belief is a barrier preventing many young girls from consuming the milk they need to reach their bone mass potential and is not supported by research. In a study conducted in Utah, 9- to 13-year-old girls who increased their calcium intake to recommended levels by eating more milk, yogurt, and cheese (no fat level specified) had an increased rate of bone mineralization, but did not gain weight or increase body fatness compared to girls who followed their normal diet [99]. Similarly, 12-year-old girls who consumed an additional two cups of either whole or low-fat milk per day gained bone mineral density, but not weight or fat mass compared to the control group [91]. A longitudinal study conducted among children ages 2 to 8 years found that a high intake of calcium and dairy foods was associated with lower body fat [100]. Additional studies showing that dairy food intake does not cause excessive weight gain and may reduce body fat in children are discussed in Chapter 7.

Parents of girls in particular need to be very careful not to criticize their children about their weight or communicate through their own actions that outward appearance is of greater importance than health. Doing so increases the likelihood that children will restrict their dietary intake and develop nutritional deficiencies.

9.4.3.2 School Meals

Dairy foods, such as milk, yogurt, and cheese, are an important component of meals and snacks offered in the school lunch and breakfast programs, as well as other federal child nutrition programs [101]. In 2003 an estimated 5.4 billion half-pints of fluid milk were served in child nutrition programs in schools: 4.0 billion half-pints in the National School Lunch Program (NSLP), 1.2 billion half-pints in the School Breakfast Program (SBP), and 108 million half-pints in the Special Milk Program (SMP) [102]. The SMP allows children to purchase milk at a reduced price or receive it free. As a result of the Child Nutrition and WIC Reauthorization Act signed into law (P.L.108 to 265) on June 30, 2004, schools are required to offer fluid milk (e.g., flavored or unflavored whole milk, low-fat milk, fat-free (skim) milk, or cultured buttermilk) in a variety of fat levels and are no longer constrained by prior year preferences as they had been in the past [103]. This change both increases local schools' options and ensures that students will have more than one fat level from which to choose. In addition, for the first time, schools are encouraged to offer flavored milk and lactose-free milk [103]. Although children participating in the NSLP or the SBP are given a choice of milk, as a result of the "offer vs. serve" option they can decide not to select milk. The "offer vs. serve" option is required in senior high schools and permitted at the discretion of school authorities for younger grade levels [101]. Yogurt may be used to meet all or part of the meat/meat alternate requirement in child feeding programs. Four ounces of yogurt equals one ounce of the meat/meat alternate requirement [104].

Findings from USDA's School Nutrition Dietary Assessment-II Study [105]. indicate that, during the 1998 to 1999 school year, elementary and secondary lunches exceeded the calcium standard (i.e., 25% for breakfast and 30% for lunch) by providing 58% and 40%, respectively, of the daily amount of calcium recommended. Elementary and secondary school breakfasts also exceeded the standard by providing 43% and 29%, respectively, of the daily recommended amount of calcium. More than 95% of the school lunch menus and 80% of the school breakfast menus included two or more types of milk.

Consuming milk or milk products at breakfast (whether at home or at school) is an important way for schoolchildren to meet their daily calcium needs [106]. Studies have shown that children who participate in the SBP have higher intakes of milk and several nutrients (e.g., calcium, phosphorus, magnesium, protein, thiamin, riboflavin) at breakfast and over a 24-hour period than nonparticipants who have breakfast at home or skip this meal [107,108]. Recognizing the benefits of a nutritious breakfast for children, the U.S. government established the School Breakfast Program in 1975. An evaluation of the program in the 1980s revealed that breakfast participants had superior intakes of milk-related nutrients, such as calcium, phosphorus, riboflavin, and protein, and had higher overall nutrient intakes over 24 hours than breakfast skippers [109]. A longitudinal study of almost 2400 African American and white girls ages 9 to 10 years at baseline found that those who frequently ate breakfast had higher calcium and fiber intakes and a lower body mass index than those who infrequently consumed this meal [110].

The Food Research and Action Center (FRAC) estimates that almost 9.6 million low-income schoolchildren who participate in school lunch go without school breakfast — even though the 2004 to 2005 school year marked the largest increase in SBP participation since 1994 to 1995 [111]. Expansion of the breakfast program into more schools, and greater student participation within schools by integrating breakfast into the school day, for example, would likely improve schoolchildren's calcium and nutritional status.

School lunch also contributes significantly to a child's intake of calcium and milk products. Compared to nonparticipants, NSLP participants consumed more milks and vegetables at lunch and fewer sweets and snack foods [112]. Evidence indicates that participating in the NSLP improves students' intakes of vitamins and minerals at lunch and over 24 hours [112].

In a nationwide sample of more than 2000 children ages 5 to 17, only those who drank milk at the noon meal met or exceeded 33% of the 1989 Recommended Dietary Allowance (RDA) for calcium for that meal or the recommended amount of calcium over the whole day [113]. Those who drank other beverages at lunch, such as soft drinks, juice, tea, or fruit drinks, failed to meet their calcium recommendations. When milk was included in the noon meal, intakes of vitamin A, vitamin E, calcium, and zinc were highest both for that meal and for the total day [89]. When the nutrient contributions of five meal components (entrée, milk, vegetable/fruit, grain/bread, and miscellaneous, such as condiments) of school lunches were examined, researchers found that milk provided the most calcium and protein per 100 kcal and per penny [89].

Children need to select and consume milk at breakfast and lunch in order to meet the current recommendations for calcium for 9- to 18-year-olds (1300 mg/day). An informal analysis of one week's worth of sample school lunch and breakfast menus indicated that a child must consume an 8-ounce serving of milk at breakfast to meet the 25% of the current recommendation for calcium (325 mg) required of this meal. However, even if children consumed 8 ounces of milk with lunch, this meal may fall short of the one-third of the current recommendation for calcium (433 mg) required for this meal [114].

While school breakfast and lunch programs have largely been successful at promoting healthy eating among children, the availability of competitive foods (many of which are high energy, low-nutrient foods and beverages) from vending machines and à la carte programs may have an adverse affect on the quality of foods children consume at school [115]. This now is being addressed. As part of the Child Nutrition and WIC Reauthorization Act of 2004, each school district participating in federal meal programs (e.g., school breakfast and/or lunch) must establish a local school wellness policy by the beginning of the 2006 to 2007 school year [103].

Children's low intake of milk and milk products and dairy food nutrients such as calcium, as well as dairy's health benefits (e.g., in bone health) are among the reasons to make dairy foods a part of school wellness policies [37,65,108]. Promoting the consumption of nutrient-rich, low-fat and nonfat dairy foods in the cafeteria, in vending, and through à la carte sales is a good way to reduce the consumption of empty-calorie beverages and foods. In the past, barriers to consumption of milk at school included (1) temperature problems (milk not cold enough), (2) lack of colorful, eye-catching packaging, and (3) taste. The New Look of School Milk program, initiated by the National Dairy Council (NDC), addresses these barriers by providing cold milk in a variety of flavors, in colorful single-serve plastic containers, and merchandised in attractive retail-style coolers throughout the school. This program was launched after a pilot test involving 100,000 students in 146 elementary and secondary schools, sponsored by the NDC and the School Nutrition Association, found that offering milk served cold in single-serve plastic containers in at least three flavors, and merchandising throughout the school, increased milk consumption by 37% and increased participation in the school lunch program as much as 5% [116]. More than eight in ten schools serve milk in paper cartons, but this is not the packaging preferred by students. The majority of students (71%) believed that the quality of milk in plastic bottles was better than that in paper cartons [117]. Using improvements in packaging, flavors, and merchandising milk in schools may help improve school meal participation, which in turn may help children eat more healthfully at school.

The presence of soft drink marketers in the schools encourages students to drink beverages other than milk with their meals [118,119]. According to an analysis of data collected among 1548 10-year-old children enrolled in the Bogalusa Heart Study and followed for 21 years, milk consumption was significantly lower in those who consumed medium to high amounts of sweetened beverages compared to those with lower or no intake of sweetened beverages [120]. Leading soft drink manufacturers in the United States are offering monetary incentives to school districts in return for exclusive contracts to provide products and advertising within schools. However, milk vending is protected by the new child nutrition law which says that an exclusive beverage contract can't be used to limit a school's ability to sell milk anywhere on school property or at school events [121]. The American Heart Association's dietary recommendations for children and adolescents, endorsed by the AAP, encourages schools to improve nutrition and reduce the prevalence of overweight in children by working to "make predominantly healthful foods available at school and school functions by influencing food and beverage contracts, adapt marketing techniques to influence students to make healthy choices, and restrict in-school availability of and marketing of poor food choices" [122,123]. In addition, the ADA supports nutrition integrity in schools, and recommends that only foods that make a significant contribution to children's nutritional needs, such as low-fat milk and yogurt, be available wherever and whenever food is served in schools [118].

The AAP issued a position statement outlining nutritional concerns regarding soft drink consumption in schools, which calls for district-wide policy restricting the sale of soft drinks in schools [124]. Potential health problems associated with high intake of sweetened drinks indicated in the statement include (1) overweight or obesity attributable to additional calories in the diet, (2) displacement of milk consumption, resulting in calcium deficiency with an attendant risk of osteoporosis and fractures, and (3) dental caries and potential enamel erosion. The statement encourages school officials and parents to become well-informed about the health implications of vended drinks in school before making a decision about student access to them.

A publication by the CDC and USDA's Team Nutrition, entitled *Making It Happen! School Nutrition Success Stories*, describes how 32 schools and school districts across the United States have improved the nutritional quality of foods and beverages apart from the school meals program [125]. The success stories relate to how schools have:

- Established nutrition standards for competitive foods.
- Influenced food and beverage contracts.
- Made more healthful foods and beverages available (e.g., *Massachusetts Action for Healthy Kids* à la carte food and beverage standards to promote a healthier school environment).
- Adopted marketing techniques to promote healthful choices (e.g., those featuring dairy vending machines in Iowa that provided milk, cheese, and yogurt).
- Limited student access to competitive foods.
- Used fundraising activities and rewards that support student health.

Research is needed to determine what impact these environmental and policy changes will have on children's dietary intake from school meals and on total dietary intake over the whole day.

9.4.3.3 Flavored Milk

Flavored milks are highly nutritious beverages that increase children's enjoyment and consumption of milk, improving their nutrient intake. When children ages 6 to 12 were asked about their milk-drinking habits, 90% said they like the taste of chocolate milk, 86% said it is fun to drink, and 61% described chocolate milk as their favorite drink [117]. When given a choice of milks, the children surveyed preferred chocolate milk over white milk. An investigation of how children view milk served at school found that milk flavor strongly influences milk-drinking behavior and that the majority of children prefer chocolate milk [126]. In the School Milk Pilot Test described above, the presence of a third flavor of milk, particularly strawberry, was responsible for much of the incremental sales [116].

The nutrient content of chocolate milk — whole, 2% reduced-fat, 1% low-fat, and nonfat — is similar to that of the corresponding unflavored milk [127]. The major difference is an increased carbohydrate and calorie content in chocolate milk due to the addition of sucrose and other nutritive

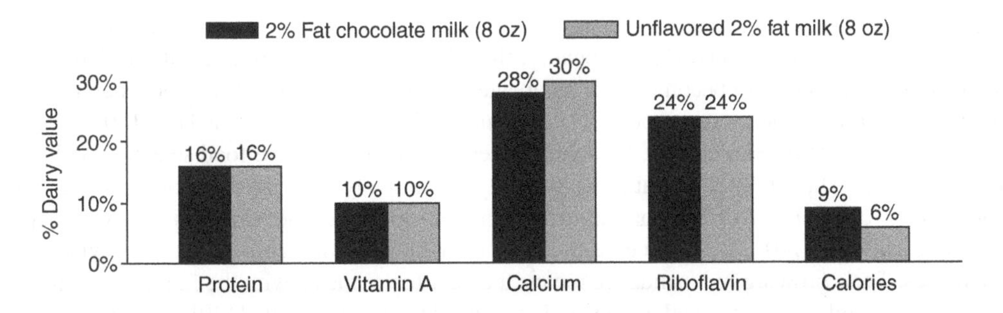

FIGURE 9.2 Nutrient comparison of flavored and unflavored milk. (Courtesy of the National Dairy Council®.)

sweeteners [127]. In general, chocolate flavored milk provides about 60 calories more per 8-ounce serving than do their unflavored counterparts [127]. Despite concerns related to the sugar content of flavored milks, a recent analysis of national eating trends indicates that flavored milk contributes little (2.2%) to children's and adolescents' intake of added sugars [128]. Carbonated soft drinks account for the largest share of added sugar (24%) in their diets [128]. The 2005 *Dietary Guidelines for Americans* as well as the ADA recognizes that small amounts of sugars added to nutrient dense foods, such as breakfast cereals and reduced-fat milk products, may increase a person's nutrient intake by enhancing the palatability of these foods without contributing excessive calories [45,129].

A study of nearly 4000 school-aged children and adolescents found that those who drank flavored milk, such as chocolate milk, consumed more total milk and fewer soft drinks and fruit drinks than children who did not drink flavored milk [130]. Also, flavored milk consumers had high calcium intakes but not a higher percent of energy from total fat and added sugars intake than non-consumers of flavored milk [130]. This study's findings support earlier suggestions that providing chocolate milk as part of school lunch programs may increase children's milk and calcium intakes [131]. A retrospective analysis of the diets of more than 3000 children ages 6 to 17 found a positive effect on children's overall diets when they chose flavored milks and yogurts instead of sodas and sweetened drinks [132]. The AAP, in a policy statement on soft drinks in schools, encourages pediatricians to work to eliminate sweetened drinks in school and instead recommend more nutritious beverage choices including low-fat white or flavored milk [133]. In a 2006 report on calcium and bone health, the AAP encourages pediatricians to support children's increased consumption of flavored and unflavored milk, yogurt, and cheese to meet their calcium requirements [23].

Chocolate milk is just as nutritious as white milk (Figure 9.2), and research has shown that the sweeteners do not cause hyperactivity [134] or tooth decay [135], and that the calcium is just as well absorbed as from white milk [136]. In addition, chocolate milk may be better tolerated than white milk for people with lactose intolerance [137] — and it is nutritionally superior to soft drinks and fruit drinks. For these reasons government and health organizations, such as the USDA, the AAP, and the ADA support the consumption of flavored milk to meet calcium and other nutrient needs [23,45,129].

9.5 ADOLESCENCE

9.5.1 CHARACTERISTICS

The adolescent period is characterized by rapid physical growth as well as maturational changes. The adolescent "growth spurt" which begins at the onset of puberty contributes 15% to adult height, 50% to adult weight, and 45% to adult skeletal mass [138]. It typically occurs between the ages of 10 and 13 in girls and 2 years later in boys. A nutritionally adequate diet is needed for growth, but the rate of growth is influenced by a number of factors including genetics, physical activity age, gender, and endocrine balance [139]. Socially, the adolescent moves from a state of dependence upon parents and family to become more independent and self-directing. The peer group becomes more important as a source of support, self-esteem, and behavioral standards [138,140].

Various aspects of teen culture, lifestyle, and environment influence food selection and nutritional status. As the adolescent matures physically, cognitively, and psychosocially, focus shifts from family food habits to peer group influence, and eventually to the adolescent's own independent food patterns [140]. Teens receive much of their nutrition information from television and magazines. Their growing independence means they eat fewer meals with the family and eat more meals in fast food restaurants and at concession stands at sporting events [140]. Changes in eating patterns as children become adolescents and young adults can result in an overall decrease in diet quality [141]. For example, as children get older they tend to decrease their milk consumption and increase their intake of less nutritious beverages, such as carbonated soft drinks and fruit drinks [142,143].

Data from the National Heart, Lung, and Blood Institute Growth and Health Study found that fast food intake increases with age in both African American and white adolescent girls and is associated with poor diet quality [144]. In contrast, the frequency of family meals among adolescents is positively associated with higher diet quality, including an increased intake of calcium and calcium-rich foods [145].

9.5.2 Importance of Adequate Dairy Food/Calcium Intake

9.5.2.1 Peak Bone Mass

Optimizing the amount of bone laid down during the adolescent period appears to be the most effective strategy for reducing the risk of osteoporosis (porous bones) later in life [23,146,147]. The most opportune time to initiate efforts to increase calcium intake is during the 5-year period from 11 to 16 years of age, since this is when a substantial part of bone accretion takes place [148]. By age 18 in girls and 20 in boys, about 85% to 90% of final adult bone mass is acquired [147]. However, efforts to improve calcium intake may need to begin even earlier to be successful as mentioned in the previous section on school-aged children.

Several nutrients are involved in the production and maintenance of bone, such as calcium, protein, phosphorus, vitamins D, C, and K, fluoride, copper, manganese, and zinc [147,149]. The composition of bone is mainly calcium, phosphorus, and protein. Milk and milk products are the main sources of calcium and other nutrients involved in bone development. The proportions of calcium and phosphorus in dairy foods are optimal for skeletal growth and development [150]. An analysis of data from NHANES 1999 to 2002 indicated that milk consumption frequency and milk intake (measured as grams of milk, or protein, or calcium from milk) significantly predicted height in adolescents ages 12 to 18 years, along with age, sex, household income, and ethnicity [151].

Calcium and vitamin D are critically important for bone mineral accrual during adolescence; however, dietary calcium intake has declined over the past several decades among adolescents, and up to 54% of teens have inadequate blood levels of vitamin D [152]. The decline in consumption of dairy foods and vitamin D-fortified milk in particular has contributed to this problem [152,153].

A British study of 80 adolescent girls found that bone mineral density and bone mineral content increased in those who consumed an additional daily pint of milk for 18 months [91]. A study of adolescent girls 12 to 14 years old in China demonstrated that increasing milk intake increased bone mineral content and bone mineral density, and milk was a better nutritional determinant of bone mineral content than intake of any single milk nutrient [154]. In a 12-week randomized clinical trial in the United States, whole body bone mineral density was significantly higher in adolescent boys (13 to 17 years of age) who drank 3 servings a day of milk while participating in a strength training program compared with boys who drank 100% fruit juice [155]. The researchers suggested that this beneficial effect on bone was most likely due to the additional calcium and/or vitamin D consumed by the milk drinkers.

Further support for a positive effect of calcium and dairy products on bone health in adolescents is provided by findings from a study of two groups of adolescent girls (15 to 18 years) [156]. One group was part of a randomized double-blind, placebo-controlled clinical trial with calcium supplements, and the other group was part of an observational study in which calcium was provided by dairy products. Both calcium and dairy products improved bone mass accrual, leading to a higher peak bone mass. While calcium influenced volumetric bone density, dairy products had an additional impact on bone growth and bone expansion, perhaps due to the calcium and protein content of dairy products [156]. Interventions to increase dietary calcium intake should occur in mid-puberty, when the skeleton is most responsive [157].

Health professional organizations including the AAP23 and the ADA42, as well as the U.S. Surgeon General [60], recognize the importance of calcium and calcium-rich foods such as milk, cheese, and yogurt for both child and adolescent bone health.

9.5.2.2 Nutritional Status

Milk supplies calcium, as well as eight other essential nutrients that contribute to the nutritional status of teens. In an analysis of more than 4000 children ages 2 to 5, 6 to 11, and 12 to 17 participating in the CSFII 1994 to 96, milk consumption was positively associated with the likelihood of achieving recommended intakes of vitamin A, folate, vitamin B_{12}, calcium, and magnesium intakes in all age strata [143]. In an earlier analysis of calcium consumption and food sources of calcium in the United States, Fleming and Heimbach compared the nutrient profiles of teenage girls (13 to 18 years) who drank milk with those who did not (Table 9.8) [158]. Milk-drinkers consumed 80% more calcium, 59% more vitamin B_{12}, 56% more riboflavin, 38% more folate, 35% more vitamin A, 24% more of each vitamin B_6 and potassium, and 22% more magnesium than did nonmilk-drinking teenagers [158]. An analysis of data from the Bogalusa Heart Study, reporting longitudinal trends in calcium intake and food sources, found that at age

TABLE 9.8
Nutrient Density of Diets of Teenage Girls 13 to 18 Years Who Use and Do Not Use Milk

Nutrient	Mean Intake (d-1000 kcal) per day per 1000 kcal		(Users — Nonusers)/ Nonusers (%)
	Users of Fluid Milk	Nonusers of Fluid Milk	
Fat (*g*)	41	42	
Protein (*g*)	38	36	
Vitamin *A, RE*	475	351	35
Folate (μg)	121	88	38
Riboflavin (*mg*)	1.03	0.66	56
Vitamin B6 (*mg*)	0.78	0.63	24
Vitamin B-12 (μg)	2.57	1.62	59
Calcium (*mg*)	495	275	80
Magnesium (*mg*)	117	96	22
Potassium (*mg*)	1232	994	24

1987 to 1988 Nationwide Food Consumption Survey Weighted Data.

Source: From Fleming, K. H. and Heimbach, J. T., *J. Nutr.*, 124, 1426s, 1994. With permission.

TABLE 9.9
Calcium Recommendations for Adolescents

Age	Calcium (mg/d)
9 to 18 Years	1300
Pregnancy/lactation <18 years	1300

Source: From Dietary Reference Intakes, National Academy of Sciences, 1997.

10 and in young adulthood, milk was the major source of calcium [120]. An analysis of the nutrient contribution of dairy foods to Americans' diets found that higher intakes of total dairy and milk were associated with statistically significant and often large increases in the intake of several nutrients, including calcium, magnesium, potassium, zinc, iron, vitamin A, riboflavin, and folate [159]. Dairy foods contributed 62% of the calcium to the diets of children under 19 years [159].

9.5.3 Dairy Food/Calcium Recommendations and Consumption

The National Academy Sciences (NAS) recommends that children ages 9 to 18 consume 1300 mg of calcium per day to maximize calcium retention [5]. This amount of calcium is the equivalent of about 4 servings of milk, cheese, or yogurt, which the AAP recommends for adolescents to meet their calcium needs (Table 9.9) [23]. Although other foods — such as green vegetables, nuts, and dried beans — may supply up to 300 mg of calcium in the overall diet of the average American, these foods are not routinely eaten by teenagers. Therefore, AAP's recommendation relies primarily on dairy foods to supply calcium in the teen diet. The 2005 *Dietary Guidelines for Americans* recognizes the low calcium intakes among adolescents, and recommends 3 servings of low-fat or nonfat milk, cheese, or yogurt per day for adolescents [45].

Unfortunately, many teens do not consume enough calcium. Among boys ages 14 to 18 years, 69% do not meet or exceed their calcium intake recommendation of 1300 mg/day (AI), while 91% of girls that age do not meet or exceed their recommended calcium intake [37]. Boys 14 to 18 years have a median usual calcium intake (50th percentile) of 1094 mg/day, while girls of that age have a median usual calcium intake of 753 mg/day [37]. An evaluation of food sources of calcium for adolescent females published in 1997 reports that calcium intakes in girls ages 11 to 18 have "declined over time, with age, and appear to be related to a decline in fluid milk consumption" [160]. The situation is the same today. On average, teenage boys ages 12 to 19 years are consuming 2.4 servings per day of milk or milk products (1.5 servings of fluid milk), while girls are consuming 1.7 dairy servings (1 serving of fluid milk) [65].

9.5.4 Issues Affecting Dairy Consumption

9.5.4.1 Lack of Knowledge

A study conducted in more than 1000 ninth grade students found that most are aware that dietary calcium "is healthy" (98%), it "strengthens bones" (92%), and it "prevents osteoporosis" (51%) [161]. However, only 19% knew how much calcium was recommended for their age group, and only 10% knew the calcium content of various dairy products. The authors concluded that this lack of information may contribute to adolescents' suboptimal intake of calcium. In fact, adolescents who are aware of the link between calcium intake and bone health have higher calcium intakes [162]. A study among adolescent girls in grades 6 through 10 in southwestern Michigan found that these girls had limited knowledge of the risk factors for osteoporosis, calcium-rich foods, dietary calcium requirements, or the type of exercise needed to maximize bone mineral density [163]. However, sometimes even though they may know about healthy foods and healthy eating, adolescents frequently consumed foods they perceived as unhealthy [164]. Parents, teachers, and health care providers need to talk with teens about calcium recommendations and food sources then assist them in translating their knowledge into increased consumption of Milk Group foods.

9.5.4.2 Eating Away from Home

Fully 72% of teenage boys (12 to 19 years) and 64% of teenage girls eat away from home on any given day, according to a USDA survey [165]. However, milk is most often consumed at home, rather than away from home. Only about one-third of milk-drinkers report away-from-home usage [166]. More than half of young teens surveyed said they would rather not drink milk in a restaurant [167]. Fast food intake is associated with a low intake of milk and a high intake of soft drinks [168,170]. Since family meals are generally higher in calcium and calcium-rich foods [145], the trend toward greater away-from-home eating may be contributing to the low calcium and milk intake of adolescents. However, the recent introduction of milk with flavor options in plastic containers at quick-serve restaurants may help to increase away-from-home milk consumption.

9.5.4.3 Image

For teens, in particular, milk-drinking is linked to images of home and family, which may be at odds with teens' need for peer approval and independence. Researchers in Toronto found that adolescent girls categorized milk as a "healthy food" which was associated in their minds with home and family, while "junk foods" were associated with peers and independence [169]. As children get older, drinking milk, especially at school, is often not considered to be "cool" [170]. However, if a teen's peers drink milk, he/she is also likely to consume this beverage [171]. Therefore, it is important for any nutrition intervention to identify and address the functional meaning of foods in the teen culture in order to bring about more healthful food choices.

9.5.4.4 Substituting Other Beverages for Milk

There is some evidence that adolescents may be substituting fruit juice and soft drinks for milk — putting them at greater risk for deficiencies of bone-building nutrients [23]. Soft drink consumption has risen dramatically over the 20 years between 1977 and 1978 and 1994 to 1998, especially among teens (Figure 9.3) [172]. Over that same time period, milk consumption has declined (Figure 9.4) [172]. A study examining the trends in beverage consumption among females ages 12 to 19 years, found that milk intakes decreased by 36%, whereas that of sodas and fruit drinks almost doubled from the late 1970s to the mid 1990s [173]. At 12 years of age, 78% of those studied drank milk and had the lowest daily soda intake (276 g or about 9 ounce), while at age 19 years, only 36% drank milk and drank a high daily amount of soda (423 g or about 14 ounces). Those who did not drink milk had inadequate intakes of vitamin A, folate, calcium, phosphorus, and magnesium [173].

A multisite longitudinal study of more than 2300 African American and white girls evaluated changes in beverage consumption over a period of 10 years [174]. Girls entered the National Heart, Lung, and Blood Institute Growth and Health Study at ages 9 or 10 and were followed until age 19 years. For girls of both races, milk consumption decreased by more than 25% and soda consumption increased almost threefold during the course of this 10-year study. In addition, the authors report, "Increasing soda consumption predicted the greatest increase of BMI and the lowest increase in calcium intake" [174].

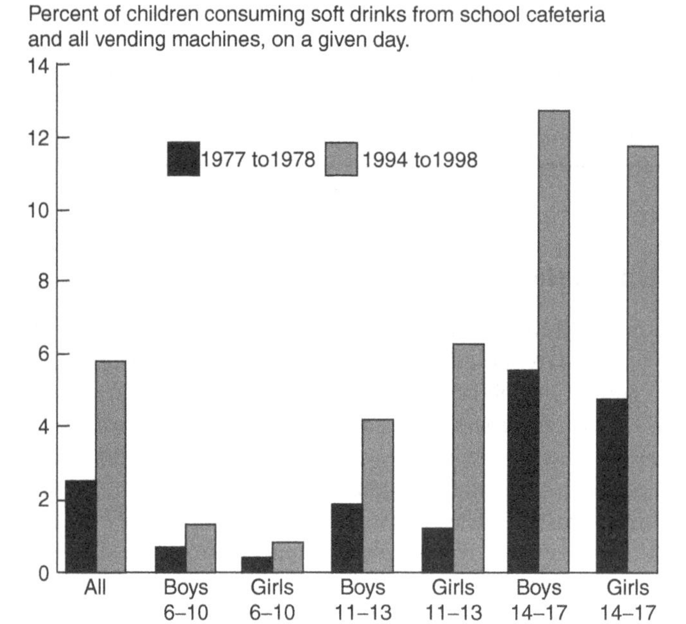

FIGURE 9.3 Soft drink consumption rising, especially for teenagers.

According to an analysis of data collected among 1548 10-year-old children enrolled in the Bogalusa Heart Study and followed for 21 years, milk consumption was significantly lower in those who consumed medium to high amounts of sweetened beverages compared to those with lower or no intake of sweetened beverages [120].

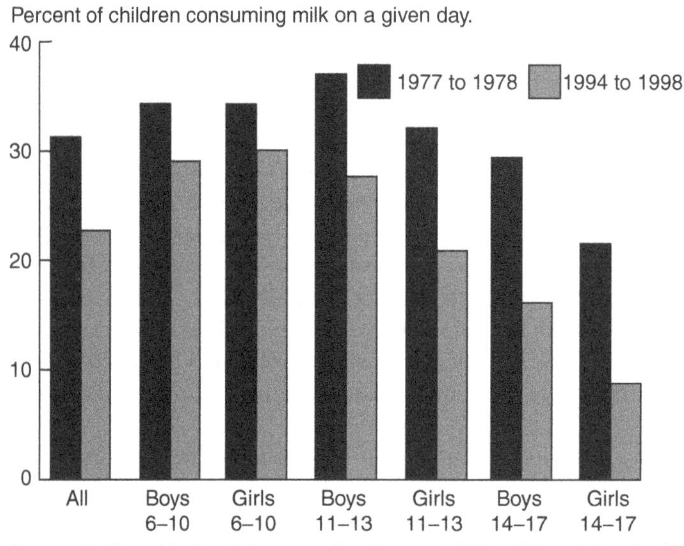

FIGURE 9.4 Milk consumption declining, especially for teenagers.

Research has shown that soft drinks can have short-term consequences as well. Researchers found a strong association between carbonated beverage consumption (particularly colas containing phosphoric acid) and the occurrence of bone fractures in 14-year-old girls [175]. They found, however, that a high intake of dietary calcium was protective.

As discussed earlier, the AAP issued a position statement outlining nutritional concerns regarding soft drink consumption in schools, which calls for district-wide policy restricting the sale of soft drinks in schools [133].

When parents of adolescents were interviewed by telephone about eating habits and the home food environment, the availability of soft drinks in the home was associated with reduced dairy intake [176]. Among boys, serving milk at meals was positively associated with dairy intake. Parental intake of dairy foods was associated with dairy intake in both adolescent boys and girls.

9.5.4.5 Body Image/Weight Concerns

The misperception that milk and other dairy foods are fattening, coupled with strong societal pressures to be thin, prevents many young people, especially teenage girls and young women, from consuming the amounts of calcium-rich dairy foods that would provide the amount of calcium needed for bone health [162,171]. According to a study of more than 34,000 Minnesota students in grades 7 through 12, dieting and dissatisfaction with body weight are strongly linked to low intake of dairy foods [162].

The AAP report on optimizing bone health and calcium intakes recognizes that the preoccupation to being thin and the misconception that all dairy foods are fattening is a barrier to adequate calcium intake among 12- to 19-year-olds [23]. The report states that adolescents and parents may not be aware that low-fat milk contains the same amount of calcium as whole milk.

Fear of obesity, which leads to excessive dieting, may adversely affect an adolescent's growth and development [177]. Dieting teenage girls tend to have poor eating habits (i.e., skipping meals) and low intakes of nutrients, particularly calcium and iron. Despite all the dieting by adolescents, rates of obesity continue to rise. Studies conducted among restrained and unrestrained eaters indicate that on-and-off dieting produces little if any weight loss. On the contrary, an expert in eating behavior warns that dieting frequently results in feelings of psychological deprivation that result in binge eating [178]. By willfully training oneself not to eat in response to internal hunger signals, the dieter becomes susceptible to other signals to eat. Since dietary restraint is often counterproductive, the author recommends that individuals who are of normal weight (up to a Body Mass Index [BMI] of 25 to 27) avoid food restrictions. Instead, they should be advised to establish a healthful lifestyle that incorporates moderate exercise, and a balanced diet without restrictions of any particular food. Even those who are obese should be taught to incorporate their favorite foods into more moderate levels of intake, while increasing energy expenditure with physical activity [179].

The prevention of chronic dieting and other eating disorders could be included as part of a comprehensive health education program in schools. Programs to change dieting and eating behaviors need to address both psychological (body image) and cognitive issues (nutrition knowledge/attitudes).

Research has examined the relationship between calcium/dairy food intake and body weight/-body fat in children and adolescents, with a few of these studies including overweight children or adolescents [180]. Findings from a cross-sectional study of 323 Asian and white adolescents (ages 9 to 14 years) in Hawaii found that total calcium and dairy calcium, but not nondairy calcium, were associated with lower body fat after adjusting for other factors [181]. For the entire group, 1 milk serving was associated with a decrease of approximately 0.78 mm in iliac skinfold thickness, whereas soda intake was positively associated with body weight. In the Asian children, 1 serving of milk was associated with a 1.89 mm smaller iliac skinfold thickness.

A recent longitudinal study of more than 12,000 children aged 9 to 14 years found that children who reported consuming more than 3 servings of milk/day experienced gains in BMI greater than those who drank smaller amounts over the 3-year period [182]. However, when adjusted for total calorie intake, these associations were no longer statistically significant. The researchers concluded that calorie intake was the most important predictor of weight gain in this study [182].

Other studies have shown that increasing calcium or dairy intake has no effect on body weight or fat in children and adolescents [91,99,183]. Data from the Massachusetts Institute of Technology (MIT) Growth and Development Study, a longitudinal study that followed 196 nonobese premenarcheal girls 8 to 12 years old until 4 years postmenarche, found no association between intake of calcium or dairy foods and body mass index or percent body fat [183].

The 2005 *Dietary Guidelines for Americans* states that "adults and children should not avoid milk and milk products because of concerns that these foods lead to weight gain" [45]. Further research is needed to determine if consumption of recommended servings of dairy foods as part of a nutritionally balanced diet helps to prevent and/or treat overweight in children and adolescents — or helps provide a healthier body composition which is lower in body fat and higher in lean body mass.

9.5.5 Groups at Risk for Low Consumption of Dairy Foods

9.5.5.1 Vegetarians

Adolescents are increasingly expressing interest in following a vegetarian diet and lifestyle for a variety of reasons, including an increased sensitivity about animals. Adolescent vegetarians (especially males) are at greater risk than others for using unhealthy and extreme weight control behaviors [184]. According to a 2000 Roper poll, two percent of teenagers (ages 13 to 17) never eat meat, fish, or poultry. Six percent of 6 to 17 year olds do not eat meat [185]. About one-third to one-half of teen vegetarians (0.5% of all teens) are vegan (do not eat meat, fish, fowl, dairy, or eggs) [185]. Health professionals are concerned that teenage girls who avoid all dairy products are at risk for low peak bone density and, eventually, osteoporosis [186]. See Chapter 5 for more information on the bone health of vegetarians. The AAP notes that lacto-vegetarian teens who consume even a modest amount of milk and milk products have normal growth and development and rarely have nutrient deficiencies [187].

9.5.5.2 Pregnant Teens

Adequate calcium intake to maximize peak bone mass is particularly important for pregnant teens since their bone mass is still increasing [188,189]. Significantly greater bone losses have been reported in pregnant [190]. and lactating [191]. adolescents than in women. The NAS recommends 1300 mg of calcium daily for both pregnant and lactating teens [5]. This is the equivalent of 4 servings of milk, yogurt, or cheese.

Longitudinal changes in bone mass from lactation to postweaning were evaluated in ten adolescent mothers ages 15 to 18 years in Brazil who habitually consumed less than 500 mg of calcium per day [192]. The results showed that while these adolescent mothers with low calcium intakes recovered from lactation-associated bone loss after weaning, the rate of bone accretion may not be sufficient to attain peak bone mass at maturity. A study in Mexico evaluating the bone density and bone turnover in adolescent women 9 months postpartum had similar findings [193].

The first study to measure fractional calcium absorption in pregnant adolescents found that its average was 53% (similar to that of pregnant adults), and was higher during the third trimester of pregnancy than in the early postpartum period [194]. Despite maximal increases in intestinal calcium absorption, the degree of calcium retention achieved by these adolescents was not sufficient to support calculated rates of fetal calcium accretion and still allow for skeletal accretion in the adolescent. Although the average calcium intake of these adolescents approached the recommended level, 33% of the adolescents had spinal bone density scores that met the definition of osteopenia or osteoporosis. Higher calcium intakes were related to significantly higher estimated calcium balance during pregnancy and lactation [194].

Adequate dairy food intake during pregnancy can help pregnant teens preserve bone mass and achieve an adequate nutrient intake. Chan and colleagues compared bone mineral content after 16 weeks of lactation between adolescents who consumed at least 1600 mg of calcium per day (primarily as dairy foods) and those who consumed their usual 900 mg of calcium daily [195]. The group who consumed their usual diet experienced a 10% decrease in bone mineral content, while those consuming the high calcium diet maintained bone mineral. By increasing their dairy food intake, those in the experimental group also increased their intake of nutrients including calcium and protein.

The available evidence suggests that pregnancy and lactation in adolescent adversely affect their acquisition of bone mass, particularly when calcium intake is low [189]. More studies are needed to assess the impact of pregnancy and lactation during adolescence to maternal bone mass later in life.

9.5.6 Strategies to Improve Consumption

Choosing to eat a healthful diet is a behavior influenced by a complex interaction between environmental factors and the personality and behavioral factors of an individual [196]. To be successful, nutrition education programs to increase consumption of dairy foods need to recognize and address these factors. Adolescents can understand abstract nutrition concepts, such as cause/effect. Therefore, evaluation of their own diets and eating behavior patterns is very useful at this age [197]. They exhibit independence in food choices, recognize conflicts between taste and health (taste will dominate decisions), and they understand nutritional concepts [198]. Components of nutrition interventions that may encourage behavioral change include (1) teaching adolescents how to respond to the media and social pressures, (2) helping adolescents make the connection between food and health, and (3) letting adolescents identify potential problem areas and set goals for more healthful behavior [197].

Programs with successful outcomes for adolescents have tended to be behaviorally based, using methods such as Social Cognitive Theory (SCT) for the developmental framework [199]. SCT is a model in which behavior, personal factors, and environmental influences continuously interact. It is important to address environmental issues, since adolescents, while gaining in independence, are not completely in control of their behavior (i.e., they intend to eat more dairy foods, but these foods are not available at home). Since parental food intake is associated with adolescent food intake, most effective interventions also include a home component that extends the interventional efforts to the family [199]. Parental presence at the evening meal was positively associated with adolescents' higher consumption of fruits, vegetables, and dairy foods, according to an analysis conducted among more than 18,000 adolescents enrolled in the National Longitudinal Study of Adolescent Health [200].

Cultural factors can also influence the consumption of milk and milk products. Focus groups were conducted among multiethnic (Asian, Hispanic, and white) girls ages 1 to 12 years and 16 to 17 years, recruited from public schools in ten states, to identify factors that influenced consumption of dairy foods [201]. Results showed that a barrier to milk consumption, particularly among older girls and Asian groups, was the low expectation within families for drinking milk. Many controlled their own beverage choices, and milk, even if liked, was only one option. Milk was associated with breakfast consumption, school lunches, cereal, and desserts; white girls had the most positive reactions to milk and Hispanic girls the most negative. Across all ethic groups milk was associated with bone health and strength, which were perceived as being attributes more important to boys. The types of dairy foods preferred differed by ethnicity. White girls liked milk served cold, whereas Asian girls preferred milk warm and sweetened in combination with other beverages. Hispanic girls preferred milk in the form of shakes, puddings, and flan. These findings suggest that to improve calcium intake among teens, interventions should include a family component, stress the benefits of milk for girls, focus on breakfast, and take taste preferences into consideration [201].

In response to the critically low calcium intakes among adolescents, the NICHD has sponsored a publicly funded calcium awareness campaign, "Milk Matters". The campaign educates pediatricians, other health care professionals, children and adolescents 11 to 15 years, and their parents about the importance of calcium for building strong bones and a healthy body. The campaign is designed to help prevent the next generation from suffering the effects of osteoporosis.

While the campaign encourages children and teens to consume a variety of calcium-rich foods, the emphasis is on drinking more milk. The NICHD believes that milk is the best source of calcium for three reasons: (1) it is already a part of most American diets, (2) the calcium from milk is easily absorbed by the body, and (3) along with calcium, milk provides several other essential nutrients — including vitamin D, potassium, and magnesium — essential for bone growth.

An interactive Web site on calcium for teenagers, Clueless in the Mall, increased knowledge and positive attitudes about calcium among youth ages 11 to 15 years [202]. The program (no longer available on the Internet) was based on an educational model that addressed predisposing factors (knowledge and attitudes related to calcium), reinforcing factors (providing continuing reward or incentive to continue the target behavior, i.e., encouragement from parents, teachers, physicians), and enabling factors (resources and skills needed to realize the target behavior, i.e., reading food labels, recipes). High school students who tested the Web site commented, "I had no idea that the most important time for my bone development was now," and "I am going to go home and drink some milk."

9.6 ADULTS

9.6.1 Characteristics

The main physiologic characteristic of adulthood is stability. In general, the cells of most tissues are catabolized (broken down) and replaced at about the same rate. Over time, however, breakdown slightly exceeds replacement, and there are small changes in structure and function. The adult reaches maximum strength, endurance, and agility about 5 years after maximum height is attained, and most body systems reach their peak efficiency and optimum function before age 30 years [203]. Physiologic maturity is defined as the completion of skeletal growth, as characterized by achievement of maximum height and formation of peak bone mass.

9.6.2 Dairy Food/Calcium Recommendations and Consumption

Adequate calcium intake throughout the adult years is important for maintaining bone mass between the time peak bone mass has been reached (about age 30) and menopause in women or about age 50 in men. (See Chapter 5 for more details on research in this area.) The NAS currently recommends that adult men and women ages 25 to 50 years consume 1000 mg of calcium per day (Table 9.10) [5]. This is the equivalent of about 3 servings of milk, yogurt, or cheese, which the 2005 *Dietary Guidelines of Americans* recommends for everyone 9 years and older [45].

Many American adults are not meeting current recommendations for calcium or dairy food intake. At all ages, males consume greater amounts of calcium than females, presumably due to their higher caloric intake. The median usual calcium intake of males ages 19 to 30 years and 31 to 50 years is 1034 mg/day and 961 mg/day, respectively — with about 47% and 54% of these age groups, respectively, not meeting or exceeding their calcium recommendation [37]. Though women

TABLE 9.10
Calcium Recommendations for Adults

Age	Calcium (mg/d)
19 to 30 Years	1000
31 to 50 Years	1000
Pregnancy/lactation 19 to 50 years	1000

Source: From Dietary Reference Intakes, National Academy of Sciences, 1997.

are consuming more calcium than in past years, a majority do not meet recommended intake levels. According to NHANES 2001 to 2002, the median usual calcium intakes for women ages 19 to 30 and 31 to 50 years are 755 mg/day and 722 mg/day, respectively — with 79% and 85%, respectively, not meeting or exceeding their calcium recommendation [37].

The trend is the same for milk and milk products, where consumption tends to be higher in males than females. For example, adult males ages 20 to 29, 30 to 39, and 40 to 49 years consume an average of 2, 1.9, and 1.8 servings of milk, cheese, and yogurt, while women consume an average of only 1.5 (ages 20 to 39) and 1.3 (ages 40 to 49) servings [65]. Women are consuming only half of the 3 servings of milk and milk products recommended by the 2005 *Dietary Guidelines for Americans* [45].

Data from the Bogalusa Heart Study, a long-term epidemiologic study assessing the influence of dairy product consumption on the dietary intakes of more than 1200 biracial (white and African American) adults 20 to 38 years, revealed that dairy product consumption has a major influence on their vitamin and mineral intakes [204]. Intakes of calcium, magnesium, potassium, zinc, sodium, folate, thiamin, riboflavin, and vitamins B_6, B_{12}, A, D, and E were higher with a greater number of dairy products consumed (Table 9.11).

Forty-eight percent of adults consumed 1 serving or less of dairy products per day, 32% consumed 2 servings, 12% consumed 3 servings, and 8% consumed 4 or more servings per day. African American men and women consumed significantly less total dairy products (1.27 and 1.19 servings, respectively) than white men and white women. Less than 10% of adults who consumed 2 servings or less of dairy products consumed the recommended amount of calcium, while 78% and 99% of those who consumed 3, or 4 or more servings, respectively, met the calcium recommendation [204].

9.6.3 Milk Group Foods and the Reduction of Chronic Disease Risk

A prolonged low calcium intake has been linked to the development of several chronic diseases, including osteoporosis, hypertension, and cancer [205,206]. Experts have proposed that disease occurs either when the body's adaptation to low intakes is inadequate to maintain the calcium regulatory system or when the constant, forced, adaptive response itself produces adverse consequences [206].

9.6.3.1 Osteoporosis

Although the bone mass of the hip and vertebrae peaks in late adolescence, the long bones continue to slowly increase in mass well into the third decade [207]. After bone mass has peaked, the bones grow wider. This process is called consolidation. Physical activity, particularly resistance training, may help prevent both bone and muscle loss associated with aging [203].

TABLE 9.11
Vitamin and Mineral Intake among Four Dairy Consumption Groups Surveyed in the Bogalusa Heart Study (1995 to 1996)

Nutrient	Servings of Dairy Products ≤1 (n=611)	2 (n=409)	3 (n=144)	≧4 (n=102)	P for Trend
Least-square mean					
Calcium (mg)	568.6[a]	770.0[a]	1025.7[a]	1421.0[a]	0.0001
Iran (mg)	101.4	101.3	102.1	98.6	
Magnesium (mg)	237.3[a]	248.0[a]	271.9[a]	301.0[a]	0.0001
Phosphorous (mg)	6.0	5.9	6.0	6.0	
Potassium (mg)	2252.6[a]	2319.1[a]	2436.4[a]	2804.5[a]	0.0001
Sodium (mg)	2501.5[a]	2573.9[a]	2685.9[a]	2539.6[a]	0.01
Zinc (mg)	11.6[a]	12.8[a]	14.7[a]	14.8[a]	0.0001
Vitamin C (mg)	123.0[a]	122.8[a]	117.6[a]	149.6[a]	
Thiamin	1.7[a]	1.8[a]	1.9[a]	2.0[a]	0.0001
Riboflavin	1.8[a]	2.1[a]	2.5[a]	3.0[a]	0.0001
Niacin (mg)	22.8	23.3	24.9[a]	23.5	
Vitamin B-6 (mg)	2.0[a]	2.1[a]	2.4[a]	2.4[a]	0.001
Folate (μg)	283.2[a]	309.7[a]	352.6[a]	367.3[a]	0.0001
Vitamin A (IU)	8047.3	8324.3	9020.3	9454.2	0.01
Vitamin D (IU)	240.9[a]	312.1[a]	397.6[a]	528.5[a]	0.0001
Vitamin E (mg)	11.9	12.9	15.1	14.4	
Vitamin B-12 (μg)	6.7[a]	7.3[a]	8.3[a]	8.5[a]	0.001

Model adjusted for total energy intako, age, body mass index, income, physical activity level outside of work, ethnicity, sex, and ethnicity × sex.

[a] Indicate significant mean difference.

Source: From Rajeshwari, R. et al., *J. Am. Dietetic Anoc.* 105, 1391, 2005.

Although reduced bone mass leading to osteoporosis has many contributing causes (i.e., genetic predisposition, inactivity, excessive alcohol use, cigarette smoking), poor nutrition, particularly a low calcium/dairy food intake throughout life can substantially increase the risk of osteoporosis and fracture [60]. The 2004 U.S. Surgeon General's Report on Bone Health and Osteoporosis recommends lifestyle changes for all Americans, including participating in regular physical activity and consumption of calcium- and vitamin D-rich foods such as dairy foods [60].

A state of calcium deficiency exists when calcium intakes are so low that the body can no longer conserve enough calcium (by increasing absorption and/or decreasing excretion) to maintain serum-ionized calcium levels. Calcium stored in bone is the most vulnerable to the effects of calcium deficiency. Calcium deficiency leads to parathyroid hormone-mediated release of calcium from bone to maintain the serum level of ionized calcium — a higher physiological priority. This deficiency state, over time, leads to bone fragility and risk of fracture [205]. Chapter 5 reviews the scientific evidence illustrating the positive influence of lifelong adequate intake of calcium and dairy foods on adult bone density.

9.6.3.2 Hypertension

At least 65 million adults or nearly one-third (31.3%) of the U.S. adult population has hypertension [208]. In 1980, McCarron and colleagues hypothesized that chronic calcium deficiency may lead to hypertension [209]. In subsequent intervention trials, calcium supplementation successfully reduced blood pressure in participants who had low serum ionized calcium, and elevated parathyroid hormone and 1,25-dihydroxy vitamin D levels [210]. These conditions are consequences of and adaptations to restricted calcium intake. Parathyroid hormone and 1,25-dihydroxy vitamin D are thought to increase blood pressure through increases in intracellular free calcium and in muscle tone [210]. These observations serve to confirm the hypothesis that at least some cases of hypertension are secondary to the adaptive response to conserve calcium in a calcium-deficient state [206]. Other studies showed that diets high in calcium, potassium, and magnesium — nutrients abundantly supplied by fruits, vegetables, and dairy foods — may also be effective in reducing hypertension. Two meta-analyses found calcium to be significantly effective in reducing blood pressure in normotensive and hypertensive individuals, and in preventing pregnancy-induced hypertension and preeclampsia [211,212].

The DASH (Dietary Approaches to Stop Hypertension) Trial, studied the effects of dietary patterns on blood pressure — both in hypertensive and normotensive populations. The results demonstrated that a combination diet, low in fat and rich in fruits, vegetables, and low-fat dairy products, can substantially lower blood pressure [213]. The DASH diet findings have been reconfirmed by findings from the DASH-Sodium study [214]. This multicenter, randomized controlled trial found that a low-fat diet rich in low-fat dairy products, fruits, and vegetables and low in sodium lowered blood pressure in adults with and without hypertension. The DASH diet lowered blood pressure at all sodium levels tested (3400, 2400, or 1500 mg/day). A smaller, but significant reduction occurred when subjects consumed the DASH diet at the lowest sodium level [214]. The DASH diet is an attractive option for individuals seeking to control blood pressure, as it may replace or reduce the need for drug treatment for some patients.

The National Heart, Lung, and Blood Institute, in its most recent (7th) Report of the Joint National Committee on Prevention, Evaluation, and Treatment of High Blood Pressure, ranks the DASH diet as the most effective nutritional intervention ahead of sodium restriction [215]. A scientific statement from the American Heart Association recognizes that dietary factors have a prominent and likely predominant role in regulating blood pressure and endorses the DASH dietary pattern as one of the lifestyle modifications to prevent and treat hypertension [216]. The 2005 *Dietary Guidelines for Americans* recognizes the DASH diet as an eating pattern that can be used interchangeably with the USDA food pattern to meet nutrient requirements and promote health [45].

Of the other nutrients in milk that lower blood pressure, potassium and magnesium have been the most researched. According to several studies, increasing dietary potassium or the dietary potassium-to-sodium ratio modestly lowers blood pressure, particularly in individuals whose diets are high in sodium and relatively low in potassium [217–219]. The U.S. Food and Drug Administration (FDA) has approved a health claim for the reduction of high blood pressure and stroke for foods that are good sources of potassium [220]. Foods making this claim must contain at least 350 mg of potassium per serving, have no more than 140 mg of sodium per serving, and be low in fat, saturated fat, and cholesterol [220]. Nonfat milk qualifies to make this claim. A meta-analysis of twenty randomized clinical trials found that increasing magnesium intake resulted in a small, significant reduction in systolic blood pressure and a nonsignificant trend for reduction of diastolic blood pressure, in a dose-responsive manner [221].

Based on an analysis of research over the past two decades, researchers estimate that consuming a healthful diet containing 3 to 4 servings of dairy foods a day would lead to a 40% reduction in the prevalence of mild to moderate hypertension, resulting in first-year health care cost savings of $14 billion with cumulative savings of $70 billion at 5 years [222]. Additional information on dairy foods and hypertension is found in Chapter 3.

9.6.3.3 Cancer

Cancer is the second leading cause of death in the United States (after heart disease), responsible for one out of every four deaths [223]. Both genetic and environmental factors contribute to this disease. Among environmental factors, about one-third of cancer deaths are estimated to be related to poor nutrition and physical inactivity, including overweight or obesity [223].

Epidemiologic research as well as studies in animals and humans indicate that dairy foods and/or their components have a protective effect against cancer. Several components in dairy foods, specifically calcium and vitamin D, bacterial cultures (e.g., *Lactobacillus acidophilus*), a class of fatty acids known as conjugated dienoic derivatives of linoleic acid (CLA), sphingolipids, butyric acid, and milk proteins may protect against cancer [224–231].

Colon cancer in susceptible persons may be the unfortunate result of adaptation to a low calcium intake [206]. It is theorized that on a high-calcium diet, much of the unabsorbed calcium (75% to 85%) remains in the intestinal lumen, where it forms insoluble complexes with bile acids and unabsorbed fatty acids, and protects the mucosal lining of the colon from their toxic effects. Conversely, on a low-calcium diet, the body adapts by increasing calcium absorption, leaving less unabsorbed calcium reaching the colon to complex with irritant acids. This increases the likelihood that the cells lining the colon will be damaged, proliferate, and progress toward cancer [232].

Based on a review of 30 case-controlled or cohort studies of dairy foods and colorectal cancer using a meta-analytical approach, Norat and Riboli concluded that "there is some epidemiological evidence that the consumption of total dairy products, and in particular milk, may be associated to a modest reduction in colorectal cancer risk" [233]. An inverse association was found between milk intake and colorectal cancer in cohort studies, whereas case-controlled studies provided heterogeneous results. No clear association was found between cheese or yogurt intake and colorectal cancer [233].

Most clinical trials have indirectly assessed the effects of calcium or dairy food intake on colorectal cancer by measuring colonic cell proliferation [234]. or the formation of adenomatous polyps [235]. In addition, calcium or dairy foods may also reduce the risk of colon cancer by decreasing the cytotoxicity of fecal water [236].

The National Medical Association (NMA), in a consensus report, recommends that the American public as a whole and African Americans in particular consume 3 to 4 servings/day of low-fat milk, cheese, and/or yogurt to help reduce the risk of certain chronic diseases including colon cancer [237]. Based on a review of the science, researchers conservatively estimated that consuming 3 to 4 servings of dairy foods/day could reduce the risk of colorectal cancer by 5% annually after 3 years, resulting in health care cost savings of $75 billion over 5 years [222].

With respect to breast cancer, there is evidence from experimental animal studies that dairy food components reduce the risk of this cancer [238]. However, epidemiological evidence supporting an association between consumption of milk or specific types of dairy products and risk of breast cancer is limited [238]. Regarding prostate cancer risk, there is mixed epidemiological evidence that dairy foods or dairy food components are associated with it [239]. A clinical trial of calcium supplementation as well as reviews of vitamin D and calcitriol, the most active metabolite of vitamin D, indicate that these nutrients may protect against prostate cancer [240–242]. For more detailed information on dairy foods and cancer and additional research needs, see Chapter 4.

9.6.3.4 Overweight/Obesity

Nearly two-thirds (65.1%) of adults 20 years of age and older are overweight (BMI of 25 to 29.9) or obese (BMI of 30 or greater), according to NHANES 1999 to 2002 [243]. In adults 20 to 39 years, the highest prevalence of overweight and obesity occurs among Mexican American men (64.8%) and both non-Hispanic Black (70.3%) and Mexican American women (61.8%). Non-Hispanic Black women in this age group have the highest prevalence of obesity (46.6%) and extreme obesity (11.8% with a BMI >40) [243].

The main goals for adult weight loss and management is to reduce body weight, maintain a lower body weight over the long term, and prevent further weight gain (a minimum goal) [244]. For obese adults, even modest weight loss of about 10% of body weight lost over a period of 6 months can reduce disease risk factors (i.e., elevated blood pressure, blood glucose, and blood lipids). The prevention of further weight gain is very important. For overweight adults (BMI 25 to 29.9) who do not have other risk factors, the prevention of weight gain is an appropriate goal [244].

Recent randomized clinical trials have demonstrated that overweight or obese adults who consumed recommended daily intakes of dairy products/calcium as part of a balanced calorie-restricted diet lost significantly more body weight and body fat than those who consumed a balanced, reduced-calorie diet with little or no dairy foods. This finding has been demonstrated in both males and females, whites, and African Americans [245–247]. A recent clinical trial in African American adults found that consuming 3 servings of milk, cheese, or yogurt per day not only enhanced body weight/fat loss and helped preserve lean body mass when dieting, but also improved body composition (i.e., reduced total body and trunk fat and increased lean body mass) and metabolic profile during weight maintenance compared to low intakes of dairy products [247]. Research shows that dairy foods exert a significantly greater effect on body weight and body fat compared to calcium supplements or low-dairy diets [245].

Further support for a role of calcium and dairy products in weight management in adults comes from observational studies, although factors such as the level of baseline calcium or dairy intake, gender, and body weight appear to influence this relationship. These studies are discussed in several reviews [248–251].

Research from *in vitro* and experimental animal studies indicates that dietary calcium and other dairy components (e.g., protein, branched-chain amino acids, bioactives) may regulate energy metabolism and obesity risk [250,251]. There is also evidence that an adequate intake of dairy foods increases fat oxidation in humans [252,253].

It should be noted that the beneficial effect of dairy food/calcium intake on body weight and fat appears to be most effective under certain circumstances, such as during calorie restriction, in those who are overweight or obese, and in those who have a low baseline dairy food/calcium intake (1 serving of dairy foods per day) [254]. Consuming more than the optimal 3 servings of dairy foods per day is unlikely to result in further significant weight loss.

The 2005 *Dietary Guidelines for Americans* states, "Adults and children should not avoid milk and milk products because of concerns that these foods lead to weight gain" [45]. After reviewing the science available at the time, the 2005 Dietary Guidelines Advisory Committee report concluded there was insufficient evidence on which to base a more definitive statement regarding the intake of milk products and management of body weight [53]. It states the need for large-scale randomized trials or controlled feeding studies designed explicitly to test the effect of intake of milk group foods or calcium on body weight. See Chapter 7 for more detailed information on dairy foods and weight management.

Since the sequelae of low dairy food/calcium intake appear to increase the risk of several chronic diseases, and several components of dairy foods are potentially protective, it makes sense for health practitioners to encourage a lifelong adequate intake (3 to 4 servings) of milk, cheese, and yogurt.

9.6.4 Special Needs of Women

9.6.4.1 Pregnancy and Lactation

During pregnancy a woman's requirement for calcium increases by approximately 33% [255]. Adequate calcium is needed to maintain maternal bone density, to mineralize infant bone, to regulate blood pressure, and to supply a readily available source of calcium in breast milk during lactation. Over the course of pregnancy, a remarkable series of physiological adjustments occur to preserve maternal bone mass, while providing for the skeletal growth of the fetus. Thus, under normal conditions and adequate calcium intake, pregnancy exerts little influence on net bone mineral content, even when calcium intake is not increased [256]. Both biochemical and clinical data suggest that increased calcium needs during pregnancy are met primarily by an increase in calcium absorption (by 50% or more) and by increased bone turnover. Although the hormones responsible for triggering these changes are still under investigation, production of 1,25-dihydroxy vitamin D may almost double, stimulating the synthesis of calcium binding protein and an increased intestinal absorption of calcium [257].

The demand for calcium during lactation can be twice that of pregnancy. Lactating women secrete 240 to 320 mg of calcium daily in breast milk [257]. The major source of calcium for milk secretion appears to be maternal bone. Studies have shown, however, that increased intestinal absorption and renal retention of calcium in the postweaning period facilitate the recovery of bone lost during pregnancy and/or lactation — and that transient bone loss during lactation does not seem to increase a woman's risk of osteoporotic fracture in later years [258–260]. However, calcium supplementation during this time may be beneficial. Kalkwarf et al. found that lactating women who received a calcium supplement of 1000 mg/day postweaning (12 months after delivery) had a 5.9% increase in spinal bone density, which was significantly greater than the 4.4% increase in those who received a placebo [261].

The NAS 1997 Dietary Reference Intake report concluded that "the maternal skeleton is not used as a reserve for fetal calcium needs provided that dietary calcium intake is sufficient for maximizing bone accretion rates in the nonpregnant state" [5]. Therefore, it recommends a calcium intake during pregnancy and lactation no higher than for nonpregnant women of the same age (Table 9.12). Data on the calcium intake of pregnant and lactating women, presented in the NAS report on Dietary Reference Intakes, shows that while half (median intake) are meeting the recommended intake of 1000 mg/day, many are not (Table 9.11). According to the report, roughly two-thirds of pregnant adolescents and one-third of pregnant adults are not meeting their AI for calcium [5]. It should be noted that although the data was statistically adjusted to account for day-to-day variation of the small number of women sampled, it is less reliable than the data for females in general. Current available calcium intake data excludes pregnant and lactating females [37].

The previous *Healthy People* objectives for the nation (*HP 2000*) included the goal that "at least 50 percent of pregnant and lactating women will consume at least 3 or more servings daily of calcium-rich foods." According to USDA data (CSFII 1985 to 86) that was submitted to provide a baseline for the HP 2000 goal, only 24% of pregnant and/or lactating women met the goal [262]. Rather than improving over time, the 1995 to 1996 *Healthy People 2000 Review* reported that only

TABLE 9.12
Current Calcium Intake of Females

	Calcium (mg) Percentiles		
	5th	**50th**	**95th**
9 to 13 Years (200)	486	889	1452
14 to 18 Years (169)	348	413	1293
19 to 30 Years (302)	300	612	1116
31 to 50 Years (590)	297	606	1082
51 to 70 Years (510)	294	571	1001
>70 Years (221)	277	517	860
Pregnancy (33)	656	1154	1729
Lactation (16)	794	1050	1324

Source: From Food and Nutrition Board/Institute of Medicine, *Dietary Reference Intakes, Calcium, Phosphorus, Magnesium, Vitamin D, and Fluoride*, National Academy Press, Washington, D.C., 1997.

22% of pregnant and/or lactating women were meeting the goal [263]. However, the *Healthy People* objectives no longer include a specific calcium and/or dairy intake goal for pregnant women. Instead, the goal in *Healthy People 2010* is to increase to 74% (from 45%) the proportion of persons ages 2 years and older who meet dietary recommendations for calcium — which applies to pregnant women as well [264].

A low intake of calcium during pregnancy and lactation (defined by NAS as 600 mg/day or less) has been associated with biochemical indices of bone resorption in the mother [265,266], low bone density in the infant [267,268], reduced calcium in breast milk [269], and increased exposure of the fetus and breast-fed infant to lead mobilized from bone [270,271]. A study of calcium kinetics across pregnancy and lactation in a group of Brazilian women with calcium intakes less than 500 mg/day, 50% of which was provided by dairy products, found that a more positive bone calcium balance was significantly associated with higher calcium intake during early and late pregnancy [266]. The authors say that increasing calcium intake in women with habitually low calcium intakes may minimize bone calcium losses across pregnancy [266].

There is evidence that adequate calcium intake is important for maintaining normal blood pressure during pregnancy and in preventing preeclampsia or its complications [212,272,273]. A meta-analysis of fourteen randomized trials found that calcium supplementation during pregnancy reduced the incidence of pregnancy-induced hypertension by 70% and preeclampsia by 62% [212]. However, the results of the Calcium for Preeclampsia Prevention (CPEP) trial, conducted among over 4500 pregnant women at five U.S. medical centers, found only a slightly beneficial, but not statistically significant, effect of 2000 mg of supplemental calcium on preeclampsia, pregnancy-associated hypertension, or other adverse outcomes of pregnancy [274]. It is difficult to reconcile these conflicting results. It may be that increasing calcium intake may be most important when baseline calcium intake is low (CPEP participants had an average calcium intake of 1000 mg/d), or for those at the highest risk for preeclampsia, such as women with diabetes or who are pregnant with twins. Most recently, a randomized placebo-controlled, double-blinded trial among more than 8000 pregnant women — recruited from clinics in populations with average calcium intakes less than 600 mg per day (Egypt, Argentina, Peru, East London, South Africa, and Vietnam) — found that supplementation with 1.5 g of calcium per day did not prevent preeclampsia, but did reduce its severity, as well as maternal morbidity and neonatal mortality [273]. Calcium supplementation reduced preeclampsia by 10%, but this was not statistically significant. Supplementation with 1.5 g of calcium per day did reduce the most serious complications of preeclampsia, significantly, by 25%. In addition, calcium supplementation reduced preterm delivery (primary outcome) and early preterm delivery (a secondary outcome), among mothers 20 years old or less [273].

There is some evidence that ensuring adequate vitamin D status during pregnancy may help prevent preeclampsia [275]. Preeclampsia is suggested to be the result of material breakdown of immune tolerance to the fetus. The fact that preeclampsia is characterized by marked changes in vitamin D metabolism, and evidence that the immunomodulatory properties of the hormonal form of vitamin D (1,25$(OH)_2D$) may play a key role in maintaining immunological tolerance in pregnancy, support this hypothesis. Well-controlled clinical trials using vitamin D and calcium supplementation are needed to clarify the possible role of vitamin D intake and status in the prevention and treatment of preeclampsia [275].

Vitamin D sufficiency during pregnancy may also be an important factor influencing bone content and future risk of fracture in the offspring [276,277]. Longitudinal study of the effect of maternal vitamin D status during pregnancy on childhood skeletal growth at age 9 found that maternal vitamin D insufficiency during late pregnancy was associated with a deficit in bone size and bone mineral content of the children, without effects on childhood height or lean mass [277]. This effect was independent of the children's milk intake or physical activity level.

Pregnant women should be encouraged to consume the recommended 3 servings of milk and other dairy foods daily to provide calcium, vitamin D, and other nutrients needed for their own health and for optimal fetal development. One study reported that females of child-bearing age (14 to 50 years) were about half as likely as their male counterparts to meet vitamin D recommendations from food sources [278]. However, there is no evidence that pregnant women need vitamin D intakes above amounts routinely required to prevent deficiency among nonpregnant women [279]. Milk is voluntarily fortified with 400 IU of vitamin D per quart. Two cups of vitamin D-fortified milk will meet the requirement for vitamin D of women of childbearing age [5].

9.6.4.2 Premenstrual Syndrome (PMS)

A diet rich in dairy foods or dairy food nutrients may be beneficial in alleviating symptoms and preventing premenstrual syndrome (PMS), a condition occurring in about 8% to 20% of women of childbearing age [280]. Results of clinical trials indicate that increasing calcium intake by about 1000 to 1300 mg/day substantially alleviates PMS symptoms [281–286]. For example, in a multicenter trial, researchers found that women ages 18 to 45 who received 1200 mg of calcium/day reported a 48% decrease in premenstrual symptoms (cramping, bloating, food cravings, irritability) when compared to those who received a placebo [282].

Studies show that intake of milk, cheese, and yogurt is associated with fewer PMS symptoms [282,283,287]. In addition to reducing PMS symptoms, consuming calcium and vitamin D in foods may help prevent PMS from developing in the first place [280]. In a recent case-control investigation, researchers compared the diets and supplement use of 1057 women ages 27 to 44 years who reported developing PMS over the course of 10 years with that in 1968 women who reported no or minimal PMS symptoms during the same period [280]. High calcium and vitamin D intake from food (but not supplements) — equivalent to about 4 servings of fat-free or low-fat milk or low-fat yogurt — was associated with a significantly lower risk of PMS compared to intake of 1 serving or less a day [280].

9.6.4.3 Other Potential Health Benefits

Researchers recently found that hip and spine bone loss associated with oral contraceptive use was reduced in women using oral contraceptives who consumed dairy products containing at least 1000 mg of calcium per day [288]. Use of oral contraceptives without adequate calcium intake may prevent young women from reaching peak bone mass and increase their risk of osteoporosis in later life. In this 1-year study, 154 women ages 18 to 30 years (oral contraceptive users and nonusers) with low dietary calcium intakes (<800 mg/day) were randomized to one of three diet intervention groups: control (<800 mg calcium/day), medium dairy (1000 to 1100 mg calcium/day), or high dairy (1200 to 1300 mg calcium/day) [288]. At the end of the year, women consuming the medium or high dairy diets had significantly higher bone mineral density in their hips and spines compared to the low dairy group. Oral contraceptive users consuming low calcium diets lost bone at both spine and hip sites compared to nonusers, but this loss was prevented with the medium or high dairy intakes [288]. Findings of this study indicate that women taking oral contraceptives should consume dairy products at levels necessary to achieve recommended intakes of calcium to optimize their bone health [288].

Fermented dairy products or dairy products containing probiotics (i.e., live microorganisms that confer a health benefit) may help protect against urinary tract infections in women, according to a case-controlled study that evaluated dietary and other risk factors for urinary tract infections [289]. Women who consumed fermented milk products such as yogurt and certain cheeses three or more times a week had a 79% lower incidence of urinary tract infections compared to those who ate these dairy foods once a week or less [289]. More studies are needed to confirm this benefit.

9.6.5 Strategies to Improve Intake of Dairy Foods

Reversing the decline in intake of calcium-rich dairy foods, especially milk consumption, is one of the two major challenges dietitians and other health professionals face as they work as agents for behavior change, concluded participants at a multidisciplinary seminar, "Changing Behaviors to Optimize Women's Health" [290]. The other major challenge highlighted by this seminar was helping women of all ages change their attitudes about their bodies. This second challenge influences the first, since concerns about body weight can influence milk and dairy food intake. At this seminar, nutrition professionals were encouraged to build partnerships with patients, understand the patient, start where the patient is, and concentrate on small changes for success [290].

Knowledge of personal characteristics associated with either meeting or not meeting dairy food/calcium recommendations is useful for developing nutrition education programs. A survey of factors influencing milk and milk product consumption among both young and elderly New Zealand women with low calcium intakes, found that among the younger women (ages 19 to 23), the main reasons given for low consumption of dairy foods were a "change in lifestyle" (i.e., leaving the family home) and "health reasons," primarily weight reduction and lowering fat intake [291]. Nearly one-third of the younger women reported that the reason they did not consume dairy foods other than milk (e.g., yogurt or cheese) was their concern for calorie/fat intake and body weight. The authors conclude that education for younger women should emphasize the availability of low-fat versions of dairy foods and that weight control does not require the exclusion of Milk Group foods from the diet. All but one of the young women in the above-mentioned study said they would be willing to make changes in their diets if it would improve their health. Of the women surveyed, 86% said they would drink more milk, 55% and 64% said they would eat more cheese or low-fat cheese, respectively, and 91% said they would eat more yogurt, if it would improve their health [291].

Focus groups were conducted in Virginia among 39 white women ages 30 to 55 years to gain insight into their thoughts and feelings about dairy foods [292]. Overall, the women knew that dairy foods were a good source of calcium and important for preventing osteoporosis. However, many used calcium supplements or vitamin/mineral supplements to help meet calcium requirements — and most thought dairy foods were high in fat.

A study of 2261 women (not pregnant or lactating) who participated in USDA's 1990 to 91 Continuing Survey of Food Intakes by Individuals — Diet and Health Knowledge Survey, identified several factors positively associated with meeting the RDA for calcium from food sources [293]. According to this study, women who met or exceeded the RDA for calcium were more likely to work part-time, take vitamin-mineral supplements, report avoidance of whole milk only, be aware of a relationship between calcium intake and health, and to report a higher number of milk group servings as being recommended daily. Women who met calcium recommendations also met recommendations for magnesium, vitamin E, vitamin B_6, iron, and vitamin A, but the other women did not. This confirms earlier research showing that women who had low intakes of calcium also had low intakes of several other vitamins and minerals [294]. This data emphasizes the need for health professionals to continue to communicate the benefits of dairy foods for bone health, blood pressure maintenance, reduction of cancer risk, and nutrient adequacy of the diet — particularly to adult women.

A nationally representative consumer survey conducted in 1997 found that adult milk drinkers fall into three categories — those who drink milk at several meal occasions, those who drink milk at only one meal, and those who are "light" milk drinkers or use it only on cereal [295]. People in all three of these groups have common motivations for drinking milk. They like the taste of milk, they believe that milk is needed for strong bones at every stage of life, and they believe milk to be compatible with food. However, they have barriers to drinking milk in certain situations. For example, they may feel that milk is incompatible with certain foods, they may prefer another beverage with a particular meal, and they note that milk is not readily available when they are eating away from home. Health professionals can help their clients increase their intake of milk and milk products by identifying the behavioral routines and attitudes of their clients, and suggesting new ways to include these foods with their meals. For example, a person who only consumes milk with a sandwich at lunch may be encouraged to add a café latte at breakfast, or a carton of yogurt as a between-meal snack.

First and foremost, communicating the many health benefits of Milk Group foods will help motivate clients to increase their intake. Nutrition education, conducted either in a group or private counseling session, or communicated through articles in consumer publications, may help bring dairy food intake closer to the recommended level. The 3-A-Day of Dairy program (www.3aday.org), a nutrition-based marketing and education campaign helps consumers know what constitutes a serving of dairy foods, and how many servings are needed to meet calcium recommendations. The 3-A-Day of Dairy program is supported by leading health organizations, including the AAP, the ADA, the American Academy of Family Physicians, and the NMA. The U.S. Surgeon General's Report on Bone Health and Osteoporosis contains examples of community-based interventions and communication tools and messages that can be used with populations of various ages [60].

9.7 OLDER ADULTS

9.7.1 CHARACTERISTICS

As adults age they experience a gradual functional decline in many physiological processes and changes in body composition. A majority of older adults enjoy good health, but no two people age in exactly the same way, and older adults are a remarkably diverse group [296]. Aging is associated with slow declines in weight, bone mass (Figure 9.5), lean body mass, and gains in adipose tissue. For example, muscle mass declines approximately 2% to 3% per decade, contributing to a reduced basal metabolic rate. Resistance training can help preserve fat-free mass and increase muscular strength in the elderly. Likewise, adequate calcium and vitamin D intakes can help slow age-related bone loss [296]. Several of the physiological changes of aging influence the intake and metabolism of bone-related nutrients, increasing the older adult's need for these nutrients and the susceptibility to bone loss. For example, as physical activity and lean body mass decline with age, so do energy needs and food intake. Reduced food intake in the elderly contributes to low intakes of bone-related nutrients, including calcium, vitamin D, phosphorus, and protein [297]. Calcium absorption and the renal conservation of calcium decreases with aging, increasing its requirement. Reduced sun

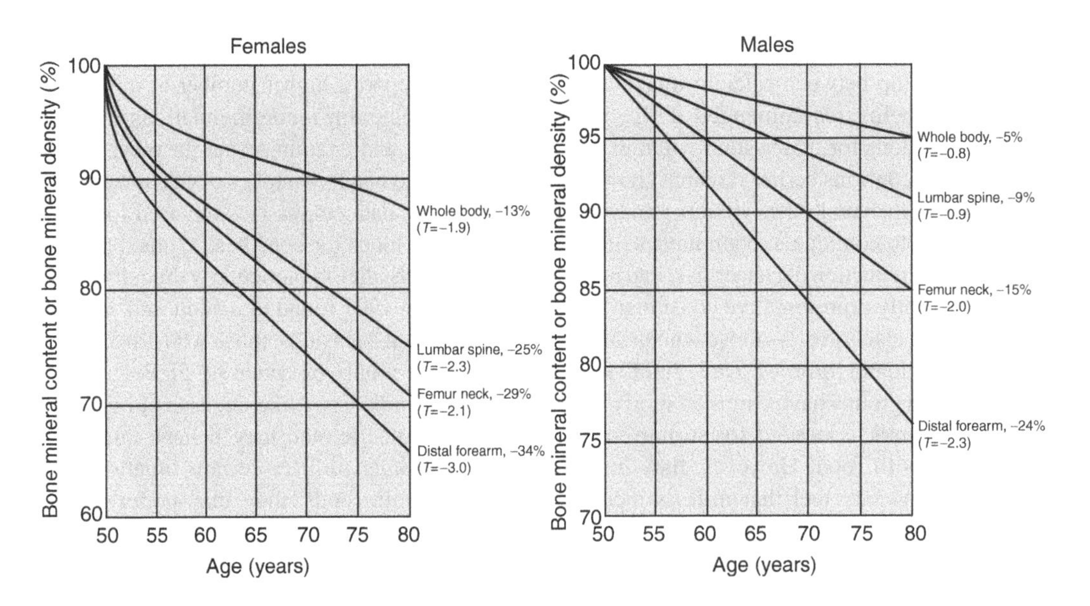

FIGURE 9.5 Percentage loss of bone at four different sites as a function of age in men and women. (From FAO Food, Nutrition, and Agriculture Division, *Food, Nutrition, and Agriculture: Calcium throughout Life,* 20, 15, 1997. With permission.)

TABLE 9.13
Calcium Recommendations for Older Adults

Age	Calcium (mg/d)	Vitamin D (IU)
51 to 70 Years	1200	400
>70 Years	1200	600

Source: From Dietary Reference Intakes, National Academy of Sciences, 1997.

exposure, impaired renal conversion of the circulating form of vitamin D [25(OH)D] to the active form [1,25(OH)$_2$D], and partial intestinal resistance to the active form of vitamin D, increases the requirement of vitamin D with age (Table 9.13). Adequate vitamin D status is needed for optimal calcium absorption. All of these changes contribute to the deterioration of calcium, phosphorus, vitamin D, and protein nutriture often seen in older adults [297].

In addition, absorption of naturally-occurring vitamin B_{12} (milk is a good source) decreases after age 50. Therefore, individuals over age 50 should be encouraged to meet their RDA for vitamin B_{12} by eating foods fortified with B_{12} or by taking the crystalline form of vitamin B_{12} supplements [53].

9.7.2 Milk Group Foods and the Reduction of Chronic Disease Risk

9.7.2.1 Osteoporosis

Osteoporosis affects an enormous number of people, with the incidence expected to rise with increasing life expectancy and the increasing number of older Americans in the population [298]. Eighty percent of those affected are women; however, one in two women and one in four men over age 50 will have an osteoporosis-related fracture in their lifetime [299]. Twenty percent of non-Hispanic white and Asian women ages 50 and older are estimated to have osteoporosis, while 5% of African Americans and 10% of Hispanics have the disease [299]. The National Osteoporosis Foundation released guidelines for the physician in the prevention and treatment of osteoporosis. The guidelines include universal recommendations for adequate intake of calcium and vitamin D, regular weight-bearing exercise, and the avoidance of tobacco use and alcohol abuse [298]. Many older women take bone active pharmacologic agents, such as bisphosphonates, to prevent or treat osteoporosis and low bone mass. These agents depend on adequate intakes of calcium phosphorus, vitamin D and protein to be effective — nutrients abundant in dairy foods that are often lacking in the diets of older women [300]. Chapter 5 has additional information on osteoporosis risk in this age group.

9.7.2.1.1 Dairy Foods and Calcium

The NAS recognizes that the calcium requirement increases with age (Table 9.13). In 1997, the NAS recommended 1200 mg of calcium daily for adults over age 50 [5]. In 2003, the National Osteoporosis Foundation recommended that physicians encourage a calcium intake of at least 1200 mg daily for all their patients, both to prevent and treat osteoporosis [298]. They state that calcium-rich foods should be the primary source of calcium, and that calcium supplements be used only when "an adequate dietary intake cannot be achieved" [298].

Many older adults (50+) fail to meet their AI of 1200 mg/day of calcium — which is equivalent to about 4 servings from the Milk Group. Calcium intakes continue to decline with advancing age. According to NHANES 2001 to 2002 nutrient intake data, among men ages 51 to 70 and 71+, half (50th percentile) consumed less than 813 mg and 771 mg of calcium per day, respectively. Eighty-four percent and 88% of men in these age groups, respectively, did not meet or exceed the recommended amount of calcium [37]. Older women consumed even less calcium than older men. Among women ages 51 to 70 and 71+, half (50th percentile) consumed less than 661 mg and 613 mg of calcium per day, respectively. Ninety-five percent and 96% of women at these ages, respectively, did not meet or exceed the recommended amount of calcium [37]. On average, both older men and women (ages 70 and over) consumed little more than 1 serving from the Milk Group each day [65]. This national consumption data shows that many older adults are not consuming the recommended amount of calcium they need to maintain bone health and minimize bone loss that occurs with aging.

Since nutritional status clearly influences the rate of physiological and functional declines with age, such a large calcium deficit in the elderly population is likely to accelerate rates of bone loss and increase the risk of fracture and disability [301]. Conversely, clinical trials in which older adults were given calcium and/or vitamin D supplements (1000 to 1700 mg of calcium per day) have demonstrated a significant reduction in age-related bone loss, and incidence of fractures [302–304]. Increasing adults' dietary calcium in the form of foods (e.g., yogurt, milk) has been demonstrated to decrease bone resorption, the first step in reducing fragility [305], as well as in maintaining bone density [306,307]. Consuming a yogurt snack three times a day significantly improved postmenopausal women's intake of calcium and other nutrients (e.g., riboflavin, vitamin B_{12}, potassium, protein) and decreased their rate of bone resorption, as indicated by urinary excretion of *N*-telopeptide, according to a randomized controlled clinical trial [306]. In another study of healthy older adults with habitually low intakes of dairy foods, those who consumed 3 servings of fat-free or low-fat milk as part of their daily diet for 12 weeks experienced a significant decrease in bone resorption compared to those who maintained their usual diets [307]. According to a recent cross-sectional study, higher consumption of dairy foods was associated with increased hip bone mineral density in older men [308]. A 2-year randomized controlled study of 149 men over age 50 found that supplementation with calcium- and vitamin D-fortified milk (providing an additional 1000 mg of calcium and 800 IU of vitamin D_3 per day) effectively suppressed PTH (parathyroid hormone) and stopped or slowed bone loss at several clinically relevant sites such as the femoral neck, total hip, and the ultradistal radius [309].

A review of the calcium needs of adults over 65 years of age concludes that increasing daily calcium intake (e.g., from 1300 to 1700 mg/day) will reduce osteoporotic fracture risk by 30% to 50% [310]. "Many of the features of the calcium economy in the older adult which we had once attributed to age, turn out to be manifestations of calcium privation," states world-renowned calcium researcher Dr. Robert Heaney [297].

9.7.2.1.2 Vitamin D

Because of the vital role vitamin D plays in calcium absorption, poor vitamin D status profoundly affects bone and mineral metabolism, increasing the risk of osteomalacia and fracture [301]. In addition, vitamin D deficiency can cause muscle weakness, increasing the risk of falling and fractures [311,312]. There is emerging scientific evidence linking vitamin D deficiency with an increased risk of type 1 diabetes, multiple sclerosis, rheumatoid arthritis, hypertension, cardiovascular heart disease, and many common cancers [311,312]. Many older adults are deficient in vitamin D as indicated by low blood levels of the circulating form, 25-hydroxy vitamin D, especially those who are homebound or institutionalized [313]. Deficiency is a combined result of a lack of exposure to sunlight, the age-related decrease in both cutaneous and endogenous synthesis of vitamin D, and a low dietary intake of vitamin D.

Vitamin D-fortified milk is one of the few dietary sources of vitamin D, although some cheeses and yogurts are also fortified with vitamin D; milk is voluntarily fortified to a level of 400 IU per quart. However, older adults consume little milk and even less yogurt. Men over age 50 consume about a cup of milk daily, while women that age consume slightly less than one cup [37]. Less than 10% of older adults (51 to 70 years old) and no more than 2% of the elderly (older than 70 years old) met vitamin D requirements from food sources alone, according to data from CSFII 1994 to 1996, 1998 and NHANES III [314]. Even after considering vitamin D intake from dietary supplements, up to 90% of older individuals still did not consume adequate amounts of vitamin D [314].

A number of studies indicate that increasing the vitamin D intake of older adults (either alone or with calcium) reduces bone loss and risk of fractures [302,304,315,316]. Calcium and vitamin D supplementation resulted in a 29% reduction in hip fracture among those who took 80% of the study medication in the Women's Health Initiative, a 7-year clinical trial among more than 36,000 postmenopausal women [316]. According to a meta-analysis of 25 randomized controlled trials in postmenopausal women, vitamin D significantly reduced spine fractures and showed a trend toward reduced incidence of nonspine fractures [317].

The recommendations for vitamin D intake for older adults is two to three times higher than that for younger adults and children. Currently, 400 IU/day is recommended for adults ages 51 to 70, and 600 IU is recommended for adults over age 70 (Table 9.13) [5].

Vitamin D status is assessed by measuring the serum level of 25(OH)D. It is now recognized that maintaining a serum level of 25(OH)D at 80 nmol/L (32 ng/L) or greater is needed to improve muscle strength and bone mineral density in adults [311]. Figure 9.6 shows that three-fourths of women ages 60 to 79 have serum levels of 25(OH)D below 80 nmol/L [318]. Experts are calling on the medical community to make screening for vitamin D deficiency part of the routine physical examination for all adults and children [311].

Older adults can satisfy their vitamin D needs by exposing their arms and legs or hands, face and arms, to sunlight for 5 to 15 minutes per day during the spring, the summer, and the fall [311]. Those who choose to get a little more sunlight by walking outdoors should apply sunscreen after the initial exposure. However, older adults as a whole are more likely than younger persons to apply sunscreen, wear more clothing, and get insufficient vitamin D synthesis from sunlight.

In the absence of any sun exposure, vitamin D investigators now say that 1000 IU of vitamin D a day is necessary to maintain the blood level of 25(OH)D between 80 and 100 nmol/L, which can be achieved with diet and supplements [311,312]. One investigator estimates that it would require a vitamin D intake of 2600 IU per day to ensure that 97.5% of older women have 25(OH)D levels at or above desirable levels [318]. Currently, the Upper Limit for vitamin D intake (2000 IU) prevents

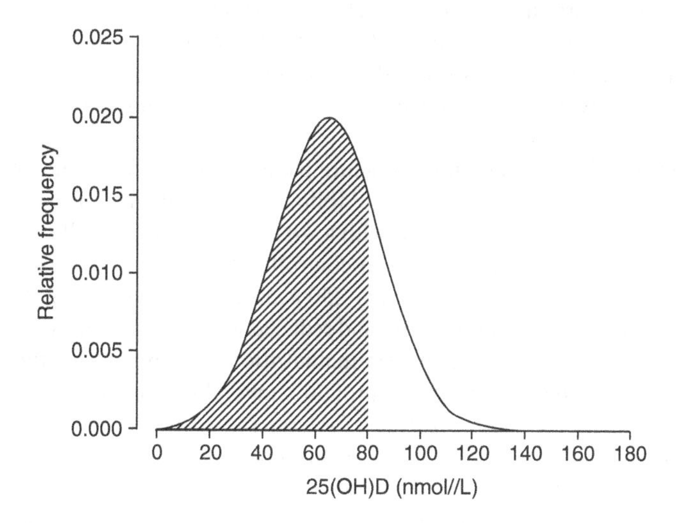

FIGURE 9.6 Approximation of the NHANES distribution of serum 25(OH)D values in women aged 60 to 79 years. (From Heaney, R. P., *J. Nutr.*,136, 1123, 2006.)

such a recommendation. Older adults can meet their vitamin D needs by judicious sun exposure and consuming the recommended amount of vitamin D-fortified milk — though vitamin D supplementation may be needed to meet their high vitamin D requirements. Additional information on vitamin D and bone health is available in Chapter 5.

9.7.2.1.3 Protein

Protein is an important structural component of bone. By weight, bone tissue is 70% mineral (primarily calcium and phosphorus), 22% protein, and 8% water [319]. High protein intake may increase urinary calcium excretion, but whether or not calcium balance is adversely affected is uncertain due in large part to the presence of other dietary constituents. Controversial findings regarding protein's role in bone health may be explained in large part by failure to consider the presence of other nutrients in the protein food source or total diet [320,321].

New findings, particularly in older adults, suggest that increasing dietary protein benefits bone health [322–326]. For example, in a 3-year prospective study of more than 30,000 postmenopausal women who participated in the Iowa Women's Health Study, higher protein intake, particularly animal protein, was associated with a 70% reduction in hip fractures, even after controlling for major confounding variables [322]. Similarly, when dietary protein (mostly animal protein) and bone mineral density were examined in a 4-year follow-up study of older men and women from the Framingham Osteoporosis study, higher protein intake was associated with increased bone mineral density of the femoral neck and spine [323]. Also, dietary protein and total hip bone mineral density were positively associated in a study of postmenopausal women in the NHANES III survey [324]. High intakes of total and animal protein were significantly associated with increased bone mineral density of the hip and total body in older women, but not in older men, in a 4-year prospective study of 960 participants of the Rancho Bernardo study in California [325]. When the relationship between intake of various nutrients and bone mineral density was examined in a cross-sectional study of 136 healthy postmenopausal women, intake of protein was positively associated with bone mineral density/content of the total body, hip, and hand [326].

Although protein intake in adults is usually more than sufficient, in older adults it is often low [297]. Epidemiological studies have associated low protein intakes in older adults with low bone mineral density, high rates of bone loss, and increased risk of hip fractures [322–324,327]. For example, a low protein diet was significantly associated with low hip bone mineral density in non-Hispanic white women participating in the NHANES III survey [324]. Similarly, low levels of protein were significantly associated with higher rates of bone loss at the hip and spine in elderly women in the Framingham Osteoporosis study [323]. Increased risk of hip fractures was found in older women in the Iowa Women's Health study who consumed the lowest amounts of protein [322].

Protein malnutrition is prevalent in hip fracture patients. For example, in a recent study of 225 postmenopausal women in Minnesota who were followed for an average of 16 years, a decrease in both total and animal protein was associated with a 44% increased risk of all osteoporotic fractures [327]. In a randomized, double-blind, placebo-controlled trial, elderly persons with hip fracture who were given a protein supplement supplying 250 kcals and 20 g of protein (90% milk proteins) had less bone loss, improved muscle strength, and reduced length of stay in a rehabilitation hospital [328]. It is unclear whether preventing protein malnutrition will prevent fracture.

Although the mechanism(s) is unknown, protein's favorable effect on bone may be explained by its ability to provide the necessary substrates for bone formation and remodeling [329]. Another possibility is that dietary protein may increase the production of insulin-like growth factor-1 (IGF-1), a hormone that stimulates bone formation [330,331].

Tufts University researchers recently found that the association between protein intake and bone mineral density in older adults depended on calcium intake [332]. Milk is a unique source of protein because its calcium content is high in relation to its protein content, with a calcium-to-protein ratio of approximately 36:1 [333]. Because protein exists in close association with other nutrients in the diet (e.g., calcium, phosphorus, magnesium, vitamin D, potassium, etc.), the overall dietary pattern impacts protein's effect on bone health [320].

Some have suggested that older adults utilize protein less efficiently, so need more protein per kilogram of body weight than younger adults [334]. The Institute of Medicine (IOM) recommends that adults consume 10% to 35% of total calories from protein [335]. Dairy foods, meat, and eggs provide high quality protein, as well as many other essential nutrients needed by older adults.

9.7.2.2 Hypertension

An age-related rise in hypertension is very common among older Americans. As in younger patients, hypertension therapy — as outlined in the 7th Report of the Joint National Committee on Prevention, Detection, Evaluation, and Treatment of High Blood Pressure — should begin with lifestyle modifications that include consuming adequate amounts of calcium, magnesium, and potassium in a diet rich in low-fat dairy foods, fruits, and vegetables, as exemplified in the DASH diet [215]. Because of the high risk associated with elevated blood pressure in the elderly, the beneficial effects of dietary changes should translate into substantial reduction in cardiovascular risk [215]. See a more complete discussion in the adult section of this chapter, and in Chapter 3.

9.7.2.3 Cancer

The risk of developing cancer increases with age, as does the risk of all chronic diseases. Emerging research in this area is showing a protective benefit for dairy foods and/or their components in reducing the risk of some cancers. See discussion in the adult section of this chapter, and in Chapter 4.

9.7.2.4 Overweight/Obesity

There is little evidence that weight should change as adults age. However, NHANES 1999 to 2002 reports that adults age 60 and older have a higher prevalence of overweight and obesity than younger adults. Mexican Americans are an exception; prevalence of overweight and obesity decreases after age 40 to 59 years [244]. In general, adults gain weight until the sixth decade, then there is a gradual decline, typically 10% between 70 and 80 years old. NHANES data do not report these older ages separately. While the proportion of body fat increases through middle age, after age 65 body fat typically decreases [296].

Though energy needs decline, the requirements for many nutrients, including calcium, vitamin D, and protein may increase. Older adults need to carefully select nutrient-dense foods, such as fruits, vegetables, and low-fat dairy foods to meet their nutritional needs with fewer calories [296]. See the adult section of this chapter and Chapter 7 for more information on the contribution of dairy foods to a healthy weight in adults.

9.7.3 Strategies to Improve Intake of Dairy Foods

Many older Americans would benefit by increasing their intake of milk and milk products to recommended levels. Attention to diet and nutrition tends to increase steadily with age. A survey found that persons age 65 said "I am very careful about the foods I eat" more often than younger persons [166]. Even a brief educational intervention resulted in a significantly increased calcium intake in persons over age 60 [336].

Adults over age 65 may be the biggest challenge for the nutrition professional who wants to encourage clients to meet calcium recommendations with food. Adults over age 65 have higher calcium requirements, but lower energy needs compared to younger adults. Therefore, nutrition education for the elderly should focus on the value of high quality, nutrient-dense foods, with lower energy density [301]. Due to reduced physical activity, older persons are at greater risk for becoming overweight even though their food and nutrient intake may be declining [337]. It is important to encourage the overweight elderly to increase physical activity as they are able and to include adequate amounts of low-fat and nonfat dairy foods as part of a healthy, lower-calorie diet. However, when told to reduce their intake of dietary fat, some older adults may restrict their dairy food intake, rather than choose lower fat versions [338]. Educational materials for dietary fat reduction should contain balanced eating messages to prevent the restriction of nutrient-dense dairy foods.

Looking at the attributes of older adults who consume dairy foods and the characteristics that influence their intake can aid in the development of effective education strategies. A study involving one hundred postmenopausal women over age 50, recruited from three Midwestern churches, evaluated how attitudes toward health promotion affect osteoporosis preventive behaviors, such as calcium intake and exercise [339]. The investigators found that women who perceived greater benefits and fewer barriers to calcium intake tended to consume a greater amount of milk. Women who consumed the most calcium-rich foods perceived themselves as more self-efficacious (believed their actions could influence their health), believed health was internally controlled or influenced by significant others (such as physicians), perceived themselves to be in good health, and perceived fewer barriers to calcium intake. The authors conclude that "Effective education about osteoporosis prevention needs to emphasize the required daily calcium amount for postmenopausal women, provide examples of the calcium content of calcium-rich foods, educate women about supplements, assess and address individual barriers, explain benefits, and use research findings to support information provided" [339]. A cross-sectional survey of older adults with hypertension, who participated in a Pennsylvania pharmaceutical assistance program, found that daily intake of dairy foods was more prevalent among women and whites as well as those who exhibited certain health-conscious behaviors, such as exercising and not smoking, and those who spent more time with others [340]. The authors conclude that practitioners should focus educational efforts on men, African Americans, and those who do not practice other health-related behaviors, as well as those who have little social support [340].

Several barriers to adequate dairy food intake have been identified in older adults, including perceived lactose intolerance, misinformation about dairy foods, and culturally-based food patterns. A telephone survey of 495 older adults ages 60 to 94 years found that total milk consumption was positively influenced by consumption of milk during youth and negatively influenced by a perception of milk intolerance, though lactose maldigestion had not been clinically diagnosed [341]. Lactose intolerance, whether perceived or real, does not require dairy avoidance. Chapter 8 has more information about lactose intolerance and simple dietary strategies that can be used to improve tolerance to dairy foods.

Nutrition education to increase calcium and dairy consumption is especially important in African American older adults, many of whom believe the myth that African Americans don't get osteoporosis [342]. In fact, there are 300,000 documented cases of osteoporosis among African American women, who have a lower calcium and dairy food intake than the balance of the population [342]. Nutrition educators need to understand the barriers to increasing dairy intake among older African Americans, which include past negative experiences, limited availability, culturally-based food consumption patterns, and lifestyle [342]. A low intake of calcium and other nutrients put African Americans at an increased risk for chronic diseases. The NMA, an African American physician's group, recommends that African Americans consume 3 to 4 servings of dairy foods daily to reduce their risk of osteoporosis, hypertension, overweight, and colon cancer [343]. Research has shown that lactose maldigesters, including African Americans, can consume at least one cup of milk without experiencing symptoms, and tolerance can be improved by consuming milk with a meal, choosing yogurt or hard cheeses, or using lactose-reduced products or lactase supplements [344]. There is a strong need for nutrition education of elderly African Americans that clearly spells out practical, culturally-specific, innovative approaches to incorporating dairy products into their daily diet [342].

In a study of New Zealand women with low calcium intakes, a major barrier to improving calcium/dairy food intake in elderly women was the common misperception that increasing the intake of milk or milk products will have either no effect or an adverse effect on health [291]. The health reasons mentioned by the older women included lowering fat and cholesterol intake, kidney stones, asthma, and pancreatic problems. Thirteen percent of all participants (young and older) reported they had been advised by their doctors not to consume milk or milk products. The elderly women said their doctors advised against consuming dairy foods to reduce cholesterol intake or mucus production, to ameliorate kidney or pancreatic problems, or for the management of bronchitis, diabetes, or a heart condition. The authors conclude, "There is a need to actively counter misconceptions concerning the adverse effects of milk or milk products on medical conditions, particularly amongst elderly women" [291]. Several articles included in a supplement to the *Journal of the American College of Nutrition* provide science-based information to help health professionals address a number of misperceptions and myths about dairy foods [10,321,344,345]. Older Americans should be encouraged to use food first, rather than supplements, to meet their calcium needs, as older adults often have low intakes of several nutrients that milk and milk products can supply [346]. For those who are not able to consistently obtain enough calcium from dairy foods, a judicious use of calcium-fortified foods or a calcium supplement is preferable to neglecting the difference.

Clinical interventions have demonstrated that dairy food intake can be increased in older adults [347,348]. In a 6-month home-based nutrition intervention to increase fruit, vegetable, and calcium-rich food consumption, seventy adults older than age 69 years were randomly assigned to a nutrition education group or an exercise group (placebo) [348]. Compared with the exercise group, the nutrition education group increased their self-reported intake of fruits/vegetables and dairy foods by 1 serving per day, which resulted in significantly higher intake of vitamin A, vitamin C, folate, beta-carotene, alpha-carotene, lutein, lycopene, protein, calcium, and phosphorus [348]. Factors that encouraged compliance in participants included record keeping, continuous monitoring, and positive reinforcement.

A 4-year longitudinal study among 64 postmenopausal women in Australia demonstrated the value of fat-free (skim) milk at improving diet quality [347]. When compared to the women who took a calcium supplement (1000 mg/day in addition to diet), those who increased their calcium intake to 1600 mg/day with fat-free milk also significantly increased their intakes of protein, potassium, magnesium, phosphorus, riboflavin, thiamin and zinc. The participants did so without increasing their total fat or saturated fat intake. In an accompanying editorial, Robert Heaney, M.D., calcium researcher from Creighton University in Omaha, Nebraska, emphasizes, "Diets low in calcium are typically low in other nutrients, too. When you drink milk, you're getting an entire nutrient package" [349]. He states that some nutrition practitioners have a "defeatist attitude toward encouraging increased milk consumption and a too easy acceptance of supplements" [349].

Based on the documented concerns of older adults, nutrition initiatives to increase the consumption of calcium-rich foods might contain the following elements:

- Design educational materials to appeal to both men and women. A survey of more than 400 older Americans (ages 55 to 89) found no gender-related differences in health concerns or behaviors. Eighty-five percent of older married men shopped for food and 84% cooked at least part of the time [350].
- Present information about the benefits of milk and milk products for reducing the risk of several chronic diseases — including osteoporosis, hypertension, overweight, and cancer — and improving the quality of their latter years. Actively counter any misinformation they may have received about adverse health effects of milk.

- Compare the calcium, fat, and calorie content of various calcium-rich foods. Weight control ranked second among the diet concerns of the elderly [350]. Provide clients with sample high-calcium, low-calorie menus; help them customize the menus to their own taste preferences.
- Discuss how milk, yogurt, and cheese can improve the nutrient adequacy of the total diet. In a screening initiative designed to identify older adults at nutritional risk, over one-third said they ate few fruits and vegetables, and drank little milk [351]. A majority of those surveyed had inadequate calcium intakes and 40% had inadequate intakes of vitamin A — both nutrients provided by dairy foods.
- Discuss the client's attitudes toward health promotion in general and barriers to the intake of milk and milk products. Strategize with the client to overcome these barriers.

9.8 CONCLUSION

An adequate intake of milk and milk products as part of a healthy, balanced diet is needed throughout the lifespan to promote health. Milk, yogurt, and cheese contain a high calcium content, substantial amounts of other essential nutrients, and health-promoting components. Because of their unique nutritional package, dairy foods contribute significantly to the nutritional adequacy of the diets of children and adults. Research has established the benefit of dairy foods for reducing the risk of chronic diseases such as osteoporosis, hypertension, and possibly some cancers. Results from human clinical trials suggest that dairy foods, with their unique nutritional profile, may be more effective than a single nutrient (i.e. calcium, potassium, magnesium, vitamin D) for reducing the risk of hypertension and colon cancer.

Unfortunately, the consumption of dairy foods by many Americans is grossly inadequate — particularly among females and the elderly. Although educational efforts are important for all age groups, children in particular deserve special attention. Increasing dairy food consumption to recommended levels in children and adolescents — along with regular physical activity — appears to be the most effective strategy for reducing the risk of osteoporosis later in life. It affords the best chance to influence peak bone mass and to establish eating habits that will continue throughout life. To turn this tide, we will need a concerted effort of governmental agencies, industry, individual health professionals, and the media to educate consumers about the important health benefits of milk and milk products, and also to address personal and social barriers to their consumption.

REFERENCES

1. Mitchell, M. K., *Nutrition during Infancy Nutrition Across the Lifespan*, W.B. Saunders Company, Philadelphia, PA, p. 209, 2003.
2. American Academy of Pediatrics, Breast-feeding and the use of human milk, *Pediatrics*, 115 (2), 496, 2005.
3. Committee on Nutrition, American Academy of Pediatrics, Breast-feeding, in *Pediatric Nutrition Handbook*, 5th ed., Kleinman, R. E., Ed., American Academy of Pediatrics, Elk Grove Village, 1L, p. 55, 2004.
4. Position of the American dietetic association: promoting and supporting breast-feeding, *J. Am. Diet. Assoc.*, 105, 810–818, 2005.
5. Food and Nutrition Board/Institute of Medicine, *Dietary Reference Intakes, Calcium, Phosphorus, Magnesium, Vitamin D, and Fluoride*, National Academy Press, Washington, D.C., 1997.
6. American Academy of Pediatrics, Formula feeding of term infants, In *Pediatric Nutrition Handbook*, 5th ed., Kleinman, R. E., Ed., American Academy of Pediatrics, Elk Grove Village, IL, 2004, chap. 4.

7. Code of Federal Regulations, title 21, Parts 106 and 107., U.S. Government Printing Office, Washington, D.C., 1999.
8. Congressional Record, 99th Congress 2nd Session, Senate S 14042-14047, U.S. Government Printing Office, Washington, D.C., 132 (130), 1986.
9. American Academy of Pediatrics, Committee on nutrition, the use of whole cow's milk in infancy, *Pediatrics*, 89, 1105, 1992.
10. Crittenden, R. G. and Bennett, L. E., Cow's milk allergy: a complex disorder, *J. Am. Coll. Nutr.*, 24 (6), 582S, 2005.
11. Committee on Nutrition, American Academy of Pediatrics, Food sensitivity, in *Pediatric Nutrition Handbook,* 5th ed., Kleinman, R. E., Ed., American Academy of Pediatrics, Elk Grove Village, IL, 2004, chap. 34.
12. Thong, B.-H. and Hourihane, J. B., Monitoring of EgE-mediated food allergy in childhood, *Acta Paediatr.*, 93, 759, 2004.
13. Host, A., Cow's milk allergy, *J. Royal Soc. Med.*, 90 (suppl. 30), 34, 1997.
14. Committee on Nutrition, American Academy of Pediatrics, Food sensitivity, in *Pediatric Nutrition Handbook,* 5th ed., Kleinman, R. E., Ed., American Academy of Pediatrics, Elk Grove Village, IL, 605, 2004.
15. Zeiger, R. S., Dietary manipulations in infants and their mothers and the natural course of atopic disease, *Pediatr. Allergy Immunol.*, 5 (suppl. 1), 33, 1994.
16. Baumgartner, M. et al., Brown.Controlled trials investigating the use of one partially hydrolyzed whey formula for dietary prevention of atopic manifestations until 60 months of age: an overview using meta-analytical methods, *Nutr. Res.*, 18 (8), 1425, 1998.
17. Chandra, R. K., Five-year follow up of high risk infants with family history of allergy exclusively breast-fed or fed partial whey hydrolysate, soy and conventional cow's milk formulas, *Nutr. Res.*, 18 (8), 1395, 1998.
18. Fritsche, R., Induction of oral tolerance to cow's milk proteins in rats fed with a whey protein hydrolysate, *Nutr. Res.*, 18 (8), 1335, 1998.
19. Halken, S. and Host, A., Prevention of allergic disease: exposure to food allergens and dietetic intervention, *Pediatr. Allergy Immunol.*, 7, 102, 1996.
20. Committee on Nutrition, American Academy of Pediatrics, Complementary Feeding, in *Pediatric Nutrition Handbook*, 5th ed., Kleinman, R. E., Ed., American Academy of Pediatrics, Elk Grove Village, IL, 2004, chap. 6.
21. World Health Organization, *Infant and Young Child Nutrition*, Geneva, Switzerland, 54th World Health Assembly, 54.2, 2001.
22. Stang, J., Improving the eating patterns of infants and toddlers, *J. Am. Diet. Assoc.*, 106, S7, 2006.
23. Greer, F., Optimizing bone health and calcium intakes of infants, children, and adolescents, *Pediatrics*, 117 (2), 578, 2006.
24. Butte, N. et al., The start healthy feeding guidelines for infants and toddlers, *J. Am. Diet. Assoc.*, 104 (3), 442, 2004.
25. Mitchell, M. K., Nutrition during infancy, *Nutrition Across the Lifespan*, W. B. Saunders Company, Philadelphia, PA, 240, 2003.
26. Guerin-Danan, C. et al., Milk fermented with yogurt cultures and lactobacillus casei compared with yogurt and gelled milk: influence on intestinal microflora in healthy infants, *Am. J. Clin. Nutr.*, 67, 111, 1998.
27. Pettifor, J., Rickets and vitamin D deficiency in children and adolescents, *Endo. Metab. Clin. Nutr. Am.*, 34 (3), 537–553, vii, 2005.
28. Mitchell, M. K., Nutrition during growth, *Nutrition Across the Lifespan*, W.B. Saunders Company, Philadelphia, PA, 290, 2003.
29. Pettifor, J., Nutritional rickets: deficiency of vitamin D, calcium, or both? *Am. J. Clin. Nutr.*, 80 (suppl. 6), 1725S, 2004.
30. Committee on Nutrition, American Academy of Pediatrics, Vitamins, In *Pediatric Nutrition Handbook*, 5th ed., Kleinman, R. E., Ed., American Academy of Pediatrics, Elk Grove Village, IL, 347, 2004.
31. Alouf, B. and Grigalonis, M., Incidental finding of vitamin-D deficient rickets in an otherwise healthy infant–a reappraisal of current vitamin-D supplementation guidelines, *J. Nat. Med. Assoc.*, 97 (8), 1170, 2005.

32. Committee on Nutrition, American Academy of Pediatrics, Feeding the Child, in *Pediatric Nutrition Handbook*, 5th ed., Kleinman, R. E., Ed., American Academy of Pediatrics, Elk Grove Village, Illinois, 2004, chap. 7.
33. Mitchell, M. K., Nutrition during growth: preschool through preadolescence, *Nutrition Across the Lifespan*, W. B. Saunders, Philadelphia, PA, 2003, chap. 9.
34. Ryan, C. and Dwyer, J., The Toddler's smorgasbord: common table foods and dietary guidance for children aged 13 to 24 months, *Nutr. Today*, 38 (5), 164, 2003.
35. Fox, M. K. et al., Sources of energy and nutrients in the diets of infants and toddlers, *J. Am. Diet. Assoc.*, 106, S28, 2006.
36. Briefel, R. et al., Feeding infants and toddlers study: characteristics and usual nutrient intake of hispanic and non-hispanic infants and toddlers, *J. Am. Diet. Assoc.*, 106, S84, 2006.
37. Moshfegh, A., Goldman, J., and Cleveland, L., *What We Eat in America, NHANES 2001–2002: Usual Nutrient Intakes from Food Compared to Dietary Reference Intakes*, U.S. Department of Agriculture, Agricultural Research Service,www.ars.usda.gov/foodsurvey, September 2005.
38. Fox, M. K. et al., Average portions of foods commonly eaten by infants and toddlers in the United States, *J. Am. Diet. Assoc.*, 106, S66, 2006.
39. Ziegler, P. et al., Nutrient intakes and food patterns of toddlers' lunches and snacks: influence of location, *J. Am. Die. Assoc.*, 106, S124, 2006.
40. Birch, L. L., Children's food acceptance patterns, *Nutr. Today*, 31 (6), 234, 1997.
41. Patrick, H. et al., The benefits of authoritative feeding style: care giver feeding styles and children's food consumption patterns, *Appetite*, 44 (2), 243, 2005.
42. Position, ADA, Dietary guidance for healthy children aged 2 to 11 years, *J. Am. Diet. Assoc.*, 104, 660, 2004.
43. USDA, Center for Nutrition and Policy Promotion, The Food Guide Pyramid for Young Children, 2003, http://www.usda.gov/cnpp/KidsPyra/ (Accessed on February 22, 2006).
44. Pugliese, M. T. et al., Parental health beliefs as a cause of nonorganic failure to thrive, *Pediatrics*, 80, 175, 1987.
45. U. S. Department of Agriculture/Department of Health and Human Services, *Dietary Guidelines for Americans 2005*, 6th ed., *Home and Garden Bulletin No. 232*, U. S. Government Printing Office, Washington, D.C., January 2005.
46. Zlotkin, S. H., A review of the canadian nutrition recommendations update: dietary fat and children, *J. Nutr.*, 126, 1022, 1996.
47. Smith, M. M. and Lifshitz, F., Excess fruit juice consumption as a contributing factor in nonorganic failure to thrive, *Pediatrics*, 93 (3), 438, 1994.
48. Dennison, B. A., Rockwell, H. L., and Baker, S. L., Excess fruit juice consumption by preschool-aged children is associated with short stature and obesity, *Pediatrics*, 99 (1), 15, 1997.
49. Skinner, J. D. et al., Fruit juice intake is not related to children's growth, *Pediatrics*, 103 (1), 58, 1999.
50. Newby, P. K. et al., Beverage consumption is not associated with changes in weight and body mass index among low-income preschool children in North Dakota, *J. Am. Diet. Assoc.*, 104 (7), 1086, 2004.
51. Marshall, T. A. et al., Diet quality in young children is influenced by beverage consumption, *J. Am. Coll. Nutr.*, 24 (1), 65, 2005.
52. American Academy of Pediatrics, The use and misuse of fruit juice in pediatrics, *Pediatrics*, 107, 1210, 2001.
53. Dietary Guidelines Advisory Committee Report, http://www.health.gov/DietaryGuidelines/dga2005/report/, 2005.
54. Centers for Disease Control and Prevention, Blood lead levels, United States, 1999 to 2002, *Morbidity Mortality Weekly Report*, 54(20): 513, 2005.
55. Miller, G. D. and Groziak, S., Essential and nonessential mineral interactions, in *Handbook of Human Toxicology*, Massaro, E. J., Miller, G. D., Kang, Y. J., Morgan, D. L., Rodgers, K. E., and Schardein, J. L., Eds., CRC Press, Boca Raton, FL, July, 1997.
56. Haan, M. N., Gerson, M., and Zishka, B. A., Identification of children at risk for lead poisoning: an evaluation of routine pediatric blood lead screening in an HMO-insured population, *Pediatrics*, 97 (1), 79, 1996.

57. Centers for Disease Control and Prevention, *Screening Young Children for Lead Poisoning: Guidance for State and Local Public Health Officials*, Centers for Disease Control and Prevention, Atlanta, GA, 1997.
58. Sargent, J. D., The role of nutrition in the prevention of lead poisoning in children, *Pediatric Annals*, 23 (11), 636, 1994.
59. Institute of Medicine, *Food Marketing to Children and Youth: Threat or Opportunity?* National Academy Press, http://www.nap.edu/catalog/11514.html, December 2005.
60. U.S. Department of Health and Human Services, *Bone Health and Osteoporosis: A Report of the Surgeon General*, U.S. Department of Health and Human Services, Office of the Surgeon General, Rockville, MD, www.surgeongeneral.gov/library, 2004.
61. Abrams, S. A. and Stuff, J. E., Calcium metabolism in girls: current dietary intakes lead to low rates of calcium absorption and retention during puberty, *Am. J. Clin. Nutr.*, 60, 739, 1994.
62. Bounds, W. et al., The relationship of dietary and lifestyle factors to bone mineral indexes in children, *J. Am. Diet. Assoc.*, 105, 735, 2005.
63. Kalkwarf, H. J., Khoury, J. C., and Lanphear, B. P., Milk intake during childhood and adolescence, adult bone density, and osteoporotic fractures in U.S. women, *Am. J. Clin. Nutr.*, 77, 257, 2003.
64. Teegarden, D. et al., Previous milk consumption is associated with greater bone density in young women, *Am. J. Clin. Nutr.*, 69, 1014, 1999.
65. U.S. Department of Agriculture, Community Nutrition Research Group, Agricultural Research Service, Pyramid Servings Intakes in the United States, 1999–2002, http://www.barc.usda.gov/bhnrc/cnrg/, Table set 3.0, March 2005.
66. Lau, E. M. C. et al., Benefits of milk powder supplementation on bone accretion in chinese children, *Osteopor. Internal.*, 15, 654, 2004.
67. Du, X. et al., School-milk intervention trial enhances growth and bone mineral accretion in Chinese girls aged 10–12 years in Beijing, *Br. J. Nutr.*, 92, 159, 2004.
68. Fisher, J. O. et al., Meeting calcium recommendations during middle childhood reflects mother-daughter beverage choices and predicts bone mineral status, *Am. J. Clin. Nutr.*, 79, 698, 2004.
69. Black, R. E. et al., Children who avoid drinking cow milk have low dietary calcium intakes and poor bone health, *Am. J. Clin. Nutr.*, 76, 675, 2002.
70. Goulding, A. et al., Children who avoid drinking cow's milk are at increased risk for prepubertal bone fractures, *J. Am. Diet. Assoc.*, 104 (2), 250, 2004.
71. Goulding, A. et al., Bone mineral density in girls with forearm fractures, *J. Bone Min. Res.*, 13, 143, 1998.
72. Khosla, S. et al., Incidence of childhood distal forearm fractures over 30 years: a population-based study, *J. Am. Med. Assoc.*, 290, 1479, 2003.
73. National Center for Health Statistics, *Health United States, 2005*, with Chartbook on Trends in the Health of Americans, Hyattsville, MD, Table 85, 2005.
74. Kashket, S. and DePaola, D., Cheese consumption and the development and progression of dental caries, *Nutr. Rev.*, 60 (4), 97, 2002.
75. Bowen, W. H. and Pearson, S. K., Effect of milk on cariogenesis, *Caries Res.*, 27, 461, 1993.
76. Levy, S. M. et al., Fluoride, beverages and dental caries in the primary dentition, *Caries Res.*, 37 (3), 157, 2003.
77. Vacca-Smith, A. M. et al., The effect of milk and casein proteins on the adherence of *Streptococcus mutans* to saliva-coated hydroxyapatite, *Arch. Oral Biol.*, 39 (12), 1063, 1994.
78. Greenby, T. H. et al., Dental caries-protective agents in milk and milk products: investigations *in vitro*, *J. Dent.*, 29 (2), 83, 2001.
79. Aimutis, W. R., Bioactive properties of milk proteins with particular focus on anticariogenesis, *J. Nutr.*, 134 (4), 989S, 2004.
80. Comelli, E. M., Guggenheim, B., Stingele, R., and Neeser, J-R. , Selection of dairy bacterial strains as probiotics for oral health, *Eur. J. Oral Sci.*, 110 (3), 218, 2002.
81. Paolino, V. J. and Kashket, S., Inhibition of cocoa extracts of biosynthesis of extracellular polysaccharide by human oral bacteria, *Arch. Oral Biol.*, 30 (4), 359, 1985.
82. Palmer, C. A., Important relationships between diet, nutrition, and oral health, *Nutr. Clin. Care*, 4 (1), 4, 2001.
83. Nunn, J., Nutrition and dietary challenges in oral health, *Nutrition*, 17, 426, 2001.

84. American Academy of Pediatrics, Nutrition and oral health, in *Pediatric Nutrition Handbook*, 5th ed., Kleinman, R. E., Ed., American Academy of Pediatrics, Elk Grove Village, IL, 790, 2004.
85. Cook, A. J. and Friday, J. E., Food mixture or ingredient sources for dietary calcium: shifts in food group contributions using four grouping protocols, *J. Am. Diet. Assoc.*, 103, 1513, 2003.
86. Subar, A. F. et al., Dietary sources of nutrients among U.S. children, 1989–1991, *Pediatrics*, 102 (4), 913, 1998.
87. Bowman, S. A., Beverage choices of young females: changes and impact on nutrient intakes, *J. Am. Diet. Assoc.*, 102, 1234, 2002.
88. Johnson, R. K., Frary, C., and Wang, M. Q., The nutritional consequences of flavored-milk consumption by school-aged children and adolescents in the United States, *J. Am. Diet. Assoc.*, 102 (6), 853, 2002.
89. Johnson, R. K., Panely, C., and Wang, M. Q., The association between noon beverage consumption and the diet quality of school-age children, *J. Child Nutr. Manag.*, 22, 95, 1998.
90. Juanita, L. E. et al., Maternal resources, parenting, and dietary patterns among rural African American children in single-parent families, *Public Health Nurs.*, 19 (2), 104, 2002.
91. Cadogan, J., Eastell, R., Jones, N. et al., Milk intake and bone mineral acquisition in adolescent girls: randomised, controlled intervention trial, *Br. Med. J.*, 315, 1255, 1997.
92. Lappe, J. M., Rafferty, K. A., Davies, K. M. et al., Girls on a high-calcium diet gain weight at the same rate as girls on a normal diet: a pilot study, *J. Am. Diet. Assoc.*, 104, 1361, 2004.
93. U.S. Department of Agriculture, *MyPyramid for Kids*, September 2005. http://www.mypyramid.gov/kids/index.html (accessed on March 2006).
94. National Institute of Child Health Development (NICHD), Milk Matters, http://www.nichd.nih.gov/milk/.
95. Panley, C. V., Johnson, R. K., and Wang, M. Q., Predictors of milk consumption in U.S. school-aged children: evidence from the 1994–1995 USDA continuing survey of food intakes by individuals, *J. Am. Diet. Assoc*, 98 (9), A.52, 1998.
96. Fisher, J. O. et al., Maternal milk consumption predicts the tradeoff between milk and soft drinks in young girls' diets, *J. Nutr.*, 131, 246, 2001.
97. Johnson, R. K., Panely, C. V., and Wang, M. Q., Associations between the milk mothers drink and the milk consumed by their school-aged children, *Fam. Econom. Nutr. Rev.*, 13 (1), 27, 2001.
98. Dairy Management, Inc., *Consumer Segmentation Study*, 1997.
99. Chan, G. M., Hoffman, K., and McMurry, M., Effects of dairy products on bone and body composition in pubertal girls, *J. Pediatrics*, 126, 551, 1995.
100. Skinner, J. D. et al., Predictors of children's body mass index: a longitudinal study of diet and growth in children aged 2–8 y, *Int. J. Obes. Relat. Metab. Disord.*, 28 (4), 476, 2004.
101. U.S. Department of Agriculture, Food and Nutrition Service. Nutrition Assistance Programs Home Page, www.fns.usda.gov/tn/Resources/offer_v_serve.html (Accessed october 11, 2006).
102. International Dairy Foods Association, *Dairy Facts, 2004 Edition*, International Dairy Foods Association, Washington, D.C., p. 91, 2004.
103. Child Nutrition and WIC Reauthorization Act of 2004 (P.L. 108–265, signed June 30, 2004), Sec. 102.
104. U.S. Department of Agriculture, Food and consumer service, *Fed. Registr.*, 62 (44), 10187, 1997.
105. U.S. Department of Agriculture, *School Nutrition Dietary Assessment Study–II, January 2001*, www.fns.usda.gov/oane (accessed on March 2006).
106. Nicklas, T. A., O'Neil, C., and Myers, L., The importance of breakfast consumption to nutrition of children, adolescents, and young adults, *Nutr. Today*, 39 (1), 30, 2004.
107. Gleason, P., Suitor, C. Children's diets in the mid-1990s: dietary intake and its relationship with school meal participation. *Nutrition Assistance Program Report Series*, Report No. CN-01-CD1, www.fns.usda.gov/oane, January 2001.
108. Nicklas, T. A. J., Calcium intake trends and health consequences from childhood through adulthood, *J. Am. Coll. Nutr.*, 22 (5), 340, 2003.
109. Hanes, S., Vermeersch, J., and Gale, S., The national evaluation of school nutrition programs: program impact on dietary intake, *Am. J. Clin. Nutr.*, 40, 390, 1984.
110. Affenito, S. G. et al., Breakfast consumption by African–American and white adolescent girls correlates positively with calcium and fiber intake and negatively with body mass index, *J. Am Diet. Assoc.*, 105, 938, 2005.

111. Food Research and Action Center, School Breakfast Scorecard: 2005, December 2005, http://www.frac.org/ (accessed March 2006).
112. Fox, M. K., Hamilton, W., and Lin, B-H., *Effects of Food Assistance and Nutrition Programs on Nutrition and Health. Volume 4, Executive Summary of the Literature Review*, Food Assistance and Nutrition Research Report No. 19–4, U.S. Department of Agriculture, Washington, D.C., November 2004.
113. Shanklin, C. W. and Wie, S., Nutrient contribution per 100 kcal and per penny for the 5 meal components in school lunch: entrée, milk, vegetable/fruit, bread/grain, and miscellaneous, *J. Am. Diet. Assoc.*, 101 (11), 1358, 2001.
114. Groziak, S.M., Boning up on calcium, *School Foodservice and Nutrition*, 23, November, 1998.
115. Patrick, H. and Nicklas, T. A., A review of family and social determinants of children's eating patterns and diet quality, *J. Am. Coll. Nutr.*, 24 (2), 83, 2005.
116. National Dairy Council and American School Food Service Association, The School Milk Pilot Test, Beverage Marketing Corporation for National Dairy Council and American School Food Service Association, 2002, www.nationaldairycouncil.org.
117. *2005 Kids Milk Tracking Study*, Wave V, GFK Custom Research, Inc., October 2005.
118. Position of the American Dietetic Association, local support for nutrition integrity in schools. *J. Am. Diet. Assoc.* 106 (1), 122, 2006.
119. Lin, B-H., Ralston, K., *Competitive Foods: Soft Drinks vs. Milk*, U.S. Department of Agriculture, Economic Research Service, Food Assistance and Nutrition Research Report, Number 34–7, July 2003.
120. Rajeshwari, R. et al., Secular trends in children's sweetened beverage consumption (1994): The Bogalusa Heart Study, *J. Am. Diet. Assoc.*, 105, 208, 1973.
121. Public Law 108-265, Sec. 102 (42 USC 1754).
122. Gidding, S. S. et al., Dietary recommendations for children and adolescents: a guide for practitioners, consensus statement from the American Heart Association, *Circulation*, 112, 2061, 2005.
123. American Academy of Pediatrics, Endorsed policy statement, dietary recommendations for children and adolescents: a guide for practitioners, *Pediatrics*, 117 (2), 544, 2006.
124. American Academy of Pediatrics, Committee on School Health, Soft drinks in schools, *Pediatrics*, 113, 152, 2004.
125. Food and Nutrition Service, U.S. Department of Agriculture, Centers for Disease Control and Prevention, U.S. Department of Health and Human Services, and U.S. Department of Education, FNS-374, *Making it Happen! School Nutrition Success Stories*, Alexandria, VA, January 2005.
126. Conners, P., Bednar, C., and Klammer, S., Cafeteria factors that influence milk-drinking behaviors of elementary schoolchildren: grounded theory approach, *J. Nutr. Edu.*, 33, 31, 2001.
127. U.S. Department of Agriculture, Agricultural Research Service. 2005, *USDA National Nutrient Database for Standard Reference, Release 18*, Nutrient Data Laboratory Home Page, www.ars.usda.gov/ba/bhnrc/ndl (accessed on October 7, 2005).
128. NPD Group's National Eating Trends and Nutrient Intake Databases, *Flavored Milk: Sugar in a Kid's/Teen's Diet*, September 14, 2005.
129. Position of the American Dietetic Association, Use of nutritive and non-nutritive sweeteners, *J. Am. Diet. Assoc.*, 104 (2), 255, 2004.
130. Johnson, R. K., Frary, C., and Wang, M. Q., The nutritional consequences of flavored milk consumption by school-aged children and adolescents in the United States, *J. Am. Diet. Assoc.*, 102, 853, 2002.
131. Garey, J. G., Chan, M. M., and Parlia, S. R., Effect of fat content and chocolate flavoring of milk on meal consumption and acceptability by schoolchildren, *J. Am. Diet. Assoc.*, 90, 719, 1990.
132. Frary, C. D., Johnson, R. K., and Wang, M. Q., Children and adolescents' choices of foods and beverages high in added sugars are associated with intakes of key nutrients and food groups, *J. Adol. Health*, 34, 56, 2004.
133. American Academy of Pediatrics, Committee on School Health, Soft drinks in schools, *Pediatrics*, 113, 152, 2004.
134. Wolraich, M. L., Wilson, D. B., and White, J. W., The effect of sugar on behavior or cognition in children: a meta-analysis, *J. Am. Med. Assoc.*, 274 (20), 1617, 1995.
135. Bowen, W. J. and Pearson, S. K., Effect of milk on cariogenesis, *Caries Res.*, 27, 461, 1993.

136. Recker, R. R., Bammi, A., Barger-Lux, M. J., and Heaney, R. P., Calcium absorbability from milk products, an imitation milk, and calcium carbonate, *Am. J. Clin. Nutr.*, 47, 93, 1988.
137. Lee, C. M. and Hardy, C. M., Cocoa feeding and human lactose intolerance, *Am. J. Clin. Nutr.*, 49 (5), 840, 1989.
138. Gong, E. J., and Heald, F. P., Diet, nutrition, and adolescence, in *Modern Nutrition in Health and Disease*, 8th ed., Shils, M. E., Olsen, J. A., and Shike, M., Ed., Lea & Febiger, Philadelphia, PA, pp. 759–769, 1994.
139. Wotecki, C. E. and Filer, L. J., Dietary issues and nutritional status of American children, in *Child, Health, Nutrition, and Physical Activity*, Ceung, L. W. Y. and Richmond, J. B., Eds., Human Kinetics, Champaign, IL, pp. 3–40, 1995.
140. Mitchell, M.K., Nutrition during adolescence, in *Nutrition Across the Lifespan*, W.B. Saunders Company, Philadelphia, PA, 2003, chap. 11.
141. Demory-Luce, D. et al., Changes in food group consumption patterns from childhood to young adulthood: The Bogalusa Heart Study, *J. Am. Diet. Assoc.*, 104 (11), 1684, 2004.
142. Nicklas, T. A. et al., Children's food consumption patterns have changed over two decades (1973–1994): The Bogalusa Heart Study, *J. Am. Diet. Assoc.*, 104, 1127, 2004.
143. Ballew, C., Kuester, S., and Gillespie, C., Beverage choices affect adequacy of children's nutrient intakes, *Arch. Pediatr. Adolesc. Med.*, 154 (11), 8, 2000.
144. Schmidt, M. et al., Fast-food intake and diet quality in black and white girls: The National Heart Lung, and Blood Institute Growth and Health Study, *Arch. Pediatr. Adolesc. Med.*, 159 (7), 626, 2005.
145. Neumark-Sztainer, D. et al., Family meal patterns: associations with sociodemographic characteristics and improved dietary intake among adolescents, *J. Am. Diet. Assoc.*, 103 (3), 317, 2003.
146. Weaver, C. M., Peacock, M., Martin, B. R., Plawecki, K. L., and McCabe, G. P., Calcium retention estimated from indicators of skeletal status in adolescent girls and young women, *Am. J. Clin. Nutr.*, 64, 67, 1996.
147. Heaney, R. P. et al., Peak bone mass, *Osteoporos. Int.*, 11, 985, 2000.
148. Gunnes, M., Bone mineral density in the cortical and trabecular distal forearm in healthy children and adolescents, *Acta Paediatr.*, 83, 463, 1994.
149. Ilich, J. Z. and Kerstetter, J. E., Nutrition in bone health revisited: a story beyond calcium, *J. Am. Coll. Nutr.*, 19 (6), 715, 2000.
150. Huth, P. J., DiRienzo, D. B., and Miller, G. D., Major scientific advances with dairy foods in nutrition and health, *J. Dairy Sci.*, 89, 1207, 2006.
151. Wiley, A. S., Does milk make children grow? Relationships between milk consumption and height in NHANES 1999–2002, *Am. J. Hum. Biol.*, 17, 425, 2005.
152. Harkness, L. S. and Bonny, A. E., Calcium and vitamin D status in the adolescent: key roles for bone, body weight, glucose tolerance, and estrogen biosynthesis, *J. Pediatr. Adolesc. Gynecol.*, 18 (5), 305, 2005.
153. Tylavsky, F. A. et al., Vitamin D, parathyroid hormone, and bone mass in adolescents, *J. Nutr.*, 135 (11), 2735S, 2005.
154. Du, X. Q. et al., Milk consumption and bone mineral content in Chinese adolescent girls, *Bone*, 30, 521, 2002.
155. Volek, J. S. et al., Increasing fluid milk favorably affects bone mineral density responses to resistance training in adolescent boys, *J. Am. Diet. Assoc.*, 103, 1353, 2003.
156. Matkovic, V. et al., Nutrition influences skeletal development from childhood to adulthood: a study of hip, spine, and forearm in adolescent females, *J. Nutr.*, 134, 701S, 2004.
157. Wang, M-C. et al.Diet in midpuberty and sedentary activity in prepuberty predict peak bone mass, *Am. J. Clin. Nutr.*, 77, 495, 2003.
158. Fleming, K. H. and Heimback, J. T., Consumption of calcium in the U.S.: food sources and intake levels, *J. Nutr.*, 124, 1426S, 1994.
159. Weinberg, L. G., Berner, L. A., and Groves, J. E., Nutrient contributions of dairy foods in the United States, Continuing Survey of Food Intakes by Individuals, 1994–1996, 1998, *J. Am. Diet. Assoc.*, 104, 895, 2004.
160. Albertson, A. M., Tobelmann, R. C., and Marquart, L., Estimated dietary calcium intake and food sources for adolescent females: 1980–1992, *J. Adol. Health*, 20, 20, 1997.

161. Harel, Z., Riggs, S., Vaz, R., White, L., and Menzies, G., Adolescents and calcium: what they do and do not know and how much they consume, *J. Adolesce. Health*, 22, 225, 1998.
162. Neumark-Sztainer, D. et al., Correlates of inadequate consumption of dairy products among adolescents, *J. Nutr. Edu.*, 29, 12, 1997.
163. Martin, J. T. et al., Female adolescents' knowledge of bone health promotion behaviors and osteoporosis risk factors, *Orthop. Nurs.*, 23 (4), 235, 2004.
164. Croll, J. K., Neumark-Sztainer, D., and Story, M., Healthy eating: what does it mean to adolescents? *J. Nutr. Edu.*, 33 (4), 193, 2001.
165. U.S. Department of Agriculture, Agricultural Research Service, Data tables: Results from USDA's 1994–1996 Continuing Survey of Food Intakes by Individuals and 1994–1996 Diet and Health Knowledge Survey, 1997.
166. Dairy Management, Inc., *Attitude and Usage Trends Study*, 1998.
167. Teenage Research Unlimited, National Teen Nutrition Quantitative Research Final Report, June 1996.
168. Bowman, S. A. et al., Effects of fast food consumption on energy intake and diet quality among children in a national household survey, *Pediatrics*, 113, 112, 2004.
169. Chapman, G. and Maclean, H., "Junk food" and "healthy food": meanings of food in adolescent women's culture, *J. Nutr. Ed.*, 25 (3), 108, 1993.
170. Neumark-Sztainer, D. et al., Factors influencing food choices of adolescents: findings from focus group discussions with adolescents, *J. Am. Diet. Assoc.*, 99, 929, 1999.
171. Barr, S. I., Associations of social and demographic variables with calcium intakes of high school students, *J. Am. Diet., Assoc.*, 94, 260, 1994.
172. Lin, B-H., Ralston, K., *Competitive Foods: Soft Drinks vs. Milk*, United States Department of Agriculture, Economic Research Service, Food Assistance and Nutrition Research Report Number 34–7, July 2003.
173. Bowman, S. A., Beverage choices of young females: changes and impact on nutrient intakes, *J. Am. Diet. Assoc.*, 102, 1234, 2002.
174. Streigel-Moore, R. H. et al., Correlates of beverage intake in adolescent girls: The National Heart, Lung, and Blood Institute Growth and Health Study, *J. Pediatr.*, 148, 183, 2006.
175. Wyshak, G. and Frisch, R. E., Carbonated beverages, dietary calcium, the dietary calcium/phosphorus ratio and bone fractures in girls and boys, *J. Adoles. Health*, 15, 210, 1994.
176. Hanson, N. I. et al., Associations between parental report of the home food environment and adolescent intakes of fruits, vegetables, and dairy foods, *Pub. Health Nutr.*, 8 (1), 77, 2005.
177. Pugliese, M. T., Lifshitz, F., Grad, G., Fort, P., and Marks-Katz, M., Fear of obesity: a cause of short stature and delayed puberty, *N. Engl. J. Med.*, 309, 513, 1983.
178. Polivy, J., Psychological consequences of food restriction, *J. Am. Diet. Assoc.*, 96, 589, 1996.
179. Epstein, L. H., Coleman, K. J., and Myers, M. D., Exercise in treating obesity in children and adolescents, *Med. Sci. Sports Exer.*, 28 (4), 428, 1996.
180. Huang, T. T. K. and McCrory, M. A., Dairy intake, obesity, and metabolic health in children and adolescents: knowledge and gaps, *Nutr. Rev.*, 63, 71, 2005.
181. Novotny, R. et al., Dairy, calcium and body composition of multiethnic youth, *J. Nutr.*, 134, 2004, 1905.
182. Berkey, C. S. et al., Milk, Dairy fat, dietary calcium, and weight gain: a longitudinal study of adolescents, *Arch. Pediatr. Adolesc. Med.*, 159, 543, 2005.
183. Phillips, S. et al., Dairy food consumption and body weight and fatness studied longitudinally over the adolescent period, *Int. J. Obes. Relat. Metab. Disord.*, 27 (9), 1106, 2003.
184. Perry, C. L. et al., Characeristics of vegetarian adolescents in a multiethnic urban population, *J. Adolesc. Health*, 29 (6), 406, 2001.
185. Vegetarian Resource Group, How many teens are vegetarian? How many kids don't eat meat? *Veg. J.*, January/February, 2001, http://www.vrg.org/journal/vj2001jan/2001janteen.htm (accessed September 28, 2006).
186. Tatiana R., More teenagers forsaking meat: Diet's shortcomings draw concern, advice on healthy nutrition, *Boston Globe*, December 7, 1997.
187. The American Academy of Pediatrics, Nutritional aspects of vegetarian diets, in *Pediatric Nutrition Handbook*, 5th ed., Kleinman, R. E., Ed., American Academy of Pediatrics, Elk Grove Village, IL, 2003, chap. 12.

188. Story, M. and Alton, I., Nutrition issues and adolescent pregnancy, *Nutr. Today*, 30 (4), 142, 1995.
189. Bezerra, F. F. and Donangelo, C. M., Pregnancy and lactation in adolescents: possible implications for calcium metabolism and bone mass, *Curr. Nutr. Food Sci.*, I, 265, 2005.
190. Sowers, M. F. et al., Bone loss in adolescent and adult pregnant women, *Obstet. Gynecol.*, 96, 189, 2000.
191. Chan, G. M. et al., Bone mineral status of lactating mothers of different ages, *J. Clin., Endocrinol. Metab.*, 144, 438, 1982.
192. Bezerra, F. F. et al., Bone mass is recovered from lactation to postweaning in adolescent mothers with low calcium intakes, *Am. J. Clin. Nutr.*, 80, 1322, 2004.
193. Casanueva, E. et al., Bone mineral density and bone turnover in adolescent mothers after lactation, *Adv. Exp. Med. Biol.*, 554, 341, 2004.
194. O'Brien, K. O. et al., Calcium absorption is significantly higher in adolescents during pregnancy than in the early postpartum period, *Am. J. Clin. Nutr.*, 78, 1188, 2003.
195. Chan, G. M., McMurry, M., Westover, K., Engelbert-Fenton, K., and Thomas, M. R., Effects on increased dietary calcium intake upon the calcium and bone mineral status of lactating adolescent and adult women, *Am. J. Clin. Nutr.*, 46, 319, 1987.
196. Backman, D. R. et al., Psychosocial predictors of healthful dietary behavior in adolescents, *J. Nutr. Edu. Behav.*, 34, 184, 2002.
197. Lytle, L., *Nutrition Education for School-aged Children: A Review of Research*, prepared for U.S. Department of Agriculture, Food and Consumer Service, Office of Analysis and Evaluation, September, 1994.
198. Sigman-Grant, M., Strategies for counseling adolescents, *J. Am. Diet. Assoc.*, 102 (3), S32, 2002.
199. Hoelscher, D. et al., Designing effective nutrition interventions for adolescents, *J. Am. Diet. Assoc.*, 102 (3), 52, 2002.
200. Videon, T. M. and Manning, C. K., Influences on adolescent eating paterns: the importance of family meals, *J. Adolsc. Health*, 32 (5), 365, 2003.
201. Auld, G. et al., Perspectives on intake of calcium-rich foods among Asian, Hispanic, and white preadolescent and adolescent females, *J. Nutr. Edu. Behav.*, 34 (5), 242, 2002.
202. Reed, D. B. et al., Clueless in the Mall: a web site on calcium for teens, *J. Am. Diet. Assoc.*, 102 (3), S73, 2002.
203. Mitchell, M. K., Adult years, *Nutrition Across the Lifespan*, 2nd ed., W. B. Saunders, Philadelphia, PA, 2003, chap. 12.
204. Rajeshwari, R. et al., The nutritional impact of dairy product consumption on dietary intakes of adults 1995–1996: The Bogalusa Heart Study, *J. Am. Diet. Assoc.*, 105, 1391, 2005.
205. Heaney, R. P. and Barger-Lux, J., Low calcium intake: the culprit in many chronic diseases, *J. Dairy Sci.*, 77, 1155, 1994.
206. McCarron, D. A., Lipkin, M., Rivlin, R. S., and Heaney, R. P., Dietary calcium and chronic diseases, *Med. Hypoth.*, 31, 265, 1990.
207. Haapasalo, H., Kannus, P., Sievanen, H., Pasanen, M., Uusi-Rasi, K., Heinonen, A., Oja, P., and Vuori, I., Development of mass, density, and estimated mechanical characteristics of bones in Caucasian females, *J. Bone Min. Res.*, 11, 1751, 1996.
208. Fields, L. E. et al., The burden of adult hypertension in the United States 1999 to: a rising tide, *Hypertension*, 44, 1, 2004.
209. McCarron, D. A., Pingree, P. A., Rubin, R. J., Gaucher, S. M., Molitch, M., and Krutzik, S., Enhanced parathyroid function in essential hypertension: a homeostatic response to a urinary calcium leak, *Hypertension*, 2, 162, 1980.
210. Sowers, J. R., Zemel, M. B., Zemel, P. C., and Standley, R. P., Calcium metabolism and dietary calcium in salt sensitive hypertension, *Am. J. Hypertens.*, 4, 557, 1991.
211. Bucher, H. C. et al., Effects of dietary calcium supplementation on blood pressure: a meta-analysis of randomized controlled trials, *J. Am. Med. Assoc.*, 275 (13), 1016, 1996.
212. Bucher, H. C. et al., Effect of calcium supplementation on pregnancy-induced hypertension and preeclampsia: a meta-analysis of randomized controlled trials, *J. Am. Med. Assoc.*, 275 (14), 1113, 1996.

213. Appel, L. J., Moore, T. J., Obarzanek, E., Vollmer, W. M., Svetkey, L. P., Sacks, F. M., Bray, G. A. et al., A clinical trial of the effects of dietary patterns on blood pressure, *N. Engl. J. Med*, 336, 1117, 1997.
214. Sacks, F. M. et al., for the DASH-Sodium Collaborative Research Group, Effects on blood pressure of reduced dietary sodium and the Dietary Approaches to Stop Hypertension (DASH) diet, *N. Engl. J. Med.*, 344, 3, 2001.
215. Chobanian, A. V. et al., The Seventh Report of the Joint National Committee on Prevention, Detection, Evaluation, and Treatment of High Blood Pressure, *J. Am. Med. Assoc.*, 289, 2560, 2003.
216. Appel, L. J. et al., Dietary approaches to prevent and treat hypertension: a scientific statement from the American Heart Association, *Hypertension*, 47, 296, 2006.
217. Whelton, P. K. et al., Effects of oral potassium on blood pressure: meta-analysis of randomized controlled clinical trials, *J. Am. Med. Assoc.*, 277, 1624, 1997.
218. Drueke, T. B., Roles of sodium and potassium in the development and management of hypertension, *Nutr. Clin. Care*, 2, 292, 1999.
219. Sacks, F. M. et al., Effect on blood pressure of potassium, calcium, and magnesium in women with low habitual intake, *Hypertension*, 31 (1), 131, 1998.
220. U.S. Food and Drug Administration, Health Claim Notification for Potassium Containing Foods, October 31, 2000, http://vm.cfsan.fda.gov/~dms/hclm-k.html (accessed October 30, 2005).
221. Jee, S. H. et al., The effect of magnesium supplementation on blood pressure: a meta-analysis of randomized clinical trials, *Am. J. Hypertens.*, 15, 691, 2002.
222. McCarron, D. A. and Heaney, R. P., Estimated health care savings associated with adequate dairy food intake, *Am. J. Hypertens.*, 17, 88, 2004.
223. American Cancer Society, Cancer Facts & Figures, American Cancer Society, Atlanta, GA, 2005.
224. Parodi, P. W., A role for milk proteins in cancer prevention, *Aust. J. Dairy Technol.*, 53, 37, 1998.
225. Parodi, P. W., Conjugated linoleic acid and other anticarcinogenic agents of bovine milk fat, *J. Dairy Sci.*, 82, 1339, 1999.
226. Parodi, P. W., Cow's milk components with anti-cancer potential, *Austr. J. Dairy Technol.*, 56, 65, 2001.
227. Parodi, P. W., Anti-cancer agents in milkfat, *Aust. J. Dairy Technol.*, 58, 114, 2003.
228. Parodi, P. W., Milk fat in human nutrition, *Austr. J. Dairy Technol.*, 59, 3, 2004.
229. German, J. B. and Dillard, C. J., Composition, structure and absorption of milk lipids: a source of energy, fat-soluble nutrients and bioactive molecules, *Crit. Rev. Food Sci. Nutr.*, 46, 57, 2006.
230. Holt, P. R., Calcium, vitamin D, and cancer, in *Calcium in Human Health*, Weaver, C. M., and Heaney, R. P. Eds., Humana Press, Totowa, NJ, 2006, chap. 25.
231. Garland, C. F. et al., The role of vitamin D in cancer prevention, *Am. J. Publ. Health*, 96, 252, 2006.
232. Govers, M. J. A. P., Termont, D. S. M. L., and Van der Meer, R., Mechanism of the antiproliferative effect of milk mineral and other calcium supplements on colonic epithelium, *Cancer Res.*, 54, 95, 1994.
233. Norat, T. and Riboli, E., Dairy products and colorectal cancer: a review of possible mechanisms and epidemiological evidence, *Eur. J. Clin. Nutr.*, 57, 1, 2003.
234. Holt, P. R. et al., Modulation of abnormal colonic epithelial cell proliferation and differentiation by lowfat dairy foods, *J. Am. Med. Assoc.*, 280 (12), 1074, 1998.
235. Baron, J. A. et al., Calcium supplements for the prevention of colorectal adenomas, *N. Engl. J. Med.*, 340 (2), 101, 1999.
236. Govers, M. J. A. P. et al., Calcium in milk products precipitates intestinal fatty acids and secondary bile acids and thus inhibits colonic cytotoxicity in man, *Cancer Res.*, 56, 3270, 1996.
237. Wooten, W. J. and Price, W., Consensus Report of the National Medical Association, The role of dairy and dairy nutrients in the diet of African Americans, *J. National Med. Assoc.*, 96 (suppl. to December 2004), 1s, 2004.
238. Moorman, P. G. and Terry, P. D., Consumption of dairy product and the risk of breast cancer: a review of the literature, *Am. J. Clin. Nutr.*, 80, 5, 2004.
239. Dagnelie, P. C. et al., Diet, anthropometric measures and prostate cancer risk: a review of prospective cohort and intervention studies, *BJU Int.*, 93, 1139, 2004.
240. Baron, J. A., Risk of prostate cancer in a randomized clinical trial of calcium supplementation, *Cancer Epidemiol. Biomarkers Prev.*, 14, 586, 2005.

241. Chen, T. C. and Holick, M. F., Vitamin D and prostate cancer prevention and treatment, *Trends Endocrinol. Metab.*, 14, 423, 2003.
242. Trump, D. L. et al., Anti-tumor activity of calcitriol: pre-clinical and clinical studies, *J. Steroid Biochem. Mol. Biol.*, 89–90, 519, 2004.
243. Hedley, A. A. et al., Prevalence of overweight and obesity among U.S. children, adolescents, and adults, 1999–2002, *JAMA*, 291, 2847, 2004.
244. National Institutes of Health, The Practical Guide, Identification, Evaluation and Treatment of Overweight and Obesity in Adults, NIH Publication No. 00-4084, October 2000.
245. Zemel, M. B. et al., Calcium and dairy acceleration of weight and fat loss during energy restriction in obese adults, *Obes. Res.*, 12, 582, 2004.
246. Zemel, M. B. et al., Dairy augmentation of total and central fat loss in obese subjects, *Int. J. Obes. Relat. Metab. Disord.*, 29, 391, 2005.
247. Zemel, M. B. et al., Effects of calcium and dairy on body composition and weight loss in African-American adults, *Obes. Res.*, 13, 1218, 2005.
248. Teegarden, D. J., Calcium intake and reduction in weight or fat mass, *J. Nutr.*, 133, 249s, 2003.
249. Parikh, S. J. and Yanovski, J. A., Calcium intake and adiposity, *Am. J. Clin. Nutr.*, 77, 281, 2003.
250. Zemel, M. B., Role of calcium and dairy products in energy partitioning and weight management, *Am. J. Clin. Nutr.*, 79, 907s, 2004.
251. Zemel, M. B., Calcium and dairy modulation of obesity risk, *Obesity Res.*, 13 (1), 192, 2005.
252. Gunther, C. W. et al., Fat oxidation and its relation to serum parathyroid hormone in young women enrolled in a 1-y dairy calcium intervention, *Am. J. Clin. Nutr.*, 82 (6), 1228, 2005.
253. Melanson, E. L. et al., Effect of low- and high-calcium dairy-based diets on macronutrient oxidation in humans, *Obes. Res.*, 13 (12), 2102, 2005.
254. Zemel, M. B., The role of dairy foods in weight management, *J. Am. College Nutr.*, 24 (6), 537S, 2005.
255. Repke, J. T., Calcium homeostasis in pregnancy, *Clin. Obstet. Gynecol.*, 37 (1), 59, 1994.
256. Pitkin, R. M., Calcium metabolism in pregnancy and the perinatal period: a review, *Am. J. Obstet. Gynecol.*, 151, 99, 1985.
257. King, J. C. Halloran, B. P., Huq, N. Diamond, T., and Buckendahl, P. E., Calcium metabolism during pregnancy and lactation, *Mechanisms Regulating Lactation and Infant Nutrient Utilization*, Wiley-Liss, Inc., New York, 129–146, 1992.
258. Kalkwarf, H. J. and Specker, B. L., Bone mineral loss during lactation and recovery after weaning, *Obstet. Gynecol.*, 86, 26, 1995.
259. Cross, N. A. et al., Calcium homeostasis and bone metabolism during pregnancy, lactation, and postweaning: a longitudinal study, *Am. J. Clin. Nutr.*, 61, 514, 1995.
260. Kalkwarf, H. J., Lactation and maternal bone health, in *Protecting Infants through Human Milk*, Pickering, et al., Eds., Kluwer Academic/Plenum Publishers, Netherlands/New York, 2004.
261. Kalkwarf, H. J. et al., The effect of calcium supplementation on bone density during lactation and after weaning, *N. Engl. J. Med.*, 337 (8), 523, 1997.
262. U.S. Department of Health and Human Services, Public Health Service, *Healthy People 2000 National Health Promotion and Disease Prevention Objectives*, DHHS Publication No. (PHS) 91-50212, September 1990.
263. U.S. Department of Health and Human Services, Public Health Service, Healthy People 2000 Review 1995–1996, Public Health Service, Hyattsville, MD, 1996.
264. Office of Disease Prevention and Health Promotion, U.S. Department of Health and Human Services, Healthy People Midcourse Review http://www.healthypeople.gov/data/midcourse/comments/ (accessed March 28, 2006).
265. Donangelo, C. M. et al., Calcium homeostasis during pregnancy and lactation in primiparous and multiparous women with sub-adequate calcium intakes, *Nutr. Res.*, 16 (10), 1631, 1996.
266. O'Brien, K. O. et al., Bone calcium turnover during pregnancy and lactation in women with low calcium diets is associated with calcium intake and circulating insulin-like growth factor 1 concentrations, *Am. J. Clin. Nutr.*, 83, 317, 2006.
267. Raman, L., Rajalskshmi, K., Krishnamachari, K. A. V. R., and Sastry, J. C., Effect of calcium supplementation to undernourished mothers during pregnancy on the bone density of the neonates, *Am. J. Clin. Nutr.*, 31, 466, 1978.

268. Koo, W. W. et al., Maternal calcium supplementation and fetal bone mineralization, *Obstet. Gynecol.*, 94, 577, 1999.
269. Ortega, R. M. et al., Calcium levels in maternal milk: relationships with calcium intake during the third trimester of pregnancy, *Br. J. Nutr.*, 79, 501, 1998.
270. Gulson, B. L. et al., Mobilization of lead from the skeleton during the postnatal period is larger than during pregnancy, *J. Lab. Clin. Med.*, 131, 324, 1998.
271. Gulson, B. L. et al., Blood lead changes during pregnancy and postpartum with calcium supplementation, *Environ. Health Pers.*, 112 (15), 1499, 2004.
272. Repke, J. T. and Villar, J., Pregnancy-induced hypertension and low birth weight: the role of calcium, *Am. J. Clin. Nutr.*, 54, 237S, 1991.
273. Villar, J. et al., World Health Organization randomized trial of calcium supplementation among low calcium intake pregnant women, *Am. J. Obstet. Gynecol.*, 194, 639, 2006.
274. Levine, R. J. et al., Trial of calcium for prevention of preeclampsia, *New Engl. J. Med.*, 337 (2), 69, 1997.
275. Hypponen, E., Vitamin D for the prevention of preeclapsia? A hypothesis, *Nutr. Rev.*, 63 (7), 225, 2005.
276. Cooper, C., Developmental origins of osteoporotic fracture: the role of maternal vitamin D insufficiency, *J. Nutr.*, 135, 2728S, 2005.
277. Javaid, M. K. et al., Maternal vitamin D status during pregnancy and childhood bone mass at age 9 years: a longitudinal study, *Lancet*, 367, 36, 2006.
278. Moore, C. et al., Vitamin D intake in the United States, *J. Am. Diet. Assoc.*, 104, 980, 2004.
279. Specker, B., Vitamin D requirements during pregnancy, *Am. J. Clin. Nutr.*, 80 (suppl.), 1740S, 2004.
280. Bertone-Johnson, E. R. et al., Calcium and vitamin D intake and risk of incident premenstrual syndrome, *Arch. Intern. Med.*, 165, 1246, 2005.
281. Thy-Jacobs, S. et al., Calcium supplementation in premenstrual syndrome: a randomized crossover trial, *J. Gen. Int. Med.*, 4, 183, 1989.
282. Thy-Jacobs, S., Starkey, P., Bernstein, D., and Tian, J., Calcium carbonate and the premenstrual syndrome: effects on premenstrual and menstrual symptoms, *Am. J. Obstet. Gynecol.*, 179, 444, 1998.
283. Thys-Jacobs, S., Micronutrients and the premenstrual syndrome: the case for calcium, *J. Am. Coll. Nutr.*, 19, 220, 2000.
284. Penland, J. G. and Johnson, P. E., Dietary calcium and manganese effects on menstrual cycle symptoms, *Am. J. Obstet. Gynecol.*, 168, 1417, 1993.
285. Bendich, A., Dietary calcium and manganese effects on menstrual cycle symptoms, *J. Am. Coll. Nutr.*, 19, 3, 2000.
286. Bendich, A., Micronutrients in women's health and immune function, *Nutrition*, 17 (10), 858, 2001.
287. Derman, O. et al., Premenstrual syndrome and associated symptoms in adolescent girls, *Eur. J. Obstet. Gynecol. Reprod. Biol.*, 116, 201, 2004.
288. Teegarden, D. et al., Dietary calcium intake protects women consuming oral contraceptives from spine and hip bone loss, *J. Clin. Endocrinol. Metab.*, 90 (9), 5127, 2005.
289. Kontiokari, T. et al., Dietary factors protecting women from urinary tract infection, *Am. J. Clin. Nutr.*, 77, 600, 2003.
290. Fahm, E. G. and Jocelyn, J., Changing behaviors to optimize women's health: a multidisciplinary seminar, *J. Am. Diet. Assoc.*, 98 (7), 818, 1998.
291. Horwath, C. C. et al., Factors influencing milk and milk product consumption in young and elderly women with low calcium intakes, *Nutr. Res.*, 15 (12), 1735, 1995.
292. Hagy, L. F., Brochetti, D., and Duncan, S. E., Focus groups identified women's perceptions of dairy foods, *J. Women Aging*, 12 (3-4), 99, 2000.
293. Guthrie, J. F., Dietary patterns and personal characteristics of women consuming recommended amounts of calcium, *Family Econ. Nutr. Rev.*, 9 (3), 1, 1996.
294. Barger-Lux, M. J. et al., Nutritional correlates of low calcium intake, *Clin. Appl. Nutr.*, 2 (4), 39, 1992.
295. Dairy Management, Inc., *Consumer Segmentation Study*, 1997.
296. Mitchell, M. K., Aging and older adults, *Nutrition Across the Lifespan*, W. B. Saunders, Philadelphia, PA, 2003, chap. 13.

297. Heaney, R. P., Age considerations in nutrient needs for bone health: older adults, *J. Am. Coll. Nutr.*, 15 (6), 575, 1996.
298. National Osteoporosis Foundation, Physician's Guide to Prevention and Treatment of Osteoporosis, National Osteoporosis Foundation, Washington, D.C., 2003, http://www.nof.org/physguide/ (accessed on March 30, 2006).
299. Fast facts on osteoporosis, National Osteoporosis Foundation, 2006 www.nof.org/osteoporosis/diseasefacts/ (accessed on March 30, 2006).
300. Heaney, R. P., Constructive interactions among nutrients and bone-active pharmacologic agents with principal emphasis on calcium, phosphorus, vitamin D and protein, *J. Am. Coll. Nutr.*, 20 (5 suppl.), 403S, 2001.
301. Blumberg, J., Nutritional needs of seniors, *J. Am. Coll. Nutr.*, 16 (6), 517, 1997.
302. Chapuy, M. C. et al., Vitamin D_3 and calcium to prevent hp fractures in elderly women, *N. Engl. J. Med.*, 327, 1637, 1992.
303. Aloia, J. F. et al., Calcium supplementation with and without hormone replacement therapy to prevent postmenopausal bone loss, *Ann. Intern. Med.*, 120, 97, 1994.
304. Dawson-Hughes, B. et al., Effect of calcium and vitamin D supplementation on bone density in men and women 65 years of age or older, *N. Engl. J. Med.* i, 337 (10), 670, 1997.
305. Heaney, R. P., Is the paradigm shifting? *Bone*, 33, 457, 2003.
306. Heaney, R. P., Rafferty, K., and Dowell, M. S., Effect of yogurt on a urinary marker of bone resorption in postmenopausal women, *J. Am. Diet. Assoc.*, 102, 1672, 2002.
307. Heaney, R. P. et al., Dietary changes favorably affect bone remodeling in older adults, *J. Am. Diet. Assoc.*, 99, 1228, 1999.
308. McCabe, L. D. et al., Dairy intakes affect bone density in the elderly, *Am. J. Clin. Nutr.*, 80, 1066, 2004.
309. Daley, R. M. et al., Calcium- and vitamin D3-fortified milk reduces bone loss at clinically relevant skeletal sites in older men: a 2-year randomized controlled trial, *J. Bone Miner. Res.*, 21, 397, 2006.
310. Heaney, R. P., Calcium needs of the elderly to reduce fracture risk, *J. Am. Coll. Nutr.*, 20, 192s, 2001.
311. Holick, M. F., The vitamin D epidemic and its health consequences, *J. Nutr*, 135, 2739S, 2005.
312. Holick, M. F., Sunlight and vitamin D for bone health and prevention of autoimmune diseases, cancer, and cardiovascular disease, *Am. J. Clin. Nutr.*, 80 (suppl.), 1678S, 2004.
313. Dawson-Hughes, B., Harris, S. S., and Dallal, G. E., Plasma calcidiol, season, and serum parathyroid hormone concentrations in healthy elderly men and women, *Am. J. Clin. Nutr.*, 65 (1), 67, 1997.
314. Moore, C. et al., Vitamin D intake in the United States, *J. Am. Diet. Assoc.*, 104, 980, 2004.
315. Dawson-Hughes, B. et al., Rates on bone loss in postmenopausal women randomly assigned to one of two dosages of vitamin D, *Am. J. Clin. Nutr.*, 61 (5), 1140, 1995.
316. Jackson, R. D. et al., Calcium plus vitamin D supplementation and the risk of fractures, *N. Engl. J. Med.*, 354, 669, 2006.
317. Papadimitropoulos, E. et al., Meta-analyses of therapies for postmenopausal osteoporosis, VIII: meta-analysis of the efficacy of vitamin D treatment in preventing osteoporosis in postmenopausal women, *Endocr. Rev.*, 23, 560, 2002.
318. Heaney, R. P., Barriers to optimizing vitamin D3 intake for the elderly, *J. Nutr.*, 136, 1123, 2006.
319. Dawson-Hughes, B., Interaction of dietary calcium and protein in bone health in humans, *J. Nutr.*, 133, 852S, 2003.
320. Massey, L. K., Dietary animal and plant protein and human bone health: a whole foods approach, *J. Nutr.*, 133, 862S, 2003.
321. Bonjour, J.-P., Dietary protein: an essential nutrient for bone health, *J. Am. Coll. Nutr.*, 24 (6), 526S, 2005.
322. Munger, R. G., Cerhan, J. R., and Chiu, B. C.-H., Prospective study of dietary protein intake and risk of hip fracture in postmenopausal women, *Am. J. Clin. Nutr.*, 69, 147, 1999.
323. Hannan, M. T. et al., Effect of dietary protein on bone loss in elderly men and women: the Framingham Osteoporosis Study, *J. Bone Miner. Res.*, 15, 2504, 2000.
324. Kerstetter, J. E., Looker, A. C., and Insogna, K. L., Low dietary protein and low bone density, *Calc. Tissue Int.*, 66, 313, 2000.
325. Promislow, J. H. E. et al., Protein consumption and bone mineral density in the elderly: the Rancho Bernardo Study, *Am. J. Epidemiol.*, 155, 636, 2002.

326. Ilich, J. Z., Brownbill, R. A., and Tamborini, L., Bone and nutrition in elderly women: protein, energy, and calcium as main determinants of bone, *Eur. J. Clin. Nutr.*, 57, 554, 2003.
327. Melton, L. J. et al., Relative contributions of bone density, bone turnover, and clinical risk factors to long-term fracture prediction, *J. Bone Miner. Res.*, 18, 312, 2003.
328. Schurch, M-A. et al., Protein supplements increase serum insulin-like growth factor-I levels and attenuate proximal femur bone loss in patients with recent hip fracture, *Ann. Int. Med.*, 128, 801, 1998.
329. Roughead, Z. K., Is the interaction between dietary protein and calcium destructive or constructive for bone? *J. Nutr.*, 133, 866S, 2003.
330. Rizzoli, R. et al., Protein intake and bone disorders in the elderly, *Joint Bone Spine*, 68, 383, 2001.
331. Ammann, P. S. et al., Protein undernutrition-induced bone loss is associated with decreased IGF-I levels and estrogen deficiency, *J. Bone Miner. Res.*, 15, 683, 2000.
332. Dawson-Hughes, B. and Harris, S. S., Calcium intake influences the association of protein intake with rates of bone loss in elderly men and women, *Am. J. Clin. Nutr.*, 75, 773, 2002.
333. Burckhardt, P., Dawson-Hughes, B., and Heaney, R. P., Eds., *Nutritional Aspects of Osteoporosis*, Academic Press, San Diego, CA, p. 55, 2001.
334. Campbell, W. W. et al., Increased protein requirements in the elderly: new data and retrospective reassessments, *Am. J. Clin. Nutr.*, 60, 501, 1994.
335. Institute of Medicine of the National Academies, *Dietary Reference Intakes, Energy, Carbohydrate, Fiber, Fat, Fatty Acids, Cholesterol, Protein, and Amino Acids*, National Academy Press, Washington, D.C., 2002.
336. Constans, T. et al., Effects of nutrition education on calcium intake in the elderly, *J. Am. Diet. Assoc.*, 94 (4), 447, 1994.
337. Jensen, G. L. and Rogers, J., Obesity in older persons, *J. Am. Diet. Assoc.*, 98 (11), 1308, 1998.
338. Greene, G. W., The relationship between dietary change over 18 months and the aging process, *J. Am. Diet. Assoc*, 98 (9), A–69, 1998.
339. Ali, N. S. and Twibell, R. K., Health promotion and osteoporosis prevention among postmenopausal women, *Prev. Med.*, 24, 528, 1995.
340. Lancaster, K. J., Characteristics influencing daily consumption of fruits and vegetables and lowfat dairy products in older adults with hypertension, *J. Nutr. Elderly*, 23 (4), 4, 2004.
341. Elbon, S. M., Johnson, M. A., and Fischer, J. G., Milk consumption in older Americans, *Am. J. Pub. Health*, 88 (5), 1221, 1998.
342. Bronner, Y. I. et al., Models for nutrition education to increase consumption of calcium and dairy products among African Americans, *J. Nutr.*, 136, 1103, 2006.
343. Wooten, W. J. and Price, W., The role of dairy and dairy nutrients in the diet of African Americans, *J. Nat. Med. Assoc*, 96 (12), 1S, 2004.
344. Byers, K. G. and Savaiano, D. A., The myth of increased lactose intolerance in African Americans, *J. Am. Coll. Nutr.*, 24 (6), 569S, 2005.
345. Wuthrich, B. et al., Milk consumption does not lead to mucus production or occurrence of asthma, *J. Am. Coll. Nutr.*, 24 (6), 547S, 2005.
346. Miller, G. D., Jarvis, J. K., and McBean, L. D., The importance of meeting calcium needs with foods, *J. Am. Coll. Nutr.*, 20 (2), 168S, 2001.
347. Devine, A., Prince, R. L., and Roma, B., Nutritional effect of calcium supplementation by skim milk powder or calcium tablets on total nutrient intake in postmenopausal women, *Am. J. Clin. Nutr.*, 64, 731, 1996.
348. Bernstein, M. A. et al., A home-based nutrition intervention to increase consumption of fruits, vegetables, and calcium-rich foods in community dwelling elders, *J. Am. Diet. Assoc.*, 102, 1421, 2002.
349. Heaney, R. P., Food: what a surprise! *Am. J. Clin. Nutr.*, 64, 791, 1996.
350. Goldberg, J. P., Gershoff, S. N., and McGandy, R. B., Appropriate topics for nutrition education for the elderly, *J. Nutr. Edu.*, 22, 303, 1990.
351. Posner, B. M. et al., Nutrition and health risks in the elderly: the nutrition screening initiative, *Am. J. Pub. Health*, 83, 972, 1993.

Index

D

N

O

P